SAUNDERS

2006
HCPCS Level II

SAUNDERS

2006
HCPCS Level II

Carol J. Buck, MS, CPC, CPC-H, CCS-P

Program Director (Ret.), Medical Secretary Programs
Northwest Technical College
East Grand Forks, Minnesota

SAUNDERS
ELSEVIER

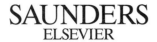

11830 Westline Industrial Drive
St. Louis, Missouri 63146

SAUNDERS 2006 HCPCS LEVEL II

ISBN-13: 978-1-4160-3248-9
ISBN-10: 1-4160-3248-7

Notice

Knowledge and best practice in this field are constantly changing. As new research and experience broaden our knowledge, changes in practice, treatment and drug therapy may become necessary or appropriate. Readers are advised to check the most current information provided (i) on procedures featured or (ii) by the manufacturer of each product to be administered, to verify the recommended dose or formula, the method and duration of administration, and contraindications. It is the responsibility of the practitioner, relying on their own experience and knowledge of the patient, to make diagnoses, to determine dosages and the best treatment for each individual patient, and to take all appropriate safety precautions. To the fullest extent of the law, neither the Publisher nor the Author assumes any liability for any injury and/or damage to persons or property arising out or related to any use of the material contained in this book.

Previous edition copyrighted 2005, 2004, 2003, 2002, 2001, 2000 by Elsevier, Inc.

ISBN-13: 978-1-4160-3248-9

ISBN-10: 1-4160-3248-7

Publishing Director: Andrew Allen
Senior Acquisitions Editor: Susan Cole
Developmental Editor: Beth LoGiudice
Associate Developmental Editor: Josh Rapplean
Publishing Services Manager: Melissa Lastarria
Designer: Andrea Lutes

Printed in the United States of America.

Last digit is the print number: 9   8   7   6   5   4   3   2

CONTENTS

GUIDE TO USING THE SAUNDERS 2006 HCPCS Level II

Medical coding has long been a part of the health care profession. Through the years medical coding systems have become more complex and extensive. Today, medical coding is an intricate and immense process that is present in every health care setting. The increased use of electronic submissions for health care services only increases the need for coders who understand the coding process.

Saunders 2006 HCPCS Level II was developed to help meet the needs of students preparing for a career in medical coding.

All material adheres to the latest government versions available at the time of printing.

Annotated

Throughout this text revisions and additions are indicated by the following symbols:

- ◀▥▶ **Revised:** Revisions within the line or code from the previous edition are indicated by the black arrow.
- ◀▶ **New:** Additions to the previous edition are indicated by the color triangle.

HCPCS Symbols

- ⊙ **Special coverage instructions** apply to these codes. Usually these special coverage instructions are included in the Medicare Carrier Manual (MCM) select references in Appendix A or in the Coverage Issues Manual (CIM) in Appendix B.
- ◆ **Not covered by or valid for Medicare** is indicated by the diamond. Usually the reason for the exclusion is included in the Medicare Carrier Manual (MCM) select references in Appendix A or in the Coverage Issues Manual (CIM) in Appendix B.
- ∗ **Carrier discretion** is an indication that you must contact the individual third-party payors to find out the coverage available for codes identified by this symbol.

SYMBOLS AND CONVENTIONS

HCPCS Symbols

Special coverage instructions apply to these codes. Usually these instructions are included in the Medicare Carrier Manual (MCM) select references in Appendix A or in the Coverage Issues Manual (CIM) in Appendix B of this text.

→ ✷ **L3540** Miscellaneous shoe additions, sole, full
MCM 2079, CIM 70-3

Medicare Carrier Manual (MCM) and Coverage Issues Manual (CIM) give instructions regarding use of the code. MCM and CIM select references are located in the appendices of this text.

Not covered by or valid for Medicare is indicated by the diamond. Usually the reason for the exclusion is included in the Medicare Carrier Manual (MCM) references in Appendix A or in the Coverage Issues Manual (CIM) in Appendix B of this text.

→ ◆ **A5074** Pouch, urinary; with faceplate attached; plastic or rubber
MCM 2130

Carrier discretion is an indication that you must contact the individual third-party payors to find out the coverage available for these codes.

→ ✱ **A6154** Wound pouch, each

Indicates **new** information or a new code.

→ ▶ **A4614** Peak expiratory flow rate meter, hand held

Indicates a **revision** within the line or code.

→ ⇒ **J0270** Injection alprostadil, per 1.25 mcg

HCPCS 2006 New/Revised/Deleted Codes and Modifiers

2006 HCPCS quarterly updates will be posted on the companion website
(http://evolve.elsevier.com/Buck/hcpcs) when available

NEW CODES/MODIFIERS

AQ	A6538	A9563	E2219	J1751	L0625	L3977	Q0489	Q9959	
BL	A6539	A9564	E2220	J1752	L0626	L3978	Q0490	Q9960	
CR	A6540	A9565	E2221	J1945	L0627	L5703	Q0491	Q9961	
FB	A6541	A9566	E2222	J2278	L0628	L5858	Q0492	Q9962	
GR	A6542	A9567	E2223	J2325	L0629	L5971	Q0493	Q9963	
GS	A6543	A9698	E2224	J2425	L0630	L6621	Q0494	Q9964	
J1	A6544	B4185	E2225	J2503	L0631	L6677	Q0495	S0133	
J2	A6549	C2637	E2226	J2504	L0632	L6883	Q0496	S0142	
J3	A9275	C9224	E2371	J2513	L0633	L6884	Q0497	S0143	
P1	A9281	C9225	E2372	J2805	L0634	L6885	Q0498	S0145	
P2	A9282	C9723	G0235	J2850	L0635	L7400	Q0499	S0146	
P3	A9535	C9724	G0372	J3285	L0636	L7401	Q0500	S0197	
P4	A9536	C9725	G0375	J3355	L0637	L7402	Q0501	S0198	
P5	A9537	E0170	G0376	J3471	L0638	L7403	Q0502	S0265	
P6	A9538	E0171	G0378	J3472	L0639	L7404	Q0503	S0595	
QR	A9539	E0172	G0379	J7188	L0640	L7405	Q0504	S0613	
A0998	A9540	E0485	G9033	J7189	L0859	L7600	Q0505	S0625	
A4218	A9541	E0486	G9041	J7306	L2034	L8609	Q0510	S2068	
A4233	A9542	E0641	G9042	J7318	L2387	L8623	Q0511	S2075	
A4234	A9543	E0642	G9043	J7341	L3671	L8624	Q0512	S2076	
A4235	A9544	E0705	G9044	J7620	L3672	L8680	Q0513	S2077	
A4236	A9545	E0762	J0132	J7627	L3673	L8681	Q0514	S2078	
A4363	A9546	E0764	J0133	J7640	L3702	L8682	Q0515	S2079	
A4411	A9547	E0911	J0278	J8498	L3763	L8683	Q4079	S2114	
A4412	A9548	E0912	J0365	J8515	L3764	L8684	Q4080	S2117	
A4604	A9549	E1392	J0480	J8540	L3765	L8685	Q9945	S2900	
A5120	A9550	E1812	J0795	J8597	L3766	L8686	Q9946	S3005	
A5512	A9551	E2207	J0881	J9025	L3905	L8687	Q9947	S3626	
A5513	A9552	E2208	J0882	J9027	L3913	L8688	Q9948	S3854	
A6457	A9553	E2209	J0885	J9175	L3919	L8689	Q9949	S8270	
A6513	A9554	E2210	J0886	J9225	L3921	Q0480	Q9950	S8940	
A6530	A9555	E2211	J1162	J9264	L3933	Q0481	Q9951	V2788	
A6531	A9556	E2212	J1265	K0730	L3935	Q0482	Q9952		
A6532	A9557	E2213	J1430	L0491	L3961	Q0483	Q9953		
A6533	A9558	E2214	J1451	L0492	L3967	Q0484	Q9954		
A6534	A9559	E2215	J1566	L0621	L3971	Q0485	Q9955		
A6535	A9560	E2216	J1567	L0622	L3973	Q0486	Q9956		
A6536	A9561	E2217	J1640	L0623	L3975	Q0487	Q9957		
A6537	A9562	E2218	J1675	L0624	L3976	Q0488	Q9958		

REVISED CODES/MODIFIERS

Change in	A4306	Payment	A4414	A9505	A6550	A9699	J7344	L3215
Administrative	A4421	Change	A4415	A9507	A7032	B4149	J7350	L3216
Data Field	A4458	E0463		A9508	A7033	C2634	J7626	L3217
TS	A4554	E0464	Both	A9510	A9512	C2635	K0669	L3219
A4244	A4632	E0550	Administrative	A9524	A9516	E0116	L1832	L3221
A4245	A4932	E0560	and Long	A9526	A9517	E0637	L1843	L3222
A4246	A6025	E0616	Description		A9521	E0638	L1844	L3230
A4247	A6412	L8010	Change	Long	A9528	E0935	L1845	L3906
A4281	B4100		A4641	Description	A9529	E0971	L1846	L3923
A4282	E0203	Short	A4642	Change	A9530	E1038	L2036	
A4283	E0240	Description	A9500	A4215	A9531	E1039	L2037	
A4284	E0761	Change	A9502	A4216	A9532	J7340	L2038	
A4285	L3031	A4409	A9503	A4372	A9600	J7342	L2405	
A4286	Q3001	A4410	A9504	A4630	A9605	J7343	L3170	
A4305								

DELETED CODES/MODIFIERS

QB	C1305	C9418	E0996	G0210	G0347	K0104	L8100	Q3002
QQ	C1775	C9419	E1000	G0211	G0348	K0106	L8110	Q3003
QU	C9000	C9420	E1001	G0212	G0349	K0415	L8120	Q3004
A4254	C9007	C9421	E1019	G0213	G0350	K0416	L8130	Q3005
A4260	C9008	C9422	E1021	G0214	G0351	K0452	L8140	Q3006
A4643	C9009	C9423	E1025	G0215	G0353	K0600	L8150	Q3007
A4644	C9013	C9424	E1026	G0216	G0354	K0618	L8160	Q3008
A4645	C9102	C9425	E1027	G0217	G0355	K0619	L8170	Q3009
A4646	C9103	C9426	E1210	G0218	G0356	K0620	L8180	Q3010
A4647	C9105	C9427	E1211	G0220	G0357	K0628	L8190	Q3011
A4656	C9112	C9428	E1212	G0221	G0358	K0629	L8195	Q3012
A5119	C9123	C9429	E1213	G0222	G0359	K0630	L8200	Q4054
A5509	C9126	C9430	E1239	G0223	G0360	K0631	L8210	Q4055
A5511	C9127	C9431	G0030	G0224	G0361	K0632	L8220	Q4075
A6551	C9128	C9432	G0031	G0225	G0362	K0633	L8230	Q4076
A9511	C9129	C9433	G0032	G0226	G0363	K0634	L8239	Q4077
A9513	C9200	C9435	G0033	G0227	G0369	K0635	L8620	Q9941
A9514	C9201	C9436	G0034	G0228	G0370	K0636	Q0136	Q9942
A9515	C9202	C9437	G0035	G0229	G0371	K0637	Q0137	Q9943
A9519	C9203	C9438	G0036	G0230	G0374	K0638	Q0187	Q9944
A9520	C9205	C9439	G0037	G0231	J0880	K0639	Q1001	S0016
A9522	C9206	C9440	G0038	G0232	J1563	K0640	Q1002	S0071
A9523	C9211	C9704	G0039	G0233	J1564	K0641	Q2001	S0072
A9525	C9212	C9713	G0040	G0234	J1750	K0642	Q2002	S0107
A9533	C9218	C9718	G0041	G0242	J2324	K0643	Q2003	S0114
A9534	C9223	C9719	G0042	G0244	J7051	K0644	Q2005	S0118
B4184	C9226	C9720	G0043	G0252	J7317	K0645	Q2006	S0158
B4186	C9400	C9721	G0044	G0253	J7320	K0646	Q2007	S0159
C1079	C9401	C9722	G0045	G0254	J7616	K0647	Q2008	S0168
C1080	C9402	E0169	G0046	G0258	J7617	K0648	Q2011	S0173
C1081	C9403	E0752	G0047	G0263	K0064	K0649	Q2012	S2082
C1082	C9404	E0754	G0110	G0264	K0066	K0670	Q2013	S2090
C1083	C9405	E0756	G0111	G0279	K0067	K0671	Q2014	S2091
C1091	C9410	E0757	G0112	G0280	K0068	K0731	Q2018	S2215
C1092	C9411	E0758	G0113	G0296	K0074	K0732	Q2019	S8004
C1093	C9413	E0759	G0114	G0336	K0075	L0860	Q2020	S8095
C1122	C9414	E0953	G0115	G0338	K0076	L1750	Q2021	S8434
C1200	C9415	E0954	G0116	G0345	K0078	L2039	Q2022	T2006
C1201	C9417	E0972	G0125	G0346	K0102	L3963	Q3000	

HCPCS 2006: LEVEL II NATIONAL CODES

HCPCS Quarterly Updates available on the companion website at:
http://evolve.elsevier.com/Buck/hcpcs

DISCLAIMER

Every effort has been made to make this text complete and accurate, but no guarantee, warranty, or representation is made for its accuracy or completeness. It is based on the Centers for Medicare and Medicaid Services Healthcare Common Procedure Coding System (HCPCS).

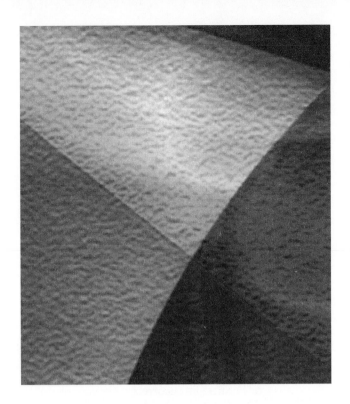

PART I

Introduction

HCPCS Quarterly Updates available
on the companion website at:
http://evolve.elsevier.com/Buck/hcpcs

The Centers for Medicare and Medicaid Services (CMS) (formerly Health Care Financing Administration [HCFA]) Healthcare Common Procedure Coding System (HCPCS) is a collection of codes and descriptors that represent procedures, supplies, products, and services that may be provided to Medicare beneficiaries and to individuals enrolled in private health insurance programs. The codes are divided as follows:

Level I: Codes and descriptors copyrighted by the American Medical Association's (AMA's) Current Procedural Terminology, ed. 4 (CPT-4). Five-position numeric codes primarily represent physician services.

Level II: Five-position alpha-numeric codes representing primarily items and nonphysician services that are not represented in the Level I codes. Codes and descriptors copyrighted by the American Dental Association's (ADA's) Current Dental Terminology, (CDT-5), are five-position alpha-numeric codes comprising the D series. **This book does not contain codes D0100 through D9999.** They can be purchased from the ADA. All other Level II codes and descriptors are approved and maintained jointly by the Alpha-Numeric Editorial Panel.

Level III: The CMS has eliminated Level III local codes. See Program Memorandum AB-02-113.

Headings are provided as a means of grouping similar or closely related items. The placement of a code under a heading does not indicate additional means of classification, nor does it relate to any health insurance coverage categories.

HCPCS also contains modifiers, which are two-position codes and descriptors used to indicate that a service or procedure that has been performed has been altered by some specific circumstance but not changed in its definition or code. Modifiers are grouped by the three levels. Level I modifiers and descriptors are copyrighted by the AMA. Modifiers in the D series are copyrighted by the ADA. **This book does not contain D series modifiers.** They are available directly from the ADA.

HCPCS is designed to promote uniform reporting and statistical data collection of medical procedures, supplies, products, and services.

HCPCS Disclaimer

Inclusion or exclusion of a procedure, supply, product, or service does not imply any health insurance coverage or reimbursement policy.

HCPCS makes as much use as possible of generic descriptions, but the inclusion of brand names to describe devices or drugs is intended only for indexing purposes; it is not meant to convey endorsement of any particular product or drug.

Updating HCPCS

The primary updates are made annually.

Legend
✿	Special coverage instructions
◆	Not covered by or valid for Medicare
✳	Carrier discretion
◀▶	New
◀▥▥▶	Revised

The revised symbol is placed in front of items with data, payment, or miscellaneous changes.

LEVEL II NATIONAL MODIFIERS

* A1   Dressing for one wound
* A2   Dressing for two wounds
* A3   Dressing for three wounds
* A4   Dressing for four wounds
* A5   Dressing for five wounds
* A6   Dressing for six wounds
* A7   Dressing for seven wounds
* A8   Dressing for eight wounds
* A9   Dressing for nine or more wounds
◎ AA   Anesthesia services performed personally by anesthesiologist
◎ AD   Medical supervision by a physician: more than four concurrent anesthesia procedures
         MCM 3350.5
* AE   Registered dietician
* AF   Specialty physician
* AG   Primary physician
◎ AH   Clinical psychologist
         MCM 2150, MCM 5112
◎ AJ   Clinical social worker
         MCM 2152, MCM 5113
* AK   Non-participating physician
◎ AM   Physician, team member service
         MCM 4105.7, Cross Reference QM
* AP   Determination of refractive state was not performed in the course of diagnostic ophthalmological examination
▶* AQ   Physician providing a service in an unlisted health professional shortage area (HPSA)
* AR   Physician provider services in physician scarcity area
* AS   Physician assistant, nurse practitioner, or clinical nurse specialist services for assistant at surgery
* AT   Acute treatment (this modifier should be used when reporting service 98940, 98941, 98942*)
* AU   Item furnished in conjunction with a urological, ostomy, or tracheostomy supply
* AV   Item furnished in conjunction with a prosthetic device, prosthetic or orthotic
* AW   Item furnished in conjunction with a surgical dressing
* AX   Item furnished in conjunction with dialysis services
* BA   Item furnished in conjunction with parenteral enteral nutrition (PEN) services
▶* BL   Special acquisition of blood and blood products
* BO   Orally administered nutrition, not by feeding tube

* BP   The beneficiary has been informed of the purchase and rental options and has elected to purchase the item.
* BR   The beneficiary has been informed of the purchase and rental options and has elected to rent the item.
* BU   The beneficiary has been informed of the purchase and rental options and after 30 days has not informed the supplier of his/her decision.
* CA   Procedure payable only in inpatient setting when performed emergently on an outpatient who expires prior to admission
* CB   Service ordered by a renal dialysis facility (RDF) physician as part of the ESRD beneficiary's dialysis benefit, is not part of the composite rate, and is separately reimbursable
* CC   Procedure code change. (Use CC when the procedure code submitted was changed either for administrative reasons or because an incorrect code was filed.)
   CD   AMCC test has been ordered by an ESRD facility or MCP physician that is part of the composite rate and is not separately billable
   CE   AMCC test has been ordered by an ESRD facility or MCP physician that is a composite rate test but is beyond the normal frequency covered under the rate and is separately reimbursable based on medical necessity
   CF   AMCC test has been ordered by an ESRD facility or MCP physician that is not part of the composite rate and is separately billable
▶* CR   Catastrophe/Disaster related
* FP   Service provided as part of family planning program
* E1   Upper left eyelid
* E2   Lower left eyelid
* E3   Upper right eyelid
* E4   Lower right eyelid
◎ EJ   Subsequent claim for a defined course of therapy (e.g., EPO, sodium hyaluronate, infliximab
◎ EM   Emergency reserve supply (for end state renal disease [ESRD] benefit only)
* EP   Service provided as part of Medicaid early periodic screening diagnosis and treatment (EPSDT) program
* ET   Emergency services
* EY   No physician or other licensed health care provider order for this item or service
* F1   Left hand, second digit
* F2   Left hand, third digit
* F3   Left hand, fourth digit
* F4   Left hand, fifth digit
* F5   Right hand, thumb

✳ F6	Right hand, second digit
✳ F7	Right hand, third digit
✳ F8	Right hand, fourth digit
✳ F9	Right hand, fifth digit
✳ FA	Left hand, thumb
▶◆ FB	Item provided without cost to provider, supplier or practitioner (examples, but not limited to: covered under warranty, replaced due to defect, free samples)
✳ FP	Service provided as part of family planning program
✳ G1	Most recent URR reading of less than 60
✳ G2	Most recent URR reading of 60 to 64.9
✳ G3	Most recent URR reading of 65 to 69.9
✳ G4	Most recent URR reading of 70 to 74.9
✳ G5	Most recent URR reading of 75 or greater
✳ G6	ESRD patient for whom less than six dialysis sessions have been provided in a month
⊙ G7	Pregnancy resulting from rape or incest or pregnancy certified by physician as life threatening MCM 2005.1, CIM 35-99
✳ G8	Monitored anesthesia care (MAC) for deep complex, complicated, or markedly invasive surgical procedure
✳ G9	Monitored anesthesia care patient who has history of severe cardio-pulmonary condition
✳ GA	Waiver of liability statement on file
✳ GB	Claims being resubmitted for payment because it is no longer covered under a global payment demonstration
⊙ GC	This service has been performed in part by a resident under the direction of a teaching physician. MCM 3350.5, MCM 4116
⊙ GE	This service has been performed by a resident without the presence of a teaching physician under the primary care exception. MCM 4116
GF	Non-physician (e.g., nurse practitioner (NP), certified registered nurse anesthetists (CRNA), certified registered nurse (CRN), clinical nurse specialist (CNS), physician assistant (PA) services in a critical access hospital
✳ GG	Performance and payment of a screening mammogram and diagnostic mammogram on the same patient, same day
✳ GH	Diagnostic mammogram converted from screening mammogram on same day
✳ GJ	"Opt out" physician or practitioner emergency or urgent service
✳ GK	Actual item/service ordered by physician, item associated with GA or GZ modifier
✳ GL	Medically unnecessary upgrade provided instead of standard item, no charge, no Advance Beneficiary Notice (ABN)
✳ GM	Multiple patients on one ambulance trip
✳ GN	Services delivered under an outpatient speech-language pathology plan of care
✳ GO	Services delivered under an outpatient occupational therapy plan of care
✳ GP	Services delivered under an outpatient physical therapy plan of care
✳ GQ	Via asynchronous telecommunications system
▶✳ GR	This service was performed in whole or in part by a resident in a department of Veterans' Affairs medical center or clinic, supervised in accordance with VA policy
▶⊙ GS	Dosage of EPO or darbepoetin alfa has been reduced 25% of preceding month's dosage MCM 4273.1
⊙ GT	Via interactive audio and video telecommunication systems
⊙ GV	Attending physician not employed or paid under arrangement by the patient's hospice provider MCM 4175-5
⊙ GW	Service not related to the hospice patient's terminal condition MCM 4175-5
◆ GY	Item or service statutorily excluded or does not meet the definition of any Medicare benefit
◆ GZ	Item or service expected to be denied as not reasonable or necessary MCM 2000
◆ H9	Court-ordered
◆ HA	Child/adolescent program
◆ HB	Adult program, non geriatric
◆ HC	Adult program, geriatric
◆ HD	Pregnant/parenting women's program
◆ HE	Mental health program
◆ HF	Substance abuse program
◆ HG	Opioid addiction treatment program
◆ HH	Integrated mental health/substance abuse program
◆ HI	Integrated mental health and mental retardation/developmental disabilities program
◆ HJ	Employee assistance program
◆ HK	Specialized mental health programs for high-risk populations
◆ HL	Intern
◆ HM	Less than bachelor degree level
◆ HN	Bachelor's degree level
◆ HO	Master's degree level
◆ HP	Doctoral level
◆ HQ	Group setting
◆ HR	Family/couple with client present
◆ HS	Family/couple without client present

◆ HT   Multi-disciplinary team

◆ HU   Funded by child welfare agency

◆ HV   Funded state addictions agency

◆ HW   Funded by state mental health agency

◆ HX   Funded by county/local agency

◆ HY   Funded by juvenile justice agency

◆ HZ   Funded by criminal justice agency

▶ ✳ J1   Competitive acquisition program no-pay submission for a prescription number

▶ ✳ J2   Competitive acquisition program, restocking of emergency drugs after emergency administration

▶ ✳ J3   Competitive acquisition program (CAP), drug not available through CAP as written, reimbursed under average sales price methodology

✳ JW   Drug amount discarded/not administered to any patient

✳ K0   Lower extremity prosthesis functional Level 0 does not have the ability or potential to ambulate or transfer safely with or without assistance and a prosthesis does not enhance their quality of life or mobility

✳ K1   Lower extremity prosthesis functional Level 1 has the ability or potential to use a prosthesis for transfers or ambulation on level surfaces at fixed cadence. Typical of the limited and unlimited household ambulator.

✳ K2   Lower extremity prosthesis functional Level 2 has the ability or potential for ambulation with the ability to traverse low level environmental barriers such as curbs, stairs or uneven surfaces. Typical of the limited community ambulator.

✳ K3   Lower extremity prosthesis functional Level 3 has the ability or potential for ambulation with variable cadence. Typical of the community ambulator who has the ability to traverse most environmental barriers and may have vocational, therapeutic, or exercise activity that demands prosthetic utilization beyond simple locomotion.

✳ K4   Lower extremity prosthesis functional Level 4 has the ability or potential for prosthetic ambulation that exceeds the basic ambulation skills, exhibiting high impact, stress, or energy levels, typical of the prosthetic demands of the child, active adult, or athlete.

✳ KA   Add on option/accessory for wheelchair

✳ KB   Beneficiary requested upgrade for ABN, more than 4 modifiers identified on claim

✳ KC   Replacement of special power wheelchair interface

KD   Drug or biological infused through DME

KF   Item designated by FDA as Class III device

✳ KH   Durable medical equipment prosthetics and orthotics supplies (DMEPOS) item, initial claim, purchase or first month rental

✳ KI   DMEPOS item, second or third month rental

✳ KJ   DMEPOS item, parenteral enteral nutrition (PEN) pump or capped rental, months four to fifteen

✳ KM   Replacement of facial prosthesis including new impression/moulage

✳ KN   Replacement of facial prosthesis using previous master model

✳ KO   Single drug unit dose formulation

✳ KP   First drug of a multiple drug unit dose formulation

✳ KQ   Second or subsequent drug of a multiple drug unit dose formulation

✳ KR   Rental item, billing for partial month

◎ KS   Glucose monitor supply for diabetic beneficiary not treated with insulin

✳ KX   Specific required documentation on file

✳ KZ   New coverage not implemented by managed care

✳ LC   Left circumflex coronary artery

✳ LD   Left anterior descending coronary artery

✳ LL   Lease/rental (use the LL modifier when durable medical equipment [DME] rental is to be applied against the purchase price)

✳ LR   Laboratory round trip
CIM 65-7

◎ LS   Food and Drug Administration (FDA)–monitored intraocular lens implant

✳ LT   Left side (used to identify procedures performed on the left side of the body)

✳ MS   Six-month maintenance and servicing fee for reasonable and necessary parts and labor, which are not covered under any manufacturer or supplier warranty

✳ NR   New when rented (use the NR modifier when DME which was new at the time of rental is subsequently purchased)

✳ NU   New equipment

▶ ✳ P1   A normal healthy patient

▶ ✳ P2   A patient with mild systemic disease

▶ ✳ P3   A patient with severe systemic disease

▶ ✳ P4   A patient with severe systemic disease that is a constant threat to life

▶ ✳ P5   A moribund patient who is not expected to survive without the operation

▶ ✳ P6   A declared brain-dead patient whose organs are being removed for donor purposes

✳ PL   Progressive addition lenses

✳ Q2   HCFA/ORD demonstration project procedure/service

* Q3   Live kidney donor surgery and related services

* Q4   Service for ordering/referring physician qualifies as a service exemption

☼ Q5   Service furnished by a substitute physician under a reciprocal billing arrangement
MCM 3060.6

☼ Q6   Service furnished by a locum tenens physician
MCM 3060.7

* Q7   One Class A finding

* Q8   Two Class B findings

* Q9   One Class B and two Class C findings

* QA   FDA investigational device exemption

QB   Deleted 12/31/05

* QC   Single channel monitoring

* QD   Recording and storage in solid state memory by a digital recorder

* QE   Prescribed amount of oxygen is less than 1 liter per minute (LPM)

* QF   Prescribed amount of oxygen exceeds 4 LPM and portable oxygen is prescribed

* QG   Prescribed amount of oxygen is greater than 4 LPM

* QH   Oxygen-conserving device is being used with an oxygen delivery system

☼ QJ   Services/items provided to a prisoner or patient in state or local custody, however the state or local government, as applicable, meets the requirements in 42 CFR 411.4 (B)

☼ QK   Medical direction of two, three, or four concurrent anesthesia procedures involving qualified individuals
MCM 3350.5

* QL   Patient pronounced dead after ambulance called

* QM   Ambulance service provided under arrangement by a provider of services

* QN   Ambulance service furnished directly by a provider of services

☼ QP   Documentation is on file showing that the laboratory test(s) was ordered individually or ordered as a CPT-recognized panel other than automated profile codes 80002 to 80019,* G0058, G0059, and G0060
MCM 7517.1

QQ   Deleted 12/31/05

▶ QR   Item or service provided in a Medicare specified study

☼ QS   Monitored anesthesia care service
MCM 150181

* QT   Recording and storage on tape by an analog tape recorder

QU   Deleted 12/31/05

☼ QV   Item or service provided as routine care in a Medicare qualifying clinical trial
CIM 30-1

* QW   CLIA-waived test

* QX   Certified registered nurse anesthetist (CRNA) service: with medical direction by a physician

☼ QY   Medical direction of one CRNA by an anesthesiologist
MCM 3350.5

* QZ   CRNA service: without medical direction by a physician

* RC   Right coronary artery

* RD   Drug provided to beneficiary, but not administered "incident-to"

* RP   Replacement and repair (RP may be used to indicate replacement of DME or orthotic and prosthetic devices that have been in use for sometime.) The claim shows the code for the part, followed by the *RP* modifier and the charge for the part.

* RR   Rental (use the RR modifier when DME is to be rented)

* RT   Right side (used to identify procedures performed on the right side of the body

♦ SA   Nurse practitioner rendering service in collaboration with a physician

♦ SB   Nurse midwife

♦ SC   Medically necessary service or supply

♦ SD   Services provided by registered nurse with specialized, highly technical home infusion training

♦ SE   State and/or federally funded programs/services

* SF   Second opinion ordered by a professional review organization (PRO) per Section 9401, P.L. 99-272 (100% reimbursement/no Medicare deductible or coinsurance)

* SG   Ambulatory surgical center (ASC) facility service

♦ SH   Second concurrently administered infusion therapy

♦ SJ   Third or more concurrently administered infusion therapy

♦ SK   Member of high risk population (use only with codes for immunization)

♦ SL   State supplied vaccine

♦ SM   Second surgical opinion

♦ SN   Third surgical opinion

♦ SQ   Item ordered by home health

♦ SS   Home infusion services provided in the infusion suite of the IV therapy provider

♦ ST   Related to trauma or injury

♦ SU   Procedure performed in physician's office (to denote use of facility and equipment)

♦ SV   Pharmaceuticals delivered to patient's home but not utilized

	SW	Services provided by a certified diabetic educator
◆	SY	Persons who are in close contact with member of high-risk population (use only with codes for immunization)
✳	T1	Left foot, second digit
✳	T2	Left foot, third digit
✳	T3	Left foot, fourth digit
✳	T4	Left foot, fifth digit
✳	T5	Right foot, great toe
✳	T6	Right foot, second digit
✳	T7	Right foot, third digit
✳	T8	Right foot, fourth digit
✳	T9	Right foot, fifth digit
✳	TA	Left foot, great toe
✳	TC	Technical component (Under certain circumstances, a charge may be made for the technical component alone. Under those circumstances the technical component charge is identified by adding modifier TC to the usual procedure number. Technical component charges are institutional charges and not billed separately by physicians. However, portable x-ray suppliers only bill for technical component and should utilize modifier TC. The charge data from portable x-ray suppliers will then be used to build customary and prevailing profiles.)
◆	TD	RN
◆	TE	LPN/LVN
◆	TF	Intermediate level of care
◆	TG	Complex/high-tech level of care
◆	TH	Obstetrical treatment/services, prenatal or postpartum
◆	TJ	Program group, child, and/or adolescent
◆	TK	Extra patient or passenger, non-ambulance
◆	TL	Early intervention/individualized family services plan (IFSP)
◆	TM	Individualized education program (IEP)
◆	TN	Rural/outside providers customary service area
◆	TP	Medical transport, unloaded vehicle
◆	TQ	Basic life support (BLS) transport by a volunteer ambulance provider
◆	TR	School-based IEP services provided outside the public school district responsible for the student
➠✳	TS	Follow-up service
◆	TT	Individualized service provided to more than one patient in same setting
◆	TU	Special payment rate, overtime
◆	TV	Special payment rates, holidays/weekends
◆	TW	Back-up equipment
◆	U1	Medicaid Level of Care 1, as defined by each State
◆	U2	Medicaid Level of Care 2, as defined by each State
◆	U3	Medicaid Level of Care 3, as defined by each State
◆	U4	Medicaid Level of Care 4, as defined by each State
◆	U5	Medicaid Level of Care 5, as defined by each State
◆	U6	Medicaid Level of Care 6, as defined by each State
◆	U7	Medicaid Level of Care 7, as defined by each State
◆	U8	Medicaid Level of Care 8, as defined by each State
◆	U9	Medicaid Level of Care 9, as defined by each State
◆	UA	Medicaid Level of Care 10, as defined by each State
◆	UB	Medicaid Level of Care 11, as defined by each State
◆	UC	Medicaid Level of Care 12, as defined by each State
◆	UD	Medicaid Level of Care 13, as defined by each State
✳	UE	Used DME
◆	UF	Services provided in the morning
◆	UG	Services provided in the afternoon
◆	UH	Services provided in the evening
◆	UJ	Services provided at night
◆	UK	Services provided on behalf of the client to someone other than the client (collateral relationship)
✳	UN	Two patients served
✳	UP	Three patients served
✳	UQ	Four patients served
✳	UR	Five patients served
✳	US	Six or more patients served
✳	VP	Aphakic patient

Ambulance Modifiers

Modifiers that are used on claims for ambulance services are created by combining two alpha characters. Each alpha character, with the exception of X, represents an origin (source) code or a destination code. The pair of alpha codes creates one modifier. The first position alpha-code = origin; the second position alpha-code = destination. On form HCFA-1491, used to report ambulance services, Item 12 should contain the origin code and Item 13 should contain the destination code. Origin and destination codes and their descriptions are as follows:

D   Diagnostic or therapeutic site other than *P* or *H* when these are used as origin codes

E   Residential, domiciliary, custodial facility (other than an 1819 facility)

G   Hospital-based dialysis facility (hospital or hospital related)

H   Hospital

I   Site of transfer (e.g., airport or helicopter pad) between modes of ambulance transport

✿ **Special coverage instructions**   ◆ **Not covered by or valid for Medicare**   ✳ **Carrier discretion**   ◀▶ **New**   ➠➠ **Revised**

J   Non–hospital-based dialysis facility
N   Skilled nursing facility (SNF) (1819 facility)
P   Physician's office (includes HMO non-hospital facility, clinic, etc.)
R   Residence
S   Scene of accident or acute event
X   Destination code only. Intermediate stop at physician's office en route to the hospital (includes non-hospital facility, clinic, etc.)

TRANSPORT SERVICES INCLUDING AMBULANCE (A0000-A0999)

◆ A0021   Ambulance service, outside state per mile, transport (Medicaid only)
Cross Reference A0030
◆ A0080   Non-emergency transportation: per mile—vehicle provided by volunteer (individual or organization), with no vested interest
◆ A0090   Non-emergency transportation, per mile—vehicle provided by individual (family member, self, neighbor), with vested interest
◆ A0100   Non-emergency transportation: taxi
◆ A0110   Non-emergency transportation and bus, intra or inter state carrier
◆ A0120   Non-emergency transportation: minibus, mountain area transports, or other transportation systems
◆ A0130   Non-emergency transportation: wheelchair van
◆ A0140   Non-emergency transportation and air travel (private or commercial), intra or inter state
◆ A0160   Non-emergency transportation: per mile—caseworker or social worker
◆ A0170   Transportation: ancillary: parking fees, tolls, other
◆ A0180   Non-emergency transportation: ancillary: lodging—recipient
◆ A0190   Non-emergency transportation: ancillary: meals—recipient
◆ A0200   Non-emergency transportation: ancillary: lodging—escort
◆ A0210   Non-emergency transportation: ancillary: meals—escort
∗ A0225   Ambulance service, neonatal transport, base rate, emergency transport, one way
∗ A0380   BLS mileage (per mile)
Cross Reference A0425
∗ A0382   BLS routine disposable supplies
∗ A0384   BLS specialized service disposable supplies; defibrillation (used by advanced life support [ALS] ambulances and BLS ambulances in jurisdictions where defibrillation is permitted in BLS ambulances)

∗ A0390   ALS mileage (per mile)
Cross Reference A0425
∗ A0392   ALS specialized service disposable supplies; defibrillation (to be used only in jurisdictions where defibrillation cannot be performed in BLS ambulances)
∗ A0394   ALS specialized service disposable supplies; intravenous (IV) drug therapy
∗ A0396   ALS specialized service disposable supplies; esophageal intubation
∗ A0398   ALS routine disposable supplies
∗ A0420   Ambulance waiting time (ALS or BLS), one half (½) hour increments

Waiting Time Table

Units	Time	Units	Time
1	½ to 1 hrs.	6	3 to 3½ hrs.
2	1 to 1½ hrs.	7	3½ to 4 hrs.
3	1½ to 2 hrs	8	4 to 4½ hrs.
4	2 to 2½ hrs.	9	4½ to 5 hrs.
5	2½ to 3 hrs.	10	5 to 5½ hrs.

∗ A0422   Ambulance (ALS or BLS) oxygen and oxygen supplies, life-sustaining situation
∗ A0424   Extra ambulance attendant, ALS or BLS or air (fixed or rotary winged); (requires medical review)
∗ A0425   Ground mileage, per statute mile
∗ A0426   Ambulance service, advanced life support, non-emergency transport, Level 1 (ALS1)
∗ A0427   Ambulance service, advanced life support, emergency transport, Level 1 (ALS1-Emergency)
∗ A0428   Ambulance service, BLS, non-emergency transport
∗ A0429   Ambulance service, basic life support, emergency transport (BLS-Emergency)
∗ A0430   Ambulance service, conventional air services, transport, one way (fixed wing)
∗ A0431   Ambulance service, conventional air services, transport, one way (rotary wing)
∗ A0432   Paramedic intercept (PI), rural area, transport furnished by a volunteer ambulance company, which is prohibited by state law from billing third-party payers
∗ A0433   Advanced life support, Level 2 (ALS2)
∗ A0434   Specialty care transport (SCT)
∗ A0435   Fixed wing air mileage, per statute mile
∗ A0436   Rotary wing air mileage, per statute mile
∗ A0800   Ambulance transport provided between the hours of 7 pm and 7 am
◆ A0888   Noncovered ambulance mileage, per mile (e.g., for miles traveled beyond closest appropriate facility)
MCM 2125
▶◆ A0998   Ambulance response and treatment, no transport
◎ A0999   Unlisted ambulance service
MCM 2120.1, MCM 2125

MEDICAL AND SURGICAL SUPPLIES (A4000-A8999)

◆ A4206 Syringe with needle, sterile 1 cc, each

◆ A4207 Syringe with needle, sterile 2 cc, each

◆ A4208 Syringe with needle, sterile 3 cc, each

◆ A4209 Syringe with needle, sterile 5 cc or greater, each

◆ A4210 Needle-free injection device, each
CIM 60-9

⊙ A4211 Supplies for self-administered injections
MCM 2049

✳ A4212 Non-coring needle or stylet with or without catheter

◆ A4213 Syringe, sterile, 20 cc or greater, each

⇒ ◆ A4215 Needle, sterile, any size, each

⇒ ⊙ A4216 Sterile water, saline and/or dexrose (diluent), 10 ml
MCM 2049

⊙ A4217 Sterile water/saline, 500 ml
MCM 2049

▶ ⊙ A4218 Sterile saline or water, metered dose dispenser, 10 ml

⊙ A4220 Refill kit for implantable infusion pump
CIM 60-14

✳ A4221 Supplies for maintenance of drug infusion catheter, per week (list drug separately)

✳ A4222 Infusion supplies for external drug infusion pump, per cassette or bag (list drug separately)

◆ A4223 Infusion supplies not used with external infusion pump, per cassette or bag (list drugs separately)
CIM 60-14

⊙ A4230 Infusion set for external insulin pump, non-needle cannula type
CIM 60-14

⊙ A4231 Infusion set for external insulin pump, needle type
CIM 60-14

◆ A4232 Syringe with needle for external insulin pump, sterile, 3 cc
CIM 60-14

▶ ✳ A4233 Replacement battery, alkaline (other than J cell), for use with medically necessary home blood glucose monitor owned by patient, each

▶ ✳ A4234 Replacement battery, alkaline, J cell, for use with medically necessary home blood glucose monitor owned by patient, each

▶ ✳ A4235 Replacement battery, lithium, for use with medically necessary home blood glucose monitor owned by patient, each

▶ ✳ A4236 Replacement battery, silver oxide, for use with medically necessary home blood glucose monitor owned by patient, each

⇒ ◆ A4244 Alcohol or peroxide, per pint

⇒ ◆ A4245 Alcohol wipes, per box

⇒ ◆ A4246 Betadine or pHisoHex solution, per pint

⇒ ◆ A4247 Betadine or iodine swabs/wipes, per box

✳ A4248 Chlorhexidine containing antiseptic, 1 ml

◆ A4250 Urine test or reagent strips or tablets (100 tablets or strips)
MCM 2100

⊙ A4253 Blood glucose test or reagent strips for home blood glucose monitor, per 50 strips
CIM 60-11

A4254 Deleted 12/31/05

⊙ A4255 Platforms for home blood glucose monitor, 50 per box
CIM 60-11

⊙ A4256 Normal, low and high calibrator solution/chips
CIM 60-11

✳ A4257 Replacement lens shield cartridge for use with laser skin piercing device, each

⊙ A4258 Spring-powered device for lancet, each
CIM 60-11

⊙ A4259 Lancets, per box of 100
CIM 60-11

A4260 Deleted 12/31/05

◆ A4261 Cervical cap for contraceptive use
Medicare Statute 1862a1

⊙ A4262 Temporary, absorbable lacrimal duct implant, each

⊙ A4263 Permanent, long-term, non-dissolvable lacrimal duct implant, each
MCM 15030

⊙ A4265 Paraffin, per pound
CIM 60-9

◆ A4266 Diaphragm for contraceptive use

◆ A4267 Contraceptive supply, condom, male, each

◆ A4268 Contraceptive supply, condom, female, each

◆ A4269 Contraceptive supply, spermicide (e.g., foam, gel), each

✳ A4270 Disposable endoscope sheath, each

✳ A4280 Adhesive skin support attachment for use with external breast prosthesis, each

⇒ ◆ A4281 Tubing for breast pump, replacement

⇒ ◆ A4282 Adapter for breast pump, replacement

⇒ ◆ A4283 Cap for breast pump bottle, replacement

⇒ ◆ A4284 Breast shield and splash protector for use with breast pump, replacement

⇒ ◆ A4285 Polycarbonate bottle for use with breast pump, replacement

⇒ ◆ A4286 Locking ring for breast pump, replacement

✳ A4290 Sacral nerve stimulation test lead, each

Vascular Catheters

⊕ A4300 Implantable access catheter, (e.g., venous, arterial, epidural subarachnoid, or peritoneal, etc.) external access
MCM 2130

∗ A4301 Implantable access total; catheter, port/reservoir (e.g., venous, arterial, epidural, or subarachnoid, peritoneal etc.)

➡∗ A4305 Disposable drug delivery system, flow rate of 50 ml or greater per hour

➡∗ A4306 Disposable drug delivery system, flow rate of 5 ml or less per hour

Incontinence Appliances and Care Supplies

⊕ A4310 Insertion tray without drainage bag and without catheter (accessories only)
MCM 2130

⊕ A4311 Insertion tray without drainage bag with indwelling catheter, Foley type, two-way latex with coating (Teflon, silicone, silicone elastomer or hydrophilic, etc.)
MCM 2130

⊕ A4312 Insertion tray without drainage bag with indwelling catheter, Foley type, two-way, all silicone
MCM 2130

⊕ A4313 Insertion tray without drainage bag with indwelling catheter, Foley type, three-way, for continuous irrigation
MCM 2130

⊕ A4314 Insertion tray with drainage bag with indwelling catheter, Foley type, two-way latex with coating (Teflon, silicone, silicone elastomer or hydrophilic, etc.)
MCM 2130

⊕ A4315 Insertion tray with drainage bag with indwelling catheter, Foley type, two-way, all silicone
MCM 2130

⊕ A4316 Insertion tray with drainage bag with indwelling catheter, Foley type, three-way, for continuous irrigation
MCM 2130

⊕ A4320 Irrigation tray with bulb or piston syringe, any purpose
MCM 2130

∗ A4321 Therapeutic agent for urinary catheter irrigation

⊕ A4322 Irrigation syringe, bulb or piston, each
MCM 2130

⊕ A4326 Male external catheter specialty type with integral collection chamber, each
MCM 2130

⊕ A4327 Female external urinary collection device; metal cup, each
MCM 2130

⊕ A4328 Female external urinary collection device; pouch, each
MCM 2130

⊕ A4330 Perianal fecal collection pouch with adhesive, each
MCM 2130

∗ A4331 Extension drainage tubing, any type, any length, with connector/adaptor, for use with urinary leg bag or urostomy pouch, each

∗ A4332 Lubricant, individual sterile packet, each

∗ A4333 Urinary catheter anchoring device, adhesive skin attachment, each

∗ A4334 Urinary catheter anchoring device, leg strap, each

⊕ A4335 Incontinence supply; miscellaneous
MCM 2130

⊕ A4338 Indwelling catheter; Foley type, two-way latex with coating (Teflon, silicone, silicone elastomer, or hydrophilic, etc.), each
MCM 2130

⊕ A4340 Indwelling catheter; specialty type (e.g., coudé, mushroom, wing, etc.), each
MCM 2130

⊕ A4344 Indwelling catheter, Foley type, two-way, all silicone, each
MCM 2130A

⊕ A4346 Indwelling catheter; Foley type, three-way for continuous irrigation, each
MCM 2130

∗ A4348 Male external catheter with integral collection compartment, extended wear, (e.g., two per month)

⊕ A4349 Male external catheter, with or without adhesive, disposable, each
CIM 60-9

⊕ A4351 Intermittent urinary catheter; straight tip, with or without coating (Teflon, silicone, silicone elastomer, or hydrophilic, etc.), each
MCM 2130

⊕ A4352 Intermittent urinary catheter; coudé (curved) tip, with or without coating (Teflon, silicone, silicone elastomeric, or hydrophilic, etc.), each
MCM 2130

∗ A4353 Intermittent urinary catheter, with insertion supplies

⊕ A4354 Insertion tray with drainage bag but without catheter
MCM 2130

⊕ A4355 Irrigation tubing set for continuous bladder irrigation through a three-way indwelling Foley catheter, each
MCM 2130

External Urinary Supplies

⊛ A4356   External urethral clamp or compression device (not to be used for catheter clamp), each
MCM 2130

⊛ A4357   Bedside drainage bag, day or night, with or without anti-reflux device, with or without tube, each
MCM 2130

⊛ A4358   Urinary drainage bag, leg or abdomen, vinyl, with or without tube, with straps, each
MCM 2130

⊛ A4359   Urinary suspensory without leg bag, each
MCM 2130

Ostomy Supplies

⊛ A4361   Ostomy faceplate, each
MCM 2130A

⊛ A4362   Skin barrier; solid, 4 × 4 or equivalent; each
MCM 2130

▶⊛ A4363   Ostomy clamp, any type, replacement only, each

∗ A4364   Adhesive, liquid or equal, any type, per ounce (oz)

∗ A4365   Adhesive remover wipes, any type, per 50

∗ A4366   Ostomy vent, any type, each

⊛ A4367   Ostomy belt, each
MCM 2130A

∗ A4368   Ostomy filter, any type, each

∗ A4369   Ostomy skin barrier, liquid (spray, brush, etc.), per oz

∗ A4371   Ostomy skin barrier, powder, per oz

➠⊛ A4372   Ostomy skin barrier, solid 4 × 4 or equivalent, standard wear, with built-in convexity, each
MCM 2130

∗ A4373   Ostomy skin barrier, with flange (solid, flexible, or accordion), with built-in convexity, any size, each
MCM 2130

∗ A4375   Ostomy pouch, drainable, with faceplate attached, plastic, each

∗ A4376   Ostomy pouch, drainable, with faceplate attached, rubber, each

∗ A4377   Ostomy pouch, drainable, for use on faceplate, plastic, each

∗ A4378   Ostomy pouch, drainable, for use on faceplate, rubber, each

∗ A4379   Ostomy pouch, urinary, with faceplate attached, plastic, each

∗ A4380   Ostomy pouch, urinary, with faceplate attached, rubber, each

∗ A4381   Ostomy pouch, urinary, with faceplate attached, plastic, each

∗ A4382   Ostomy pouch, urinary, for use on faceplate, heavy plastic, each

∗ A4383   Ostomy pouch, urinary, for use on faceplate, rubber, each

∗ A4384   Ostomy faceplate equivalent, silicone ring, each

∗ A4385   Ostomy skin barrier, solid 4 × 4 or equivalent, extended wear, without built-in convexity, each

∗ A4387   Ostomy pouch closed, with barrier attached, with built-in convexity (1 piece), each
MCM 2130

∗ A4388   Ostomy pouch, drainable, with extended wear barrier attached (1 piece), each
MCM 2130

∗ A4389   Ostomy pouch, drainable, with barrier attached, with built-in convexity (1 piece), each
MCM 2130

∗ A4390   Ostomy pouch, drainable, with extended wear barrier attached, with built-in convexity (1 piece), each

∗ A4391   Ostomy pouch, urinary, with extended wear barrier attached (1 piece), each
MCM 2130

∗ A4392   Ostomy pouch, urinary, with standard wear barrier attached, with built-in convexity (1 piece), each

∗ A4393   Ostomy pouch, urinary, with extended wear barrier attached, with built-in convexity (1 piece), each

∗ A4394   Ostomy deodorant for use in ostomy pouch, liquid, per fluid ounce

∗ A4395   Ostomy deodorant for use in ostomy pouch, solid, per tablet

∗ A4396   Ostomy belt with peristomal hernia support

⊛ A4397   Irrigation supply; sleeve, each
MCM 2130

⊛ A4398   Ostomy irrigation supply; bag, each
MCM 2130A

⊛ A4399   Ostomy irrigation supply; cone/catheter, including brush
MCM 2130A

⊛ A4400   Ostomy irrigation set
MCM 2130

⊛ A4402   Lubricant, per ounce
MCM 2130

⊛ A4404   Ostomy ring, each
MCM 2130

⊛ A4405   Ostomy skin barrier, non-pectin based, paste, per ounce
MCM 2130

⊛ A4406   Ostomy skin barrier, pectin-based, paste, per ounce
MCM 2130

⊛ A4407 Ostomy skin barrier, with flange (solid, flexible, or accordion), extended wear, with built-in convexity, 4 × 4 inches or smaller, each
MCM 2130

⊛ A4408 Ostomy skin barrier, with flange (solid, flexible or accordion), extended wear, with built-in convexity, larger than 4 × 4 inches, each
MCM 2130

⊛ A4409 Ostomy skin barrier, with flange (solid, flexible or accordion), extended wear, without built-in convexity, 4 × 4 inches or smaller, each
MCM 2130

⊛ A4410 Ostomy skin barrier, with flange (solid, flexible or accordion), extended wear, without built-in convexity, larger than 4 × 4 inches, each
MCM 2130

▶⊛ A4411 Ostomy skin barrier, solid 4 × 4 or equivalent, extended wear, with built-in convexity, each

▶⊛ A4412 Ostomy pouch, drainable, high output, for use on a barrier with flange (2 piece system), without filter, each
MCM 2130

⊛ A4413 Ostomy pouch, drainable, high output, for use on a barrier with flange (2 piece system), with filter, each
MCM 2130

⊛ A4414 Ostomy skin barrier, with flange (solid, flexible or accordion), without built-in convexity, 4 × 4 inches or smaller, each
MCM 2130

⊛ A4415 Ostomy skin barrier, with flange (solid, flexible or accordion), without built-in convexity, larger than 4 × 4 inches, each
MCM 2130

∗ A4416 Ostomy pouch, closed, with barrier attached, with filter (1 piece), each

∗ A4417 Ostomy pouch, closed, with barrier attached, with built-in convexity, with filter (1 piece), each

∗ A4418 Ostomy pouch, closed; without barrier attached, with filter (1 piece), each

∗ A4419 Ostomy pouch, closed; for use on barrier with non-locking flange, with filter (2 piece), each

∗ A4420 Ostomy pouch, closed; for use on barrier with locking flange (2 piece), each

➡ ⊛ A4421 Ostomy supply; miscellaneous
MCM 2130

⊛ A4422 Ostomy absorbent material (sheet/pad/crystal packet) for use in ostomy pouch to thicken liquid stomal output, each
MCM 2130

∗ A4423 Ostomy pouch, closed; for use on barrier with locking flange, with filter (2 piece), each

∗ A4424 Ostomy pouch, drainable, with barrier attached, with filter (1 piece), each

∗ A4425 Ostomy pouch, drainable; for use on barrier with non-locking flange, with filter (2 piece system), each

∗ A4426 Ostomy pouch, drainable; for use on barrier with locking flange (2 piece system), each

∗ A4427 Ostomy pouch, drainable; for use on barrier with locking flange, with filter (2 piece system), each

∗ A4428 Ostomy pouch, urinary, with extended wear barrier attached, with faucet-type tap with valve (1 piece), each

∗ A4429 Ostomy pouch, urinary, with barrier attached, with built-in convexity, with faucet-type tap with valve (1 piece), each

∗ A4430 Ostomy pouch, urinary, with extended wear barrier attached, with built-in convexity, with faucet-type tap with valve (1 piece), each

∗ A4431 Ostomy pouch, urinary; with barrier attached, with faucet-type tap with valve (1 piece), each

∗ A4432 Ostomy pouch, urinary; for use on barrier with non-locking flange, with faucet-type tap with valve (2 piece), each

∗ A4433 Ostomy pouch, urinary; for use on barrier with locking flange (2 piece), each

∗ A4434 Ostomy pouch, urinary; for use on barrier with locking flange, with faucet-type tap with valve (2 piece), each

Miscellaneous Supplies

⊛ A4450 Tape, non-waterproof, per 18 square inches
MCM 2130

⊛ A4452 Tape, waterproof, per 18 square inches
MCM 2130

⊛ A4455 Adhesive remover or solvent (for tape, cement or other adhesive), per ounce
MCM 2130

➡ ◆ A4458 Enema bag with tubing, reusable

∗ A4462 Abdominal dressing holder, each
MCM 2130

∗ A4465 Non-elastic binder for extremity

⊛ A4470 Gravlee jet washer
MCM 2320, CIM 50-4

⊛ A4480 VABRA aspirator
MCM 2320, CIM 50-4

∗ A4481 Tracheostoma filter, any type, any size, each

∗ A4483 Moisture exchanger, disposable, for use with invasive mechanical ventilation

◆ A4490 Surgical stockings above knee length, each
MCM 2079, MCM 2133, CIM 60-9

◆ A4495 Surgical stockings thigh length, each
MCM 2079, MCM 2133, CIM 60-9

◆ A4500 Surgical stockings below knee length, each
MCM 2079, MCM 2133, CIM 60-9

◆ A4510 Surgical stockings full length, each
MCM 2079, MCM 2133, CIM 60-9

◆ A4520 Incontinence garment, any type, (e.g., brief, diaper), each

☺ A4550 Surgical trays
MCM 15030

➡☺ A4554 Disposable underpads, all sizes
MCM 2130, CIM 60-9

✱ A4556 Electrodes, (e.g., apnea monitor), per pair

✱ A4557 Lead wires, (e.g., apnea monitor), per pair

◆ A4558 Conductive paste or gel

✱ A4561 Pessary, rubber, any type

✱ A4562 Pessary, non-rubber, any type

✱ A4565 Slings

◆ A4570 Splint
MCM 2079

◆ A4575 Topical hyperbaric oxygen chamber, disposable
CIM 35-10

◆ A4580 Cast supplies (e.g., plaster)
MCM 2079

◆ A4590 Special casting material (e.g., fiberglass)

✱ A4595 Electrical stimulators supplies, 2-lead, per month (e.g. tens, NMES)
CIM 45-25

Supplies for Respiratory and Oxygen Equipment

▶✱ A4604 Tubing with integrated heating element for use with positive airway pressure device

✱ A4605 Tracheal suction catheter, closed system, each

✱ A4606 Oxygen probe for use with oximeter device, replacement

✱ A4608 Transtracheal oxygen catheter, each

✱ A4611 Battery, heavy duty; replacement for patient-owned ventilator

✱ A4612 Battery cables; replacement for patient-owned ventilator

✱ A4613 Battery charger; replacement for patient-owned ventilator

✱ A4614 Peak expiratory flow rate meter, hand-held

☺ A4615 Cannula, nasal
MCM 3312, CIM 60-4

☺ A4616 Tubing (oxygen), per foot
MCM 3312, CIM 60-4

☺ A4617 Mouth piece
MCM 3312, CIM 60-4

☺ A4618 Breathing circuits
MCM 3312, CIM 60-4

☺ A4619 Face tent
MCM 3312, CIM 60-4

☺ A4620 Variable concentration mask
MCM 3312, CIM 60-4

◆ A4623 Tracheostomy, inner cannula
MCM 2130, CIM 65-16

✱ A4624 Tracheal suction catheter, any type, other than closed system, each

✱ A4625 Tracheostomy care kit for new tracheostomy

✱ A4626 Tracheostomy cleaning brush, each

◆ A4627 Spacer, bag or reservoir, with or without mask, for use with metered dose inhaler
MCM 2100

✱ A4628 Oropharyngeal suction catheter, each

✱ A4629 Tracheostomy care kit for established tracheostomy

Supplies for Other Durable Medical Equipment

➡☺ A4630 Replacement batteries; medically necessary, transcutaneous electrical stimulator, owned by patient
CIM 65-8

➡◆ A4632 Replacement battery for external infusion pump, any type, each

✱ A4633 Replacement bulb/lamp for ultraviolet light therapy system, each

✱ A4634 Replacement bulb for therapeutic light box, tabletop model

☺ A4635 Underarm pad, crutch, replacement, each
CIM 60-9

☺ A4636 Replacement, handgrip, cane, crutch, or walker, each
CIM 60-9

☺ A4637 Replacement, tip, cane, crutch, walker, each
CIM 60-9

✱ A4638 Replacement battery for patient-owned ear pulse generator, each

✱ A4639 Replacement pad for infrared heating pad system, each

☺ A4640 Replacement pad for use with medically necessary alternating pressure pad owned by patient
MCM 4107.6, CIM 60-9

Supplies for Radiological Procedures

➡✱ A4641 Radiopharmaceutical, diagnostic, not otherwise classified

➡✱ A4642 Indium In-111 satumomab pendetide, diagnostic, per study dose, up to 6 millicurie

A4643 Deleted 12/31/05
A4644 Deleted 12/31/05
A4645 Deleted 12/31/05
A4646 Deleted 12/31/05
A4647 Deleted 12/31/05

✱ A4649 Surgical supply, miscellaneous

Supplies for End Stage Renal Disease

NOTE: For DME items for ESRD see procedures codes E1550 to E1699.

- ✪ A4651 Calibrated microcapillary tube, each
MCM 4270
- ✪ A4652 Microcapillary tube sealant
MCM 4270
- ✻ A4653 Peritoneal dialysis catheter anchoring device, belt, each
- A4656 Deleted 12/31/05
- ✪ A4657 Syringe, with or without needle, each
MCM 4270
- ✪ A4660 Sphygmomanometer/blood pressure apparatus with cuff and stethoscope
MCM 4270
- ✪ A4663 Blood pressure cuff only
MCM 4270
- ◆ A4670 Automatic blood pressure monitor
MCM 4270, CIM 50-42
- ✪ A4671 Disposable cycler set used with cycler dialysis machine, each
MCM 4270
- ✪ A4672 Drainage extension line, sterile, for dialysis, each
MCM 4270
- ✪ A4673 Extension line with easy lock connectors, used with dialysis
MCM 4270
- ✪ A4674 Chemicals/antiseptics solution used to clean/sterilize dialysis equipment, per 8 oz
MCM 4270
- ✪ A4680 Activated carbon filters for hemodialysis, each
MCM 4270, CIM 55-1
- ✪ A4690 Dialyzers (artificial kidneys) all types, all sizes, for hemodialysis, each
MCM 4270
- ✪ A4706 Bicarbonate concentrate, solution, for hemodialysis, per gallon
MCM 4270
- ✪ A4707 Bicarbonate concentrate, powder, for hemodialysis, per packet
MCM 4270
- ✪ A4708 Acetate concentrate solution, for hemodialysis, per gallon
MCM 4270
- ✪ A4709 Acid concentrate, solution, for hemodialysis, per gallon
MCM 4270
- ✪ A4714 Treated water (deionized, distilled, reverse osmosis) for peritoneal dialysis, per gallon
MCM 4270, CIM 55-1
- ✪ A4719 "Y set" tubing for peritoneal dialysis
MCM 4270
- ✪ A4720 Dialysate solution, any concentrate of dextrose, fluid volume greater than 249 cc, but less than or equal to 999 cc, for peritoneal dialysis
MCM 4270
- ✪ A4721 Dialysate solution, any concentrate of dextrose, fluid volume greater than 999 cc, but less than or equal to 1999 cc, for peritoneal dialysis
MCM 4270
- ✪ A4722 Dialysate solution, any concentrate of dextrose, fluid volume greater than 1999 cc, but less than or equal to 2999 cc, for peritoneal dialysis
MCM 4270
- ✪ A4723 Dialysate solution, any concentrate of dextrose, fluid volume greater than 2999 cc, but less than or equal to 3999 cc, for peritoneal dialysis
MCM 4270
- ✪ A4724 Dialysate solution, any concentrate of dextrose, fluid volume greater than 3999 cc, but less than or equal to 4999 cc, for peritoneal dialysis
MCM 4270
- ✪ A4725 Dialysate solution, any concentrate of dextrose, fluid volume greater than 4999 cc, but less than or equal to 5999 cc, for peritoneal dialysis
MCM 4270
- ✪ A4726 Dialysate solution, any concentrate of dextrose, fluid volume greater than 5999 cc, for peritoneal dialysis
MCM 4270
- ✻ A4728 Dialysate solution, non-dextrose containing, 500 ml
- ✪ A4730 Fistula cannulation set for hemodialysis, each
MCM 4270
- ✪ A4736 Topical anesthetic, for dialysis, per gram
MCM 4270
- ✪ A4737 Injectable anesthetic, for dialysis, per 10 ml
MCM 4270
- ✪ A4740 Shunt accessories for hemodialysis, any type, each
MCM 4270
- ✪ A4750 Blood tubing, arterial or venous for hemodialysis, each
MCM 4270
- ✪ A4755 Blood tubing, arterial and venous combined, for hemodialysis, each
MCM 4270
- ✪ A4760 Dialysate solution test kit, for peritoneal dialysis, any type, each
MCM 4270
- ✪ A4765 Dialysate concentrate, powder, additive for peritoneal dialysis, per packet
MCM 4270

⊛ A4766 Dialysate concentrate, solution, additive for peritoneal dialysis, per 10 ml
MCM 4270

⊛ A4770 Blood collection tube, vacuum, for dialysis, per 50
MCM 4270

⊛ A4771 Serum clotting time tube, for dialysis, per 50
MCM 4270

⊛ A4772 Blood glucose test strips, for dialysis, per 50
MCM 4270

⊛ A4773 Occult blood test strips, for dialysis, per 50
MCM 4270

⊛ A4774 Ammonia test strips, for dialysis, per 50
MCM 4270

⊛ A4802 Protamine sulfate, for hemodialysis, per 50 mg
MCM 4270

⊛ A4860 Disposable catheter tips for peritoneal dialysis, per 10

⊛ A4870 Plumbing and/or electrical work for home dialysis equipment

⊛ A4890 Contracts, repair and maintenance, for hemodialysis equipment
MCM 2100.4

⊛ A4911 Drain bag/bottle, for dialysis, each

⊛ A4913 Miscellaneous dialysis supplies, not otherwise specified

⊛ A4918 Venous pressure clamp, for hemodialysis, each

⊛ A4927 Gloves, non-sterile, per 100

⊛ A4928 Surgical mask, per 20

⊛ A4929 Tourniquet for dialysis, each

⊛ A4930 Gloves, sterile, per pair

∗ A4931 Oral thermometer, reusable, any type, each

➠◆ A4932 Rectal thermometer, reusable, any type, each

Additional Ostomy Supplies

⊛ A5051 Ostomy pouch, closed; with barrier attached (1 piece), each
MCM 2130

⊛ A5052 Ostomy pouch, closed; without barrier attached (1 piece), each
MCM 2130

⊛ A5053 Ostomy pouch, closed; for use on faceplate, each
MCM 2130

⊛ A5054 Ostomy pouch, closed; for use on barrier with flange (2 piece), each
MCM 2130

⊛ A5055 Stoma cap
MCM 2130

⊛ A5061 Ostomy pouch, drainable; with barrier attached (1 piece), each
MCM 2130

⊛ A5062 Ostomy pouch, drainable; without barrier attached (1 piece), each
MCM 2130

⊛ A5063 Ostomy pouch, drainable; for use on barrier with flange (2 piece), each
MCM 2130

⊛ A5071 Ostomy pouch, urinary; with barrier attached (1 piece), each
MCM 2130

⊛ A5072 Ostomy pouch, urinary; without barrier attached (1 piece), each
MCM 2130

⊛ A5073 Ostomy pouch, urinary; for use on barrier with flange (2 piece), each
MCM 2130

⊛ A5081 Continent device; plug for continent stoma
MCM 2130

⊛ A5082 Continent device; catheter for continent stoma
MCM 2130

⊛ A5093 Ostomy accessory; convex insert
MCM 2130

Additional Incontinence Appliances/Supplies

⊛ A5102 Bedside drainage bottle with or without tubing, rigid or expandable, each
MCM 2130

⊛ A5105 Urinary suspensory; with leg bag, with or without tube
MCM 2130

⊛ A5112 Urinary leg bag; latex
MCM 2130

⊛ A5113 Leg strap; latex, replacement only, per set
MCM 2130

⊛ A5114 Leg strap; foam or fabric, replacement only, per set
MCM 2130

Supplies for Either Incontinence or Ostomy Appliances

A5119 Deleted 12/31/05

▶⊛ A5120 Skin barrier, wipes or swabs, each
MCM 2130

⊛ A5121 Skin barrier; solid, 6 × 6 or equivalent, each
MCM 2130

⊛ A5122 Skin barrier; solid, 8 × 8 or equivalent, each
MCM 2130

⊛ A5126 Adhesive or non-adhesive; disc or foam pad
MCM 2130

☼ A5131 Appliance cleaner, incontinence and ostomy appliances, per 16 oz
MCM 2130

∗ A5200 Percutaneous catheter/tube anchoring
device, adhesive skin attachment

Diabetic Shoes, Fitting and Modifications

☼ A5500 For diabetics only, fitting (including follow-up), custom preparation and sup-
ply of off-the-shelf depth-inlay shoe
manufactured to accommodate multi-
density insert(s), per shoe
MCM 2134

☼ A5501 For diabetics only, fitting (including follow-up), custom preparation and sup-
ply of shoe molded from cast(s) of patient's foot (custom molded shoe), per
shoe
MCM 2134

☼ A5503 For diabetics only, modification (including fitting) of off-the-shelf depth-inlay
shoe or custommolded shoe with roller
or rigid rocker bottom, per shoe
MCM 2134

☼ A5504 For diabetics only, modification (including fitting) of off-the-shelf depth-inlay
shoe or custom-molded shoe with
wedge(s), per shoe
MCM 2134

☼ A5505 For diabetics only, modification (including fitting) of off-the-shelf depth-inlay
shoe or custom-molded shoe with
metatarsal bar, per shoe
MCM 2134

☼ A5506 For diabetics only, modification (including fitting) of off-the-shelf depth-inlay
shoe or custom-molded shoe with offset heel(s), per shoe
MCM 2134

☼ A5507 For diabetics only, not otherwise specified modification (including fitting) of
off-the-shelf depth-inlay shoe or custom-molded shoe, per shoe
MCM 2134

∗ A5508 For diabetics only, deluxe feature of
off-the-shelf depth-inlay shoe or custom-molded shoe, per shoe

A5509 Deleted 12/31/05

☼ A5510 For diabetics only, direct formed, compression molded to patient's foot without external heat source, multiple-den-
sity insert(s) prefabricated, per shoe
MCM 2134

A5511 Deleted 12/31/05

▶∗ A5512 For diabetics only, multiple density insert, direct formed, molded to foot after
external heat source of 230 degrees
Fahrenheit or higher, total contact with
patient's foot, including arch, base layer
minimum of 1/4 inch material of shore
a 35 durometer or 3/16 inch material of
shore a 40 durometer (or higher), prefabricated, each

▶∗ A5513 For diabetics only, multiple density insert, custom molded from model of patient's foot, total contact with patient's
foot, including arch, base layer minimum of 1/4 inch material of shore a 35
durometer or 3/16 inch material of
shore a 40 durometer (or higher), includes arch filler and other shaping material, custom fabricated, each

Dressings

∗ A6000 Non-contact wound warming wound
cover for use with the non-contact wound
warming device and warming card

∗ A6010 Collagen based wound filler, dry form,
per gram of collagen

☼ A6011 Collagen based wound filler, gel/paste,
per gram of collagen
MCM 2079

∗ A6021 Collagen dressing, pad size 16 square
inch (in²) or less, each

∗ A6022 Collagen dressing, pad size more than
16 in² but less than or equal to 48 in²,
each

∗ A6023 Collagen dressing, pad size more than
48 in², each

∗ A6024 Collagen dressing wound filler, per 6 in

⇒◆ A6025 Gel sheet for dermal or epidermal application, (e.g., silicon, hydrogel, other),
each

∗ A6154 Wound pouch, each

∗ A6196 Alginate or other fiber gelling dressing,
wound cover, pad size 16 in² or less,
each dressing

∗ A6197 Alginate or other fiber gelling dressing,
wound cover, pad size more than 16
in², but less than or equal to 48 in²,
each dressing

∗ A6198 Alginate or other fiber gelling dressing,
wound cover, pad size more than 48
in², each dressing

∗ A6199 Alginate or other fiber gelling dressing,
wound filler, per 6 in

∗ A6200 Composite dressing, pad size 16 in² or
less, without adhesive border, each
dressing

* A6201 Composite dressing, pad size more than 16 in^2 but less than or equal to 48 in^2, without adhesive border, each dressing

* A6202 Composite dressing, pad size more than 48 in^2, without adhesive border, each dressing

* A6203 Composite dressing, pad size 16 in^2 or less, with any size adhesive border, each dressing

* A6204 Composite dressing, pad size more than 16 in^2 but less than or equal to 48 in, with any size adhesive border, each dressing

* A6205 Composite dressing, pad size more than 48 in^2, with any size adhesive, each dressing

* A6206 Contact layer, 16 in^2 or less, each dressing

* A6207 Contact layer, more than 16 in^2 but less than or equal to 48 in^2, each dressing

* A6208 Contact layer, more than 48 in^2, each dressing

* A6209 Foam dressing, wound cover, pad size 16 in^2 or less, without adhesive border, each dressing

* A6210 Foam dressing, wound cover, pad size more than 16 in^2 but less than or equal to 48 in^2, without adhesive border, each dressing

* A6211 Foam dressing, wound cover, pad size more than 48 in^2, without adhesive border, each dressing

* A6212 Foam dressing, wound cover, pad size 16 in^2 or less, with any size adhesive border, each dressing

* A6213 Foam dressing, wound cover, pad size more than 16 in^2 but less than or equal to 48 in^2, with any size adhesive border, each dressing

* A6214 Foam dressing, wound cover, pad size more than 48 in^2, with any size adhesive border, each dressing

* A6215 Foam dressing, wound filler, per gram

* A6216 Gauze, non-impregnated, non-sterile, pad size 16 in^2 or less, without adhesive border, each dressing

* A6217 Gauze, non-impregnated, non-sterile, pad size more than 16 in^2 but less than or equal to 48 in^2, without adhesive border, each dressing

* A6218 Gauze, non-impregnated, non-sterile, pad size more than 48 in^2, without adhesive border, each dressing

* A6219 Gauze, non-impregnated, pad size 16 in^2 or less, with any size adhesive border, each dressing

* A6220 Gauze, non-impregnated, pad size more than 16 in^2 but less than or equal to 48 in^2, with any size adhesive border, each dressing

* A6221 Gauze, non-impregnated, pad size more than 48 in^2, with any size adhesive border, each dressing

* A6222 Gauze, impregnated, other than water, normal saline or hydrogel, pad size 16 in^2 or less, without adhesive border, each dressing

* A6223 Gauze, impregnated, with other than water, normal saline or hydrogel, pad size more than 16 in^2 but less than or equal to 48 in^2, without adhesive border, each dressing

* A6224 Gauze, impregnated, other than water or normal saline or hydrogel, pad size more than 48 in^2, without adhesive border, each dressing

* A6228 Gauze, impregnated, water or normal saline, pad size 16 in^2 or less, without adhesive border, each dressing

* A6229 Gauze, impregnated, water or normal saline, pad size more than 16 in^2 but less than or equal to 48 in^2, without adhesive border, each dressing

* A6230 Gauze, impregnated, water or normal saline, pad size more than 48 in^2, without adhesive border, each dressing

* A6231 Gauze, impregnated, hydrogel, for direct wound contact, pad size 16 in^2 or less, each dressing

* A6232 Gauze, impregnated, hydrogel, for direct wound contact, pad size greater than 16 in^2, but less than or equal to 48 in^2, each dressing

* A6233 Gauze, impregnated, hydrogel, for direct wound contact, pad size more than 48 in^2, each dressing

* A6234 Hydrocolloid dressing, wound cover, pad size 16 in^2 or less, without adhesive border, each dressing

* A6235 Hydrocolloid dressing, wound cover, pad size more than 16 in^2 but less than or equal to 48 in^2, without adhesive border, each dressing

* A6236 Hydrocolloid dressing, wound cover, pad size more than 48 in^2, without adhesive border, each dressing

* A6237 Hydrocolloid dressing, wound cover, pad size 16 in^2 or less, with any size adhesive border, each dressing

* A6238 Hydrocolloid dressing, wound cover, pad size more than 16 in^2 but less than or equal to 48 in^2, with any size adhesive border, each dressing

* A6239 Hydrocolloid dressing, wound cover, pad size more than 48 in^2, with any size adhesive border, each dressing

* A6240 Hydrocolloid dressing, wound filler, paste, per fluid ounce

* A6241 Hydrocolloid dressing, wound filler, dry form, per gram

○ **Special coverage instructions** ◆ **Not covered by or valid for Medicare** * **Carrier discretion** ◀▶ **New** ⬅▬▬➡ **Revised**

* A6242 Hydrogel dressing, wound cover, pad size 16 in^2 or less, without adhesive border, each dressing

* A6243 Hydrogel dressing, wound cover, pad size more than 16 in^2 but less than or equal to 48 in^2, without adhesive border, each dressing

* A6244 Hydrogel dressing, wound cover, pad size more than 48 in^2, without adhesive border, each dressing

* A6245 Hydrogel dressing, wound cover, pad size 16 in^2 or less, with any size adhesive border, each dressing

* A6246 Hydrogel dressing, wound cover, pad size more than 16 in^2 but less than or equal to 48 in^2, with any size adhesive border, each dressing

* A6247 Hydrogel dressing, wound cover, pad size more than 48 in^2, with any size adhesive border, each dressing

* A6248 Hydrogel dressing, wound filler, gel, per fluid ounce

* A6250 Skin sealants, protectants, moisturizers, ointments, any type, any size

* A6251 Specialty absorptive dressing, wound cover, pad size 16 in^2 or less, without adhesive border, each dressing

* A6252 Specialty absorptive dressing, wound cover, pad size more than 16 in^2 but less than or equal to 48 in^2, without adhesive border, each dressing

* A6253 Specialty absorptive dressing, wound cover, pad size more than 48 in^2, without adhesive border, each dressing

* A6254 Specialty absorptive dressing, wound cover, pad size 16 in^2 or less, with any size adhesive border, each dressing

* A6255 Specialty absorptive dressing, wound cover, pad size more than 16 in^2 but less than or equal to 48 in^2, with any size adhesive border, each dressing

* A6256 Specialty absorptive dressing, wound cover, pad size more than 48 in^2, with any size adhesive border, each dressing

* A6257 Transparent film, 16 in^2 or less, each dressing

* A6258 Transparent film, more than 16 in^2 but less than or equal to 48 in^2, each dressing

* A6259 Transparent film, more than 48 in^2, each dressing

* A6260 Wound cleansers, any type, any size

* A6261 Wound filler, not elsewhere classified, gel/paste, per fluid ounce

* A6262 Wound filler, not elsewhere classified, dry form, per gram

* A6266 Gauze, impregnated, other than water normal saline, or zinc paste, any width, per linear yard
MCM 2079

* A6402 Gauze, non-impregnated, sterile, pad size 16 in^2 or less, without adhesive border, each dressing

* A6403 Gauze, non-impregnated, sterile, pad size more than 16 in^2, less than or equal to 48 in^2, without adhesive border, each dressing

* A6404 Gauze, non-impregnated, sterile, pad size more than 48 in^2, without adhesive border, each dressing

* A6407 Packing strips, non-impregnated, up to 2 inches in width, per linear yard

☯ A6410 Eye pad, sterile, each
MCM 2079

☯ A6411 Eye pad, non-sterile, each
MCM 2079

⇒ ◆ A6412 Eye patch, occlusive, each

* A6441 Padding bandage, non-elastic, non-woven/non-knitted, width greater than or equal to three inches and less than five inches, per yard

* A6442 Conforming bandage, non-elastic, knitted/woven, non-sterile, width less than three inches, per yard

* A6443 Conforming bandage, non-elastic, knitted/woven, non-sterile, width greater than or equal to three inches and less than five inches, per yard

* A6444 Conforming bandage, non-elastic, knitted/woven, non-sterile, width greater than or equal to 5 inches, per yard

* A6445 Conforming bandage, non-elastic, knitted/woven, sterile, width less than three inches, per yard

* A6446 Conforming bandage, non-elastic, knitted/woven, sterile, width greater than or equal to three inches and less than five inches, per yard

* A6447 Conforming bandage, non-elastic, knitted/woven, sterile, width greater than or equal to five inches, per yard

* A6448 Light compression bandage, elastic, knitted/woven, width less than three inches, per yard

* A6449 Light compression bandage, elastic, knitted/woven, width greater than or equal to three inches and less than five inches, per yard

* A6450 Light compression bandage, elastic, knitted/woven, width greater than or equal to five inches, per yard

* A6451 Moderate compression bandage, elastic, knitted/woven, load resistance of 1.25 to 1.34 foot pounds at 50% maximum stretch, width greater than or equal to three inches and less than five inches, per yard

* A6452 High compression bandage, elastic, knitted/woven, load resistance greater than or equal to 1.35 foot pounds at 50% maximum stretch, width greater than or equal to three inches and less than five inches, per yard

* A6453 Self-adherent bandage, elastic, non-knitted/non-woven, width less than three inches, per yard

* A6454 Self-adherent bandage, elastic, non-knitted/non-woven, width greater than or equal to three inches and less than five inches, per yard

* A6455 Self-adherent bandage, elastic, non-knitted/non-woven, width greater than or equal to five inches, per yard

* A6456 Zinc paste impregnated bandage, non-elastic, knitted/woven, width greater than or equal to three inches and less than five inches, per yard

▶* A6457 Tubular dressing with or without elastic, any width, per linear yard

⊛ A6501 Compression burn garment, bodysuit (head to foot), custom fabricated
MCM 2079

⊛ A6502 Compression burn garment, chin strap, custom fabricated
MCM 2079

⊛ A6503 Compression burn garment, facial hood, custom fabricated
MCM 2079

⊛ A6504 Compression burn garment, glove to wrist, custom fabricated
MCM 2079

⊛ A6505 Compression burn garment, glove to elbow, custom fabricated
MCM 2079

⊛ A6506 Compression burn garment, glove to axilla, custom fabricated
MCM 2079

⊛ A6507 Compression burn garment, foot to knee length, custom fabricated
MCM 2079

⊛ A6508 Compression burn garment, foot to thigh length, custom fabricated
MCM 2079

⊛ A6509 Compression burn garment, upper trunk to waist including arm openings (vest), custom fabricated
MCM 2079

⊛ A6510 Compression burn garment, trunk, including arms down to leg openings (leotard), custom fabricated
MCM 2079

⊛ A6511 Compression burn garment, lower trunk including leg openings (panty), custom fabricated
MCM 2079

⊛ A6512 Compression burn garment, not otherwise classified
MCM 2079

▶* A6513 Compression burn mask, face and/or neck, plastic or equal, custom fabricated

GRADIENT COMPRESSION STOCKINGS (A6530-A6549)

▶◆ A6530 Gradient compression stocking, below knee, 18–30 mmHg, each
CIM 60-9

▶⊛ A6531 Gradient compression stocking, below knee, 30–40 mmHg, each
MCM 2079

▶⊛ A6532 Gradient compression stocking, below knee, 40–50 mmHg, each

▶◆ A6533 Gradient compression stocking, thigh length, 18–30 mmHg, each
MCM 2133, CIM 60-9

▶◆ A6534 Gradient compression stocking, thigh length, 30–40 mmHg, each
MCM 2133, CIM 60-9

▶◆ A6535 Gradient compression stocking, thigh length, 40–50 mmHg, each
MCM 2133, CIM 60-9

▶◆ A6536 Gradient compression stocking, full length/chap style, 18–30 mmHg, each
MCM 2133, CIM 60-9

▶◆ A6537 Gradient compression stocking, full length/chap style, 30–40 mmHg, each
MCM 2133, CIM 60-9

▶◆ A6538 Gradient compression stocking, full length/chap style, 40–50 mmHg, each
MCM 2133, CIM 60-9

▶◆ A6539 Gradient compression stocking, waist length, 18–30 mmHg, each
MCM 2133, CIM 60-9

▶◆ A6540 Gradient compression stocking, waist length, 30–40 mmHg, each
MCM 2133, CIM 60-9

▶◆ A6541 Gradient compression stocking, waist length, 40–50 mmHg, each
MCM 2133, CIM 60-9

▶◆ A6542 Gradient compression stocking, custom made
MCM 2133, CIM 60-9

▶◆ A6543 Gradient compression stocking, lymphedema
MCM 2133, CIM 60-9

▶◆ A6544 Gradient compression stocking, garter belt
MCM 2133, CIM 60-9

▶◆ A6549 Gradient compression stocking, not otherwise specified
MCM 2133, CIM 60-9

➡* A6550 Wound care set, for negative pressure wound therapy electrical pump, includes all supplies and accessories

A6551 Deleted 12/31/05

RESPIRATORY DURABLE MEDICAL EQUIPMENT, INEXPENSIVE AND ROUTINELY PURCHASED (A7700-A7509)

* A7700   Canister, disposable, used with suction pump, each
* A7001   Canister, non-disposable, used with suction pump, each
* A7002   Tubing, used with suction pump, each
* A7003   Administration set, with small volume nonfiltered pneumatic nebulizer, disposable
* A7004   Small volume nonfiltered pneumatic nebulizer, disposable
* A7005   Administration set, with small volume nonfiltered pneumatic nebulizer, non-disposable
* A7006   Administration set, with small volume filtered pneumatic nebulizer
* A7007   Large volume nebulizer, disposable, unfilled, used with aerosol compressor
* A7008   Large volume nebulizer, disposable, prefilled, used with aerosol compressor
* A7009   Reservoir bottle, nondisposable, used with large volume ultrasonic nebulizer
* A7010   Corrugated tubing, disposable, used with large volume nebulizer, 100 feet
* A7011   Corrugated tubing, non-disposable, used with large volume nebulizer, 10 feet
* A7012   Water collection device, used with large volume nebulizer
* A7013   Filter, disposable, used with aerosol compressor
* A7014   Filter, non-disposable, used with aerosol compressor or ultrasonic generator
* A7015   Aerosol mask, used with DME nebulizer
* A7016   Dome and mouthpiece, used with small volume ultrasonic nebulizer
* A7017   Nebulizer, durable, glass or autoclavable plastic, bottle type, not used with oxygen
        CIM 60-9
* A7018   Water, distilled, used with large volume nebulizer, 1000 ml
* A7025   High frequency chest wall oscillation system vest, replacement for use with patient-owned equipment, each
* A7026   High frequency chest wall oscillation system hose, replacement for use with patient-owned equipment, each
* A7030   Full face mask used with positive airway pressure device, each
* A7031   Face mask interface, replacement for full-face mask, each
➠ * A7032   Cushion for use on nasal mask interface, replacement only, each
➠ * A7033   Pillow for use on nasal cannula type interface, replacement only, pair

* A7034   Nasal interface (mask or cannula type) used with positive airway pressure device, with or without head strap
* A7035   Headgear used with positive airway pressure device
* A7036   Chinstrap used with positive airway pressure device
* A7037   Tubing used with positive airway pressure device
* A7038   Filter, disposable, used with positive airway pressure device
* A7039   Filter, non disposable, used with positive airway pressure device
* A7040   One-way chest drain valve
* A7041   Water seal drainage container and tubing for use with implanted chest tube
* A7042   Implanted pleural catheter, each
* A7043   Vacuum drainage bottle and tubing for use with implanted catheter
* A7044   Oral interface used with positive airway pressure device, each
⊚ A7045   Exhalation port with or without swivel used with accessories for positive airway devices, replacement only
        CIM 60-17
⊚ A7046   Water chamber for humidifier, used with positive airway pressure device, replacement, each
        CIM 60-17
⊚ A7501   Tracheostoma valve, including diaphragm, each
        MCM 2130
⊚ A7502   Replacement diaphragm/faceplate for tracheostoma valve, each
        MCM 2130
⊚ A7503   Filter holder or filter cap, reusable, for use in a tracheostoma heat and moisture exchange system, each
        MCM 2130
⊚ A7504   Filter for use in a tracheostoma heat and moisture exchange system, each
        MCM 2130
⊚ A7505   Housing, reusable without adhesive, for use in a heat and moisture exchange system and/or with a tracheostoma valve, each
        MCM 2130
⊚ A7506   Adhesive disc for use in a heat and moisture exchange system and/or with tracheostoma valve, any type, each
        MCM 2130
⊚ A7507   Filter holder and integrated filter without adhesive, for use in a tracheostoma heat and moisture exchange system, each
        MCM 2130
⊚ A7508   Housing and integrated adhesive, for use in a tracheostoma heat and moisture exchange system and/or with a tracheostoma valve, each
        MCM 2130

⊛ A7509 Filter holder and integrated filter housing, and adhesive, for use as a tracheostoma heat and moisture exchange system, each
MCM 2130

* A7520 Tracheostomy/laryngectomy tube, non-cuffed, polyvinylchloride (PVC), silicone or equal, each

* A7521 Tracheostomy/laryngectomy tube, cuffed, polyvinylchloride (PVC), silicone or equal, each

* A7522 Tracheostomy/laryngectomy tube, stainless steel or equal (sterilizable and reusable), each

* A7523 Tracheostomy shower protector, each
* A7524 Tracheostoma stent/stud/button, each
* A7525 Tracheostomy mask, each
* A7526 Tracheostomy tube collar/holder, each
* A7527 Tracheostomy/laryngectomy tube plug/stop, each

ADMINISTRATIVE, MISCELLANEOUS AND INVESTIGATIONAL (A9000-A9999)

NOTE: The following codes do not imply that codes in other sections are necessarily covered.

⊛ A9150 Non-prescription drugs
MCM 2050.5

◆ A9152 Single vitamin/mineral/trace element, oral, per dose, not otherwise specified

◆ A9153 Multiple vitamins, with or without minerals and trace elements, oral, per dose, not otherwise specified

◆ A9180 Pediculosis (lice infestation) treatment, topical, for administration by patient/caretaker

◆ A9270 Non-covered item or service
MCM 2303

▶◆ A9275 Home glucose disposable monitor, includes test strips

◆ A9280 Alert or alarm device, not otherwise classified
Medicare Statute 1861

▶◆ A9281 Reaching/Grabbing device, any type, any length, each
Medicare Statute 1862 SSA

▶◆ A9282 Wig, any type, each
Medicare Statute 1862 SSA

◆ A9300 Exercise equipment
MCM 2100.1, CIM 60-9

Supplies for Radiology Procedures

➡* A9500 Technetium Tc-99m sestamibi, diagnostic, per study dose, up to 40 millicurie

➡* A9502 Technetium Tc-99m tetrofosmin, diagnostic, per study dose, up to 40 millicurie

➡* A9503 Technetium Tc-99m medronate, diagnostic, per study dose, up to 30 millicurie

➡* A9504 Tchnetium Tc-99m apcitide, diagnostic, per study dose, up to 20 millicurie

➡* A9505 Thallium Tl-201 thallous chloride, diagnostic, per millicurie

➡* A9507 Indium In-111 capromab pendetide, diagnostic, per study dose, up to 10 millicurie

➡* A9508 Iodine I-131 iobenguane sulfate, diagnostic, per 0.5 millicurie

➡* A9510 Technetium Tc-99m disofenin, diagnostic, per study dose, up to 15 millicurie

A9511 Deleted 12/31/05

➡* A9512 Technetium Tc-99m pertechnetate, diagnostic, per millicurie

A9513 Deleted 12/31/05
A9514 Deleted 12/31/05
A9515 Deleted 12/31/05

➡* A9516 Iodine I-123 sodium iodide capsule(s), diagnostic, per 100 microcurie

➡* A9517 Iodine I-131 sodium iodide capsule(s), therapeutic, per millicurie

A9519 Deleted 12/31/05
A9520 Deleted 12/31/05

➡* A9521 Technetium Tc-99m exametazime, diagnostic, per study dose, up to 25 millicurie

A9522 Deleted 12/31/05
A9523 Deleted 12/31/05

➡* A9524 Iodine I-131 iodinated serum albumin, diagnostic, per 5 microcurie

A9525 Deleted 12/31/05

➡* A9526 Nitrogen N-13 ammonia, diagnostic, per study dose, up to 40 millicurie

➡* A9528 Iodine I-131 sodium iodide capsule(s), diagnostic, per millicurie

➡* A9529 Iodine I-131 sodium iodide solution, diagnostic, per millicurie

➡* A9530 Iodine I-131 sodium iodide solution, therapeutic, per millicurie

➡* A9531 Iodine I-131 sodium iodide, diagnostic, per microcurie (up to 100 microcurie)

➡* A9532 Iodine I-125 serum albumin, diagnostic, per 5 microcurie

A9533 Deleted 12/31/05
A9534 Deleted 12/31/05

▶* A9535 Injection, methylene blue, 1 ml

▶* A9536 Technetium Tc-99m depreotide, diagnostic, per study dose, up to 35 millicurie

▶* A9537 Technetium Tc-99m mebrofenin, diagnostic, per study dose, up to 15 millicurie

▶* A9538 Technetium Tc-99m pyrophosphate, diagnostic, per study dose, up to 25 millicurie

▶* A9539 Technetium Tc-99m pentetate, diagnostic, per study dose, up to 25 millicurie

▶ ✳ A9540 Technetium Tc-99m macroaggregated albumin, diagnostic, per study dose, up to 10 millicurie

▶ ✳ A9541 Technetium Tc-99m sulfur colloid, diagnostic, per study dose, up to 20 millicurie

▶ ✳ A9542 Indium In-111 ibritumomab tiuxetan, diagnostic, per study dose, up to 5 millicurie

▶ ✳ A9543 Yttrium Y-90 ibritumomab tiuxetan, therapeutic, per treatment dose, up to 40 millicurie

▶ ✳ A9544 Iodine I-131 tositumomab, diagnostic, per study dose

▶ ✳ A9545 Iodine I-131 tositumomab, therapeutic, per treatment dose

▶ ✳ A9546 Cobalt Co-57/58, cyanocobalamin, diagnostic, per study dose, up to 1 microcurie

▶ ✳ A9547 Indium In-111 oxyquinoline, diagnostic, per 0.5 millicurie

▶ ✳ A9548 Indium In-111 pentetate, diagnostic, per 0.5 millicurie

▶ ✳ A9549 Technetium Tc-99m arcitumomab, diagnostic, per study dose, up to 25 millicurie

▶ ✳ A9550 Technetium Tc-99m sodium gluceptate, diagnostic, per study dose, up to 25 millicurie

▶ ✳ A9551 Technetium Tc-99m succimer, diagnostic, per study dose, up to 10 millicurie

▶ ✳ A9552 Fluorodeoxyglucose-18 FDG, diagnostic, per study dose, up to 45 millicurie

▶ ✳ A9553 Chromium Cr-51 sodium chromate, diagnostic, per study dose, up to 250 microcurie

▶ ✳ A9554 Iodine I-125 sodium Iothalamate, diagnostic, per study dose, up to 10 microcurie

▶ ✳ A9555 Rubidium Rb-82, diagnostic, per study dose, up to 60 millicurie

▶ ✳ A9556 Gallium Ga-67 citrate, diagnostic, per millicurie

▶ ✳ A9557 Technetium Tc-99m bicisate, diagnostic, per study dose, up to 25 millicurie

▶ ✳ A9558 Xenon Xe-133 gas, diagnostic, per 10 millicurie

▶ ✳ A9559 Cobalt Co-57 cyanocobalamin, oral, diagnostic, per study dose, up to 1 microcurie

▶ ✳ A9560 Technetium Tc-99m labeled red blood cells, diagnostic, per study dose, up to 30 millicurie

▶ ✳ A9561 Technetium Tc-99m oxidronate, diagnostic, per study dose, up to 30 millicurie

▶ ✳ A9562 Technetium Tc-99m mertiatide, diagnostic, per study dose, up to 15 millicurie

▶ ✳ A9563 Sodium phosphate P-32, therapeutic, per millicurie

▶ ✳ A9564 Chromic phosphate P-32 suspension, therapeutic, per millicurie

▶ ✳ A9565 Indium In-111 pentetreotide, diagnostic, per millicurie

▶ ✳ A9566 Technetium Tc-99m fanolesomab, diagnostic, per study dose, up to 25 millicurie

▶ ✳ A9567 Technetium Tc-99m pentetate, diagnostic, aerosol, per study dose, up to 75 millicurie

⇒ ✳ A9600 Strontium Sr-89 chloride, therapeutic, per millicurie

⇒ ✳ A9605 Samarium Sm-153 lexidronamm, therapeutic, per 50 millicurie

▶ ⊙ A9698 Non-radioactive contrast imaging material, not otherwise classified, per study
MCM 15022

⇒ ✳ A9699 Radiopharmaceutical-therapeutic, not otherwise classified

⊙ A9700 Supply of injectable contrast material for use in echocardiography, per study
MCM 15360

Miscellaneous Service Component

✳ A9900 Miscellaneous DME supply, accessory, and/or service component of another HCPCS code

✳ A9901 DME delivery, set up, and/or dispensing service component of another HCPCS code

✳ A9999 Miscellaneous DME supply or accessory, not otherwise specified

ENTERAL AND PARENTERAL THERAPY (B4000-B9999)

Enteral Formulae and Enteral Medical Supplies

⊙ B4034 Enteral feeding supply kit; syringe, per day
MCM 2130, MCM 4450, CIM 65-10

⊙ B4035 Enteral feeding supply kit; pump fed, per day
MCM 2130, MCM 4450, CIM 65-10

⊙ B4036 Enteral feeding supply kit; gravity fed, per day
MCM 2130, MCM 4450, CIM 65-10

⊙ B4081 Nasogastric tubing with stylet
MCM 2130, MCM 4450, CIM 65-10

⊙ B4082 Nasogastric tubing without stylet
MCM 2130, MCM 4450, CIM 65-10

⊙ B4083 Stomach tube, Levine type
MCM 2130, MCM 4450, CIM

✳ B4086 Gastrostomy/jejunostomy tube, any material, any type, (standard or low profile), each

⇒ ◆ B4100 Food thickener, administered orally, per ounce

⊙ B4102   Enteral formula, for adults, used to replace fluids and electrolytes (e.g., clear liquids), 500 ml = 1 unit
CIM 65-10

⊙ B4103   Enteral formula, for pediatrics, used to replace fluids and electrolytes (e.g., clear liquids), 500 ml = 1 unit
CIM 65-10

⊙ B4104   Additive for enteral formula (e.g., fiber)
CIM 65-10

➠ ⊙ B4149   Enteral formula, manufactured blenderized natural foods with intact nutrients; includes proteins, fats, carbohydrates, vitamins, and minerals; may include fiber; administered through an enteral feeding tube, 100 calories = 1 unit
MCM 2130 MCM 4450 CIM 65-10

⊙ B4150   Enteral formulae; nutritionally complete with intact nutrients, includes proteins, fats, carbohydrates, vitamins and minerals, may include fiber, administered through an enteral feeding tube at 100 calories = 1 unit
MCM 2130, MCM 4450, CIM 65-10

⊙ B4152   Enteral formulae; nutritionally complete, calorically dense (equal to or greater than 1.5 kcal/ml) with intact nutrients, includes proteins, fats, carbohydrates, vitamins and minerals, may include fiber, administered through an enteral feeding tube at 100 calories = 1 unit
MCM 2130, MCM 4450, CIM 65-10

⊙ B4153   Enteral formulae; nutritionally complete, hydrolyzed proteins (amino acids and peptide chain), includes fats, carbohydrates, vitamins and minerals, may include fiber, administered through an enteral feeding tube at 100 calories = 1 unit
MCM 2130, MCM 4450, CIM 65-10

⊙ B4154   Enteral formulae; nutritionally complete, for special metabolic needs, excludes inherited disease of metabolism, includes altered composition of proteins, fats, carbohydrates, vitamins and/or minerals, may include fiber, administered through an enteral feeding tube at 100 calories = 1 unit
MCM 2130, MCM 4450, CIM 65-10

⊙ B4155   Enteral formulae; nutritionally incomplete/modular nutrients, includes specific nutrients, carbohydrates (e.g. glucose polymers), proteins/amino acids (e.g. glutamine, arginine), fat (e.g. medium chain triglycerides) or combination, administered through an enteral feeding tube at 100 calories = 1 unit
MCM 2130, MCM 4450, CIM 65-10

⊙ B4157   Enteral formula, nutritionally complete, for special metabolic needs for inherited disease of metabolism; includes proteins, fats, carbohydrates, vitamins, and minerals; may include fiber; administered through an enteral feeding tube, 100 calories = 1 unit
CIM 65-10

⊙ B4158   Enteral formula, for pediatrics, nutritionally complete with intact nutrients; includes proteins, fats, carbohydrates, vitamins, and minerals; may include fiber and/or iron; administered through an enteral feeding tube, 100 calories = 1 unit
CIM 65-10

⊙ B4159   Enteral formula, for pediatrics, nutritionally complete soy based with intact nutrients; includes proteins, fats, carbohydrates, vitamins, and minerals; may include fiber and/or iron; administered through an enteral feeding tube, 100 calories = 1 unit
CIM 65-10

⊙ B4160   Enteral formula, for pediatrics, nutritionally complete calorically dense (equal to or greater than 0.7 kcal/ml) with intact nutrients; includes proteins, fats, carbohydrates, vitamins, and minerals; may include fiber; administered through an enteral feeding tube, 100 calories = 1 unit
CIM 65-10

⊙ B4161   Enteral formula, for pediatrics, hydrolyzed/amino acids and peptide chain proteins; includes fats, carbohydrates, vitamins, and minerals; may include fiber; administered through an enteral feeding tube, 100 calories = 1 unit
CIM 65-10

⊙ B4162   Enteral formula, for pediatrics, special metabolic needs for inherited disease of metabolism; includes proteins, fats, carbohydrates, vitamins, and minerals; may include fiber; administered through an enteral feeding tube, 100 calories = 1 unit
CIM 65-10

Parenteral Nutritional Solutions and Supplies

⊙ B4164   Parenteral nutrition solution: carbohydrates (dextrose), 50% or less (500 ml = 1 unit)—home mix
MCM 2130, MCM 4450, CIM 65-10

⊙ B4168   Parenteral nutrition solution; amino acid, 3.5% (500 ml = 1 unit)—home mix
MCM 2130, MCM 4450, CIM 65-10

⊙ B4172   Parenteral nutrition solution; amino acid, 5.5% through 7% (500 ml = 1 unit)—home mix
MCM 2130, MCM 4450, CIM 65-10

⊛ B4176   Parenteral nutrition solution; amino acid, 7% through 8.5% (500 ml = 1 unit)—home mix
MCM 2130, MCM 4450, CIM 65-10

⊛ B4178   Parenteral nutrition solution: amino acid, greater than 8.5% (500 ml = 1 unit)—home mix
MCM 2130, MCM 4450, CIM 65-10

⊛ B4180   Parenteral nutrition solution; carbohydrates (dextrose), greater than 50% (500 ml = 1 unit)—home mix
MCM 2130, MCM 4450, CIM 65-10

B4184   Deleted 12/31/05

▶⊛ B4185   Parenteral nutrition solution, per 10 grams lipids

B4186   Deleted 12/31/05

⊛ B4189   Parenteral nutrition solution; compounded amino acid and carbohydrates with electrolytes, trace elements, and vitamins, including preparation, any strength, 10 to 51 gram (gm) of protein—premix
MCM 2130, MCM 4450, CIM 65-10

⊛ B4193   Parenteral nutrition solution; compounded amino acid and carbohydrates with electrolytes, trace elements, and vitamins, including preparation, any strength, 52 to 73 gm of protein—premix
MCM 2130, MCM 4450, CIM 65-10

⊛ B4197   Parenteral nutrition solution; compounded amino acid and carbohydrates with electrolytes, trace elements and vitamins, including preparation, any strength, 74 to 100 gm of protein—premix
MCM 2130, MCM 4450, CIM 65-10

⊛ B4199   Parenteral nutrition solution; compounded amino acid and carbohydrates with electrolytes, trace elements and vitamins, including preparation, any strength, over 100 gm of protein—premix

⊛ B4216   Parenteral nutrition additives (vitamins, trace elements, heparin, electrolytes) home mix, per day
MCM 2130, MCM 4450, CIM 65-10

⊛ B4220   Parenteral nutrition supply kit; premix, per day
MCM 2130, MCM 4450, CIM 65-10

⊛ B4222   Parenteral nutrition supply kit; home mix, per day
MCM 2130, MCM 4450, CIM 65-10

⊛ B4224   Parenteral nutrition administration kit, per day
MCM 2130, MCM 4450, CIM 65-10

⊛ B5000   Parenteral nutrition solution; compounded amino acid and carbohydrates with electrolytes, trace elements, and vitamins, including preparation, any strength, renal—Amirosyn-RF, NephrAmine, RenAmine—premix
MCM 2130, MCM 4450, CIM 65-10

⊛ B5100   Parenteral nutrition solution; compounded amino acid and carbohydrates with electrolytes, trace elements, and vitamins, including preparation, any strength, hepatic—FreAmine HBC, HepatAmine—premix
MCM 2130, MCM 4450, CIM 65-10

⊛ B5200   Parenteral nutrition solution; compounded amino acid and carbohydrates with electrolytes, trace elements, and vitamins, including preparation, any strength, stress—branch chain amino acids—premix
MCM 2130, MCM 4450, CIM 65-10

Enteral and Parenteral Pumps

⊛ B9000   Enteral nutrition infusion pump, without alarm
MCM 2130, MCM 4450, CIM 65-10

⊛ B9002   Enteral nutrition infusion pump, with alarm
MCM 2130, MCM 4450, CIM 65-10

⊛ B9004   Parenteral nutrition infusion pump, portable
MCM 2130, MCM 4450, CIM 65-10

⊛ B9006   Parenteral nutrition infusion pump, stationary
MCM 2130, MCM 4450, CIM 65-10

⊛ B9998   NOC for enteral supplies
MCM 2130, MCM 4450, CIM 65-10

⊛ B9999   NOC for parenteral supplies
MCM 2130, MCM 4450, CIM 65-10

C CODES FOR USE ONLY UNDER THE HOSPITAL OUTPATIENT PROSPECTIVE PAYMENT SYSTEM (C1000-C9999)

Note: C-codes are used ONLY as a part of Hospital Outpatient Prospective Payment System (OPPS) and are not to be used to report other services. C-codes are updated quarterly by the Centers for Medicare and Medicaid Services.

C1079   Deleted 12/31/05
C1080   Deleted 12/31/05
C1081   Deleted 12/31/05
C1082   Deleted 12/31/05
C1083   Deleted 12/31/05
C1091   Deleted 12/31/05
C1092   Deleted 12/31/05
C1093   Deleted 12/31/05
C1122   Deleted 12/31/05
⊛ C1178   Injection, bisulfan, per 6 mg
Medicare Statute 1833(t)
C1200   Deleted 12/31/05
C1201   Deleted 12/31/05

○ **C1300** Hyperbaric oxygen under pressure, full body chamber, per 30-minute, TVL SQ01
Medicare Statute 1833(t)

C1305 Deleted 12/31/05

○ **C1713** Anchor/Screw for opposing bone-to-bone or soft tissue-to-bone (implantable)
Medicare Statute 1833(t)

○ **C1714** Catheter, transluminal atherectomy, directional
Medicare Statute 1833(t)

○ **C1715** Brachytherapy needle
Medicare Statute 1833(t)

○ **C1716** Brachytherapy source, gold-198, per source
Medicare Statute 1833(t)

○ **C1717** Brachytherapy source, high dose rate iridium 192, per source
Medicare Statute 1833(t)

○ **C1718** Brachytherapy source, iodine 125, per source
Medicare Statute 1833(t)

○ **C1719** Brachytherapy source, non-high dose rate iridium-192, per source
Medicare Statute 1833(t)

○ **C1720** Brachytherapy source, palladium 103, per source
Medicare Statute 1833(t)

○ **C1721** Cardioverter-defibrillator, dual chamber (implantable)
Medicare Statute 1833(t)

○ **C1722** Cardioverter-defibrillator, single chamber (implantable)
Medicare Statute 1833(t)

○ **C1724** Catheter, transluminal atherectomy, rotational
Medicare Statute 1833(t)

○ **C1725** Catheter, transluminal angioplasty, non-laser (may include guidance, infusion/perfusion capability)
Medicare Statute 1833(t)

○ **C1726** Catheter, balloon dilatation, non-vascular
Medicare Statute 1833(t)

○ **C1727** Catheter, balloon tissue dissector, non-vascular (insertable)
Medicare Statute 1833(t)

○ **C1728** Catheter, brachytherapy seed administration
Medicare Statute 1833(t)

○ **C1729** Catheter, drainage
Medicare Statute 1833(t)

○ **C1730** Catheter, electrophysiology, diagnostic, other than 3D mapping (19 or fewer electrodes)
Medicare Statute 1833(t)

○ **C1731** Catheter, electrophysiology, diagnostic, other than 3D mapping (20 or more electrodes)
Medicare Statute 1833(t)

○ **C1732** Catheter, electrophysiology, diagnostic/ablation, 3D or vector mapping
Medicare Statute 1833(t)

○ **C1733** Catheter, electrophysiology, diagnostic/ablation, orther than 3D or vector mapping, other than cool-tip
Medicare Statute 1833(t)

○ **C1750** Catheter, hemodialysis, long term
Medicare Statute 1833(t)

○ **C1751** Catheter, infusion, inserted peripherally, centrally or midline (other than hemodialysis)
Medicare Statute 1833(t)

○ **C1752** Catheter, hemodialysis, short term
Medicare Statute 1833(t)

○ **C1753** Catheter, intravascular ultrasound
Medicare Statute 1833(t)

○ **C1754** Catheter, intradiscal
Medicare Statute 1833(t)

○ **C1755** Catheter, instraspinal
Medicare Statute 1833(t)

○ **C1756** Catheter, pacing transesophageal
Medicare Statute 1833(t)

○ **C1757** Catheter, thrombectomy/embolectomy
Medicare Statute 1833(t)

○ **C1758** Catheter, ureteral
Medicare Statute 1833(t)

○ **C1759** Catheter, intracardiac echocardiography
Medicare Statute 1833(t)

○ **C1760** Closure device, vascular (implantable/insertable)
Medicare Statute 1833(t)

○ **C1762** Connective tissue, human (includes fascia lata)
Medicare Statute 1833(t)

○ **C1763** Connective tissue, non-human (includes synthetic)
Medicare Statute 1833(t)

○ **C1764** Event recorder, cardiac (implantable)
Medicare Statute 1833(t)

○ **C1765** Adhesion barrier
Medicare Statute 1833 (t)

○ **C1766** Introduction/sheath, guiding, intracardiac electrophysiological steerable, other than peel-away
Medicare Statute 1833(t)

○ **C1767** Generator, neurostimulator (implantable)
Medicare Statute 1833(t)

○ **C1768** Graft, vascular
Medicare Statute 1833(t)

○ **C1769** Guidewire
Medicare Statute 1833(t)

○ **C1770** Imaging coil, magnetic reasonance (insertable)
Medicare Statute 1833(t)

○ **C1771** Repair device, urinary, incontinence, with sling graft
Medicare Statute 1833(t)

⊘ C1772   Infusion pump, programmable (implantable)
Medicare Statute 1833(t)

⊘ C1773   Retrieval device, insertable (used to retrieve fractured medical devices)
Medicare Statute 1833(t)

C1774   Deleted 12/31/03

C1775   Deleted 12/31/05

⊘ C1776   Joint device (implantable)
Medicare Statute 1833(t)

⊘ C1777   Lead, cardioverter-defibrillator, endocardial single coil (implantable)
Medicare Statute 1833(t)

⊘ C1778   Lead, neurostimulator (implantable)
Medicare Statute 1833(t)

⊘ C1779   Lead, pacemaker, trasvenous VDD single pass
Medicare Statute 1833(t)

⊘ C1780   Lens, intraocular (new technology)
Medicare Statute 1833(t)

⊘ C1781   Mesh (implantable)
Medicare Statute 1833(t)

⊘ C1782   Morcellator
Medicare Statute 1833(t)

⊘ C1783   Ocular implant, aqueous drainage assist device
Medicare Statute 1833(t)

⊘ C1784   Ocular device, intraoperative, detached retina
Medicare Statute 1833(t)

⊘ C1785   Pacemaker, dual chamber, rate-responsive (implantable)
Medicare Statute 1833(t)

⊘ C1786   Pacemaker, single chamber, rate-responsive (implantable)
Medicare Statute 1833(t)

⊘ C1787   Patient programmer, neurostimulator
Medicare Statute 1833(t)

⊘ C1788   Port, indwelling (implantable)
Medicare Statute 1833(t)

⊘ C1789   Prosthesis, breast (implantable)
Medicare Statute 1833(t)

⊘ C1813   Prosthesis, penile, inflatable
Medicare Statute 1833(t)

⊘ C1814   Retinal tamponade device, silicone oil
Medicare Statute 1833(t)

⊘ C1815   Prosthesis, urinary sphincter (implantable)
Medicare Statute 1833(t)

⊘ C1816   Receiver and/or transmitter, neurostimulator (implantable)
Medicare Statute 1833(t)

⊘ C1817   Septal defect implant system, intracardiac
Medicare Statute 1833(t)

⊘ C1818   Integrated keratoprosthesic
Medicare Statute 1833(t)

⊘ C1819   Surgical tissue localization and excision device (implantable)
Medicare Statute 1833(t)

⊘ C1874   Stent, coated/covered, with delivery system
Medicare Statute 1833(t)

⊘ C1875   Stent, coated/covered, without delivery system
Medicare Statute 1833(t)

⊘ C1876   Stent, non-coated/non-covered, with delivery system
Medicare Statute 1833(t)

⊘ C1877   Stent, non-coated/non-covered, without delivery system
Medicare Statute 1833(t)

⊘ C1878   Material for vocal cord medialization, synthetic (implantable)
Medicare Statute 1833(t)

⊘ C1879   Tissue marker (implantable)
Medicare Statute 1833(t)

⊘ C1880   Vena cava filter
Medicare Statute 1833(t)

⊘ C1881   Dialysis access system (implantable)
Medicare Statute 1833(t)

⊘ C1882   Cardioverter-defibrillator, other than single or dual chamber (implantable)
Medicare Statute 1833(t)

⊘ C1883   Adaptor/Extension, pacing lead or neurostimulator lead (implantable)
Medicare Statute 1833(t)

⊘ C1884   Embolization protection system
Medicare Statute 1833(t)

⊘ C1885   Catheter, transluminal angioplasty, laser
Medicare Statute 1833(t)

⊘ C1887   Catheter, guiding (may include infusion/perfusion capability)
Medicare Statute 1833(t)

⊘ C1888   Catheter, ablation, non-cardiac, endovascular (implantable)
Medicare Statute 1833(t)

⊘ C1891   Infusion pump, on-programmable, permanent (implantable)
Medicare Statute 1833(t)

⊘ C1892   Introducer/sheath, guiding, intracardiac electrophysiological, fixed-curve, peel-away
Medicare Statute 1833(t)

⊘ C1893   Introducer/Sheath, guiding, intracardiac electrophysiological, fixed-curve, other than peel-away
Medicare Statute 1833(t)

⊘ C1894   Introducer/Sheath, other than guiding, intracardiac electrophysiological, non-laser
Medicare Statute 1833(t)

⊘ C1895   Lead, cardioverter-defibrillator, endocardial dual coil (implantable)
Medicare Statute 1833(t)

⊘ C1896   Lead, cardioverter-defibrillator, other than endocardial single or dual coil (implantable)
Medicare Statute 1833(t)

⊘ C1897   Lead, neurostimulator test kit (implantable)
Medicare Statute 1833(t)

⊙ C1898 Lead, pacemaker, other than transvenous VDD single pass
Medicare Statute 1833(t)

⊙ C1899 Lead, pacemaker/cardioverter-defibrillator combination (implantable)
Medicare Statute 1833(t)

⊙ C1900 Lead, left ventricular coronary venous system
Medicare Statute 1833(t)

⊙ C2614 Probe, percutaneous lumbar disectomy
Medicare Statute 1833(t)

⊙ C2615 Sealant, pulmonary, liquid
Medicare Statute 1833(t)

⊙ C2616 Brachytherapy source, yttrium-90, per source
Medicare Statute 1833(T)

⊙ C2617 Stent, non-coronary, temporary, without delivery system
Medicare Statute 1833(t)

⊙ C2618 Probe, cryoablation
Medicare Statute 1833(t)

⊙ C2619 Pacemaker, dual chamber, non-rate-responsiveness (implantable)
Medicare Statute 1833(t)

⊙ C2620 Pacemaker, single chamber, non-rate-responsiveness (implantable)
Medicare Statute 1833(t)

⊙ C2621 Pacemaker, other than single or dual chamber (implantable)
Medicare Statute 1833(t)

⊙ C2622 Prosthesis, penile, non-inflatable
Medicare Statute 1833(t)

⊙ C2625 Stent, non-coronary, temporary, with delivery system
Medicare Statute 1833(t)

⊙ C2626 Infusion pump, non-programmable, temporary (implantable)
Medicare Statute 1833(t)

⊙ C2627 Catheter, suprapubic/cystoscopic
Medicare Statute 1833(t)

⊙ C2628 Catheter, occlusion
Medicare Statute 1833(t)

⊙ C2629 Introducer/Sheath, other than guiding, intracaradiac electrophysiological, laser
Medicare Statute 1833(t)

⊙ C2630 Catheter, electrophysiology, diagnostic/ablation, other than 3D or vector mapping, cool-tip
Medicare Statute 1833(t)

⊙ C2631 Repair device, urinary, incontinence, without sling graft
Medicare Statute 1833(t)

⊙ C2632 Brachytherapy solution, iodine-125, per millicurie
Medicare Statute 1833(t)

⊙ C2633 Brachytherapy source, Cesium-131, per source
Medicare Statute 1833(t)

⇒ ⊙ C2634 Brachytherapy source, high activity, iodine-125, greater than 1.01 millicurie (NIST), per source
Medicare Statute 1833(t)

⇒ ⊙ C2635 Brachytherapy source, high activity, paladium-103, greater than 2.2 millicurie (NIST), per source
Medicare Statute 1833(t)

⊙ C2636 Brachytherapy linear source, high activity, paladium-103, per 1 mm

▶ ⊙ C2637 Brachytherapy source, Ytterbium-169, per source
Medicare Statute 1833(t)

⊙ C8900 Magnetic resonance angiography (MRA) with contrast, abdomen
Medicare Statute 1833(t)(2)

⊙ C8901 MRA without contrast, abdomen
Medicare Statute 1833(t)(2)

⊙ C8902 MRA without contrast followed by with contrast, abdomen
Medicare Statute 1833(t)(2)

⊙ C8903 Magnetic resonance imaging (MRI) with contrast, breast; unilateral
Medicare Statute 1833(t)(2)

⊙ C8904 MRI without contrast, breast; unilateral
Medicare Statute 1833(t)(2)

⊙ C8905 MRI without contrast followed by with contrast, breast; unilateral
Medicare Statute 1833(t)(2)

⊙ C8906 MRI with contrast, breast; bilateral
Medicare Statute 1833(t)(2)

⊙ C8907 MRI without contrast, breast; bilateral
Medicare Statute 1833(t)(2)

⊙ C8908 MRI without contrast followed by with contrast, breast; bilateral
Medicare Statute 1833(t)(2)

⊙ C8909 MRA with contrast, chest (excluding myocardium)
Medicare Statute 1833(t)(2)

⊙ C8910 MRA without contrast, chest (excluding myocardium)
Medicare Statute 1833(t)(2)

⊙ C8911 MRA without contrast followed by with contrast, chest (excluding myocardium)
Medicare Statute 1833(t)(2)

⊙ C8912 MRA with contrast, lower extremity
Medicare Statute 1833(t)(2)

⊙ C8913 MRA without contrast, lower extremity
Medicare Statute 1833(t)(2)

⊙ C8914 MRA without contrast followed by with contrast, lower extremity
Medicare Statute 1833(t)(2)

⊙ C8918 Magnetic resonance angiography with contrast, pelvis
Medicare Statute 430 BIPA

⊙ C8919 Magnetic resonance angiography without contrast, pelvis
Medicare Statute 430 BIPA

⊕ C8920   Magnetic resonance angiography without contrast followed by with contrast, pelvis
      Medicare Statute 430 BIPA

C9000   Deleted 12/31/05

⊕ C9003   Palivizumab-RSV-IGM, per 50 mg
      Medicare Statute 1833(t)

C9007   Deleted 12/31/05

C9008   Deleted 12/31/05

C9009   Deleted 12/31/05

C9013   Deleted 12/31/05

C9102   Deleted 12/31/05

C9103   Deleted 12/31/05

C9105   Deleted 12/31/05

C9112   Deleted 12/31/05

⊕ C9113   Injection, pantoprazole sodium, per vial
      Medicare Statute 1833(t)

⊕ C9121   Injection, argatroban, per 5 mg Medicare Statute 1833(t)

C9123   Deleted 12/31/05

C9126   Deleted 12/31/05

C9200   Deleted 12/31/05

C9201   Deleted 12/31/05

C9202   Deleted 12/31/05

C9203   Deleted 12/31/05

C9205   Deleted 12/31/05

C9206   Deleted 12/31/05

C9211   Deleted 12/31/05

C9212   Deleted 12/31/05

C9218   Deleted 12/31/05

⊕ C9219   Mycophenolic acid, oral, per 180 mg

⊕ C9220   Sodium hyaluronate per 30 mg dose, for intra-articular injection

⊕ C9221   Acellular dermal tissue matrix, per 16 cm^2

⊕ C9222   Decellularized soft tissue scaffold, per 1 cc

▶ ⊕ C9224   Injection, galsulfase, per 5 mg
      Medicare Statute 621 MMA

▶ ⊕ C9225   Injection, fluocinolone acetonide intravitreal implant, per 0.59 mg
      Medicare Statute 621 MMA

⊕ C9399   Unclassified drugs or biologicals

C9400   Deleted 12/31/05

C9401   Deleted 12/31/05

C9402   Deleted 12/31/05

C9403   Deleted 12/31/05

C9404   Deleted 12/31/05

C9405   Deleted 12/31/05

C9410   Deleted 12/31/05

C9411   Deleted 12/31/05

C9413   Deleted 12/31/05

C9414   Deleted 12/31/05

C9415   Deleted 12/31/05

C9417   Deleted 12/31/05

C9418   Deleted 12/31/05

C9419   Deleted 12/31/05

C9420   Deleted 12/31/05

C9421   Deleted 12/31/05

C9422   Deleted 12/31/05

C9423   Deleted 12/31/05

C9424   Deleted 12/31/05

C9425   Deleted 12/31/05

C9426   Deleted 12/31/05

C9427   Deleted 12/31/05

C9428   Deleted 12/31/05

C9429   Deleted 12/31/05

C9430   Deleted 12/31/05

C9431   Deleted 12/31/05

C9432   Deleted 12/31/05

C9433   Deleted 12/31/05

C9435   Deleted 12/31/05

C9436   Deleted 12/31/05

C9437   Deleted 12/31/05

C9438   Deleted 12/31/05

C9439   Deleted 12/31/05

C9704   Deleted 12/31/05

C9713   Deleted 12/31/05

⊕ C9716   Creations of thermal anal lesions by radiofrequency energy
      Medicare Statute 1833(t)

C9718   Deleted 12/31/05

C9719   Deleted 12/31/05

C9720   Deleted 12/31/05

C9721   Deleted 12/31/05

C9722   Deleted 12/31/05

▶ ⊕ C9723   Dynamic infrared blood perfusion imaging (DIRI)
      Medicare Statute 1833(t)

▶ ⊕ C9724   Endoscopic full-thickness plication in the gastric cardia using endoscopic plication system (EPS); includes endoscopy
      Medicare Statute 1833(t)

▶ ⊕ C9725   Placement of endorectal intracavitary applicator for high intensity brachytherapy
      Medicare Statute 1833(t)

DENTAL PROCEDURES (D0000-D9999)

Codes D0100-D9999 are dental codes copyrighted to the ADA. A copy of the Current Dental Terminology (CDT), which contains all of the dental codes, can be purchased from the ADA.

DURABLE MEDICAL EQUIPMENT (E0100-E9999)

Canes

⊕ E0100   Cane, includes canes of all materials, adjustable or fixed, with tip
      MCM 2100.1, CIM 60-3, CIM 60-9

⊕ E0105   Cane, quad or three prong, includes canes of all materials, adjustable or fixed, with tips
      MCM 2100.1, CIM 60-9, CIM 60-15

Crutches

⊙ E0110   Crutches, forearm, includes crutches of various materials, adjustable or fixed, pair, complete with tips and handgrips
MCM 2100.1, CIM 60-9

⊙ E0111   Crutches, forearm, includes crutches of various materials, adjustable or fixed, each, with tips and handgrips
MCM 2100.1, CIM 60-9

⊙ E0112   Crutches, underarm, wood, adjustable or fixed, pair, with pads, tips and handgrips
MCM 2100.1, CIM 60-9

⊙ E0113   Crutches, underarm, wood, adjustable or fixed, each, with pads, tips and handgrip
MCM 2100.1, CIM 60-9

⊙ E0114   Crutches, underarm, other than wood, adjustable or fixed, pair, with pads, tips and handgrips
MCM 2100.1, CIM 60-9

➠ ⊙ E0116   Crutch, underarm, other than wood, adjustable or fixed, with pads, tip, handgrip, with or without shock absorber, each
MCM 2100.1, CIM 60-9

⊙ E0117   Crutch, underarm, articulating, spring assisted, each
MCM 2100.1

∗ E0118   Crutch substitute, lower leg platform, with or without wheels, each

Walkers

⊙ E0130   Walker, rigid (pickup), adjustable or fixed height
MCM 2100.1, CIM 60-9

⊙ E0135   Walker, folding (pickup), adjustable or fixed height
MCM 2100.1, CIM 60-9

⊙ E0140   Walker, with trunk support, adjustable or fixed height, any type
MCM 2100.1, CIM 60-9

⊙ E0141   Walker, rigid, wheeled, adjustable or fixed height
MCM 2100.1, CIM 60-9

     E0142   Deleted 12/31/02

⊙ E0143   Walker, folding, wheeled, adjustable or fixed height
MCM 2100.1, CIM 60-9

⊙ E0144   Walker, enclosed, four-sided framed, rigid or folding, wheeled, with posterior seat
MCM 2100.1, CIM 60-9

⊙ E0147   Walker, heavy duty, multiple braking system, variable wheel resistance
MCM 2100.1, CIM 60-9

∗ E0148   Walker, heavy duty, without wheels, rigid or folding, any type, each

∗ E0149   Walker, heavy duty, wheeled, rigid or folding, any type

∗ E0153   Platform attachment, forearm crutch, each

∗ E0154   Platform attachment, walker, each

∗ E0155   Wheel attachment, rigid pick-up walker, per pair

Attachments

∗ E0156   Seat attachment, walker

∗ E0157   Crutch attachment, walker, each

∗ E0158   Leg extensions for a walker, per set of four (4)

∗ E0159   Brake attachment for wheeled walker, replacement, each

Commodes

⊙ E0160   Sitz type bath or equipment, portable, used with or without commode
CIM 60-9

⊙ E0161   Sitz type bath or equipment, portable, used with or without commode, with faucet attachment/s
CIM 60-9

⊙ E0162   Sitz bath chair
CIM 60-9

⊙ E0163   Commode chair, stationary, with fixed arms
MCM 2100.1, CIM 60-9

⊙ E0164   Commode chair, mobile, with fixed arms
MCM 2100.1, CIM 60-9

⊙ E0165   Commode chair, stationary, with detachable arms
MCM 2100.1 CIM 60-9

⊙ E0166   Commode chair, mobile, with detachable arms
MCM 2100.1, CIM 60-9

⊙ E0167   Pail or pan for use with commode chair
CIM 60-9

∗ E0168   Commode chair, extra wide and/or heavy duty, stationary or mobile, with or without arms, any type, each

     E0169   Deleted 12/31/05

▶ ∗ E0170   Commode chair with integrated seat lift mechanism, electric, any type

▶ ∗ E0171   Commode chair with integrated seat lift mechanism, non-electric, any type

▶ ◆ E0172   Seat lift mechanism placed over or on top of toilet, any type
Medicare Statute 186 SSA

∗ E0175   Foot rest, for use with commode chair, each

Decubitus Care Equipment

- ☺ E0180   Pressure pad, alternating with pump
  MCM 4107.6, CIM 60-9
- ☺ E0181   Pressure pad, alternating with pump, heavy duty
  MCM 4107.6, CIM 60-9
- ☺ E0182   Pump for alternating pressure pad
  MCM 4107.6, CIM 60-9
- ☺ E0184   Dry pressure mattress
  MCM 4107.6, CIM 60-9
- ☺ E0185   Gel or gel-like pressure pad for mattress, standard mattress length and width
  MCM 4107.6, CIM 60-9
- ☺ E0186   Air pressure mattress
  CIM 60-9
- ☺ E0187   Water pressure mattress
  CIM 60-9
- ☺ E0188   Synthetic sheepskin pad
  MCM 4107.6, CIM 60-9
- ☺ E0189   Lambswool sheepskin pad, any size
  MCM 4107.6, CIM 60-9
- ☺ E0190   Positioning cushion/pillow/wedge, any shape or size
- ✳ E0191   Heel or elbow protector, each
- ✳ E0193   Powered air flotation bed (low air loss therapy)
- ☺ E0194   Air fluidized bed
  CIM 60-19, Cross Reference Q0049
- ☺ E0196   Gel pressure mattress
  CIM 60-9
- ☺ E0197   Air pressure pad for mattress, standard mattress length and width
  CIM 60-9
- ☺ E0198   Water pressure pad for mattress, standard mattress length and width
  CIM 60-9
- ☺ E0199   Dry pressure pad for mattress, standard mattress length and width
  CIM 60-9

Heat/Cold Application

- ☺ E0200   Heat lamp, without stand (table model), includes bulb, or infrared element
  MCM 2100.1, CIM 60-9
- ✳ E0202   Phototherapy (bilirubin) light with photometer
- ⇒◆ E0203   Therapeutic lightbox, minimum 10,000 lux, table top model
- ☺ E0205   Heat lamp, with stand, includes bulb, or infrared element
  MCM 2100.1, CIM 60-9
- ☺ E0210   Electric heat pad, standard
  CIM 60-9

- ☺ E0215   Electric heat pad, moist
  CIM 60-9
- ☺ E0217   Water circulating heat pad with pump
  CIM 60-9
- ☺ E0218   Water circulating cold pad with pump
  CIM 60-9
- ✳ E0220   Hot water bottle
- ✳ E0221   Infrared heating pad system
  CIM 60-25
- ☺ E0225   Hydrocollator unit, includes pads
  MCM 2210.3, CIM 60-9
- ✳ E0230   Ice cap or collar
- ✳ E0231   Non-contact wound warming device (temperature control unit, AC adapter and power cord) for use with warming card and wound cover
- ✳ E0232   Warming card for use with the non-contact wound warming device and non-contact wound warming wound cover
- ☺ E0235   Paraffin bath unit, portable (see medical supply code A4265 for paraffin)
  MCM 2210.3, CIM 60-9
- ☺ E0236   Pump for water circulating pad
  CIM 60-9
- ☺ E0238   Non-electric heat pad, moist
  CIM 60-9
- ☺ E0239   Hydrocollator unit, portable
  MCM 2210.3, CIM 60-9
- ⇒◆ E0240   Bath/shower chair, with or without wheels, any size
  CIM 60-9

Bath and Toilet Aids

- ◆ E0241   Bath tub wall rail, each
  MCM 2100.1, CIM 60-9
- ◆ E0242   Bath tub rail, floor base
  MCM 2100.1, CIM 60-9
- ◆ E0243   Toilet rail, each
  MCM 2100.1, CIM 60-9
- ◆ E0244   Raised toilet seat
  CIM 60-9
- ◆ E0245   Tub stool or bench
  CIM 60-9
- ✳ E0246   Transfer tub rail attachment
- ☺ E0247   Transfer bench for tub or toilet with or without commode opening
  CIM 60-9
- ☺ E0248   Transfer bench, heavy duty, for tub or toilet with or without commode opening
  CIM 60-9
- ☺ E0249   Pad for water circulating heat unit
  CIM 60-9

Hospital Beds and Accessories

⊛ E0250   Hospital bed, fixed height, with any type side rails, with mattress
MCM 2100.1, CIM 60-18

⊛ E0251   Hospital bed, fixed height, with any type side rails, without mattress
MCM 2100.1, CIM 60-18

⊛ E0255   Hospital bed, variable height, high-low (hi-lo), with any type side rails, with mattress
MCM 2100.1, CIM 60-18

⊛ E0256   Hospital bed, variable height, hi-lo, with any type side rails, without mattress
MCM 2100.1, CIM 60-18

⊛ E0260   Hospital bed, semi-electric (head and foot adjustment), with any type side rails, with mattress
MCM 2100.1, CIM 60-18

⊛ E0261   Hospital bed, semi-electric (head and foot adjustment), with any type side rails, without mattress
MCM 2100.1, CIM 60-18

⊛ E0265   Hospital bed, total electric (head, foot and height adjustments), with any type side rails, with mattress
MCM 2100.1, CIM 60-18

⊛ E0266   Hospital bed, total electric (head, foot and height adjustments), with any type side rails, without mattress
MCM 2100.1, CIM 60-18

◆ E0270   Hospital bed, institutional type includes: oscillating, circulating and Stryker frame, with mattress
CIM 60-9

⊛ E0271   Mattress, innerspring
CIM 60-9, CIM 60-18

⊛ E0272   Mattress, foam rubber
CIM 60-9, CIM 60-18

◆ E0273   Bed board
CIM 60-9

◆ E0274   Over-bed table
CIM 60-9

⊛ E0275   Bed pan, standard, metal or plastic
CIM 60-9

⊛ E0276   Bed pan, fracture, metal or plastic
CIM 60-9

⊛ E0277   Powered pressure-reducing air mattress
CIM 60-9

∗ E0280   Bed cradle, any type

⊛ E0290   Hospital bed, fixed height, without side rails, with mattress
MCM 2100.1, CIM 60-18

⊛ E0291   Hospital bed, fixed height, without side rails, without mattress
MCM 2100.1, CIM 60-18

⊛ E0292   Hospital bed, variable height, hi-lo, without side rails, with mattress
MCM 2100.1, CIM 60-18

⊛ E0293   Hospital bed, variable height, hi-lo, without side rails, without mattress
MCM 2100.1, CIM 60-18

⊛ E0294   Hospital bed, semi-electric (head and foot adjustment), without side rails, with mattress
MCM 2100.1, CIM 60-18

⊛ E0295   Hospital bed, semi-electric (head and foot adjustment), without side rails, without mattress
MCM 2100.1, CIM 60-18

⊛ E0296   Hospital bed, total electric (head, foot and height adjustments), without side rails, with mattress
MCM 2100.1, CIM 60-18

⊛ E0297   Hospital bed, total electric (head, foot and height adjustments), without side rails, without mattress
MCM 2100.1, CIM 60-18

∗ E0300   Pediatric crib, hospital grade, fully enclosed

⊛ E0301   Hospital bed, heavy duty, extra wide, with weight capacity greater than 350 pounds, but less than or equal to 600 pounds, with any type side rails, without mattress
CIM 60-18

⊛ E0302   Hospital bed, extra heavy duty, extra wide, with weight capacity greater than 600 pounds, with any type side rails, without mattress
CIM 60-18

⊛ E0303   Hospital bed, heavy duty, extra wide, with weight capacity greater than 350 pounds, but less than or equal to 600 pounds, with any type side rails, with mattress
CIM 60-18

⊛ E0304   Hospital bed, extra heavy duty, extra wide, with weight capacity greater than 600 pounds, with any type side rails, with mattress
CIM 60-18

Bed Accessories

⊛ E0305   Bed side rails, half length
CIM 60-18

⊛ E0310   Bed side rails, full length
CIM 60-18

◆ E0315   Bed accessory: board, table, or support device, any type
CIM 60-9

∗ E0316   Safety enclosure frame/canopy for use with hospital bed, any type

⊛ E0325   Urinal; male, jug-type, any material
CIM 60-9

⊛ E0326   Urinal; female, jug-type, any material
CIM 60-9

✱ E0350   Control unit for electronic bowel irrigation/evacuation system

✱ E0352   Disposable pack (water reservoir bag, speculum, valving mechanism and collection bag/box) for use with the electronic bowel irrigation/evacuation system

✱ E0370   Air pressure elevator for heel

✱ E0371   Non-powered advanced pressure-reducing overlay for mattress, standard mattress length and width

✱ E0372   Powered air overlay for mattress, standard mattress length and width

✱ E0373   Non-powered advanced pressure-reducing mattress

Oxygen and Related Respiratory Equipment

⊕ E0424   Stationary compressed gaseous oxygen system, rental; includes container, contents, regulator, flowmeter, humidifier, nebulizer, cannula or mask, and tubing
MCM 4107.9, CIM 60-4

⊕ E0425   Stationary compressed gas system, purchase; includes regulator, flowmeter, humidifier, nebulizer, cannula or mask, and tubing
MCM 4107.9, CIM 60-4

⊕ E0430   Portable gaseous oxygen system, purchase; includes regulator, flowmeter, humidifier, cannula or mask, and tubing
MCM 4107.9, CIM 60-4

⊕ E0431   Portable gaseous oxygen system, rental; includes portable container, regulator, flowmeter, humidifier, cannula or mask, and tubing
MCM 4107.9, CIM 60-4

⊕ E0434   Portable liquid oxygen system, rental; includes portable container, supply reservoir, humidifier, flowmeter, refill adaptor, contents gauge, cannula or mask, and tubing
MCM 4107.9, CIM 60-4

⊕ E0435   Portable liquid oxygen system, purchase; includes portable container, supply reservoir, humidifier, flowmeter, contents gauge, cannula or mask, tubing and refill adaptor
MCM 4107.9, CIM 60-4

⊕ E0439   Stationary liquid oxygen system, rental; includes container, contents, regulator, flowmeter, humidifier, nebulizer, cannula or mask, and tubing
MCM 4107.9, CIM 60-4

⊕ E0440   Stationary liquid oxygen system, purchase; includes use of reservoir, contents indicator, regulator, flowmeter, humidifier, nebulizer, cannula or mask, and tubing
MCM 4107.9, CIM 60-4

⊕ E0441   Oxygen contents, gaseous (for use with owned gaseous stationary systems or when both a stationary and portable gaseous system are owned), 1 month's supply = 1 unit
MCM 4107.9, CIM 60-4

⊕ E0442   Oxygen contents, liquid, (for use with owned liquid stationary systems or when both a stationary and portable liquid system are owned), 1 month's supply = 1 unit
MCM 4107.9, CIM 60-4

⊕ E0443   Portable oxygen contents, gaseous, (for use only with portable gaseous systems when no stationary gas or liquid system is used), 1 month's supply = 1 unit
MCM 4107.9, CIM 60-4

⊕ E0444   Portable oxygen contents, liquid (for use only with portable liquid systems when no stationary gas or liquid system is used), 1 month's supply = 1 unit
MCM 4107.9, CIM 60-4

✱ E0445   Oximeter device for measuring blood oxygen levels non-invasively

⊕ E0450   Volume control ventilator, without pressure support mode; may include pressure control mode; used with invasive interface (e.g., tracheostomy tube)
CIM 60-9

⊕ E0455   Oxygen tent, excluding croup or pediatric tents
MCM 4107.9, CIM 60-4

✱ E0457   Chest shell (cuirass)

✱ E0459   Chest wrap

⊕ E0460   Negative pressure ventilator, portable or stationary
CIM 60-9

⊕ E0461   Volume control ventilator, without pressure support mode, may include pressure control mode, used with non-invasive interface (e.g., mask)
CIM 60-9

✱ E0462   Rocking bed, with or without side rails
CIM 60-9

➡ ✱ E0463   Pressure support ventilator with volume control mode; may include pressure control mode; used with invasive interface (e.g., tracheostomy tube)

➡ ✱ E0464   Pressure support ventilator with volume control mode; may include pressure control mode; used with non-invasive interface (e.g., mask)

⊕ E0470   Respiratory assist device, bi-level pressure capability, without backup rate feature, used with noninvasive interface, e.g., nasal or facial mask (intermittent assist device with continuous positive airway pressure device)
CIM 60-9

⊚ E0471   Respiratory assist device, bi-level pressure capability, with back-up rate feature, used with noninvasive interface, e.g., nasal or facial mask (intermittent assist device with continuous positive airway pressure device)
CIM 60-9

⊚ E0472   Respiratory assist device, bi-level pressure capability, with backup rate feature, used with invasive interface, e.g., tracheostomy tube (intermittent assist device with continuous positive airway pressure device)
CIM 60-9

⊚ E0480   Percussor, electric or pneumatic, home model
CIM 60-9

◆ E0481   Intrapulmonary percussive ventilation system and related accessories
CIM 60-21

∗ E0482   Cough stimulating device, alternating positive and negative airway pressure

∗ E0483   High frequency chest wall oscillation air-pulse generator system, (includes hoses and vest), each

∗ E0484   Oscillatory positive expiratory pressure device, non-electric, any type, each

▶∗ E0485   Oral device/appliance used to reduce upper airway collapsibility, adjustable or non-adjustable, prefabricated, includes fitting and adjustment

▶∗ E0486   Oral device/appliance used to reduce upper airway collapsibility, adjustable or non-adjustable, custom fabricated, includes fitting and adjustment

IPPB Machines

⊚ E0500   IPPB machine, all types, with built-in nebulization; manual or automatic valves; internal or external power source
CIM 60-9

Humidifiers/Nebulizers/Compressors for Use with Oxygen IPPB Equipment

⇒ ⊚ E0550   Humidifier, durable for extensive supplemental humidification during IPPB treatments or oxygen delivery
CIM 60-9

⊚ E0555   Humidifier, durable, glass or autoclavable plastic bottle type, for use with regulator or flowmeter
MCM 4107.9, CIM 60-9

⇒ ⊚ E0560   Humidifier, durable for supplemental humidification during IPPB treatment or oxygen delivery
CIM 60-9

∗ E0561   Humidifier, non-heated, used with positive airway pressure device

∗ E0562   Humidifier, heated, used with positive airway pressure device

∗ E0565   Compressor, air power source for equipment which is not self-contained or cylinder driven

⊚ E0570   Nebulizer, with compressor
MCM 4107.9, CIM 60-9

⊚ E0571   Aerosol compressor, battery powered, for use with small volume nebulizer
CIM 60-9

∗ E0572   Aerosol compressor, adjustable pressure, light duty for intermittent use

∗ E0574   Ultrasonic electronic aerosol generator with small volume nebulizer

⊚ E0575   Nebulizer, ultrasonic, large volume
CIM 60-9

⊚ E0580   Nebulizer, durable, glass or autoclavable plastic, bottle type, for use with regulator or flowmeter
MCM 4107.9, CIM 60-9

⊚ E0585   Nebulizer, with compressor and heater
MCM 4107.9, CIM 60-9

∗ E0590   Dispensing fee for covered drug administered through DME nebulizer

Suction Pump/Room Vaporizers

⊚ E0600   Respiratory such pump, home model, portable or stationary, electric
CIM 60-9

⊚ E0601   Continuous airway pressure (CPAP) device
CIM 60-17

∗ E0602   Breast pump, manual, any type

∗ E0603   Breast pump, electric (AC and/or DC), any type

∗ E0604   Breast pump, heavy duty, hospital grade, piston operated, pulsatile, vacuum suction/release cycles, vacuum regulator, supplies, transformer, electric (AC and/or DC)

⊚ E0605   Vaporizer, room type
CIM 60-9

⊚ E0606   Postural drainage board
CIM 60-9

Monitoring Equipment

⊚ E0607   Home blood glucose monitor
CIM 60-11

   ⊚ **Special coverage instructions**   ◆ **Not covered by or valid for Medicare**   ∗ **Carrier discretion**   ◀ ▶ **New**   ⇐ ⇒ **Revised**

Pacemaker Monitor

⊛ E0610 Pacemaker monitor, self-contained (checks battery depletion, includes audible and visible check systems)
CIM 50-1, CIM 60-7
⊛ E0615 Pacemaker monitor, self-contained (checks battery depletion and other pacemaker components, includes digital/visible check systems)
CIM 50-1, CIM 60-7
⟼ ✳ E0616 Implantable cardiac event recorder with memory, activator, and programmer
✳ E0617 External defibrillator with integrated electrocardiogram analysis
✳ E0618 Apnea monitor, without recording feature
✳ E0619 Apnea monitor, with recording feature
✳ E0620 Skin piercing device for collection of capillary blood, laser, each

Patient Lifts

⊛ E0621 Sling or seat, patient lift, canvas or nylon
CIM 60-9
◆ E0625 Patient lift, bathroom or toilet, not otherwise classified
CIM 60-9
⊛ E0627 Seat lift mechanism incorporated into a combination lift-chair mechanism
MCM 4107.8, CIM 60-8, Cross Reference Q0080
⊛ E0628 Separate seat lift mechanism for use with patient owned furniture—electric
MCM 4107.8, CIM 60-8, Cross Reference Q0078
⊛ E0629 Separate seat lift mechanism for use with patient owned furniture—non-electric
MCM 4107.8, Cross Reference Q0079
⊛ E0630 Patient lift, hydraulic, with seat or sling
CIM 60-9
⊛ E0635 Patient lift, electric, with seat or sling
CIM 60-9
✳ E0636 Multipositional patient support system, with integrated lift, patient accessible controls
⟼ ⊛ E0637 Combination sit to stand system, any size including pediatric, with seat lift feature, with or without wheels
CIM 60-9
⟼ ◆ E0638 Standing frame system, one position (e.g. upright, supine or prone stander), any size including pediatric, with or without wheels
CIM 60-9

◆ E0639 Patient lift, moveable from room to room with disassembly and reassembly; includes all components/accessories
◆ E0640 Patient lift, fixed system; includes all components/accessories
▶◆ E0641 Standing frame system, multi-position (e.g. three-way stander), any size including pediatric, with or without wheels
CIM 60-9
▶◆ E0642 Standing frame system, mobile (dynamic stander), any size including pediatric
CIM 60-9

Pneumatic Compressor and Appliances

⊛ E0650 Pneumatic compressor, non-segmental home model
CIM 60-16
⊛ E0651 Pneumatic compressor, segmental home model without calibrated gradient pressure
CIM 60-16
⊛ E0652 Pneumatic compressor, segmental home model with calibrated gradient pressure
CIM 60-16
⊛ E0655 Non-segmental pneumatic appliance for use with pneumatic compressor, half arm
CIM 60-16
⊛ E0660 Non-segmental pneumatic appliance for use with pneumatic compressor, full leg
CIM 60-16
⊛ E0665 Non-segmental pneumatic appliance for use with pneumatic compressor, full arm
CIM 60-16
⊛ E0666 Non-segmental pneumatic appliance for use with pneumatic compressor, half leg
CIM 60-16
⊛ E0667 Segmental pneumatic appliance for use with pneumatic compressor, full leg
CIM 60-16
⊛ E0668 Segmental pneumatic appliance for use with pneumatic compressor, full arm
CIM 60-16
⊛ E0669 Segmental pneumatic appliance for use with pneumatic compressor, half leg
CIM 60-16
⊛ E0671 Segmental gradient pressure pneumatic appliance, full leg
CIM 60-16
⊛ E0672 Segmental gradient pressure pneumatic appliance, full arm
CIM 60-16

⊛ E0673 Segmental gradient pressure pneumatic appliance, half leg
CIM 60-16

∗ E0675 Pneumatic compression device, high pressure, rapid inflation/deflation cycle, for arterial insufficiency (unilateral or bilateral system)

Ultraviolet Cabinet

∗ E0691 Ultraviolet light therapy system panel, includes bulbs/lamps, timer and eye protection; treatment area 2 square feet or less

∗ E0692 Ultraviolet light therapy system panel, includes bulbs/lamps, timer and eye protection, 4 foot panel

∗ E0693 Ultraviolet light therapy system panel, includes bulbs/lamps, timer and eye protection, 6 foot panel

∗ E0694 Ultraviolet multidirectional light therapy system in 6 foot cabinet, includes bulbs/lamps, timer and eye protection

Safety Equipment

∗ E0700 Safety equipment (e.g., belt, harness or vest)

∗ E0701 Helmet with face guard and soft interface material, prefabricated

▶ ⊛ E0705 Transfer board or device, any type, each

Restraints

∗ E0710 Restraints, any type (body, chest, wrist or ankle)

Transcutaneous and/or Neuromuscular Electrical Nerve Stimulators

⊛ E0720 TENS, two lead, localized stimulation
MCM 4107.6, CIM 35-20, CIM 35-46

⊛ E0730 Transcutaneous electrical nerve stimulation device, four or more leads, for multiple nerve stimulation
MCM 4107.6, CIM 35-20, CIM 35-46

⊛ E0731 Form fitting conductive garment for delivery of TENS or NMES (with conductive fibers separated from the patient's skin by layers of fabric)
CIM 45-25

⊛ E0740 Incontinence treatment system, pelvic floor stimulator, monitor, sensor and/or trainer
CIM 65-24

∗ E0744 Neuromuscular stimulator for scoliosis

⊛ E0745 Neuromuscular stimulator, electronic shock unit
CIM 35-77

⊛ E0746 Electromyography (EMG), biofeedback device
CIM 35-27

⊛ E0747 Osteogenesis stimulator, electrical, non-invasive, other than spinal applications
CIM 35-48

⊛ E0748 Osteogensis stimulator, electrical, non-invasive, spinal applications
CIM 35-48

⊛ E0749 Osteogenesis stimulator, electrical, surgically implanted
CIM 35-48

E0752 Deleted 12/31/05

E0754 Deleted 12/31/05

∗ E0755 Electronic salivary reflex stimulator (intra-oral/non-invasive)

E0756 Deleted 12/31/05

E0757 Deleted 12/31/05

E0758 Deleted 12/31/05

E0759 Deleted 12/31/05

⊛ E0760 Osteogenesis stimulator, low intensity ultrasound, non-invasive
CIM 35-48

�⊛ E0761 Non-thermal pulsed high frequency radio waves, high peak power electromagnetic energy treatment device

▶ ∗ E0762 Transcutaneous electrical joint stimulation device system, includes all accessories

▶ ⊛ E0764 Functional neuromuscular stimulator, transcutaneous stimulation of muscles of ambulation with computer control, used for walking by spinal cord injured, entire system, after completion of training program
CIM 35-77

∗ E0765 FDA-approved nerve stimulator, with replaceable batteries, for treatment of nausea and vomiting

⊛ E0769 Electrical stimulation or electromagnetic wound treatment device, not otherwise classified
CIM 35-102

Infusion Supplies

∗ E0776 IV pole

∗ E0779 Ambulatory infusion pump, mechanical, reusable, for infusion 8 hours or greater

⊛ **Special coverage instructions**   ◆ **Not covered by or valid for Medicare**   ∗ **Carrier discretion**   ◀▶ **New**   ◀www www▶ **Revised**

✱ E0780   Ambulatory infusion pump, mechanical, reusable, for infusion less than 8 hours

⊚ E0781   Ambulatory infusion pump, single or multiple channels, electric or battery operated with administrative equipment, worn by patient
CIM 60-14

⊚ E0782   Infusion pump, implantable, non-programmable (includes all components, e.g., pump, cathether, connectors, etc.)
CIM 60-14

⊚ E0783   Infusion pump system, implantable, programmable (includes all components, e.g., pump, catheter, connectors, etc.)
CIM 60-14

⊚ E0784   External ambulatory infusion pump, insulin
CIM 60-14

⊚ E0785   Implantable intraspinal (epidural/intrathecal) catheter used with implantable infusion pump, replacement
CIM 60-14

⊚ E0786   Implantable programmable infusion pump, replacement (excludes implantable intraspinal catheter
CIM 60-14

⊚ E0791   Parenteral infusion pump, stationary, single or multi-channel
MCM 2130, MCM 4450, CIM 65-10

Traction Equipment: All Types and Cervical

⊚ E0830   Ambulatory tract device, all types, each
CIM 60-9

⊚ E0840   Traction frame, attached to headboard, cervical traction
CIM 60-9

✱ E0849   Traction equipment, cervical, free-standing stand/frame, pneumatic, applying traction force to other than mandible

⊚ E0850   Traction stand, free-standing, cervical traction
CIM 60-9

✱ E0855   Cervical traction equipment not requiring additional stand or frame

Traction: Overdoor

⊚ E0860   Traction equipment, overdoor, cervical
CIM 60-9

Traction: Extremity

⊚ E0870   Traction frame, attached to footboard, extremity traction (e.g., Buck's)
CIM 60-9

⊚ E0880   Traction stand, free-standing, extremity traction (e.g., Buck's)
CIM 60-9

Traction: Pelvic

⊚ E0890   Traction frame, attached to footboard, pelvic traction
CIM 60-9

⊚ E0900   Traction stand, free-standing, pelvic traction (e.g., Buck's)
CIM 60-9

Trapeze Equipment, Fracture Frame and Other Orthopedic Devices

⊚ E0910   Trapeze bars, also known as patient helper, attached to bed, with grab bar
CIM 60-9

▶⊚ E0911   Trapeze bar, heavy duty, for patient weight capacity greater than 250 pounds, attached to bed, with grab bar
CIM 60-9

▶⊚ E0912   Trapeze bar, heavy duty, for patient weight capacity greater than 250 pounds, free standing, complete with grab bar
CIM 60-9

⊚ E0920   Fracture frame, attached to bed, includes weights
CIM 60-9

⊚ E0930   Fracture frame, free-standing, includes weights
CIM 60-9

⇒⊚ E0935   Continuous passive motion exercise device for use on knee only
CIM 60-9

⊚ E0940   Trapeze bar, free-standing, complete with grab bar
CIM 60-9

⊚ E0941   Gravity assisted traction device, any type
CIM 60-9

✱ E0942   Cervical head harness/halter

✱ E0944   Pelvic belt/harness/boot

✱ E0945   Extremity belt/harness

⊚ E0946   Fracture, frame, dual with cross bars, attached to bed, (e.g., Balken, Four Poster)
CIM 60-9

⊛ E0947   Fracture frame, attachments for complex pelvic traction
CIM 60-9

⊛ E0948   Fracture frame, attachments for complex cervical traction
CIM 60-9

Wheelchairs

⊛ E0950   Wheelchair accessory, tray, each
CIM 60-9

∗ E0951   Heel loop/holder, any type, with or without ankle strap, each

⊛ E0952   Toe loop/holder, any type, each

    E0953   Deleted 12/31/05

    E0954   Deleted 12/31/05

∗ E0955   Wheelchair accessory, headrest, cushioned, any type, including fixed mounting hardware, each

∗ E0956   Wheelchair accessory, lateral trunk or hip support, any type, including fixed mounting hardware, each

∗ E0957   Wheelchair accessory, medial thigh support, any type, including fixed mounting hardware, each

Wheelchair Accessories

⊛ E0958   Manual wheelchair accessory, one-arm drive attachment, each
CIM 60-9

∗ E0959   Manual wheelchair accessory, adapter for amputee, each
CIM 60-9

∗ E0960   Wheelchair accessory, shoulder harness/straps or chest strap, including any type mounting hardware

∗ E0961   Manual wheelchair accessory, wheel lock brake extension (handle), each
CIM 60-9

∗ E0966   Manual wheelchair accessory, headrest extension, each
CIM 60-9

⊛ E0967   Manual wheelchair accessory, hand rim with projections, any type, replacement only each
CIM 60-9

⊛ E0968   Commode seat, wheelchair
CIM 60-9

⊛ E0969   Narrowing device, wheelchair
CIM 60-9

◆ E0970   No. 2 footplates, except for elevating leg rest
CIM 60-9; Cross Reference K0037, K0042

▬▶ ◆ E0971   Manual wheelchair accessory, anti-tipping device, each
CIM 60-9

    E0972   Deleted 12/31/05

⊛ E0973   Wheelchair accessory, adjustable height, detachable armrest, complete assembly, each
CIM 60-9

⊛ E0974   Manual wheelchair accessory, anti-rollback device, each
CIM 60-9

∗ E0977   Wedge cushion, wheelchair

∗ E0978   Wheelchair accessory, positioning belt/safety belt/pelvic strap, each

∗ E0980   Safety vest, wheelchair

∗ E0981   Wheelchair accessory, seat upholstery, replacement only, each

∗ E0982   Wheelchair accessory, back upholstery, replacement only, each

∗ E0983   Manual wheelchair accessory, power add-on to convert manual wheelchair to motorized wheelchair, joystick control

∗ E0984   Manual wheelchair accessory, power add-on to convert manual wheelchair to motorized wheelchair, tiller control

∗ E0985   Wheelchair accessory, seat lift mechanism

∗ E0986   Manual wheelchair accessory, push activated power assist, each

∗ E0990   Wheelchair accessory, elevating leg rest, complete assembly, each
CIM 60-9

∗ E0992   Manual wheelchair accessory, solid seat insert

⊛ E0994   Arm rest, each
CIM 60-9

∗ E0995   Wheelchair accessory, calf rest/pad, each

    E0996   Deleted 12/31/05

⊛ E0997   Caster with a fork
CIM 60-9

⊛ E0998   Caster without fork
CIM 60-9

⊛ E0999   Pneumatic tire with wheel
CIM 60-9

    E1000   Deleted 12/31/05

    E1001   Deleted 12/31/05

∗ E1002   Wheelchair accessory, power seating system, tilt only

∗ E1003   Wheelchair accessory, power seating system, recline only, without shear reduction

∗ E1004   Wheelchair accessory, power seating system, recline only, with mechanical shear reduction

∗ E1005   Wheelchair accessory, power seating system, recline only, with power shear reduction

∗ E1006   Wheelchair accessory, power seating system, combination tilt and recline, without shear reduction

* E1007   Wheelchair accessory, power seating system, combination tilt and recline, with mechanical shear reduction

* E1008   Wheelchair accessory, power seating system, combination tilt and recline, with power shear reduction

* E1009   Wheelchair accessory, addition to power seating system, mechanically linked leg elevation system, including pushrod and leg rest, each

* E1010   Wheelchair accessory, addition to power seating system, power leg elevation system, including leg rest, pair

☺ E1011   Modification to pediatric-size wheelchair, width adjustment package (not to be dispensed with initial chair)
CIM 60-9

☺ E1014   Reclining back, addition to pediatric-size wheelchair
CIM 60-9

☺ E1015   Shock absorber for manual wheelchair, each
CIM 60-9

☺ E1016   Shock absorber for power wheelchair, each
CIM 60-9

☺ E1017   Heavy duty shock absorber for heavy duty or extra heavy duty manual wheelchair, each
CIM 60-9

☺ E1018   Heavy duty shock absorber for heavy duty or extra heavy duty power wheelchair, each
CIM 60-9

E1019   Deleted 12/31/05

☺ E1020   Residual limb support system for wheelchair
CIM 60-6

E1021   Deleted 12/31/05
E1025   Deleted 12/31/05
E1026   Deleted 12/31/05
E1027   Deleted 12/31/05

* E1028   Wheelchair accessory, manual swing away, retractable or removable mounting hardware for joystick, other control interface or positioning accessory

* E1029   Wheelchair accessory, ventilator tray, fixed

* E1030   Wheelchair accessory, ventilator tray, gimbaled

Rollabout Chair and Transfer System

☺ E1031   Rollabout chair, any and all types with castors 5 inches or greater
CIM 60-9

☺ E1035   Multi-positional patient transfer system, with integrated seat, operated by care giver
MCM 2100

☺ E1037   Transport chair, pediatric size
CIM 60-9

➟ ☺ E1038   Transport chair, adult size; patient weight capacity up to and including 300 pounds
CIM 60-9

➟ * E1039   Transport chair, adult size, heavy duty; patient weight capacity greater than 300 pounds

Wheelchair: Fully Reclining

☺ E1050   Fully reclining wheelchair, fixed full-length arms, swing-away detachable elevating leg rests
CIM 60-9

☺ E1060   Fully reclining wheelchair, detachable arms, desk or full-length, swing-away detachable elevating leg rests
CIM 60-9

☺ E1070   Fully reclining wheelchair, detachable arms (desk or full-length), swing-away detachable foot rests
CIM 60-9

☺ E1083   Hemi-wheelchair, fixed full-length arms, swing-away detachable elevating leg rests
CIM 60-9

☺ E1084   Hemi-wheelchair, detachable arms (desk or full-length) arms, swing-away detachable elevating leg rests
CIM 60-9

◆ E1085   Hemi-wheelchair, fixed full-length arms, swing-away detachable foot rests
CIM 60-9, Cross Reference K0002

◆ E1086   Hemi-wheelchair, detachable arms (desk or full-length), swing-away detachable foot rests
CIM 60-9, Cross Reference K0002

☺ E1087   High-strength lightweight wheelchair, fixed full-length arms, swing-away detachable elevating leg rests
CIM 60-9

☺ E1088   High-strength lightweight wheelchair, detachable arms (desk or full-length), swing-away detachable elevating leg rests
CIM 60-9

◆ E1089   High-strength lightweight wheelchair, fixed-length arms, swing-away detachable foot rests
CIM 60-9, Cross Reference K0004

◆ E1090　High-strength lightweight wheelchair, detachable arms (desk or full-length), swing-away detachable foot rests
CIM 60-9, Cross Reference K0004

✿ E1092　Wide, heavy duty wheelchair, detachable arms (desk or full-length), swing-away detachable elevating leg rests
CIM 60-9

✿ E1093　Wide, heavy duty wheelchair, detachable arms (desk or full-length) swing-away detachable foot rests
CIM 60-9

Wheelchair: Semi-reclining

✿ E1100　Semi-reclining wheelchair, fixed full-length arms, swing-away detachable elevating leg rests
CIM 60-9

✿ E1110　Semi-reclining wheelchair, detachable arms (desk or full-length), elevating leg rests
CIM 60-9

Wheelchair: Standard

◆ E1130　Standard wheelchair, fixed full-length arms, fixed or swing-away detachable foot rests
CIM 60-9, Cross Reference K0001

◆ E1140　Wheelchair, detachable arms (desk or full-length), swing-away detachable foot rests
CIM 60-9, Cross Reference K0001

✿ E1150　Wheelchair, detachable arms (desk or full-length), swing-away detachable elevating leg rests
CIM 60-9

✿ E1160　Wheelchair, fixed full-length arms, swing-away detachable elevating leg rests
CIM 60-9

✱ E1161　Manual adult size wheelchair, includes tilt in space

Wheelchair: Amputee

✿ E1170　Amputee wheelchair, fixed full-length arms, swing-away detachable elevating leg rests
CIM 60-9

✿ E1171　Amputee wheelchair, fixed full-length arms, without foot rests or leg rests
CIM 60-9

✿ E1172　Amputee wheelchair, detachable arms (desk or full-length), without foot rests or leg rests
CIM 60-9

✿ E1180　Amputee wheelchair, detachable arms (desk or full-length) swing-away detachable foot rests
CIM 60-9

✿ E1190　Amputee wheelchair, detachable arms (desk or full-length), swing-away detachable elevating leg rests
CIM 60-9

✿ E1195　Heavy duty wheelchair, fixed full-length arms, swing-away detachable elevating leg rests
CIM 60-9

✿ E1200　Amputee wheelchair, fixed full-length arms, swing-away detachable foot rests
CIM 60-9

Wheelchair: Power

E1210　Deleted 12/31/05
E1211　Deleted 12/31/05
E1212　Deleted 12/31/05
E1213　Deleted 12/31/05

Wheelchair: Special Size

✿ E1220　Wheelchair; specially sized or constructed (indicate brand name, model number, if any) and justification
CIM 60-6

✿ E1221　Wheelchair with fixed arm, foot rests
CIM 60-6

✿ E1222　Wheelchair with fixed arm, elevating leg rests
CIM 60-6

✿ E1223　Wheelchair with detachable arms, foot rests
CIM 60-6

✿ E1224　Wheelchair with detachable arms, elevating leg rests
CIM 60-6

✿ E1225　Wheelchair accessory, manual semi-reclining back (recline greater than 15 degrees, but less than 80 degrees), each
CIM 60-6

✿ E1226　Wheelchair accessory, manual fully reclining back, (recline greater than 80 degrees), each
CIM 60-6

✿ E1227　Special height arms for wheelchair
CIM 60-6

✿ E1228　Special back height for wheelchair
CIM 60-6

✳ E1229   Wheelchair, pediatric size, not otherwise specified

⊛ E1230   Power operated vehicle (three- or four-wheel non-highway); specify brand name and model number
MCM 4107.6, CIM 60-5

⊛ E1231   Wheelchair, pediatric size, tilt-in-space, rigid, adjustable, with seating system
CIM 60-9

⊛ E1232   Wheelchair, pediatric size, tilt-in-space, folding, adjustable, with seating system
CIM 60-9

⊛ E1233   Wheelchair, pediatric size, tilt-in-space, rigid, adjustable, without seating system
CIM 60-9

⊛ E1234   Wheelchair, pediatric size, tilt-in-space, folding, adjustable, without seating system
CIM 60-9

⊛ E1235   Wheelchair, pediatric size, rigid, adjustable, with seating system
CIM 60-9

⊛ E1236   Wheelchair, pediatric size, folding, adjustable, with seating system
CIM 60-9

⊛ E1237   Wheelchair, pediatric size, rigid, adjustable, without seating system
CIM 60-9

⊛ E1238   Wheelchair, pediatric size, folding, adjustable, without seating system
CIM 60-9

    E1239   Deleted 12/31/05

Wheelchair: Lightweight

⊛ E1240   Lightweight wheelchair, detachable arms (desk or full-length), swing-away detachable, elevating leg rests
CIM 60-9

◆ E1250   Lightweight wheelchair, fixed full-length arms, swing-away detachable foot rests
CIM 60-9, Cross Reference K0003

◆ E1260   Lightweight wheelchair, detachable arms (desk or full-length), swing-away detachable foot rests
CIM 60-9, Cross Reference K0003

⊛ E1270   Lightweight wheelchair, fixed full-length arms, swing-away detachable elevating leg rests
CIM 60-9

Wheelchair: Heavy Duty

⊛ E1280   Heavy duty wheelchair, detachable arms (desk or full-length), elevating leg rests
CIM 60-9

◆ E1285   Heavy duty wheelchair, fixed full-length arms, swing-away detachable foot rests
CIM 60-9, Cross Reference K0006

◆ E1290   Heavy duty wheelchair, detachable arms (desk or full-length), swing-away detachable foot rests
CIM 60-9, Cross Reference K0006

⊛ E1295   Heavy duty wheelchair, fixed full-length arms, elevating leg rests
CIM 60-9

⊛ E1296   Special wheelchair seat, height from floor
CIM 60-6

⊛ E1297   Special wheelchair seat depth, by upholstery
CIM 60-6

⊛ E1298   Special wheelchair seat depth and/or width, by construction
CIM 60-6

Whirlpool Equipment

◆ E1300   Whirlpool, portable (overtub type)
CIM 60-9

⊛ E1310   Whirlpool, non-portable (built-in type)
CIM 60-9

Repairs and Replacement Parts

⊛ E1340   Repair or nonroutine service for durable medical equipment requiring the skill of a technician, labor component, per 15 minutes
MCM 2100.4

Additional Oxygen Related Equipment

⊛ E1353   Regulator
MCM 4107.9, CIM 60-4

⊛ E1355   Stand/rack
CIM 60-4

⊛ E1372   Immersion external heater for nebulizer
CIM 60-4

⊛ E1390   Oxygen concentrator, single delivery port, capable of delivering 85 percent or greater oxygen concentration at the prescribed flow rate
CIM 60-4

⊛ E1391   Oxygen concentrator, dual delivery port, capable of delivering 85 percent or greater oxygen concentration at the prescribed flow rate, each
CIM 60-4

▶ ⊛ E1392   Portable oxygen concentrator, rental
CIM 60-4

* E1399 Durable medical equipment, miscellaneous
⊚ E1405 Oxygen and water vapor enriching system with heated delivery
MCM 4107, CIM 60-4
⊚ E1406 Oxygen and water vapor enriching system without heated delivery
MCM 4107, CIM 60-4

Artificial Kidney Machines and Accessories

⊚ E1500 Centrifuge, for dialysis
⊚ E1510 Kidney, dialysate delivery system, kidney machine, pump recirculating, air removal system, flow rate meter, power off, heater and temperature control with alarm, IV poles, pressure gauge, concentrate container
⊚ E1520 Heparin infusion pump for hemodialysis
⊚ E1530 Air bubble detector for hemodialysis, each, replacement
⊚ E1540 Pressure alarm for hemodialysis, each
⊚ E1550 Bath conductivity meter for hemodialysis, each
⊚ E1560 Blood leak detector for hemodialysis, each, replacement
⊚ E1570 Adjustable chair, for ESRD patients
⊚ E1575 Transducer protectors/fluid barriers for hemohemodialysis, any size, per 10
⊚ E1580 Unipuncture control system for hemodialysis
⊚ E1590 Hemodialysis machine
⊚ E1592 Automatic intermittent peritoneal dialysis system
⊚ E1594 Cycler dialysis machine for peritoneal dialysis
⊚ E1600 Delivery and/or installation charges for hemodialysis equipment
⊚ E1610 Reverse osmosis water purification system, for hemodialysis
CIM 55-1A
⊚ E1615 Deionizer water purification system, for hemodialysis
CIM 55-1A
⊚ E1620 Blood pump for hemodialysis replacement
⊚ E1625 Water softening system, for hemodialysis
CIM 55-1B
* E1630 Reciprocating peritoneal dialysis system
⊚ E1632 Wearable artificial kidney, each
⊚ E1634 Peritoneal dialysis clamps, each
MCM 4270
⊚ E1635 Compact (portable) travel hemodialyzer system
⊚ E1636 Sorbent cartridges, for hemodialysis, per 10
⊚ E1637 Hemostats, each
⊚ E1639 Scale, each

⊚ E1699 Dialysis equipment, not otherwise specified

Jaw Motion Rehabilitation System and Accessories

* E1700 Jaw motion rehabilitation system
* E1701 Replacement cushions for jaw motion rehabilitation system, package of 6
* E1702 Replacement measuring scales for jaw motion rehabilitation system, package of 200

Other Orthopedic Devices

* E1800 Dynamic adjustable elbow extension/flexion device, includes soft interface material
* E1801 Bi-directional static progressive stretch elbow device with range of motion adjustment, includes cuffs
* E1802 Dynamic adjustable forearm pronation/supination device, includes soft interface material
* E1805 Dynamic adjustable wrist extension/flexion device, includes soft interface material
* E1806 Bi-directional static progressive stretch wrist device with range of motion adjustment, includes cuffs
* E1810 Dynamic adjustable knee extension/flexion device, includes soft interface material
* E1811 Bi-directional static progressive stretch knee device with range of motion adjustment, includes cuffs
▶ * E1812 Dynamic knee, extension/flexion device with active resistance control
* E1815 Dynamic adjustable ankle extension/flexion device, includes soft interface material
* E1816 Bi-directional static progressive stretch ankle device with range of motion adjustment, includes cuffs
* E1818 Bi-directional static progressive stretch forearm pronation/supination device with range of motion adjustment, includes cuffs
* E1820 Replacement of soft interface material, dynamic adjustable extension/flexion device
* E1821 Replacement of soft interface material/cuffs for bi-directional static progressive stretch device
* E1825 Dynamic adjustable finger extension/flexion device, includes soft interface material

* E1830   Dynamic adjustable toe extension/flexion device, includes soft interface material

* E1840   Dynamic adjustable shoulder flexion/abduction/rotation device, includes soft interface material

* E1841   Multi-directional static progressive stretch shoulder device, with range-of-motion adjustability; includes cuffs

* E1902   Communication board, non-electronic augmentative or alternative communication device

* E2000   Gastric suction pump, home model, portable or stationary, electric

☺ E2100   Blood glucose monitor with integrated voice synthesizer
         CIM 60-11

☺ E2101   Blood glucose monitor with integrated lancing/blood sample
         CIM 60-11

* E2120   Pulse generator system for tympanic treatment of inner ear endolymphatic fluid

* E2201   Manual wheelchair accessory, nonstandard seat frame, width greater than or equal to 20 inches and less than 24 inches

* E2202   Manual wheelchair accessory, nonstandard seat frame width, 24-27 inches

* E2203   Manual wheelchair accessory, nonstandard seat frame depth, 20 to less than 22 inches

* E2204   Manual wheelchair accessory, nonstandard seat frame depth, 22 to 25 inches

* E2205   Manual wheelchair accessory, handrim without projections, any type, replacement only, each

* E2206   Manual wheelchair accessory, wheel lock assembly, complete, each

▶* E2207   Wheelchair accessory, crutch and cane holder, each

▶* E2208   Wheelchair accessory, cylinder tank carrier, each

▶* E2209   Wheelchair accessory, arm trough, each

▶* E2210   Wheelchair accessory, bearings, any type, replacement only, each

▶* E2211   Manual wheelchair accessory, pneumatic propulsion tire, any size, each

▶* E2212   Manual wheelchair accessory, tube for pneumatic propulsion tire, any size, each

▶* E2213   Manual wheelchair accessory, insert for pneumatic propulsion tire (removable), any type, any size, each

▶* E2214   Manual wheelchair accessory, pneumatic caster tire, any size, each

▶* E2215   Manual wheelchair accessory, tube for pneumatic caster tire, any size, each

▶* E2216   Manual wheelchair accessory, foam filled propulsion tire, any size, each

▶* E2217   Manual wheelchair accessory, foam filled caster tire, any size, each

▶* E2218   Manual wheelchair accessory, foam propulsion tire, any size, each

▶* E2219   Manual wheelchair accessory, foam caster tire, any size, each

▶* E2220   Manual wheelchair accessory, solid (rubber/plastic) propulsion tire, any size, each

▶* E2221   Manual wheelchair accessory, solid (rubber/plastic) caster tire (removable), any size, each

▶* E2222   Manual wheelchair accessory, solid (rubber/plastic) caster tire with integrated wheel, any size, each

▶* E2223   Manual wheelchair accessory, valve, any type, replacement only, each

▶* E2224   Manual wheelchair accessory, propulsion wheel excludes tire, any size, each

▶* E2225   Manual wheelchair accessory, caster wheel excludes tire, any size, replacement only, each

▶* E2226   Manual wheelchair accessory, caster fork, any size, replacement only, each

◆ E2291   Back, planar, for pediatric size wheelchair, including fixed attaching hardware

◆ E2292   Seat, planar, for pediatric size wheelchair, including fixed attaching hardware

◆ E2293   Back, contoured, for pediatric size wheelchair, including fixed attaching hardware

◆ E2294   Seat, contoured, for pediatric size wheelchair, including fixed attaching hardware

* E2300   Power wheelchair accessory, power seat elevation system

* E2301   Power wheelchair accessory, power standing system

* E2310   Power wheelchair accessory, electronic connection between wheelchair controller and one power seating system motor, including all related electronics, indicator feature, mechanical function selection switch, and fixed mounting hardware

* E2311   Power wheelchair accessory, electronic connection between wheelchair controller and two or more power seating system motors, including all related electronics, indicator feature, mechanical function selection switch, and fixed mounting hardware

* E2320   Power wheelchair accessory, hand or chin control interface, remote joystick or touchpad, proportional, including all related electronics, and fixed mounting hardware

✻ E2321   Power wheelchair accessory, hand control interface, remote joystick, nonproportional, including all related electronics, mechanical stop switch, and fixed mounting hardware

✻ E2322   Power wheelchair accessory, hand control interface, multiple mechanical switches, nonproportional, including all related electronics, mechanical stop switch, and fixed mounting hardware

✻ E2323   Power wheelchair accessory, specialty joystick handle for hand control interface, prefabricated

✻ E2324   Power wheelchair accessory, chin cup for chin control interface

✻ E2325   Power wheelchair accessory, sip and puff interface, nonproportional, including all related electronics, mechanical stop switch, and manual swingaway mounting hardware

✻ E2326   Power wheelchair accessory, breath tube kit for sip and puff interface

✻ E2327   Power wheelchair accessory, head control interface, mechanical, proportional, including all related electronics, mechanical direction change switch, and fixed mounting hardware

✻ E2328   Power wheelchair accessory, head control or extremity control interface, electronic, proportional, including all related electronics and fixed mounting hardware

✻ E2329   Power wheelchair accessory, head control interface, contact switch mechanism, nonproportional, including all related electronics, mechanical stop switch, mechanical direction change switch, head array, and fixed mounting hardware

✻ E2330   Power wheelchair accessory, head control interface, proximity switch mechanism, nonproportional, including all related electronics, mechanical stop switch, mechanical direction change switch, head array, and fixed mounting hardware

✻ E2331   Power wheelchair accessory, attendant control, proportional, including all related electronics and fixed mounting hardware

✻ E2340   Power wheelchair accessory, nonstandard seat frame width, 20-23 inches

✻ E2341   Power wheelchair accessory, nonstandard seat frame width, 24-27 inches

✻ E2342   Power wheelchair accessory, nonstandard seat frame depth, 20 or 21 inches

✻ E2343   Power wheelchair accessory, nonstandard seat frame depth, 22-25 inches

✻ E2351   Power wheelchair accessory, electronic interface to operate speech generating device using power wheelchair control interface

✻ E2360   Power wheelchair accessory, 22 NF non-sealed lead acid battery, each

✻ E2361   Power wheelchair accessory, 22 NF sealed lead acid battery, each, (e.g., gel cell, absorbed glassmat)

✻ E2362   Power wheelchair accessory, group 24 non-sealed lead acid battery, each

✻ E2363   Power wheelchair accessory, group 24 sealed lead acid battery, each (e.g., gel cell, absorbed glassmat)

✻ E2364   Power wheelchair accessory, U-1 non-sealed lead acid battery, each

✻ E2365   Power wheelchair accessory, U-1 sealed lead acid battery, each (e.g., gel cell, absorbed glassmat)

✻ E2366   Power wheelchair accessory, battery charger, single mode, for use with only one battery type, sealed or non-sealed, each

✻ E2367   Power wheelchair accessory, battery charger, dual mode, for use with either battery type, sealed or non-sealed, each

✻ E2368   Power wheelchair component, motor, replacement only

✻ E2369   Power wheelchair component, gear box, replacement only

✻ E2370   Power wheelchair component, motor and gear box combination, replacement only

▶ ✻ E2371   Power wheelchair accessory, group 27 sealed lead acid battery, (e.g. gel cell, absorbed glass mat), each

▶ ✻ E2372   Power wheelchair accessory, group 27 non-sealed lead acid battery, each

✻ E2399   Power wheelchair accessory, not otherwise classified interface, including all related electronics and any type mounting hardware

✻ E2402   Negative pressure wound therapy electrical pump, stationary or portable

◎ E2500   Speech generating device, digitized speech, using pre-recorded messages, less than or equal to 8 minutes recording time
CIM 60-23

◎ E2502   Speech generating device, digitized speech, using pre-recorded messages, greater than 8 minutes but less than or equal to 20 minutes recording time
CIM 60-23

◎ E2504   Speech generating device, digitized speech, using pre-recorded messages, greater than 20 minutes but less than or equal to 40 minutes recording time
CIM 60-23

⊛ E2506 Speech generating device, digitized speech, using pre-recorded messages, greater than 40 minutes recording time
CIM 60-23

⊛ E2508 Speech generating device, synthesized speech, requiring message formulation by spelling and access by physical contact with the device
CIM 60-23

⊛ E2510 Speech generating device, synthesized speech, permitting multiple methods of message formulation and multiple methods of device access
CIM 60-23

⊛ E2511 Speech generating software program, for personal computer or personal digital assistant
CIM 60-23

⊛ E2512 Accessory for speech generating device, mounting system
CIM 60-23

⊛ E2599 Accessory for speech generating device, not otherwise classified
CIM 60-23

∗ E2601 General use wheelchair seat cushion, width less than 22 inches, any depth

∗ E2602 General use wheelchair seat cushion, width 22 inches or greater, any depth

∗ E2603 Skin protection wheelchair seat cushion, width less than 22 inches, any depth

∗ E2604 Skin protection wheelchair seat cushion, width 22 inches or greater, any depth

∗ E2605 Positioning wheelchair seat cushion, width less than 22 inches, any depth

∗ E2606 Positioning wheelchair seat cushion, width 22 inches or greater, any depth

∗ E2607 Skin protection and positioning wheelchair seat cushion, width less than 22 inches, any depth

∗ E2608 Skin protection and positioning wheelchair seat cushion, width 22 inches or greater, any depth

∗ E2609 Custom fabricated wheelchair seat cushion, any size

∗ E2610 Wheelchair seat cushion, powered

∗ E2611 General use wheelchair back cushion, width less than 22 inches, any height, including any type mounting hardware

∗ E2612 General use wheelchair back cushion, width 22 inches or greater, any height, including any type mounting hardware

∗ E2613 Positioning wheelchair back cushion, posterior, width less than 22 inches, any height, including any type mounting hardware

∗ E2614 Positioning wheelchair back cushion, posterior, width 22 inches or greater, any height, including any type mounting hardware

∗ E2615 Positioning wheelchair back cushion, posterior-lateral, width less than 22 inches, any height, including any type mounting hardware

∗ E2616 Positioning wheelchair back cushion, posterior-lateral, width 22 inches or greater, any height, including any type mounting hardware

∗ E2617 Custom fabricated wheelchair back cushion, any size, including any type mounting hardware

∗ E2618 Wheelchair accessory, solid seat support base (replaces sling seat), for use with manual wheelchair or lightweight power wheelchair; includes any type mounting hardware

∗ E2619 Replacement cover for wheelchair seat cushion or back cushion, each

∗ E2620 Positioning wheelchair back cushion, planar back with lateral supports, width less than 22 inches, any height, including any type mounting hardware

∗ E2621 Positioning wheelchair back cushion, planar back with lateral supports, width 22 inches or greater, any height, including any type mounting hardware

◆ E8000 Gait trainer, pediatric size, posterior support; includes all accessories and components

◆ E8001 Gait trainer, pediatric size, upright support; includes all accessories and components

◆ E8002 Gait trainer, pediatric size, anterior support; includes all accessories and components

PROCEDURES/PROFESSIONAL SERVICES (TEMPORARY) (G0000-G9999)

NOTE: This section contains national codes assigned by CMS on a temporary basis to identify procedures/professional services.

Positron Emission Tomography Scan Code Modifiers

Effective for claims received on or after July 1, 2001, CMS will no longer require the designation of the four PET Scan modifiers (N,E,P,S) and has made the determination that no paper documentation needs to be submitted up front with PET scan claims. Documentation requirements such as physician referral and medical necessity determination are to be maintained by the provider as part of the beneficiary's medical record. (AB-02-115)

∗ G0008 Administration of influenza virus vaccine

＊ G0009 Administration of pneumococcal vaccine

＊ G0010 Administration of hepatitis B vaccine

＊ G0027 Semen analysis; presence and/or motility of sperm excluding Huhner

G0030 Deleted 3/31/05

G0031 Deleted 3/31/05

G0032 Deleted 3/31/05

G0033 Deleted 3/31/05

G0034 Deleted 3/31/05

G0035 Deleted 3/31/05

G0036 Deleted 3/31/05

G0037 Deleted 3/31/05

G0038 Deleted 3/31/05

G0039 Deleted 3/31/05

G0040 Deleted 3/31/05

G0041 Deleted 3/31/05

G0042 Deleted 3/31/05

G0043 Deleted 3/31/05

G0044 Deleted 3/31/05

G0045 Deleted 3/31/05

G0046 Deleted 3/31/05

G0047 Deleted 3/31/05

⊘ G0101 Cervical or vaginal cancer screening; pelvic and clinical breast examination

⊘ G0102 Prostate cancer screening; digital rectal examination
MCM 4182, CIM 50-55

⊘ G0103 Prostate cancer screening; prostate specific antigen test (PSA), total
MCM 4182, CIM 50-55

⊘ G0104 Colorectal cancer screening; flexible sigmoidoscopy

⊘ G0105 Colorectal cancer screening; colonoscopy on individual at high risk

⊘ G0106 Colorectal cancer screening; alternative to G0104, screening sigmoidoscopy, barium enema

⊘ G0107 Colorectal cancer screening; fecal-occult blood test, 1-3 simultaneous determinations

＊ G0108 Diabetes outpatient self-management training services, individual, per 30 minute

＊ G0109 Diabetes outpatient self-management training services, group session, two or more, per 30 minutes

G0110 Deleted 12/31/05

G0111 Deleted 12/31/05

G0112 Deleted 12/31/05

G0113 Deleted 12/31/05

G0114 Deleted 12/31/05

G0115 Deleted 12/31/05

G0116 Deleted 12/31/05

＊ G0117 Glaucoma screening for high risk patients furnished by optometrist or ophthalmologist

＊ G0118 Glaucoma screening for high risk patient furnished under direct supervision by optometrist or ophthalmologist

⊘ G0120 Colorectal cancer screening; alternative to G0105, screening colonoscopy, barium enema

⊘ G0121 Colorectal cancer screening; colonoscopy on individual not meeting criteria for high risk

◆ G0122 Colorectal cancer screening; barium enema

⊘ G0123 Screening cytopathology, cervical or vaginal (any reporting system); collected in preservative fluid, automated thin layer preparation, screening by cytotechnologist under physician supervision
CIM 50-20, Laboratory Certification: cytology

⊘ G0124 Screening cytopathology, cervical or vaginal (any reporting system); collected in preservative fluid, automated thin layer preparation, requiring interpretation by physician
CIM 50-20, Laboratory Certification: cytology

G0125 Deleted 3/31/05

⊘ G0127 Trimming of dystrophic nails, any number
MCM 2323, MCM 4120

⊘ G0128 Direct (face-to-face with patient) skilled nursing services of a registered nurse provided in a comprehensive outpatient rehabilitation facility, each 10 minutes beyond the first 5 minutes
Medicare Statute 1833a

G0129 Occupational therapy requiring the skills of a qualified occupational therapist, furnished as a component of a partial hospitalization treatment program, per day

⊘ G0130 Single energy x-ray absorptiometry (SEXA) bone density study, one or more sites; appendicular skeleton (peripheral) (e.g., radius, wrist, heel)
CIM 50-44

＊ G0141 Screening cytopathology smears, cervical or vaginal, performed by automated system, with manual rescreening requiring interpretation by physician;
Laboratory Certification: cytology

＊ G0143 Screening cytopathology, cervical or vaginal (any reporting system); collected in preservative fluid, automated thin layer preparation, with manual screening and rescreening by cytotechnologist under physician supervision;
Laboratory Certification: cytology

＊ G0144 Screening cytopathology, cervical or vaginal (any reporting system); collected in preservative fluid, automated thin layer preparation, with screening by automated system, under physician supervision; Laboratory Certification: cytology

* G0145 Screening cytopathology, cervical or vaginal (any reporting system); collected in preservative fluid, automated thin layer preparation, with screening by automated system and manual rescreening under physician supervision; Laboratory Certification: cytology

* G0147 Screening cytopathology smears, cervical or vaginal; performed by automated system under physician supervision; Laboratory Certification: cytology

* G0148 Screening cytopathology smears, cervical or vaginal; performed by automated system with manual rescreening; Laboratory Certification: cytology

* G0151 Services of physical therapist in home health setting, each 15 minutes

* G0152 Services of occupational therapist in home health setting, each 15 minutes

* G0153 Services of speech and language pathologist in home health setting, each 15 minutes

* G0154 Services of skilled nurse in home health setting, each 15 minutes

* G0155 Services of clinical social worker in home health setting, each 15 minutes

* G0156 Services of home health aide in home health setting, each 15 minutes

☺ G0166 External counterpulsation, per treatment session
CIM 35-74

* G0168 Wound closure utilizing tissue adhesive(s) only

☺ G0173 Linear accelerator-based stereotactic radiosurgery, complete course of therapy in one session

* G0175 Scheduled interdisciplinary team conference (minimum of three exclusive of patient care nursing staff) with patient present

☺ G0176 Activity therapy, such as music, dance, art or play therapies not for recreation, related to the care and treatment of patient's disabling mental health problems, per session (45 minutes or more)

☺ G0177 Training and educational services related to the care and treatment of patient's disabling mental health problems per session (45 minutes or more)

* G0179 Physician re-certification for Medicare-covered home health services under a home health plan of care (patient not present), including contacts with home health agency and review of reports of patient status required by physicians to affirm the initial implementation of the plan of care that meets patient's needs, per re-certification period

* G0180 Physician certification for Medicare-covered home health services under a home health plan of care (patient not present), including contacts with home health agency and review of reports of patient status required by physicians to affirm the initial implementation of the plan of care that meets patient's needs, per certification period

* G0181 Physician supervision of a patient receiving Medicare-covered services provided by a participating home health agency (patient not present) requiring complex and multidisciplinary care modalities involving regular physician development and/or revision of care plans, review of subsequent reports of patient status, review of laboratory and other studies, communication (including telephone calls) with other health care professionals involved in the patient's care, integration of new information into the medical treatment plan, and/or adjustment of medical therapy, within a calendar month, 30 minutes or more

* G0182 Physician supervision of a patient under a Medicare-approved hospice (patient not present) requiring complex and multidisciplinary care modalities involving regular physician development and/or revision of care plans, review of subsequent reports of patient status, review of laboratory and other studies, communication (including telephone calls) with other health care professionals involved in the patient's care, integration of new information into the medical treatment plan, and/or adjustment of medical therapy, within a calendar month, 30 minutes or more

* G0186 Destruction of localized lesion of choroid (for example, choroidal neovascularization); photocoagulation, feeder vessel technique (one or more sessions)

* G0202 Screening mammography, producing direct digital image, bilateral, all views

* G0204 Diagnostic mammography, producing direct digital image, bilateral, all views

* G0206 Diagnostic mammography, producing direct digital image, unilateral, all views

G0210 Deleted 3/31/05
G0211 Deleted 3/31/05
G0212 Deleted 3/31/05
G0213 Deleted 3/31/05
G0214 Deleted 3/31/05
G0215 Deleted 3/31/05
G0216 Deleted 3/31/05

G0217   Deleted 3/31/05
G0218   Deleted 3/31/05
⊛ G0219   PET imaging whole body melanoma; for non-covered indications
      MCM 4173 CIM 50-36
G0220   Deleted 3/31/05
G0221   Deleted 3/31/05
G0222   Deleted 3/31/05
G0223   Deleted 3/31/05
G0224   Deleted 3/31/05
G0225   Deleted 3/31/05
G0226   Deleted 3/31/05
G0227   Deleted 3/31/05
G0228   Deleted 3/31/05
G0229   Deleted 3/31/05
G0230   Deleted 3/31/05
G0231   Deleted 3/31/05
G0232   Deleted 3/31/05
G0233   Deleted 3/31/05
G0234   Deleted 3/31/05
▶◆ G0235   Pet imaging, any site, not otherwise specified
      CIM 50-36
✱ G0237   Therapeutic procedures to increase strength or endurance of respiratory muscles, face to face, one on one, each 15 minutes (includes monitoring)
✱ G0238   Therapeutic procedures to improve respiratory function, other than described by G0237, one on one, face to face, per 15 minutes (includes monitoring)
✱ G0239   Therapeutic procedures to improve respiratory function or increase strength or endurance of respiratory muscles, two or more individuals (includes monitoring)
G0242   Deleted 12/31/05
⊛ G0243   Multi-source photon stereotactic radiosurgery, delivery including collimator changes and custom plugging, complete course of treatment, all lesions
G0244   Deleted 12/31/05

LOSS OF PROTECTIVE SENSATION (LOPS)

⊛ G0245   Initial physician evaluation of a diabetic patient with diabetic sensory neuropathy resulting in a loss of protective sensation (LOPS) which must include (1) the diagnosis of LOPS; (2) a patient history; (3) a physical examination that consist of *at least* the following elements:
     a. Visual inspection of the forefoot, hindfoot and toeweb spaces
     b. Evaluation of a protective sensation

     c. Evaluation of foot structure and biomechanics
     d. Evaluation of vascular status and skin integrity
     e. Evaluation and recommendation of footwear
    4. Patient education
     CIM 50-81
⊛ G0246   Follow-up physician evaluation and management of a diabetic patient with diabetic sensory neuropathy resulting in a loss of protective sensation (LOPS) to include at least the following, (1) a patient history (2) a physical examination that includes:
     a. Visual inspection of the forefoot, hindfoot and toe web spaces
     b. Evaluation of protective sensation
     c. Evaluation of foot structure and biomechanics
     d. Evaluation of vascular status and skin integrity
     e. Evaluation and recommendation of footwear
    3. Patient education
⊛ G0247   Routine foot care by a physician of a diabetic patient with diabetic sensory neuropathy resulting in a loss of protective sensation (LOPS) to include the local care of superficial wounds (i.e. superficial to muscle and fascia) and at least the following if present: (1) local care of superficial wounds, (2) debridement of corns and calluses, and (3) trimming and debridement of nails
     CIM 50-81

"G" Codes for International Normalized Ratio Monitoring

Codes established for CIM 50.55 effective for services furnished on or after July 1, 2002. Use of the International Normalized Ratio (INR) allows physician to determine the level of anti-coagulation in a patient independent of the laboratory reagents used. Home prothrombin monitoring with the use of INR devices is only covered for patients with mechanical heart valves.

CIM reference 50-36 details coverage indications. FDG Positron Emission Tomography is a minimally invasive diagnostic procedure using positron camera (tomograph) to measure the decay of radioisotopes such as FDG, CMS determined that the benefit category for the requested indications fell under 1861(s)(3) of the Social Security Act diagnostic service.

⚙ G0248   Demonstration, at initial use, of home INR monitoring for patient with mechanical heart valve(s) who meets Medicare coverage criteria, under the direction of a physician; includes: demonstrating use and care of the INR monitor, obtaining at least one blood sample, provision of instructions for reporting home INR test results, and documentation of patient ability to perform testing.
CIM 50-55

⚙ G0249   Provision of test materials and equipment for home INR monitoring to patient with mechanical heart valve(s) who meets Medicare coverage criteria; includes provision of materials for use in the home and reporting of test results to physician; per 4 tests.
CIM 50-55

⚙ G0250   Physician review, interpretation and patient management of home INR testing for a patient with mechanical heart valve(s) who meets other coverage criteria; per 4 tests (does not require face-to-face service)
CIM 50-55

⚙ G0251   Linear accelerator based stereotactic radiosurgery, delivery including collimator changes and custom plugging, fractionated treatment, all lesions, per session, maximum five sessions per course of treatment

  G0252   Deleted 3/31/05
  G0253   Deleted 3/31/05
  G0254   Deleted 3/31/05

◆ G0255   Current perception threshold/sensory nerve conduction test, (SNCT) per limb, any nerve
CIM 50-57

⚙ G0257   Unscheduled or emergency dialysis treatment for an ESRD patient in a hospital outpatient department that is not certified as an ESRD facility

  G0258   Deleted 12/31/05

⚙ G0259   Injection procedure for sacroiliac joint; arthrography

⚙ G0260   Injection procedure for sacroiliac joint; provision of anesthetic, steroid and/or other therapeutic agent with or without arthrography

  G0263   Deleted 12/31/05
  G0264   Deleted 12/31/05

∗ G0265   Cryopreservation, freezing and storage of cells for therapeutic use, each cell line

∗ G0266   Thawing and expansion of frozen cells for therapeutic use, each aliquot

∗ G0267   Bone marrow or peripheral stem cell harvest, modification or treatment to eliminate cell type(s) (e.g. t-cells, metastatic carcinoma)

∗ G0268   Removal of impacted cerumen (one or both ears) by physician on same date of service as audiologic function testing

⚙ G0269   Placement of occlusive device into either a venous or arterial access site, post surgical or interventional procedure (e.g. angioseal plug, vascular plug)

∗ G0270   Medical nutrition therapy; reassessment and subsequent intervention(s) following second referral in same year for change in diagnosis, medical condition or treatment regimen (including additional hours needed for renal disease), individual, face to face with the patient, each 15 minutes

∗ G0271   Medical nutrition therapy, reassessment and subsequent intervention(s) following second referral in same year for change in diagnosis, medical condition, or treatment regimen (including additional hours needed for renal disease), group (2 or more individuals), each 30 minutes

∗ G0275   Renal artery angiography (unilateral or bilateral) performed at the time of cardiac catheterization, includes catheter placement, injection of dye, flush aortogram and radiologic supervision and interpretation and production of images (list separately in addition to primary procedure)

∗ G0278   Iliac artery angiography performed at the same time of cardiac catheterization, includes catheter placement, injection of dye, radiologic supervision and interpretation and production of images (list separately in addition to primary procedure)

  G0279   Deleted 12/31/05
  G0280   Deleted 12/31/05

∗ G0281   Electrical stimulation, (unattended), to one or more areas, for chronic Stage III and Stage IV pressure ulcers, arterial ulcers, diabetic ulcers, and venous stasis ulcers not demonstrating measurable signs of healing after 30 days of conventional care, as part of a therapy plan of care

∗ G0282   Electrical stimulation, (unattended), to one or more areas, for wound care other than described in G0281
CIM 35-98

∗ G0283   Electrical stimulation (unattended), to one or more areas for indication(s) other than wound care, as part of a therapy plan of care

∗ G0288   Reconstruction, computed tomographic angiography of aorta for surgical planning for vascular surgery

* G0289   Arthroscopy, knee, surgical, for removal of loose body, foreign body, debridement/shaving of articular cartilage (chondroplasty) at the time of other surgical knee arthroscopy in a different compartment of the same knee

⊙ G0290   Transcatheter placement of a drug eluting intracoronary stent(s), percutaneous, with or without other therapeutic intervention, any method; single vessel

⊙ G0291   Transcatheter placement of a drug eluting intracoronary stent(s), percutaneous, with or without other therapeutic intervention, any method; each additional vessel

⊙ G0293   Noncovered surgical procedure(s) using conscious sedation, regional, general or spinal anesthesia in a Medicare qualifying clinical trial, per day

⊙ G0294   Noncovered procedure(s) using either no anesthesia or local anesthesia only, in a Medicare qualifying clinical trial, per day

◆ G0295   Electromagnetic therapy, to one or more areas, for wound care other than described in G0329 or for other uses
CIM 35-98

   G0296   Deleted 3/31/05

* G0297   Insertion of single chamber pacing cardioverter defibrillator pulse generator

* G0298   Insertion of dual chamber pacing cardioverter defibrillator pulse generator

* G0299   Insertion or repositioning of electrode lead for single chamber pacing cardioverter defibrillator and insertion of pulse generator

* G0300   Insertion or repositioning of electrode lead(s) for dual chamber pacing cardioverter defibrillator and insertion of pulse generator

* G0302   Pre-operative pulmonary surgery services for preparation for LVRS, complete course of services, to include a minimum of 16 days of services

* G0303   Pre-operative pulmonary surgery services for preparation for LVRS, 10 to 15 days of services

* G0304   Pre-operative pulmonary surgery services for preparation for LVRS, 1 to 9 days of services

* G0305   Post-discharge pulmonary surgery services after LVRS, minimum of 6 days of services

* G0306   Complete CBC, automated (HgB, HCT, RBC, WBC, without platelet count) and automated WBC differential count
Laboratory Certification 400

* G0307   Complete CBC, automated (HgB, HCT, RBC, WBC; without platelet count)

⊙ G0308   End Stage Renal Disease (ESRD) related services during the course of treatment, for patients under 2 years of age to include monitoring for the adequacy of nutrition, assessment of growth and development, and counseling of parents; with 4 or more face-to-face physician visits per month
MCM 2230

⊙ G0309   End Stage Renal Disease (ESRD) related services during the course of treatment, for patients under 2 years of age to include monitoring for the adequacy of nutrition, assessment of growth and development, and counseling of parents; with 2 or 3 face-to-face physician visits per month
MCM 2230

⊙ G0310   End Stage Renal Disease (ESRD) related services during the course of treatment, for patients under 2 years of age to include monitoring for the adequacy of nutrition, assessment of growth and development, and counseling of parents; with 1 face-to-face physician visit per month
MCM 2230

⊙ G0311   End Stage Renal Disease (ESRD) related services during the course of treatment, for patients between 2 and 11 years of age to include monitoring for the adequacy of nutrition, assessment of growth and development, and counseling of parents; with 4 or more face-to-face physician visits per month
MCM 2230

⊙ G0312   End Stage Renal Disease (ESRD) related services during the course of treatment, for patients between 2 and 11 years of age to include monitoring for the adequacy of nutrition, assessment of growth and development, and counseling of parents; with 2 or 3 face-to-face physician visits per month
MCM 2230

⊙ G0313   End Stage Renal Disease (ESRD) related services during the course of treatment, for patients between 2 and 11 years of age to include monitoring for the adequacy of nutrition, assessment of growth and development, and counseling of parents; with 1 face-to-face physician visits per month
MCM 2230

⊛ G0314 End Stage Renal Disease (ESRD) related services during the course of treatment, for patients between 12 and 19 years of age to include monitoring for the adequacy of nutrition, assessment of growth and development, and counseling of parents; with 4 or more face-to-face physician visits per month
MCM 2230

⊛ G0315 End Stage Renal Disease (ESRD) related services during the course of treatment, for patients between 12 and 19 years of age to include monitoring for the adequacy of nutrition, assessment of growth and development, and counseling of parents; with 2 or 3 face-to-face physician visits per month
MCM 2230

⊛ G0316 End Stage Renal Disease (ESRD) related services during the course of treatment, for patients between 12 and 19 years of age to include monitoring for the adequacy of nutrition, assessment of growth and development, and counseling of parents; with 1 face-to-face physician visits per month
MCM 2230

⊛ G0317 End Stage Renal Disease (ESRD) related services during the course of treatment, for patients 20 years of age and over; with 4 or more face-to-face physician visits per month
MCM 2230

⊛ G0318 End Stage Renal Disease (ESRD) related services during the course of treatment, for patients 20 years of age and over; with 2 or 3 face-to-face physician visits per month
MCM 2230

⊛ G0319 End Stage Renal Disease (ESRD) related services during the course of treatment, for patients 20 years of age and over; with 1 face-to-face physician visit per month
MCM 2230

⊛ G0320 End stage renal disease (ESRD) related services for home dialysis patients per full month; for patients under two years of age to include monitoring for adequacy of nutrition, assessment of growth and development, and counseling of parents
MCM 2230

⊛ G0321 End stage renal disease (ESRD) related services for home dialysis patients per full month; for patients two to eleven years of age to include monitoring for adequacy of nutrition, assessment of growth and development, and counseling of parents
MCM 2230

⊛ G0322 End stage renal disease (ESRD) related services for home dialysis patients per full month; for patients twelve to nineteen years of age to include monitoring for adequacy of nutrition, assessment of growth and development, and counseling of parents
MCM 2230

⊛ G0323 End stage renal disease (ESRD) related services for home dialysis patients per full month; for patients twenty years of age and older
MCM 2230

⊛ G0324 End stage renal disease (ESRD) related services for home dialysis (less than full month), per day; for patients under two years of age
MCM 2230

⊛ G0325 End stage renal disease (ESRD) related services for home dialysis (less than full month), per day; for patients between two and eleven years of age
MCM 2230

⊛ G0326 End stage renal disease (ESRD) related services for home dialysis (less than full month), per day; for patients between twelve and nineteen years of age
MCM 2230

⊛ G0327 End stage renal disease (ESRD) related services for home dialysis (less than full month), per day; for patients twenty years of age and over
MCM 2230

⊛ G0328 Colorectal cancer screening; fecal occult blood test, immunoassay, 1-3 simultaneous
Laboratory Certification 310, 400

✱ G0329 Electromagnetic therapy, to one or more areas for chronic stage III and stage not demonstrating measurable signs of healing after 30 days of conventional care as part of a therapy plan of care

G0330 PET imaging, initial diagnosis cervical
Added to Outpatient Hospital Fee Schedule, April 1, 2005

G0331 PET imaging restage ovarian cancer
Added to Outpatient Hospital Fee Schedule, April 1, 2005

G0336 Deleted 3/31/05

✱ G0337 Hospice evaluation and counseling services, pre-election

G0338 Deleted 12/31/05

✱ G0339 Image-guided robotic linear accelerator-based stereotactic radiosurgery, complete course of therapy in one session or first session or fractionated treatment

* G0340   Image-guided robotic linear accelerator-based stereotactic radiosurgery, delivery including collimator changes and custom plugging, fractionated treatment, all lesions, per session, second through fifth sessions, maximum five sessions per course of treatment

☺ G0341   Percutaneous islet cell transplant; includes portal vein catheterization and infusion
260.3 CIM 35-82

☺ G0342   Laparoscopy for islet cell transplant; includes portal vein catheterization and infusion
CIM 35-82

☺ G0343   Laparotomy for islet cell transplant; includes portal vein catheterization and infusion
CIM 35-82

* G0344   Initial preventive physical examination; face-to-face visit, services limited to new beneficiary during the first six months of Medicare enrollment

G0345   Deleted 12/31/05
G0346   Deleted 12/31/05
G0347   Deleted 12/31/05
G0348   Deleted 12/31/05
G0349   Deleted 12/31/05
G0350   Deleted 12/31/05
G0351   Deleted 12/31/05
G0353   Deleted 12/31/05
G0354   Deleted 12/31/05
G0355   Deleted 12/31/05
G0356   Deleted 12/31/05
G0357   Deleted 12/31/05
G0358   Deleted 12/31/05
G0359   Deleted 12/31/05
G0360   Deleted 12/31/05
G0361   Deleted 12/31/05
G0362   Deleted 12/31/05
G0363   Deleted 12/31/05

* G0364   Bone marrow aspiration performed with bone marrow biopsy through the same incision on the same date of service

* G0365   Vessel mapping of vessels for hemodialysis access (services for pre-operative vessel mapping prior to creation of hemodialysis access using an autogenous hemodialysis conduit, including arterial inflow and venous outflow)

* G0366   Electrocardiogram, routine ECG with at least 12 leads; performed as a component of the initial preventive physical examination with interpretation and report

* G0367   Tracing only, without interpretation and report; performed as a component of the initial preventive physical examination

* G0368   Interpretation and report only; performed as a component of the initial preventive physical examination

G0369   Deleted 12/31/05
G0370   Deleted 12/31/05
G0371   Deleted 12/31/05

▶ ☺ G0372   Physician service required to establish and document the need for a power mobility device (use in addition to primary evaluation and management code)

G0374   Deleted 12/31/05

▶ * G0375   Smoking and tobacco use cessation counseling visit; intermediate, greater than 3 minutes up to 10 minutes

▶ * G0376   Smoking and tobacco use cessation counseling visit; intensive, greater than 10 minutes

▶ ☺ G0378   Hospital observation service, per hour

▶ ☺ G0379   Direct admission of patient for hospital observation care

* G3001   Administration and supply of tositumomab, 450 mg

☺ G9001   Coordination fee, initial rate

☺ G9002   Coordinated care fee, maintenance rate

☺ G9003   Coordinated care fee, risk adjusted high, initial

☺ G9004   Coordinated care fee, risk adjusted low, initial

☺ G9005   Coordinated care fee, risk adjusted maintenance

☺ G9006   Coordinated care fee, home monitoring

☺ G9007   Coordinated care fee, scheduled team conference

☺ G9008   Coordinated care fee, physician coordinated care oversight services

☺ G9009   Coordination care fee, risk adjustment maintenance, level 3

☺ G9010   Coordination care fee, risk adjustment maintenance, level 4

☺ G9011   Coordination care fee, risk adjustment maintenance, level 5

☺ G9012   Other specified care management services not elsewhere classified

◆ G9013   ESRD demo basic bundle Level I

◆ G9014   ESRD demo expanded bundle, including venous access and related services

◆ G9016   Smoking cessation counseling, individual, in the absence of or in addition to any other evaluation and management service, per session (6-10 minutes) (demo project code only)

* G9017   Amantadine hydrochloride, oral, per 100 mg (for use as a Medicare-approved demonstration project)

* G9018   Zanamivir, inhalation powder, administered through inhaler, per 10 mg (for use as a Medicare-approved demonstration project)

* G9019   Oseltamivir phosphate, oral, per 75 mg (for use as a Medicare-approved demonstration project)

* G9020   Rimantadine hydrochloride, oral, per 100 mg (for use as a Medicare-approved demonstration project)

* G9021   Chemotherapy assessment for nausea and/or vomiting, patient reported, performed at the time of chemotherapy administration; assessment level one: not at all (for use in a Medicare-approved demonstration project)

* G9022   Chemotherapy assessment for nausea and/or vomiting, patient reported, performed at the time of chemotherapy administration; assessment level two: a little (for use in a Medicare-approved demonstration project)

* G9023   Chemotherapy assessment for nausea and/or vomiting, patient reported, performed at the time of chemotherapy administration; assessment level three: quite a bit (for use in a Medicare-approved demonstration project)

* G9024   Chemotherapy assessment for nausea and/or vomiting, patient reported, performed at the time of chemotherapy administration; assessment level four: very much (for use in a Medicare-approved demonstration project)

* G9025   Chemotherapy assessment for pain, patient reported, performed at the time of chemotherapy administration; assessment level one: not at all (for use in a Medicare-approved demonstration project)

* G9026   Chemotherapy assessment for pain, patient reported, performed at the time of chemotherapy administration; assessment level two: a little (for use in a Medicare-approved demonstration project)

* G9027   Chemotherapy assessment for pain, patient reported, performed at the time of chemotherapy administration; assessment level three: quite a bit (for use in a Medicare-approved demonstration project)

* G9028   Chemotherapy assessment for pain, patient reported, performed at the time of chemotherapy administration; assessment level four: very much (for use in a Medicare-approved demonstration project)

* G9029   Chemotherapy assessment for lack of energy (fatigue), patient reported, performed at the time of chemotherapy administration; assessment level one: not at all (for use in a Medicare-approved demonstration project)

* G9030   Chemotherapy assessment for lack of energy (fatigue), patient reported, performed at the time of chemotherapy administration; assessment level two: a little (for use in a Medicare-approved demonstration project)

* G9031   Chemotherapy assessment for lack of energy (fatigue), patient reported, performed at the time of chemotherapy administration; assessment level three: quite a bit (for use in a Medicare-approved demonstration project)

* G9032   Chemotherapy assessment for lack of energy (fatigue), patient reported, performed at the time of chemotherapy administration; assessment level four: very much (for use in a Medicare-approved demonstration project)

▶ * G9033   Amantadine hydrochloride, oral brand, per 100 mg (for use in a Medicare-approved demonstration project)

* G9034   Zanamivir, inhalation powder, administered through inhaler, brand, per 10 mg (for use in a Medicare-approved demonstration project)

* G9035   Oseltamivir phosphate, oral, brand, per 75 mg (for use in a Medicare-approved demonstration project)

* G9036   Rimantadine hydrochloride, oral, brand, per 100 mg (for use in a Medicare-approved demonstration project)

▶ * G9041   Sensory integrative techniques to enhance sensory processing and promote adaptive responses to environmental demands, self care/home management training (e.g. activities of daily living (ADL) and compensatory training, meal preparation, safety procedures, and instructions in use of assistive technology devices/adaptive equipment), community/work reintegration training (e.g. shopping, transportation, money management, avocational activities and/or work environment modification analysis, work task analysis), direct one-on-one contact by the provider, each 15 minutes

▶ * G9042   Sensory integrative techniques to enhance sensory processing and promote adaptive responses to environmental demands, self care/home management training (e.g. activities of daily living (ADL) and compensatory training, meal preparation, safety procedures, and instructions in use of assistive technology devices/adaptive equipment), community/work reintegration training (e.g. shopping, transportation, money management, avocational activities and/or work environment modification analysis, work task analysis), direct one-on-one contact by the provider, each 15 minutes

▶ ✳ G9043 Sensory integrative techniques to enhance sensory processing and promote adaptive responses to environmental demands, self care/home management training (e.g. activities of daily living (ADL) and compensatory training, meal preparation, safety procedures, and instructions in use of assistive technology devices/adaptive equipment), community/work reintegration training (e.g. shopping, transportation, money management, avocational activities and/or work environment modification analysis, work task analysis), direct one-on-one contact by the provider, each 15 minutes

▶ ✳ G9044 Sensory integrative techniques to enhance sensory processing and promote adaptive responses to environmental demands, self care/home management training (e.g. activities of daily living (ADL) and compensatory training, meal preparation, safety procedures, and instructions in use of assistive technology devices/adaptive equipment), community/work reintegration training (e.g. shopping, transportation, money management, avocational activities and/or work environment modification analysis, work task analysis), direct one-on-one contact by the provider, each 15 minutes

ALCOHOL AND/OR DRUG SERVICES (H0001-H1005)

◆ H0001 Alcohol and/or drug assessment
◆ H0002 Behavioral health screening to determine eligibility for admission to treatment program
◆ H0003 Alcohol and/or drug screening; laboratory analysis of specimens for presence of alcohol and/or drugs
◆ H0004 Behavioral health counseling and therapy, per 15 minutes
◆ H0005 Alcohol and/or drug services; group counseling by a clinician
◆ H0006 Alcohol and/or drug services; case management
◆ H0007 Alcohol and/or drug services; crisis intervention (outpatient)
◆ H0008 Alcohol and/or drug services; sub-acute detoxification (hospital inpatient)
◆ H0009 Alcohol and/or drug services; acute detoxification (hospital inpatient)
◆ H0010 Alcohol and/or drug services; sub-acute detoxification (residential addiction program inpatient)

◆ H0011 Alcohol and/or drug services; acute detoxification (residential addiction program inpatient)
◆ H0012 Alcohol and/or drug services; sub-acute detoxification (residential addiction program outpatient)
◆ H0013 Alcohol and/or drug services; acute detoxification (residential addiction program outpatient)
◆ H0014 Alcohol and/or drug services; ambulatory detoxification
◆ H0015 Alcohol and/or drug services; intensive outpatient (treatment program that operates at least 3 hours per day and at least 3 days per week and is based on an individualized treatment plan), including assessment, counseling; crisis intervention, and activity therapies or education
◆ H0016 Alcohol and/or drug services; medical/somatic (medical intervention in ambulatory setting)
◆ H0017 Behavioral health; residential (hospital residential treatment program), without room and board, per diem
◆ H0018 Behavioral health; short-term residential (non-hospital residential treatment program), without room and board, per diem
◆ H0019 Behavioral health; long-term residential (non-medial, non-acute care in a residential treatment program where stay is typically longer than 30 days), without room and board, per diem
◆ H0020 Alcohol and/or drug services; methadone administration and/or service (provision of the drug by a licensed program)
◆ H0021 Alcohol and/or drug training service (for staff and personnel not employed by providers)
◆ H0022 Alcohol and/or drug intervention service (planned facilitation)
◆ H0023 Behavioral health outreach service (planned approach to reach a target population)
◆ H0024 Behavioral health prevention information dissemination service (one-way direct or non-direct contact with service audiences to affect knowledge or attitude)
◆ H0025 Behavioral health prevention education service (delivery of services with target population to affect knowledge, attitude, and/or behavior)
◆ H0026 Alcohol and/or drug prevention process service, community-based (delivery of services to develop skills of impactors)

◆ H0027 Alcohol and/or drug prevention environmental service (broad range of external activities geared toward modifying systems in order to mainstream prevention through policy and law)

◆ H0028 Alcohol and/or drug prevention problem identification and referral service (e.g., student assistance and employee assistance programs), does not include assessment

◆ H0029 Alcohol and/or drug prevention alternatives service (services for populations that exclude alcohol and other drug use [e.g., alcohol-free social events])

◆ H0030 Behavioral health hotline service

◆ H0031 Mental health assessment, by non-physician

◆ H0032 Mental health service plan development by non-physician

◆ H0033 Oral medication administration, direct observation

◆ H0034 Medication training and support, per 15 minutes

◆ H0035 Mental health partial hospitalization, treatment, less than 24 hours

◆ H0036 Community psychiatric supportive treatment, face-to-face, per 15 minutes

◆ H0037 Community psychiatric supportive treatment program, per diem

◆ H0038 Self-help/peer services, per 15 minutes

◆ H0039 Assertive community treatment, face-to-face, per 15 minutes

◆ H0040 Assertive community treatment program, per diem

◆ H0041 Foster care, child, non-therapeutic, per diem

◆ H0042 Foster care, child, non-therapeutic, per month?

◆ H0043 Supported housing, per diem

◆ H0044 Supported housing, per month

◆ H0045 Respite care services, not in the home, per diem

◆ H0046 Mental health services, not otherwise specified

◆ H0047 Alcohol and/or other drug abuse services, not otherwise specified

◆ H0048 Alcohol and/or other drug testing: collection and handling only, specimens other than blood

◆ H1000 Prenatal care, at-risk assessment

◆ H1001 Prenatal care, at-risk enhanced service; antepartum management

◆ H1002 Prenatal care, at-risk enhanced service; care coordination

◆ H1003 Prenatal care, at-risk enhanced service; education

◆ H1004 Prenatal care, at-risk enhanced service; follow-up home visit

◆ H1005 Prenatal care, at-risk enhanced service package (includes H1001-H1004)

◆ H1010 Non-medical family planning education, per session

◆ H1011 Family assessment by licensed behavioral health professional for state defined purposes

◆ H2000 Comprehensive multidisciplinary evaluation

◆ H2001 Rehabilitation program, per 1/2 day

◆ H2010 Comprehensive medication services, per 15 minutes

◆ H2011 Crisis intervention service, per 15 minutes

◆ H2012 Behavioral health day treatment, per hour

◆ H2013 Psychiatric health facility service, per diem

◆ H2014 Skills training and development, per 15 minutes

◆ H2015 Comprehensive community support services, per 15 minutes

◆ H2016 Comprehensive community support services, per diem

◆ H2017 Psychosocial rehabilitation services, per 15 minutes

◆ H2018 Psychosocial rehabilitation services, per diem

◆ H2019 Therapeutic behavioral services, per 15 minutes

◆ H2020 Therapeutic behavioral services, per diem

◆ H2021 Community-based wrap-around services, per 15 minutes

◆ H2022 Community-based wrap-around services, per diem

◆ H2023 Supported employment, per 15 minutes

◆ H2024 Supported employment, per diem

◆ H2025 Ongoing support to maintain employment, per 15 minutes

◆ H2026 Ongoing support to maintain employment, per diem

◆ H2027 Psychoeducational service, per 15 minutes

◆ H2028 Sexual offender treatment service, per 15 minutes

◆ H2029 Sexual offender treatment service, per diem

◆ H2030 Mental health clubhouse services, per 15 minutes

◆ H2031 Mental health clubhouse services, per diem

◆ H2032 Activity therapy, per 15 minutes

◆ H2033 Multisystemic therapy for juveniles, per 15 minutes

◆ H2034 Alcohol and/or drug abuse halfway house services, per diem

◆ H2035 Alcohol and/or other drug treatment program, per hour

◆ H2036 Alcohol and/or other drug treatment program, per diem

◆ H2037   Developmental delay prevention activities, dependent child of client, per 15 minutes

DRUGS OTHER THAN CHEMOTHERAPY (J0100-J8999)

✪ J0120   Injection, tetracycline, up to 250 mg
           MCM 2049

✳ J0128   Injection, abarelix, 10 mg
           MCM 2049

✪ J0130   Injection abciximab, 10 mg
           MCM 2049

▶ ✳ J0132 Injection, acetylcysteine, 100 mg

▶ ✳ J0133 Injection, acyclovir, 5 mg

✳ J0135   Injection, adalimumab, 20 mg
           MCM 2049

✪ J0150   Injection, adenosine, for therapeutic use, 6 mg (not to be used to report any adenosine phosphate compounds; instead use A9270)
           MCM 2049

✳ J0152   Injection, adenosine, for diagnostic use, 30 mg (not to be used to report any adenosine phosphate compounds; instead use A9270)

✪ J0170   Injection, adrenalin, epinephrine, up to 1 ml ampule
           MCM 2049

✳ J0180   Injection, agalsidase beta, 1 mg
           MCM 2049

✪ J0190   Injection, biperiden lactate, per 5 mg
           MCM 2049

✪ J0200   Injection, alatrofloxacin mesylate, 100 mg
           MCM 2049.5

✪ J0205   Injection, alglucerase, per 10 units
           MCM 2049

✪ J0207   Injection, amifostine, 500 mg
           MCM 2049

✪ J0210   Injection, methyldopate HCl, up to 250 mg
           MCM 2049

✳ J0215   Injection, alefacept, 0.5 mg

✪ J0256   Injection, alpha-1-proteinase inhibitor (human), 10 mg
           MCM 2049

✪ J0270   Injection, alprostadil, per 1.25 mcg (Code may be used for Medicare when drug administered under the direct supervision of a physician, not for use when drug is self-administered.)
           MCM 2049

✪ J0275   Alprostadil urethral suppository (Code may be used for Medicare when drug administered under the direct supervision of a physician, not for use when drug is self-administered.)
           MCM 2049

▶ ✳ J0278 Injection, amikacin sulfate, 100 mg

✪ J0280   Injection, aminophylline, up to 250 mg
           MCM 2049

✪ J0282   Injection, amiodarone HCl, 30 mg
           MCM 2049

✪ J0285   Injection, amphotericin B, 50 mg
           MCM 2049

✪ J0287   Injection, amphotericin B lipid complex, 10 mg
           MCM 2049

✪ J0288   Injection, amphotericin B cholesteryl sulfate complex, 10 mg
           MCM 2049

✪ J0289   Injection, amphotericin B liposome, 10 mg
           MCM 2049

✪ J0290   Injection, ampicillin sodium, 500 mg
           MCM 2049

✪ J0295   Injection, ampicillin sodium/sulbactam sodium, per 1.5 gm
           MCM 2049

✪ J0300   Injection, amobarbital, up to 125 mg
           MCM 2049

✪ J0330   Injection, succinylcholine chloride, up to 20 mg
           MCM 2049

✪ J0350   Injection, anistreplase, per 30 units
           MCM 2049

✪ J0360   Injection, hydralazine HCl, up to 20 mg
           MCM 2049

▶ ✪ J0365 Injection, aprotonin, 10,000 KIU
           MCM 2049

✪ J0380   Injection, metaraminol bitartrate, per 10 mg
           MCM 2049

✪ J0390   Injection, chloroquine HCl, up to 250 mg
           MCM 2049

✪ J0395   Injection, arbutamine HCl, 1 mg
           MCM 2049

✪ J0456   Injection, azithromycin, 500 mg
           MCM 2049.5

✪ J0460   Injection, atropine sulfate, up to 0.3 mg
           MCM 2049

✪ J0470   Injection, dimercaprol, per 100 mg
           MCM 2049

✪ J0475   Injection, baclofen, 10 mg
           MCM 2049

✪ J0476   Injection, baclofen 50 mcg for intrathecal trial
           MCM 2049

▶ ✪ J0480 Injection, basiliximab, 20 mg
           MCM 2049

✪ J0500   Injection, dicyclomine HCl, up to 20 mg
           MCM 2049

✪ J0515   Injection, benztropine mesylate, per 1 mg
           MCM 2049

✪ J0520   Injection, bethanechol chloride, myotonachol or urecholine, up to 5 mg
           MCM 2049

⊛ J0530 Injection, penicillin G benzathine and penicillin G procaine, up to 600,000 units
MCM 2049

⊛ J0540 Injection, penicillin G benzathine and penicillin G procaine, up to 1,200,000 units
MCM 2049

⊛ J0550 Injection, penicillin G benzathine and penicillin G procaine, up to 2,400,000 units
MCM 2049

⊛ J0560 Injection, penicillin G benzathine, up to 600,000 units
MCM 2049

⊛ J0570 Injection, penicillin G benzathine, up to 1,200,000 units
MCM 2049

⊛ J0580 Injection, penicillin G benzathine, up to 2,400,000 units
MCM 2049

∗ J0583 Injection, bivalirudin, 1 mg

⊛ J0585 Botulinum toxin type A, per unit
MCM 2049

⊛ J0587 Botulinum toxin type B, per 100 units

⊛ J0592 Injection, buprenorphine hydrochloride, 0.1 mg
MCM 2049

∗ J0595 Injection, butorphanol tartrate, 1 mg

⊛ J0600 Injection, edetate calcium disodium, up to 1000 mg
MCM 2049

⊛ J0610 Injection, calcium gluconate, per 10 ml
MCM 2049

⊛ J0620 Injection, calcium glycerophosphate and calcium lactate, per 10 ml
MCM 2049

⊛ J0630 Injection, calcitonin (salmon), up to 400 units
MCM 2049

⊛ J0636 Injection, calcitriol, 0.1 mcg
MCM 2049

∗ J0637 Injection, caspofungin acetate, 5 mg

⊛ J0640 Injection, leucovorin calcium, per 50 mg
MCM 2049

⊛ J0670 Injection, mepivacaine HCl, per 10 ml
MCM 2049

⊛ J0690 Injection, cefezolin sodium, 500 mg
MCM 2049

∗ J0692 Injection, cefepime HCl, 500 mg

⊛ J0694 Injection, cefoxitin sodium, 1 gm
MCM 2049, Cross Reference Q0090

⊛ J0696 Injection, ceftriaxone sodium, per 250 mg
MCM 2049

⊛ J0697 Injection, sterile cefuroxime sodium, per 750 mg
MCM 2049

⊛ J0698 Injection, cefotaxime sodium, per gm
MCM 2049

⊛ J0702 Injection, betamethasone acetate and betamethasone sodium phosphate, per 3 mg
MCM 2049

⊛ J0704 Injection, betamethasone sodium phosphate, per 4 mg
MCM 2049

∗ J0706 Injection, caffeine citrate, 5 mg

⊛ J0710 Injection, cephapirin sodium, up to 1 gm
MCM 2049

⊛ J0713 Injection, ceftazidime, per 500 mg
MCM 2049

⊛ J0715 Injection, ceftizoxime sodium, per 500 mg
MCM 2049

⊛ J0720 Injection, chloramphenicol sodium succinate, up to 1 gm
MCM 2049

⊛ J0725 Injection, chorionic gonadotropin, per 1,000 USP units
MCM 2049

⊛ J0735 Injection, clonidine HCl, 1 mg
MCM 2049

⊛ J0740 Injection, cidofovir, 375 mg
MCM 2049

⊛ J0743 Injection, cilastatin sodium; imipenem, per 250 mg
MCM 2049

∗ J0744 Injection, ciprofloxacin for IV infusion, 200 mg

⊛ J0745 Injection, codeine phosphate, per 30 mg
MCM 2049

⊛ J0760 Injection, colchicine, per 1 mg
MCM 2049

⊛ J0770 Injection, colistimethate sodium, up to 150 mg
MCM 2049

⊛ J0780 Injection, prochlorperazine, up to 10 mg
MCM 2049

▶⊛ J0795 Injection, corticorelin ovine triflutate, 1 μg
MCM 2049

⊛ J0800 Injection, corticotropin, up to 40 units
MCM 2049

⊛ J0835 Injection, cosyntropin, per 0.25 mg
MCM 2049

⊛ J0850 Injection, cytomegalovirus immune globulin IV (human), per vial
MCM 2049

∗ J0878 Injection, daptomycin, 1 mg

J0880 Deleted 12/31/05

▶⊛ J0881 Injection, darbepoetin alfa, 1 μg (non-ESRD use)
MCM 4273.1

▶⊛ J0882 Injection, darbepoetin alfa, 1 μg (for ESRD on dialysis)
MCM 4273.1

▶ ⊗ J0885   Injection, epoetin alfa, (for non-ESRD use), 1000 units
MCM 2049

▶ ⊗ J0886   Injection, epoetin alfa, 1000 units (for ESRD on dialysis)
MCM 4273.1

⊗ J0895   Injection, deferoxamine mesylate, 500 mg
MCM 2049, Cross Reference Q0087

⊗ J0900   Injection, testosterone enanthate and estradiol valerate, up to 1 cc
MCM 2049

⊗ J0945   Injection, brompheniramine maleate, per 10 mg
MCM 2049

⊗ J0970   Injection, estradiol valerate, up to 40 mg
MCM 2049

⊗ J1000   Injection, depo-estradiol cypionate, up to 5 mg
MCM 2049

⊗ J1020   Injection, methylprednisolone acetate, 20 mg
MCM 2049

⊗ J1030   Injection, methylprednisolone acetate, 40 mg
MCM 2049

⊗ J1040   Injection, methylprednisolone acetate, 80 mg
MCM 2049

J1050   Deleted 12/31/02

⊗ J1051   Injection, medroxyprogesterone acetate, 50 mg
MCM 2049

◆ J1055   Injection, medroxyprogesterone acetate for contraceptive use, 150 mg
Medicare Statute 1862A1

✳ J1056   Injection, medroxyprogesterone acetate/estradiol cypionate, 5 mg/ 25 mg

⊗ J1060   Injection, testosterone cypionate and estradiol cypionate, up to 1 ml
MCM 2049

⊗ J1070   Injection, testosterone cypionate, up to 100 mg
MCM 2049

⊗ J1080   Injection, testosterone cypionate, 1 cc, 200 mg
MCM 2049

⊗ J1094   Injection, dexamethasone acetate, 1 mg
MCM 2049

⊗ J1100   Injection, dexamethasone sodium phosphate, 1 mg
MCM 2049

⊗ J1110   Injection, dihydroergotamine mesylate, per 1 mg
MCM 2049

⊗ J1120   Injection, acetazolamide sodium, up to 500 mg
MCM 2049

⊗ J1160   Injection, digoxin, up to 0.5 mg
MCM 2049

▶ ⊗ J1162   Injection, digoxin immune Fab (ovine), per vial
MCM 2049

⊗ J1165   Injection, phenytoin sodium, per 50 mg
MCM 2049

⊗ J1170   Injection, hydromorphone, up to 4 mg
MCM 2049

⊗ J1180   Injection, dyphylline, up to 500 mg
MCM 2049

⊗ J1190   Injection, dexrazoxane HCl, per 250 mg
MCM 2049

⊗ J1200   Injection, diphenhydramine HCl, up to 50 mg
MCM 2049

⊗ J1205   Injection, chlorothiazide sodium, per 500 mg
MCM 2049

⊗ J1212   Injection, dimethyl sulfoxide, DMSO, 50%, 50 ml
MCM 2049, CIM 45-23

⊗ J1230   Injection, methadone HCl, up to 10 mg
MCM 2049

⊗ J1240   Injection, dimenhydrinate, up to 50 mg
MCM 2049

⊗ J1245   Injection, dipyridamole, per 10 mg
MCM 2049, MCM 15030

⊗ J1250   Injection, dobutamine HCl, per 250 mg
MCM 2049

⊗ J1260   Injection, dolasetron mesylate, 10 mg
MCM 2049

▶ ✳ J1265   Injection, dopamine HCL, 40 mg

✳ J1270   Injection, doxercalciferol, 1 mcg

⊗ J1320   Injection, amitriptyline HCl, up to 20 mg
MCM 2049

⊗ J1325   Injection, epoprostenol, 0.5 mg
MCM 2049

⊗ J1327   Injection, eptifibatide, 5 mg
MCM 2049

⊗ J1330   Injection, ergonovine maleate, up to 0.2 mg
MCM 2049

✳ J1335   Injection, ertapenem sodium, 500 mg

⊗ J1364   Injection, erythromycin lactobionate, per 500 mg
MCM 2049

⊗ J1380   Injection, estradiol valerate, up to 10 mg
MCM 2049

⊗ J1390   Injection, estradiol valerate, up to 20 mg
MCM 2049

⊗ J1410   Injection, estrogen conjugated, per 25 mg
MCM 2049

▶ ⊗ J1430   Injection, ethanolamine oleate, 100 mg
MCM 2049

⊗ J1435   Injection, estrone, per 1 mg
MCM 2049

⊗ J1436   Injection, etidronate disodium, per 300 mg
MCM 2049

⊙ J1438 Injection, etanercept, 25 mg (Code may be used for Medicare when drug administered under the direct supervision of a physician, not for use when drug is self-administered.)

⊙ J1440 Injection, filgrastim (G-CSF), 300 mcg
MCM 2049

⊙ J1441 Injection, filgrastim (G-CSF), 480 mcg
MCM 2049

⊙ J1450 Injection, fluconazole, 200 mg
MCM 2049.5

▶⊙ J1451 Injection, fomepizole, 15 mg
MCM 2049

⊙ J1452 Injection, fomivirsen sodium, intraocular, 1.65 mg
MCM 2049.3

⊙ J1455 Injection, foscarnet sodium, per 1000 mg
MCM 2049

∗ J1457 Injection, gallium nitrate, 1 mg

⊙ J1460 Injection, gamma globulin, intramuscular, 1 cc
MCM 2049

⊙ J1470 Injection, gamma globulin, intramuscular, 2 cc
MCM 2049

⊙ J1480 Injection, gamma globulin, intramuscular, 3 cc
MCM 2049

⊙ J1490 Injection, gamma globulin, intramuscular, 4 cc
MCM 2049

⊙ J1500 Injection, gamma globulin, intramuscular, 5 cc
MCM 2049

⊙ J1510 Injection, gamma globulin, intramuscular, 6 cc
MCM 2049

⊙ J1520 Injection, gamma globulin, intramuscular, 7 cc
MCM 2049

⊙ J1530 Injection, gamma globulin, intramuscular, 8 cc
MCM 2049

⊙ J1540 Injection, gamma globulin, intramuscular, 9 cc
MCM 2049

⊙ J1550 Injection, gamma globulin, intramuscular, 10 cc
MCM 2049

⊙ J1560 Injection, gamma globulin, intramuscular, over 10 cc
MCM 2049

J1563 Deleted 12/31/05
J1564 Deleted 12/31/05

⊙ J1565 Injection, respiratory syncytial virus immune globulin, IV, 50 mg
MCM 2049

▶⊙ J1566 Injection, immune globulin, intravenous, lyophilized (e.g. powder), 500 mg
MCM 2049

▶⊙ J1567 Injection, immune globulin, intravenous, non-lyophilized (e.g. liquid), 500 mg
MCM 2049

⊙ J1570 Injection, ganciclovir sodium, 500 mg
MCM 2049

⊙ J1580 Injection, Garamycin, gentamicin, up to 80 mg
MCM 2049

∗ J1590 Injection, gatifloxacin, 10 mg

⊙ J1595 Injection, glatiramer acetate, 20 mg
MCM 2049

⊙ J1600 Injection, gold sodium thiomalate, up to 50 mg
MCM 2049

⊙ J1610 Injection, glucagon HCl, per 1 mg
MCM 2049

⊙ J1620 Injection, gonadorelin HCl, per 100 mcg
MCM 2049

⊙ J1626 Injection, granisetron HCl, 100 mcg
MCM 2049

⊙ J1630 Injection, haloperidol, up to 5 mg
MCM 2049

⊙ J1631 Injection, haloperidol decanoate, per 50 mg
MCM 2049

▶⊙ J1640 Injection, hemin, 1 mg
MCM 2049

⊙ J1642 Injection, heparin sodium, (heparin lock flush), per 10 units
MCM 2049

⊙ J1644 Injection, heparin sodium, per 1000 units
MCM 2049

⊙ J1645 Injection, dalteparin sodium, per 2500 IU
MCM 2049

∗ J1650 Injection, enoxaparin sodium, 10 mg

⊙ J1652 Injection, fondaparinux sodium, 0.5 mg
MCM 2049

∗ J1655 Injection, tinzaparin sodium 1000 IU

⊙ J1670 Injection, tetanus immune globulin (human), up to 250 units
MCM 2049

▶⊙ J1675 Injection, histrelin acetate, 10 μg
MCM 2049

⊙ J1700 Injection, hydrocortisone acetate, up to 25 mg
MCM 2049

⊙ J1710 Injection, hydrocortisone sodium phosphate, up to 50 mg
MCM 2049

⊙ J1720 Injection, hydrocortisone sodium succinate, up to 100 mg
MCM 2049

⊙ J1730 Injection, diazoxide, up to 300 mg
MCM 2049

⊙ J1742 Injection, ibutilide fumarate, 1 mg
MCM 2049

⊙ J1745 Injection, infliximab, 10 mg
MCM 2049

J1750 Deleted 12/31/05

▶ ✿ J1751   Injection, iron dextran 165, 50 mg

▶ ✿ J1752   Injection, iron dextran 267, 50 mg

✳ J1756   Injection, iron sucrose, 1 mg

✿ J1785   Injection, imiglucerase, per unit
MCM 2049

✿ J1790   Injection, droperidol, up to 5 mg
MCM 2049

✿ J1800   Injection, propranolol HCl, up to 1 mg
MCM 2049

✿ J1810   Injection, droperidol and fentanyl citrate, up to 2 ml ampule
MCM 2049

✿ J1815   Injection, insulin, per 5 units
MCM 2049, CIM 60-14

✳ J1817   Insulin for administration through DME (i.e., insulin pump) per 50 units

✿ J1825   Injection, interferon beta-1a, 33 mcg
MCM 2049

✿ J1830   Injection interferon beta-1b, per 0.25 mg (Code may be used for Medicare when drug administered under the direct supervision of a physician, not for use when drug is self-administered.)
MCM 2049

✳ J1835   Injection, itraconazole, 50 mg

✿ J1840   Injection, kanamycin sulfate, up to 500 mg
MCM 2049

✿ J1850   Injection, kanamycin sulfate, up to 75 mg
MCM 2049

✿ J1885   Injection, ketorolac tromethamine, per 15 mg
MCM 2049

✿ J1890   Injection, cephalothin sodium, up to 1 gm
MCM 2049

✳ J1931   Injection, laronidase, 0.1 mg

✿ J1940   Injection, furosemide, up to 20 mg
MCM 2049

▶ ✿ J1945   Injection, lepirudin, 50 mg
MCM 2049

✿ J1950   Injection, leuprolide acetate (for depot suspension), per 3.75 mg
MCM 2049

✿ J1955   Injection, levocarnitine, per 1 gm
MCM 2049

✿ J1956   Injection, levofloxacin, 250 mg
MCM 2049

✿ J1960   Injection, levorphanol tartrate, up to 2 mg
MCM 2049

✿ J1980   Injection, hyoscyamine sulfate, up to 0.25 mg
MCM 2049

✿ J1990   Injection, chlordiazepoxide HCl, up to 100 mg
MCM 2049

✿ J2001   Injection, lidocaine HCL for intravenous infusion, 10 mg
MCM 2049

✿ J2010   Injection, lincomycin HCl, up to 300 mg
MCM 2049

✳ J2020   Injection, linezolid, 200 mg

✿ J2060   Injection, lorazepam, 2 mg
MCM 2049

✿ J2150   Injection, mannitol, 25% in 50 ml
MCM 2049

✿ J2175   Injection, meperidine HCl, per 100 mg
MCM 2049

✿ J2180   Injection, meperidine and promethazine HCl, up to 50 mg
MCM 2049

✳ J2185   Injection, meropenem, 100 mg

✿ J2210   Injection, methylergonovine maleate, up to 0.2 mg
MCM 2049

✿ J2250   Injection, midazolam HCl, per 1 mg
MCM 2049

✿ J2260   Injection milrinone lactate, 5 mg
MCM 2049

✿ J2270   Injection, morphine sulfate, up to 10 mg
MCM 2049

✿ J2271   Injection, morphine sulfate, 100 mg
MCM 2049, CIM 60-14a

✿ J2275   Injection, morphine sulfate (preservative-free sterile solution), per 10 mg
MCM 2049, CIM 60-14b

▶ ✿ J2278   Injection, ziconotide, 1 μg

✳ J2280   Injection, moxifloxacin, 100 mg

✿ J2300   Injection, nalbuphine HCl, per 10 mg
MCM 2049

✿ J2310   Injection, naloxone HCl, per 1 mg
MCM 2049

✿ J2320   Injection, nandrolone decanoate, up to 50 mg
MCM 2049

✿ J2321   Injection, nandrolone decanoate, up to 100 mg
MCM 2049

✿ J2322   Injection, nandrolone decanoate, up to 200 mg
MCM 2049

   J2324   Deleted 12/31/05

▶ ✿ J2325   Injection, nesiritide, 0.1 mg
MCM 2049

✳ J2353   Injection, octreotide, depot form for intramuscular injection, 1 mg

✳ J2354   Injection, octreotide, non-depot form for subcutaneous or intravenous injection, 25 mcg

✿ J2355   Injection, oprelvekin, 5 mg
MCM 2049

✳ J2357   Injection, omalizumab, 5 mg

✿ J2360   Injection, orphenadrine citrate, up to 60 mg
MCM 2049

✿ J2370   Injection, phenylephrine HCl, up to 1 ml
MCM 2049

✿ J2400   Injection, chloroprocaine HCl, per 30 ml
MCM 2049

⊛ J2405   Injection, ondansetron HCl, per 1 mg
          MCM 2049
⊛ J2410   Injection, oxymorphone HCl, up to 1
          mg
          MCM 2049
▶ * J2425 Injection, palifermin, 50 μg
⊛ J2430   Injection, pamidronate disodium, per 30
          mg
          MCM 2049
⊛ J2440   Injection, papaverine HCl, up to 60 mg
          MCM 2049
⊛ J2460   Injection, oxytetracycline HCl, up to 50
          mg
          MCM 2049
* J2469   Injection, palonosetron HCL, 25 mcg
⊛ J2501   Injection, paricalcitol, 1 mcg
          MCM 2049
▶ * J2503 Injection, pegaptanib sodium, 0.3 mg
▶ ⊛ J2504 Injection, pegademase bovine, 25 IU
          MCM 2049
* J2505   Injection, pegfilgrastim, 6 mg
⊛ J2510   Injection, penicillin G procaine, aque-
          ous, up to 600,000 units
          MCM 2049
▶ ⊛ J2513 Injection, pentastarch, 10% solution, 100
          ml
          MCM 2049
⊛ J2515   Injection, pentobarbital sodium, per 50
          mg
          MCM 2049
⊛ J2540   Injection, penicillin G potassium, up to
          600,000 units
          MCM 2049
⊛ J2543   Injection, piperacillin sodium/tazobac-
          tam sodium, 1/0.125 gm (1.125 gm)
          MCM 2049
⊛ J2545   Pentamidine isethionate, inhalation so-
          lution, per 300 mg, administered
          through a DME
          MCM 2049, Cross Reference Q0077
⊛ J2550   Injection, promethazine HCl, up to 50
          mg
          MCM 2049
⊛ J2560   Injection, phenobarbital sodium, up to
          120 mg
          MCM 2049
⊛ J2590   Injection, oxytocin, up to 10 units
          MCM 2049
⊛ J2597   Injection, desmopressin acetate, per 1
          mcg
          MCM 2049
⊛ J2650   Injection, prednisolone acetate, up to 1
          ml
          MCM 2049
⊛ J2670   Injection, tolazoline HCl, up to 25 mg
          MCM 2049
⊛ J2675   Injection, progesterone, per 50 mg
          MCM 2049
⊛ J2680   Injection, fluphenazine decanoate, up to
          25 mg
          MCM 2049

⊛ J2690   Injection, procainamide HCl, up to 1
          gm
          MCM 2049
⊛ J2700   Injection, oxacillin sodium, up to 250
          mg
          MCM 2049
⊛ J2710   Injection, neostigmine methylsulfate, up
          to 0.5 mg
          MCM 2049
⊛ J2720   Injection, protamine sulfate, per 10 mg
          MCM 2049
⊛ J2725   Injection, protirelin, per 250 mcg
          MCM 2049
⊛ J2730   Injection, pralidoxime chloride, up to 1
          gm
          MCM 2049
⊛ J2760   Injection, phentolamine mesylate, up to
          5 mg
          MCM 2049
⊛ J2765   Injection, metoclopramide HCl, up to
          10 mg
          MCM 2049
  J2770   Injection quinupristin/dalfopristin, 500
          mg (150/350)
          MCM 2049
⊛ J2780   Injection, ranitidine HCl, 25 mg
          MCM 2049
* J2783   Injection, rasburicase, 0.5 mg
⊛ J2788   Injection, Rho (d) immune globulin, hu-
          man, minidose, 50 mcg
          MCM 2049
⊛ J2790   Injection, Rho (D) immune globulin,
          human, full dose, 300 mcg
          MCM 2049
⊛ J2792   Injection, Rho (D) immune globulin
          (human), IV, solvent detergent, 100 IU
          MDC 2049
* J2794   Injection, risperidone, long acting, 0.5 mg
* J2795   Injection, ropivacaine HCl, 1 mg
⊛ J2800   Injection, methocarbamol, up to 10 ml
          MCM 2049
▶ * J2805 Injection, sincalide, 5 μg
⊛ J2810   Injection, theophylline, per 40 mg
          MCM 2049
⊛ J2820   Injection, sargramostim (GM-CSF), 50
          mcg
          MCM 2049
▶ ⊛ J2850 Injection, secretin, synthetic, human,
          1 μg
          MCM 2049
⊛ J2910   Injection, aurothioglucose, up to 50 mg
          MCM 2049
⊛ J2912   Injection, sodium chloride, 0.9%, per
          2 ml
          MCM 2049
⊛ J2916   Injection, sodium ferric gluconate com-
          plex in sucrose injection, 12.5 mg
          MCM 2049.2, MCM 2049.4
⊛ J2920   Injection, methylprednisolone sodium
          succinate, up to 40 mg
          MCM 2049

⊛ J2930 Injection, methylprednisolone sodium succinate, up to 125 mg
MCM 2049

⊛ J2940 Injection, somatrem, 1 mg
MCM 2049, Medicare Statute 1861s2b

⊛ J2941 Injection, somatropin, 1 mg
MCM 2049, Medicare Statute 1861s2b

⊛ J2950 Injection, promazine HCl, up to 25 mg
MCM 2049

⊛ J2993 Injection, reteplase, 18.1 mg
MCM 2049

⊛ J2995 Injection, streptokinase, per 250,000 IU
MCM 2049

⊛ J2997 Injection, alteplase recombinant, 1 mg
MCM 2049

⊛ J3000 Injection, streptomycin, up to 1 gm
MCM 2049

⊛ J3010 Injection, fentanyl citrate, 0.1 mg
MCM 2049

⊛ J3030 Injection, sumatriptan succinate, 6 mg (Code may be used for Medicare when drug administered under the direct supervision of a physician, not for use when drug is self-administered.)
MCM 2049

⊛ J3070 Injection, pentazocine 30 mg
MCM 2049

∗ J3100 Injection, tenecteplase, 50 mg

⊛ J3105 Injection, terbutaline sulfate, up to 1 mg
MCM 2049

⊛ J3110 Injection, teriparatide, 10 mcg

⊛ J3120 Injection, testosterone enanthate, up to 100 mg
MCM 2049

⊛ J3130 Injection, testosterone enanthate, up to 200 mg
MCM 2049

⊛ J3140 Injection, testosterone suspension, up to 50 mg
MCM 2049

⊛ J3150 Injection, testosterone propionate, up to 100 mg
MCM 2049

⊛ J3230 Injection, chlorpromazine HCl, up to 50 mg
MCM 2049

⊛ J3240 Injection, thyrotropin alfa, 0.9 mg provided in 1.1 mg vial
MCM 2049

∗ J3246 Injection, tirofiban HCL, 0.25 mg

⊛ J3250 Injection, trimethobenzamide HCl, up to 200 mg
MCM 2049

⊛ J3260 Injection, tobramycin sulfate, up to 80 mg
MCM 2049

⊛ J3265 Injection, torsemide, 10 mg/ml
MCM 2049

⊛ J3280 Injection, thiethylperazine maleate, up to 10 mg
MCM 2049

▶ ∗ J3285 Injection, treprostinil, 1 mg

⊛ J3301 Injection triamcinolone acetonide, per 10 mg
MCM 2049

⊛ J3302 Injection triamcinolone diacetate, per 5 mg
MCM 2049

⊛ J3303 Injection triamcinolone hexacetonide, per 5 mg
MCM 2049

⊛ J3305 Injection, trimetrexate glucuronate, per 25 mg
MCM 2049

⊛ J3310 Injection, perphenazine, up to 5 mg
MCM 2049

⊛ J3315 Injection, triptorelin pamoate, 3.75 mg
MCM 2049

⊛ J3320 Injection, spectinomycin dihydrochloride, up to 2 gm
MCM 2049

⊛ J3350 Injection, urea, up to 40 gm
MCM 2049

▶ ⊛ J3355 Injection, urofollitropin, 75 IU
MCM 2049

⊛ J3360 Injection, diazepam, up to 5 mg
MCM 2049

⊛ J3364 Injection, urokinase, 5000 IU vial
MCM 2049

⊛ J3365 Injection, IV, urokinase, 250,000 IU vial
MCM 2049, Cross Reference Q0089

⊛ J3370 Injection, vancomycin HCl, 500 mg
MCM 2049, CIM 60-14

⊛ J3396 Injection, verteporfin, 0.1 mg

⊛ J3400 Injection, triflupromazine HCl, up to 20 mg
MCM 2049

⊛ J3410 Injection, hydroxyzine HCl, up to 25 mg
MCM 2049

∗ J3411 Injection, thiamine HCl, 100 mg

∗ J3415 Injection, pyridoxine HCl, 100 mg

⊛ J3420 Injection, vitamin B-12 cyanocobalamin, up to 1000 mcg
MCM 2049, CIM 45-4

⊛ J3430 Injection, phytonadione (vitamin K), per 1 mg
MCM 2049

⊛ J3465 Injection, voriconazole, 10 mg
MCM 2049

⊛ J3470 Injection, hyaluronidase, up to 150 units
MCM 2049

▶ ⊛ J3471 Injection, hyaluronidase, ovine, preservative free, per 1 USP unit (up to 999 USP units)

▶ ⊛ J3472 Injection, hyaluronidase, ovine, preservative free, per 1000 USP units

⊛ J3475 Injection, magnesium sulfate, per 500 mg
MCM 2049

⊛ **Special coverage instructions**   ◆ **Not covered by or valid for Medicare**   ∗ **Carrier discretion**   ◀▶ **New**   ◀▥▥▷ **Revised**

⊛ J3480   Injection, potassium chloride, per 2 milliequivalents (mEq)
MCM 2049

⊛ J3485   Injection, zidovudine, 10 mg
MCM 2049

∗ J3486   Injection, ziprasidone mesylate, 10 mg

∗ J3487   Injection, zoledronic acid, 1 mg

⊛ J3490   Unclassified drugs
MCM 2049

◆ J3520   Edetate disodium, per 150 mg
CIM 35-64, CIM 45-20

⊛ J3530   Nasal vaccine inhalation
MCM 2049

◆ J3535   Drug administered through a metered dose inhaler
MCM 2050.5

◆ J3570   Laetrile, amygdalin, vitamin B-17
CIM 45-10

∗ J3590   Unclassified biologics

Miscellaneous Drugs and Solutions

⊛ J7030   Infusion, normal saline solution, 1000 cc
MCM 2049

⊛ J7040   Infusion, normal saline solution, sterile (500 ml = 1 unit)
MCM 2049

⊛ J7042   5% dextrose/normal saline (500 ml = 1 unit)
MCM 2049

⊛ J7050   Infusion, normal saline solution, 250 cc
MCM 2049

J7051   Deleted 12/31/05

⊛ J7060   5% dextrose/water (500 ml = 1 unit)
MCM 2049

⊛ J7070   Infusion, D-5-W, 1000 cc
MCM 2049

⊛ J7100   Infusion, dextran 40, 500 ml
MCM 2049

⊛ J7110   Infusion, dextran 75, 500 ml
MCM 2049

⊛ J7120   Ringer's lactate infusion, up to 1000 cc
MCM 2049

⊛ J7130   Hypertonic saline solution, 50 or 100 mEq, 20 cc vial
MCM 2049

▶ ⊛ J7188   Injection, von Willebrand factor complex, human, IU
MCM 2049.5, CIM 35.30

▶ ⊛ J7189   Factor VIIa (antihemophilic factor, recombinant), per 1 μg
MCM 2049

⊛ J7190   Factor VIII, anti-hemophilic factor (human), per IU
MCM 2049

⊛ J7191   Factor VIII, anti-hemophilic factor (porcine), per IU
MCM 2049

⊛ J7192   Factor VIII (anti-hemophilic factor recombinant), per IU
MCM 2049

⊛ J7193   Factor IX (anti-hemophilic factor, purified, non-recombinant) per IU
MCM 2049

⊛ J7194   Factor IX, complex, per IU
MCM 2049

⊛ J7195   Factor IX (anti-hemophilic factor, recombinant) per IU
MCM 2049

⊛ J7197   Anti-thrombin III (human), per IU
MCM 2049

⊛ J7198   Anti-inhibitor, per IU
MCM 2049, CIM 45-24

⊛ J7199   Hemophilia clotting factor, not otherwise classified
MCM 2049, CIM 45-24

◆ J7300   Intrauterine copper contraceptive
Medicare Statute 1862A1

◆ J7302   Levonorgestrel-releasing intrauterine contraceptive system, 52 mg
Medicare Statute 1862a1

◆ J7303   Contraceptive supply, hormone containing vaginal ring, each
Medicare Statute 1862.1

◆ J7304   Contraceptive supply, hormone containing patch, each
Medicare Statute 1862.1

▶ ◆ J7306   Levonorgestrel (contraceptive) implant system, including implants and supplies

∗ J7308   Aminolevulinic acid HCl for topical administration, 20%, single unit dosage form (354 mg)

⊛ J7310   Ganciclovir, 4.5 mg, long-acting implant
MCM 2049

J7317   Deleted 12/31/05

▶ ∗ J7318   Hyaluronan (sodium hyaluronate) or derivative, intra-articular injection, 1 mg

J7320   Deleted 12/31/05

∗ J7330   Autologous cultured chondrocytes, implant

⇒ ∗ J7340   Dermal and epidermal, (substitute) tissue of human origin, with or without bioengineered or processed elements, with metabolically active elements, per square centimeter

▶ ∗ J7341   Dermal (substitute) tissue of non-human origin, with or without other bioengineered or processed elements, with metabolically active elements, per square centimeter

⇒ ∗ J7342   Dermal (substitute) tissue of human origin, with or without other bioengineered or processed elements, with metabolically active elements, per square centimeter

---

⊛ Special coverage instructions   ◆ Not covered by or valid for Medicare   ∗ Carrier discretion   ◀ ▶ New   ⇐ ⇒ Revised

➟ * J7343 Dermal and epidermal, (substitute) tissue of non-human origin, with or without other bioengineered or processed elements, without metabolically active elements, per square centimeter

➟ * J7344 Dermal (substitute) tissue of human origin, with or without other bioengineered or processed elements, without metabolically active elements, per square centimeter

➟ * J7350 Dermal (substitute) tissue of human origin, injectable, with or without other bioengineered or processed elements, but without metabolized active elements, per 10 mg

Immunosuppressive Drugs (Includes Non-injectibles)

⊗ J7500 Azathioprine, oral, 50 mg
MCM 2049.5

⊗ J7501 Azathioprine, parenteral, 100 mg
MCM 2049

⊗ J7502 Cyclosporine, oral, 100 mg
MCM 2049.5

⊗ J7504 Lymphocyte immune globulin, anti-thymocyte globulin, equine, parenteral 250 mg
MCM 2049, CIM 45-22

⊗ J7505 Muromonab-CD3, parenteral, 5 mg
MCM 2049

⊗ J7506 Prednisone, oral, per 5 mg
MCM 2049.5

⊗ J7507 Tacrolimus, oral, per 1 mg
MCM 2049.5

⊗ J7509 Methylprednisolone oral, per 4 mg
MCM 2049.5

⊗ J7510 Prednisolone oral, per 5 mg
MCM 2049.5

* J7511 Lymphocyte immune globulin, anti-thymocyte globulin, rabbit, parenteral, 25 mg

⊗ J7513 Daclizumab, parenteral, 25 mg
MCM 2049.5

* J7515 Cyclosporine, oral, 25 mg

* J7516 Cyclosporin, parenteral, 250 mg

* J7517 Mycophenolate mofetil, oral, 250 mg

⊗ J7518 Mycophenolic acid, oral, 180 mg
MCM 2050.5 MCM 4471 MCM 5249

⊗ J7520 Sirolimus, oral, 1 mg
MCM 2049.5

⊗ J7525 Tacrolimus, parenteral, 5 mg
MCM 2049.5

⊗ J7599 Immunosuppressive drug, not otherwise classified
MCM 2049.5

Inhalation Solutions

⊗ J7608 Acetylcysteine, inhalation solution administered through DME, unit dose form, per gm
MCM 2100.5

⊗ J7611 Albuterol, inhalation solution, administered through DME, concentrated form, 1 mg
MCM 2100.5

⊗ J7612 Levalbuterol, inhalation solution, administered through DME, concentrated form, 0.5 mg
MCM 2100.5

⊗ J7613 Albuterol, inhalation solution, administered through DME, unit dose, 1 mg
MCM 2100.5

⊗ J7614 Levalbuterol, inhalation solution, administered through DME, unit dose, 0.5 mg
MCM 2100.5

J7616 Deleted 12/31/05

J7617 Deleted 12/31/05

▶⊗ J7620 Albuterol, up to 2.5 mg and ipratropium bromide, up to 0.5 mg, non-compounded inhalation solution, administered through DME
MCM 2100.5

* J7622 Beclomethasone, inhalation solution administered through DME, unit dose form, per mg

* J7624 Betamethasone, inhalation solution administered through DME, unit dose form, per mg

➟ * J7626 Budesonide inhalation solution, non-compounded, administered through DME, unit dose form, up to 0.5 mg

▶ * J7627 Budesonide, powder, compounded for inhalation solution, administered through DME, unit dose form, up to 0.5 mg

⊗ J7628 Bitolterol mesylate, inhalation solution administered through DME, concentrated form, per mg
MCM 2100.5

⊗ J7629 Bitolterol mesylate, inhalation solution administered through DME, unit dose form, per mg
MCM 2100.5

⊗ J7631 Cromolyn sodium, inhalation solution administered through DME, unit dose form, per 10 mg
MCM 2100.5

* J7633 Budesonide, inhalation solution administered through DME, concentrated form, per 0.25 milligram

⊗ J7635 Atropine, inhalation solution administered through DME, concentrated form, per mg
MCM 2100.5

⊙ J7636   Atropine, inhalation solution administered through DME, unit dose form, per mg
MCM 2100.5

⊙ J7637   Dexamethasone, inhalation solution administered through DME, concentrated form, per mg
MCM 2100.5

⊙ J7638   Dexamethasone, inhalation solution administered through DME, unit dose form, per mg
MCM 2100.5

⊙ J7639   Dornase alpha, inhalation solution administered through DME, unit dose form, per mg
MCM 2100.5

▶◆ J7640   Formoterol, inhalation solution administered through DME, unit dose form, 12 μg

∗ J7641   Flunisolide, inhalation solution administered through DME, unit dose, per mg

⊙ J7642   Glycopyrrolate, inhalation solution administered through DME, concentrated form, per mg
MCM 2100.5

⊙ J7643   Glycopyrrolate, inhalation solution administered through DME, unit dose form, per mg
MCM 2100.5

⊙ J7644   Ipratropium bromide, inhalation solution administered through DME, unit dose form, per mg
MCM 2100.5

⊙ J7648   Isoetharine HCl, inhalation solution administered through DME, concentrated form, per mg
MCM 2100.5

⊙ J7649   Isoetharine HCl, inhalation solution administered through DME, unit dose form, per mg
MCM 2100.5

⊙ J7658   Isoproterenol HCl, inhalation solution administered through DME, concentrated form, per mg
MCM 2100.5

⊙ J7659   Isoproterenol HCl, inhalation solution administered through DME, unit dose form, per mg
MCM 2100.5

⊙ J7668   Metaproterenol sulfate, inhalation solution administered through DME, concentrated form, per 10 mg
MCM 2100.5

⊙ J7669   Metaproterenol sulfate, inhalation solution administered through DME, unit dose form, per 10 mg
MCM 2100.5

∗ J7674   Methacholine chloride administered as inhalation solution through a nebulizer, per 1 mg

⊙ J7680   Terbutaline sulfate, inhalation solution administered through DME, concentrated form, per mg
MCM 2100.5

⊙ J7681   Terbutaline sulfate, inhalation solution administered through DME, unit dose form, per mg
MCM 2100.5

⊙ J7682   Tobramycin, unit dose form, 300 mg, inhalation solution, administered through DME
MCM 2100.5

⊙ J7683   Triamcinolone, inhalation solution administered through DME, concentrated form, per mg
MCM 2100.5

⊙ J7684   Triamcinolone, inhalation solution administered through DME, unit dose form, per mg
MCM 2100.5

⊙ J7699   NOC drugs, inhalation solution administered through DME
MCM 2100.5

⊙ J7799   NOC drugs, other than inhalation drugs, administered through DME
MCM 2100.5

▶⊙ J8498   Antiemetic drug, rectal/suppository, not otherwise specified
Medicare Statute 1861(s)2T

◆ J8499   Prescription drug, oral, non-chemotherapeutic, NOS
MCM 2049

⊙ J8501   Aprepitant, oral, 5 mg

⊙ J8510   Busulfan; oral, 2 mg
MCM 2049.5

▶◆ J8515   Cabergoline, oral, 0.25 mg
MCM 2049.5

⊙ J8520   Capecitabine, oral, 150 mg
MCM 2049.5

⊙ J8521   Capecitabine, oral, 500 mg
MCM 2049.5

⊙ J8530   Cyclophosphamide, oral, 25 mg
MCM 2049.5

▶⊙ J8540   Dexamethasone, oral, 0.25 mg
Medicare Statute 1861(s)2T

⊙ J8560   Etoposide, oral, 50 mg
MCM 2049.5

◆ J8565   Gefitinib, oral, 250 mg

▶⊙ J8597   Antiemetic drug, oral, not otherwise specified
Medicare Statute 1861(s)2T

⊙ J8600   Melphalan, oral, 2 mg
MCM 2049.5

⊙ J8610   Methotrexate, oral, 2.5 mg
MCM 2049.5

⊙ J8700   Temozolomide, oral, 5 mg
MCM 2049.5c

⊙ J8999   Prescription drug, oral, chemotherapeutic, NOS
MCM 2049.5

CHEMOTHERAPY DRUGS (J9000-J9999)

NOTE: These codes cover the cost of the chemotherapy drug only, not to include the administration

- ⊛ J9000   Doxorubicin HCl, 10 mg
  MCM 2049
- ⊛ J9001   Doxorubicin HCl, all lipid formulations, 10 mg
  MCM 2049
- ⊛ J9010   Alemtuzumab, 10 mg
  Medicare Statute 1833(t)
- ⊛ J9015   Aldesleukin, per single use vial
  MCM 2049
- ✳ J9017   Arsenic trioxide, 1 mg
- ⊛ J9020   Asparaginase, 10,000 units
  MCM 2049
- ▶✳ J9025   Injection, azacitidine, 1 mg
- ▶✳ J9027   Injection, clofarabine, 1 mg
- ⊛ J9031   BCG (intravesical), per instillation
  MCM 2049
- ✳ J9035   Injection, bevacizumab, 10 mg
- ⊛ J9040   Bleomycin sulfate, 15 units
  MCM 2049
- ✳ J9041   Injection, bortezomib, 0.1 mg
- ⊛ J9045   Carboplatin, 50 mg
  MCM 2049
- ⊛ J9050   Carmustine, 100 mg
  MCM 2049
- ✳ J9055   Injection, cetuximab, 10 mg
- ⊛ J9060   Cisplatin, powder or solution, per 10 mg
  MCM 2049
- ⊛ J9062   Cisplatin, 50 mg
  MCM 2049
- ⊛ J9065   Injection, cladribine, per 1 mg
  MCM 2049
- ⊛ J9070   Cyclophosphamide, 100 mg
  MCM 2049
- ⊛ J9080   Cyclophosphamide, 200 mg
  MCM 2049
- ⊛ J9090   Cyclophosphamide, 500 mg
  MCM 2049
- ⊛ J9091   Cyclophosphamide, 1 gm
  MCM 2049
- ⊛ J9092   Cyclophosphamide, 2 gm
  MCM 2049
- ⊛ J9093   Cyclophosphamide, lyophilized, 100 mg
  MCM 2049
- ⊛ J9094   Cyclophosphamide, lyophilized, 200 mg
  MCM 2049
- ⊛ J9095   Cyclophosphamide, lyophilized, 500 mg
  MCM 2049
- ⊛ J9096   Cyclophosphamide, lyophilized, 1 gm
  MCM 2049
- ⊛ J9097   Cyclophosphamide, lyophilized, 2 gm
  MCM 2049
- ✳ J9098   Cytarabine liposome, 10 mg
- ⊛ J9100   Cytarabine 100 mg
  MCM 2049
- ⊛ J9110   Cytarabine, 500 mg
  MCM 2049

- ⊛ J9120   Dactinomycin, 0.5 mg
  MCM 2049
- ⊛ J9130   Dacarbazine, 100 mg
  MCM 2049
- ⊛ J9140   Dacarbazine, 200 mg
  MCM 2049
- ⊛ J9150   Daunorubicin, HCl, 10 mg
  MCM 2049
- ⊛ J9151   Daunorubicin citrate liposomal formulation, 10 mg
  MCM 2049
- ✳ J9160   Denileukin diftitox, 300 mcg
- ⊛ J9165   Diethylstilbestrol diphosphate, 250 mg
  MCM 2049
- ⊛ J9170   Docetaxel, 20 mg
  MCM 2049
- ▶⊛ J9175   Injection, Elliott's' B solution, 1 ml
  MCM 2049
- ✳ J9178   Injection, epirubicin HCl, 2 mg
- ⊛ J9181   Etoposide, 10 mg
  MCM 2049
- ⊛ J9182   Etoposide, 100 mg
  MCM 2049
- ⊛ J9185   Fludarabine phosphate, 50 mg
  MCM 2049
- ⊛ J9190   Fluorouracil, 500 mg
  MCM 2049
- ⊛ J9200   Floxuridine, 500 mg
  MCM 2049
- ⊛ J9201   Gemcitabine HCl, 200 mg
  MCM 2049
- ⊛ J9202   Goserelin acetate implant, per 3.6 mg
  MCM 2049
- ⊛ J9206   Irinotecan, 20 mg
  MCM 2049
- ⊛ J9208   Ifosfamide, 1 gm
  MCM 2049
- ⊛ J9209   Mesna, 200 mg
  MCM 2049
- ⊛ J9211   Idarubicin HCl, 5 mg
  MCM 2049
- ⊛ J9212   Injection, interferon alfacon-1, recombinant, 1 mcg
  MCM 2049
- ⊛ J9213   Interferon, alfa-2a, recombinant, 3 million units
  MCM 2049
- ⊛ J9214   Interferon, alfa-2b, recombinant, 1 million units
  MCM 2049
- ⊛ J9215   Interferon, alfa-n3 (human leukocyte derived), 250,000 IU
  MCM 2049
- ⊛ J9216   Interferon, gamma-1B, 3 million units
  MCM 2049
- ⊛ J9217   Leuprolide acetate (for depot suspension), 7.5 mg
  MCM 2049
- ⊛ J9218   Leuprolide acetate, per 1 mg
  MCM 2049

⚙	J9219	Leuprolide acetate implant, 65 mg MCM 2049
▶ ⚙	J9225	Histrelin implant, 50 mg MCM 2049
⚙	J9230	Mechlorethamine HCl (nitrogen mustard), 10 mg MCM 2049
⚙	J9245	Injection, melphalan HCl, 50 mg MCM 2049
⚙	J9250	Methotrexate sodium, 5 mg MCM 2049
⚙	J9260	Methotrexate sodium, 50 mg MCM 2049
*	J9263	Injection, oxaliplatin, 0.5 mg
▶ *	J9264	Injection, paclitaxel protein-bound particles, 1 mg
⚙	J9265	Paclitaxel, 30 mg MCM 2049
⚙	J9266	Pegaspargase, per single dose vial MCM 2049
⚙	J9268	Pentostatin, per 10 mg MCM 2049
⚙	J9270	Plicamycin, 2.5 mg MCM 2049
⚙	J9280	Mitomycin, 5 mg MCM 2049
⚙	J9290	Mitomycin, 20 mg MCM 2049
⚙	J9291	Mitomycin, 40 mg MCM 2049
⚙	J9293	Injection, mitoxantrone HCl, per 5 mg MCM 2049
*	J9300	Gemtuzumab ozogamicin, 5 mg
*	J9305	Injection, pemetrexed, 10 mg
⚙	J9310	Rituximab, 100 mg MCM 2049
⚙	J9320	Streptozocin, 1 gm MCM 2049
⚙	J9340	Thiotepa, 15 mg MCM 2049
⚙	J9350	Topotecan, 4 mg MCM 2049
*	J9355	Trastuzumab, 10 mg
⚙	J9357	Valrubicin, intravesical, 200 mg MCM 2049
⚙	J9360	Vinblastine sulfate, 1 mg MCM 2049
⚙	J9370	Vincristine sulfate, 1 mg MCM 2049
⚙	J9375	Vincristine sulfate, 2 mg MCM 2049
⚙	J9380	Vincristine sulfate, 5 mg MCM 2049
⚙	J9390	Vinorelbine tartrate, per 10 mg MCM 2049
*	J9395	Injection, fulvestrant, 25 mg
⚙	J9600	Porfimer sodium, 75 mg MCM 2049
⚙	J9999	Not otherwise classified, anti-neoplastic drugs MCM 2049, CIM 45-16

K CODES FOR DURABLE MEDICAL EQUIPMENT: TEMPORARY CODES (K0000-K9999)

Wheelchairs

NOTE: This section contains national codes assigned by CMS on a temporary basis and for the exclusive use of the durable medical equipment regional carriers (DMERC).

*	K0001	Standard wheelchair
*	K0002	Standard hemi (low seat) wheelchair
*	K0003	Lightweight wheelchair
*	K0004	High-strength, lightweight wheelchair
*	K0005	Ultra lightweight wheelchair
*	K0006	Heavy-duty wheelchair
*	K0007	Extra heavy-duty wheelchair
*	K0009	Other manual wheelchair/base
*	K0010	Standard-weight frame motorized/power wheelchair
*	K0011	Standard-weight frame motorized/power wheelchair, with programmable control parameters for speed adjustment, tremor dampening, acceleration control and braking
*	K0012	Lightweight portable motorized/power wheelchair
*	K0014	Other motorized/power wheelchair base
*	K0015	Detachable, non-adjustable height arm rest, each
*	K0017	Detachable, adjustable height arm rest, base, each
*	K0018	Detachable, adjustable height arm rest, upper portion, each
*	K0019	Arm pad, each
*	K0020	Fixed, adjustable height arm rest, pair
*	K0037	High mount flip-up footrest, each
*	K0038	Leg strap, each
*	K0039	Leg strap, H-style, each
*	K0040	Adjustable angle footplate, each
*	K0041	Large size footplate, each
*	K0042	Standard size footplate, each
*	K0043	Foot rest, lower extension tube, each
*	K0044	Foot rest, upper hanger bracket, each
*	K0045	Foot rest, complete assembly
*	K0046	Elevating leg rests, lower extension tube, each
*	K0047	Elevating leg rests, upper hanger bracket, each
*	K0050	Ratchet assembly
*	K0051	Cam release assembly, footrest or leg rests, each
*	K0052	Swing-away, detachable foot rests, each
*	K0053	Elevating foot rests, articulating (telescoping), each
*	K0056	Seat height less than 17″ or equal to or greater than 21″ for a high-strength, lightweight, or ultra lightweight wheelchair

∗ K0064 Deleted 12/31/05
∗ K0065 Spoke protectors, each
K0066 Deleted 12/31/05
K0067 Deleted 12/31/05
K0068 Deleted 12/31/05
∗ K0069 Rear wheel assembly, complete, with solid tire, spokes or molded, each
∗ K0070 Rear wheel assembly, complete, with pneumatic tire, spokes or molded, each
∗ K0071 Front caster assembly, complete, with pneumatic tire, each
∗ K0072 Front caster assembly, complete, with semi-pneumatic tire, each
∗ K0073 Caster pin lock, each
K0074 Deleted 12/31/05
K0075 Deleted 12/31/05
K0076 Deleted 12/31/05
∗ K0077 Front caster assembly, complete, with solid tire, each
K0078 Deleted 12/31/05
∗ K0090 Rear wheel tire for power wheelchair, any size, each
∗ K0091 Rear wheel tire tube other than zero pressure for power wheelchair, any size, each
∗ K0092 Rear wheel assembly for power wheelchair, complete each
∗ K0093 Rear wheel, zero pressure tire tube (flat-free insert) for power wheelchair, any size, each
∗ K0094 Wheel tire for power base, any size, each
∗ K0095 Wheel tire tube other than zero pressure for each base, any size, each
∗ K0096 Wheel assembly for power base, complete, each
∗ K0097 Wheel zero pressure tire tube (flat-free insert) for power base, any size, each
∗ K0098 Drive belt for power wheelchair
∗ K0099 Front caster for power wheelchair, each
K0102 Deleted 12/31/05
K0104 Deleted 12/31/05
∗ K0105 IV hanger, each
K0106 Deleted 12/31/05
∗ K0108 Wheelchair component or accessory, not otherwise specified

Other

⊘ K0195 Elevating leg rests, pair (for use with capped rental wheelchair base)
CIM 60-9
K0415 Deleted 12/31/05
K0416 Deleted 12/31/05
∗ K0452 Wheelchair bearings, any type
⊘ K0455 Infusion pump used for uninterrupted parenteral administration of medication (e.g., epoprostenol or treprostinol)
CIM 60-14

⊘ K0462 Temporary replacement for patient owned equipment being repaired, any type
MCM 5102.3
K0552 Deleted 12/31/05
K0600 Deleted 12/31/05
∗ K0601 Replacement battery for external infusion pump owned by patient, silver oxide, 1.5 volt, each
∗ K0602 Replacement battery for external infusion pump owned by patient, silver oxide, 3 volt, each
∗ K0603 Replacement battery for external infusion pump owned by patient, alkaline, 1.5 volt, each
∗ K0604 Replacement battery for external infusion pump owned by patient, lithium, 3.6 volt, each
∗ K0605 Replacement battery for external infusion pump owned by patient, lithium, 4.5 volt, each
∗ K0606 Automatic external defibrillator, with integrated electrocardiogram analysis, garment type
∗ K0607 Replacement battery for automated external defibrillator, garment type only, each
∗ K0608 Replacement garment for use with automated external defibrillator, each
∗ K0609 Replacement electrodes for use with automated external defibrillator, garment type only, each
K0618 Deleted 12/31/05
K0619 Deleted 12/31/05
K0620 Deleted 12/31/05
K0628 Deleted 12/31/05
K0629 Deleted 12/31/05
K0630 Deleted 12/31/05
K0631 Deleted 12/31/05
K0632 Deleted 12/31/05
K0633 Deleted 12/31/05
K0634 Deleted 12/31/05
K0635 Deleted 12/31/05
K0636 Deleted 12/31/05
K0637 Deleted 12/31/05
K0638 Deleted 12/31/05
K0639 Deleted 12/31/05
K0640 Deleted 12/31/05
K0641 Deleted 12/31/05
K0642 Deleted 12/31/05
K0643 Deleted 12/31/05
K0644 Deleted 12/31/05
K0645 Deleted 12/31/05
K0646 Deleted 12/31/05
K0647 Deleted 12/31/05
K0648 Deleted 12/31/05
K0649 Deleted 12/31/05
➡ ∗ K0669 Wheelchair accessory, wheelchair seat or back cushion, does not meet specific code criteria or no written coding verification from SADMERC

K0670   Deleted 12/31/05
K0671   Deleted 12/31/05
▶ * K0730   Controlled dose inhalation drug delivery system

ORTHOTIC PROCEDURES (L0100-L4999)

Orthotic Devices: Spinal

Cervical

* L0100   Cranial orthosis (helmet,), with or without soft interface, molded to patient model
* L0110   Cranial orthosis (helmet), with or without soft-interface, non-molded
* L0112   Cranial cervical orthosis, congenital torticollis type, with or without soft interface material, adjustable range of motion joint, custom fabricated
* L0120   Cervical, flexible, non-adjustable (foam collar)
* L0130   Cervical, flexible, thermoplastic collar, molded to patient
* L0140   Cervical, semi-rigid, adjustable (plastic collar)
* L0150   Cervical, semi-rigid, adjustable molded chin cup (plastic collar with mandibular/occipital piece)
* L0160   Cervical, semi-rigid, wire frame occipital/mandibular support
* L0170   Cervical, collar, molded to patient model
* L0172   Cervical, collar, semi-rigid thermoplastic foam, two piece
* L0174   Cervical, collar, semi-rigid, thermoplastic foam, two piece with thoracic extension

Multiple Post Collar

* L0180   Cervical, multiple post collar, occipital/mandibular supports, adjustable
* L0190   Cervical, multiple post collar, occipital/mandibular supports, adjustable cervical bars (SOMI, Guilford, Taylor types)
* L0200   Cervical, multiple post collar, occipital/mandibular supports, adjustable cervical bars, and thoracic extension

Thoracic

* L0210   Thoracic, rib belt
* L0220   Thoracic, rib belt, custom fabricated

Thoracic-Lumbar-Sacral

Anterior-Posterior-Lateral Rotary-Control

* L0430   Spinal orthosis, anterior-posterior-lateral control, with interface material, custom fitted (Dewall posture protector only)
* L0450   TLSO, flexible, provides trunk support, upper thoracic region, produces intracavitary pressure to reduce load on the intevertebral disks with rigid stays or panel(s), includes shoulder straps and closures, prefabricated, includes fitting and adjustment
* L0452   TLSO, flexible, provides trunk support, upper thoracic region, produces intracavitary pressure to reduce load on the intervertebral disks with rigid stays or panel(s), includes shoulder straps and closures, custom fabricated
* L0454   TLSO flexible, provides trunk support, extends from sacrococcygeal junction to above t-9 vertebra, restricts gross trunk motion in the sagittal plane, produces intracavitary pressure to reduce load on the intervertebral disks with rigid stays or panel(s), includes shoulder straps and closures, prefabricated, includes fitting and adjustment
* L0456   TLSO, flexible, provides trunk support, thoracic region, rigid posterior panel and soft anterior apron, extends from the sacrococcygeal junction and terminates just inferior to the scapular spine, restricts gross trunk motion in the sagittal plane, produces intracavitary pressure to reduce load on the intervertebral disks, includes straps and closures, prefabricated, includes fitting and adjustment
* L0458   TLSO, triplanar control, modular segmented spinal system, two rigid plastic shells, posterior extends from the sacrococcygeal junction and terminates just inferior to the scapular spine, anterior extends from the symphysis pubis to the xiphoid, soft liner, restricts gross trunk motion in the sagittal, coronal, and transverse planes, lateral strength is provided by overlapping plastic and stabilizing closures, includes straps and closures, prefabricated, includes fitting and adjustment

* L0460 TLSO, triplanar control, modular segmented spinal system, two rigid plastic shells, posterior extends from the sacrococcygeal junction and terminates just inferior to the scapular spine, anterior extends from the symphysis pubis to the sternal notch, soft liner, restricts gross trunk motion in the sagittal, coronal, and transverse planes, lateral strength is provided by overlapping plastic and stabilizing closures, includes straps and closures, prefabricated, includes fitting and adjustment

* L0462 TLSO, triplanar control, modular segmented spinal system, three rigid plastic shells, posterior extends from the sacrococcygeal junction and terminates just inferior to the scapular spine, anterior extends from the symphysis pubis to the sternal notch, soft liner, restricts gross trunk motion in the sagittal, coronal, and transverse planes, lateral strength is provided by overlapping plastic and stabilizing closures, includes straps and closures, prefabricated, includes fitting and adjustment

* L0464 TLSO, triplanar control, modular segmented spinal system, four rigid plastic shells, posterior extends from sacrococcygeal junction and terminates just inferior to scapular spine, anterior extends from symphysis pubis to the sternal notch, soft liner, restricts gross trunk motion in sagittal, coronal, and transverse planes, lateral strength is provided by overlapping plastic and stabilizing closures, includes straps and closures, prefabricated, includes fitting and adjustment

* L0466 TLSO, sagittal control, rigid posterior frame and flexible soft anterior apron with straps, closures and padding, restricts gross trunk motion in sagittal plane, produces intracavitary pressure to reduce load on intervertebral disks, includes fitting and shaping the frame, prefabricated, includes fitting and adjustment

* L0468 TLSO, sagittal-coronal control, rigid posterior frame and flexible soft anterior apron with straps, closures and padding, extends from sacrococcygeal junction over scapulae, lateral strength provided by pelvic, thoracic, and lateral frame pieces, restricts gross trunk motion in sagittal, and coronal planes, produces intracavitary pressure to reduce load on intervertebral disks, includes fitting and shaping the frame, prefabricated, includes fitting and adjustment

* L0470 TLSO, triplanar control, rigid posterior frame and flexible soft anterior apron with straps, closures and padding, extends from sacrococcygeal junction to scapula, lateral strength provided by pelvic, thoracic, and lateral frame pieces, rotational strength provided by subclavicular extensions, restricts gross trunk motion in sagittal, coronal, and transverse planes, produces intracavitary pressure to reduce load on the intervertebral disks, includes fitting and shaping the frame, prefabricated, includes fitting and adjustment

* L0472 TLSO, triplanar control, hyperextension, rigid anterior and lateral frame extends from symphysis pubis to sternal notch with two anterior components (one pubic and one sternal), posterior and lateral pads with straps and closures, limits spinal flexion, restricts gross trunk motion in sagittal, coronal, and transverse planes, includes fitting and shaping the frame, prefabricated, includes fitting and adjustment

* L0480 TLSO, triplanar control, one piece rigid plastic shell without interface liner, with multiple straps and closures, posterior extends from sacrococcygeal junction and terminates just inferior to scapular spine, anterior extends from symphysis pubis to sternal notch, anterior or posterior opening, restricts gross trunk motion in sagittal, coronal, and transverse planes, includes a carved plaster or CAD-CAM model, custom fabricated

* L0482 TLSO, triplanar control, one piece rigid plastic shell with interface liner, multiple straps and closures, posterior extends from sacrococcygeal junction and terminates just inferior to scapular spine, anterior extends from symphysis pubis to sternal notch, anterior or posterior opening, restricts gross trunk motion in sagittal, coronal, and transverse planes, includes a carved plaster or CAD-CAM model, custom fabricated

* L0484 TLSO, triplanar control, two piece rigid plastic shell without interface liner, with multiple straps and closures, posterior extends from sacrococcygeal junction and terminates just inferior to scapular spine, anterior extends from symphysis pubis to sternal notch, lateral strength is enhanced by overlapping plastic, restricts gross trunk motion in the sagittal, coronal, and transverse planes, includes a carved plaster or CAD-CAM model, custom fabricated

* L0486 TLSO, triplanar control, two piece rigid plastic shell with interface liner, multiple straps and closures, posterior extends from sacrococcygeal junction and terminates just inferior to scapular spine, anterior extends from symphysis pubis to sternal notch, lateral strength is enhanced by overlapping plastic, restricts gross trunk motion in the sagittal, coronal, and transverse planes, includes a carved plaster or CAD-CAM model, custom fabricated

* L0488 TLSO, triplanar control, one piece rigid plastic shell with interface liner, multiple straps and closures, posterior extends from sacrococcygeal junction and terminates just inferior to scapular spine, anterior extends from symphysis pubis to sternal notch, anterior or posterior opening, restricts gross trunk motion in sagittal, coronal, and transverse planes, prefabricated, includes fitting and adjustment

* L0490 TLSO, sagittal-coronal control, one piece rigid plastic shell, with overlapping reinforced anterior, with multiple straps and closures, posterior extends from sacrococcygeal junction and terminates at or before the T-9 vertebra, anterior extends from symphysis pubis to xiphoid, anterior opening, restricts gross trunk motion in sagittal and coronal planes, prefabricated, includes fitting and adjustment

▶ * L0491 TLSO, sagittal-coronal control, modular segmented spinal system, two rigid plastic shells, posterior extends from the sacrococcygeal junction and terminates just inferior to the scapular spine, anterior extends from the symphysis pubis to the xiphoid, soft liner, restricts gross trunk motion in the sagittal and coronal planes, lateral strength is provided by overlapping plastic and stabilizing closures, includes straps and closures, prefabricated, includes fitting and adjustment

▶ * L0492 TLSO, sagittal-coronal control, modular segmented spinal system, three rigid plastic shells, posterior extends from the sacrococcygeal junction and terminates just inferior to the scapular spine, anterior extends from the symphysis pubis to the xiphoid, soft liner, restricts gross trunk motion in the sagittal and coronal planes, lateral strength is provided by overlapping plastic and stabilizing closures, includes straps and closures, prefabricated, includes fitting and adjustment

Sacroilliac, Lumbar, Sacral Orthosis

▶ * L0621 Sacroiliac orthosis, flexible, provides pelvic-sacral support, reduces motion about the sacroiliac joint, includes straps, closures, may include pendulous abdomen design, prefabricated, includes fitting and adjustment

▶ * L0622 Sacroiliac orthosis, flexible, provides pelvic-sacral support, reduces motion about the sacroiliac joint, includes straps, closures, may include pendulous abdomen design, custom fabricated

▶ * L0623 Sacroiliac orthosis, provides pelvic-sacral support, with rigid or semi-rigid panels over the sacrum and abdomen, reduces motion about the sacroiliac joint, includes straps, closures, may include pendulous abdomen design, prefabricated, includes fitting and adjustment

▶ * L0624 Sacroiliac orthosis, provides pelvic-sacral support, with rigid or semi-rigid panels placed over the sacrum and abdomen, reduces motion about the sacroiliac joint, includes straps, closures, may include pendulous abdomen design, custom fabricated

▶ * L0625 Lumbar orthosis, flexible, provides lumbar support, posterior extends from L-1 to below L-5 vertebra, produces intracavitary pressure to reduce load on the intervertebral discs, includes straps, closures, may include pendulous abdomen design, shoulder straps, stays, prefabricated, includes fitting and adjustment

▶ * L0626 Lumbar orthosis, sagittal control, with rigid posterior panel(s), posterior extends from L-1 to below L-5 vertebra, produces intracavitary pressure to reduce load on the intervertebral discs, includes straps, closures, may include padding, stays, shoulder straps, pendulous abdomen design, prefabricated, includes fitting and adjustment

▶ * L0627 Lumbar orthosis, sagittal control, with rigid anterior and posterior panels, posterior extends from L-1 to below L-5 vertebra, produces intracavitary pressure to reduce load on the intervertebral discs, includes straps, closures, may include padding, shoulder straps, pendulous abdomen design, prefabricated, includes fitting and adjustment

▶✳ L0628　Lumbar-sacral orthosis, flexible, provides lumbo-sacral support, posterior extends from sacrococcygeal junction to T-9 vertebra, produces intracavitary pressure to reduce load on the intervertebral discs, includes straps, closures, may include stays, shoulder straps, pendulous abdomen design, prefabricated, includes fitting and adjustment

▶✳ L0629　Lumbar-sacral orthosis, flexible, provides lumbo-sacral support, posterior extends from sacrococcygeal junction to T-9 vertebra, produces intracavitary pressure to reduce load on the intervertebral discs, includes straps, closures, may include stays, shoulder straps, pendulous abdomen design, custom fabricated

▶✳ L0630　Lumbar-sacral orthosis, sagittal control, with rigid posterior panel(s), posterior extends from sacrococcygeal junction to T-9 vertebra, produces intracavitary pressure to reduce load on the intervertebral discs, includes straps, closures, may include padding, stays, shoulder straps, pendulous abdomen design, prefabricated, includes fitting and adjustment

▶✳ L0631　Lumbar-sacral orthosis, sagittal control, with rigid anterior and posterior panels, posterior extends from sacrococcygeal junction to T-9 vertebra, produces intracavitary pressure to reduce load on the intervertebral discs, includes straps, pendulous abdomen design, prefabricated, includes fitting and adjustment

▶✳ L0632　Lumbar-sacral orthosis, sagittal control, with rigid anterior and posterior panels, posterior extends from sacrococcygeal junction to T-9 vertebra, produces intracavitary pressure to reduce load on the intervertebral discs, includes straps, closures, may include padding, shoulder straps, pendulous abdomen design, custom fabricated

▶✳ L0633　Lumbar-sacral orthosis, sagittal-coronal control, with rigid posterior frame/panel(s), posterior extends from sacrococcygeal junction to T-9 vertebra, lateral strength provided by rigid lateral frame/panels, produces intracavitary pressure to reduce load on intervertebral discs, includes straps, closures, may include padding, stays, shoulder straps, pendulous abdomen design, prefabricated, includes fitting and adjustment

▶✳ L0634　Lumbar-sacral orthosis, sagittal-coronal control, with rigid posterior frame/panel(s), posterior extends from sacrococcygeal junction to T-9 vertebra, lateral strength provided by rigid lateral frame/panel(s), produces intracavitary pressure to reduce load on intervertebral discs, includes straps, closures, may include padding, stays, shoulder straps, pendulous abdomen design, custom fabricated

▶✳ L0635　Lumbar-sacral orthosis, sagittal-coronal control, lumbar flexion, rigid posterior frame/panel(s), lateral articulating design to flex the lumbar spine, posterior extends from sacrococcygeal junction to T-9 vertebra, lateral strength provided by rigid lateral frame/panel(s), produces intracavitary pressure to reduce load on intervertebral discs, includes straps, closures, may include padding, anterior panel, pendulous abdomen design, prefabricated, includes fitting and adjustment

▶✳ L0636　Lumbar sacral orthosis, sagittal-coronal control, lumbar flexion, rigid posterior frame/panels, lateral articulating design to flex the lumbar spine, posterior extends from sacrococcygeal junction to T-9 vertebra, lateral strength provided by rigid lateral frame/panels, produces intracavitary pressure to reduce load on intervertebral discs, includes straps, closures, may include padding, anterior panel, pendulous abdomen design, custom fabricated

▶✳ L0637　Lumbar-sacral orthosis, sagittal-coronal control, with rigid anterior and posterior frame/panels, posterior extends from sacrococcygeal junction to T-9 vertebra, lateral strength provided by rigid lateral frame/panels, produces intracavitary pressure to reduce load on intervertebral discs, includes straps, closures, may include padding, shoulder straps, pendulous abdomen design, prefabricated, includes fitting and adjustment

▶✳ L0638　Lumbar-sacral orthosis, sagittal-coronal control, with rigid anterior and posterior frame/panels, posterior extends from sacrococcygeal junction to T-9 vertebra, lateral strength provided by rigid lateral frame/panels, produces intracavitary pressure to reduce load on intervertebral discs, includes straps, closures, may include padding, shoulder straps, pendulous abdomen design, custom fabricated

▶ * L0639   Lumbar-sacral orthosis, sagittal-coronal control, rigid shell(s)/panel(s), posterior extends from sacrococcygeal junction to T-9 vertebra, anterior extends from symphysis pubis to xyphoid, produces intracavitary pressure to reduce load on the intervertebral discs, overall strength is provided by overlapping rigid material and stabilizing closures, includes straps, closures may include soft interface, pendulous abdomen design, prefabricated, includes fitting and adjustment

▶ * L0640   Lumbar-sacral orthosis, sagittal-coronal control, rigid shell(s)/panel(s), posterior extends from sacrococcygeal junction to T-9 vertebra, anterior extends from symphysis pubis to xyphoid, produces intracavitary pressure to reduce load on the intervertebral discs, overall strength is provided by overlapping rigid material and stabilizing closures, includes straps, closures, may include soft interface, pendulous abdomen design, custom fabricated

Cervical-Thoracic-Lumbar-Sacral

Anterior-Posterior-Lateral Control

* L0700   Cervical-thoracic-lumbar-sacral orthosis (CTLSO), anterior-posterior-lateral control, molded to patient model (Minerva type)
* L0710   CTLSO, anterior-posterior-lateral control, molded to patient model, with interface material (Minerva type)

HALO Procedure

* L0810   HALO procedure, cervical halo incorporated into jacket vest
* L0820   HALO procedure, cervical halo incorporated into plaster body jacket
* L0830   HALO procedure, cervical halo incorporated into Milwaukee type orthosis
▶ * L0859   Addition to halo procedure, magnetic resonance image compatible systems, rings and pins, any material
   L0860   Deleted 12/31/05
* L0861   Addition to HALO procedure, replacement liner/interface material

Torso Supports

* L0960   Torso support, postsurgical support, pads for postsurgical support

Additions to Spinal Orthoses

* L0970   TLSO, corset front
* L0972   LSO, corset front
* L0974   TLSO, full corset
* L0976   LSO, full corset
* L0978   Axillary crutch extension
* L0980   Peroneal straps, pair
* L0982   Stocking supporter grips, set of four (4)
* L0984   Protective body sock, each
* L0999   Addition to spinal orthosis, not otherwise specified

Orthotic Devices: Scoliosis Procedures (L1000-L1499)

NOTE: Orthotic care of scoliosis differs from other orthotic care in that the treatment is more dynamic in nature and uses ongoing continual modification of the orthosis to the patient's changing condition. This coding structure uses the proper names, or eponyms, of the procedures because they have historic and universal acceptance in the profession. It should be recognized that variations to the basic procedures described by the founders/developers are accepted in various medical and orthotic practices throughout the country. All procedures include a model of patient when indicated.

Scoliosis: Cervical-Thoracic-Lumbar-Sacral (CTLSO) (Milwaukee)

* L1000   CTLSO (Milwaukee), inclusive of furnishing initial orthosis, including model
* L1005   Tension-based scoliosis orthosis and accessory pads, includes fitting and adjustment
* L1010   Addition to CTLSO or scoliosis orthosis, axilla sling

Correction Pads

* L1020   Addition to CTLSO or scoliosis orthosis, kyphosis pad
* L1025   Addition to CTLSO or scoliosis orthosis, kyphosis pad, floating
* L1030   Addition to CTLSO or scoliosis orthosis, lumbar bolster pad
* L1040   Addition to CTLSO or scoliosis orthosis, lumbar or lumbar rib pad
* L1050   Addition to CTLSO or scoliosis orthosis, sternal pad

* L1060 Addition to CTLSO or scoliosis orthosis, thoracic pad
* L1070 Addition to CTLSO or scoliosis orthosis, trapezius sling
* L1080 Addition to CTLSO or scoliosis orthosis, outrigger
* L1085 Addition to CTLSO or scoliosis orthosis, outrigger, bilateral with vertical extensions
* L1090 Addition to CTLSO or scoliosis orthosis, lumbar sling
* L1100 Addition to CTLSO or scoliosis orthosis, ring flange, plastic or leather
* L1110 Addition to CTLSO or scoliosis orthosis, ring flange, plastic or leather, molded to patient model
* L1120 Addition to CTLSO, scoliosis orthosis, cover for upright, each

Scoliosis: Cervical-Thoracic-Lumbar-Sacral (Low Profile)

* L1200 TLSO, inclusive of furnishing initial orthosis only
* L1210 Addition to TLSO, (low profile), lateral thoracic extension
* L1220 Addition to TLSO (low profile), anterior thoracic extension
* L1230 Addition to TLSO (low profile), Milwaukee type superstructure
* L1240 Addition to TLSO (low profile), lumbar derotation pad
* L1250 Addition to TLSO (low profile), anterior ASIS pad
* L1260 Addition to TLSO (low profile), anterior thoracic derotation pad
* L1270 Addition to TLSO (low profile), abdominal pad
* L1280 Addition to TLSO (low profile), rib gusset (elastic), each
* L1290 Addition to TLSO (low profile), lateral trochanteric pad

Other Scoliosis Procedures

* L1300 Other scoliosis procedure, body jacket molded to patient model
* L1310 Other scoliosis procedure, postoperative body jacket
* L1499 Spinal orthosis, NOS

Scoliosis: Thoracic-Hip-Knee-Ankle (THKA)

* L1500 Thoracic-hip-knee-ankle orthosis (THKAO), mobility frame (Newington, Parapodium types)
* L1510 THKAO, standing frame, with or without tray and accessories
* L1520 THKAO, swivel walker

Orthotic Devices: Lower Limb

NOTE: the procedures in L1600-L2999 are considered as *base* or *basic procedures* and may be modified by listing procedure from the Additions Sections and adding them to the base procedure.

Hip: Flexible

* L1600 Hip orthosis (HO), abduction control of hip joints, flexible, Frejka type with cover, prefabricated, includes fitting and adjustment
* L1610 HO, abduction control of hip joints, flexible, Frejka cover only, prefabricated, includes fitting and adjustment
* L1620 HO, abduction control of hip joints, flexible, Pavlik harness, prefabricated, includes fitting and adjustment
* L1630 HO, abduction control of hip joints, semi-flexible (Von Rosen type), custom fabrication
* L1640 HO, abduction control of hip joints, static, pelvic band or spreader bar, thigh cuffs, custom fabrication
* L1650 HO, abduction control of hip joints, static, adjustable, (Ilfeld type), prefabricated, includes fitting and adjustment
* L1652 Hip orthosis, bilateral thigh cuffs with adjustable abductor spreader bar, adult size, prefabricated, includes fitting and adjustment, any type
* L1660 HO, abduction control of hip joints, static, plastic, prefabricated, includes fitting and adjustment
* L1680 HO, abduction control of hip joints, dynamic, pelvic control, adjustable hip motion control, thigh cuffs (Rancho hip action type), custom fabrication
* L1685 HO, abduction control of hip joint, postoperative hip abduction type, custom fabricated
* L1686 HO, abduction control of hip joint, postoperative hip abduction type, prefabricated, includes fitting and adjustment
* L1690 Combination, bilateral, lumbar sacral, hip, femur orthosis providing adduction and internal rotation control, prefabricated, includes fitting and adjustment

Legg-Perthes

* L1700 Legg-Perthes orthosis (Toronto type), custom fabrication
* L1710 Legg-Perthes orthosis (Newington type), custom fabrication
* L1720 Legg-Perthes orthosis, trilateral (Tachdjian type), custom fabrication

© **Special coverage instructions** ◆ **Not covered by or valid for Medicare** * **Carrier discretion** ◄► **New** ◄▪▪▪▪► **Revised**

* L1730   Legg-Perthes orthosis (Scottish Rite type), custom fabrication

L1750   Deleted 12/31/05

* L1755   Legg-Perthes orthosis (Patten bottom type), custom fabrication

Knee (KO)

* L1800   Knee orthosis (KO), elastic with stays, prefabricated, includes fitting and adjustment

* L1810   KO, elastic with joints, prefabricated, includes fitting and adjustment

* L1815   KO, elastic or other elastic type material with condylar pads, prefabricated, includes fitting and adjustment

* L1820   KO, elastic with condylar pads and joints, with or without patellar control, prefabricated, includes fitting and adjustment

* L1825   KO, elastic kneecap, prefabricated, includes fitting and adjustment

* L1830   KO, immobilizer, canvas longitudinal, prefabricated, includes fitting and adjustment

* L1831   Knee orthosis, locking knee joint(s), positional orthosis, prefabricated, includes fitting and adjustment

➡ * L1832   Knee orthrosis, adjustable knee joints (unicentric or polycentric), positional orthosis, rigid support, prefabricated, includes fitting and adjustment

* L1834   KO, without knee joint, rigid, custom fabrication

* L1836   Knee orthosis, rigid, without joint(s), includes soft interface material, prefabricated, includes fitting and adjustment

* L1840   KO, derotation, medial-lateral, anterior cruciate ligament, custom fabricated

➡ * L1843   Knee orthosis, single upright, thigh and calf, with adjustable flexion and extension joint (unicentric or polycentric), medial-lateral and rotation control, with or without varus/valgus adjustment; prefabricated, includes fitting and adjustment

➡ * L1844   Knee orthosis, single upright, thigh and calf, with adjustable flexion and extension joint (unicentric or polycentric), medial-lateral and rotation control, with or without varus/valgus adjustment, custom fabricated

➡ * L1845   Knee orthrosis, double upright, thigh and calf, with adjustable flexion and extension joint (unicentric or polycentric), medial-lateral and rotation control, with or without varus/valgus adjustment, prefabricated, includes fitting and adjustment

➡ * L1846   Knee orthrosis, double upright, thigh and calf, with adjustable flexion and extension joint (unicentric or polycentric), medial-lateral and rotation control, with or without varus/valgus adjustment, custom fabricated

* L1847   Knee orthosis, double upright with adjustable joint, with inflatable air support chambers, prefabricated, includes fitting and adjustment

* L1850   KO, Swedish type, prefabricated, includes fitting and adjustment

* L1855   KO, molded plastic, thigh and calf sections, with double upright knee joints, custom fabrication

* L1858   KO, molded plastic, polycentric knee joints, pneumatic knee pads (CTI), custom fabrication

* L1860   KO, modification of supracondylar prosthetic socket, custom fabrication (SK)

* L1870   KO, double upright, thigh and calf lacers, with knee joints, custom fabrication

* L1880   KO, double upright, non-molded thigh and calf cuffs/lacers with knee joints, custom fabrication

Ankle-Foot (AFO)

* L1900   Ankle-foot orthosis (AFO), spring wire, dorsiflexion assist calf band, custom fabrication

* L1901   Ankle orthosis, elastic, prefabricated, includes fitting and adjustment (e.g. neoprene, Lycra)

* L1902   AFO, ankle gauntlet, prefabricated, includes fitting and adjustment

* L1904   AFO, molded ankle gauntlet, custom fabrication

* L1906   AFO, multiligamentus ankle support, prefabricated, includes fitting and adjustment

* L1907   AFO (ankle foot orthosis), supramalleolar with straps, with or without interface/pads, custom fabricated

* L1910   AFO, posterior, single bar, clasp attachment to shoe counter, prefabricated, includes fitting and adjustment

* L1920   AFO, single upright with static or adjustable stop (Phelps or Perlstein type), custom fabrication

* L1930   AFO, plastic or other material, prefabricated, includes fitting and adjustment

* L1932   AFO, rigid anterior tibial section, total carbon fiber or equal material, prefabricated; includes fitting and adjustment

* L1940   AFO, plastic or other material, custom fabrication

* L1945   AFO, plastic, rigid anterior tibial section (floor reaction), custom fabrication

* L1950   Ankle foot orthosis, spiral, (Institute of Rehabilitation Medicine type), plastic, custom-fabrication

* L1951   Ankle foot orthosis, spiral, (Institute of Rehabilitative Medicine type), plastic or other material, prefabricated, includes fitting and adjustment

* L1960   AFO, posterior solid ankle, plastic, custom fabrication

* L1970   AFO, plastic, with ankle joint, custom fabrication

* L1971   Ankle foot orthosis, plastic or other material with ankle joint, prefabricated, includes fitting and adjustment

* L1980   AFO, single upright free plantar dorsiflexion, solid stirrup, calf band/cuff (single bar BK orthosis), custom fabrication

* L1990   AFO, double upright free plantar dorsiflexion, solid stirrup, calf band/cuff (double bar BK orthosis), custom fabrication

Hip-Knee-Ankle-Foot (or Any Combination)

NOTE: L2000, L2020, and L2036 are base procedures to be used with any knee joint. L2010 and L2030 are to be used only with no knee joint.

* L2000   Knee-ankle-foot orthosis (KAFO), single upright, free knee, free ankle, solid stirrup, thigh and calf bands/cuffs (single bar 'AK' orthosis), custom fabrication

* L2005   Knee-ankle-foot orthosis, any material, single or double upright, stance control, automatic lock and swing phase release, mechanical activation; includes ankle joint, any type, custom fabricated

* L2010   KAFO, single upright, free ankle, solid stirrup, thigh and calf bands/cuffs (single bar AK orthosis), without knee joint, custom fabrication

* L2020   KAFO, double upright, free knee, free ankle, solid stirrup, thigh and calf bands/cuffs (double bar AK orthosis), custom fabrication

* L2030   KAFO, double upright, free ankle, solid stirrup, thigh and calf bands/cuffs (double bar AK orthosis), without knee joint, custom fabrication

▶* L2034   Knee ankle foot orthosis, full plastic, single upright, with or without free motion knee, medial lateral rotation control, with or without free motion ankle, custom fabricated

* L2035   KAFO, full plastic, static, (pediatric size), without free motion ankle, prefabricated, includes fitting and adjustment

⇒* L2036   Knee ankle foot orthosis, full plastic, double upright, with or without free motion knee, with or without free motion ankle, custom fabricated

⇒* L2037   Knee ankle foot orthosis, full plastic, single upright, with or without free motion knee, with or without free motion ankle, custom fabricated

⇒* L2038   Knee ankle foot orthosis, full plastic, with or without free motion knee, multi-axis ankle, custom fabricated

L2039   Deleted 12/31/05

Torsion Control

* L2040   Hip-knee-ankle-foot orthosis (HKAFO), torsion control, bilateral rotation straps, pelvic band/belt, custom fabrication

* L2050   HKAFO, torsion control, bilateral torsion cables, hip joint, pelvic band/belt, custom fabrication

* L2060   HKAFO, torsion control, bilateral torsion cables, ball bearing hip joint, pelvic band/belt, custom fabrication

* L2070   HKAFO, torsion control, unilateral rotation straps, pelvic band/belt, custom fabrication

* L2080   HKAFO, torsion control, unilateral torsion cable, hip joint, pelvic band/belt, custom fabrication

* L2090   HKAFO, torsion control, unilateral torsion cable, ball bearing hip joint, pelvic band/belt, custom fabrication

Fracture Orthoses

* L2106   AFO, fracture orthosis, tibial fracture cast orthosis, thermoplastic type casting material, custom fabrication

* L2108   AFO, fracture orthosis, tibial fracture cast orthosis, custom fabrication

* L2112   AFO, fracture orthosis, tibial fracture orthosis, soft, prefabricated, includes fitting and adjustment

* L2114   AFO, fracture orthosis, tibial fracture orthosis, semi-rigid, prefabricated, includes fitting and adjustment

* L2116   AFO, fracture orthosis, tibial fracture orthosis, rigid, prefabricated, includes fitting and adjustment

* L2126   KAFO, fracture orthosis, femoral fracture cast orthosis, thermoplastic type casting material, custom fabrication

* L2128   KAFO, fracture orthosis, femoral fracture cast orthosis, custom fabrication

* L2132   KAFO, fracture orthosis, femoral fracture cast orthosis, soft, prefabricated, includes fitting and adjustment

* L2134   KAFO, fracture orthosis, femoral fracture cast orthosis, semi-rigid, prefabricated, includes fitting and adjustment
* L2136   KAFO, fracture orthosis, femoral fracture cast orthosis, rigid, prefabricated, includes fitting and adjustment

Additions to Fracture Orthosis

* L2180   Addition to lower extremity fracture orthosis, plastic shoe insert with ankle joints
* L2182   Addition to lower extremity fracture orthosis, drop lock knee joint
* L2184   Addition to lower extremity fracture orthosis, limited motion knee joint
* L2186   Addition to lower extremity fracture orthosis, adjustable motion knee joint (Lerman type)
* L2188   Addition to lower extremity fracture orthosis, quadrilateral brim
* L2190   Addition to lower extremity fracture orthosis, waist belt
* L2192   Addition to lower extremity fracture orthosis, hip joint, pelvic band, thigh flange, and pelvic belt

Additions to Lower Extremity Orthosis

Shoe-Ankle-Shin-Knee

* L2200   Addition to lower extremity, limited ankle motion, each joint
* L2210   Addition to lower extremity, dorsiflexion assist (plantar flexion resist), each joint
* L2220   Addition to lower extremity, dorsiflexion and plantar flexion assist/resist, each joint
* L2230   Addition to lower extremity, split flat caliper stirrups and plate attachment
* L2232   Addition to lower extremity orthosis, rocker bottom for total contact ankle foot orthosis, for custom fabricated orthosis only
* L2240   Addition to lower extremity, round caliper and plate attachment
* L2250   Addition to lower extremity, footplate, molded to patient model, stirrup attachment
* L2260   Addition to lower extremity, reinforced solid stirrup (Scott-Craig type)
* L2265   Addition to lower extremity, long tongue stirrup
* L2270   Addition to lower extremity, varus/valgus correction (T) strap, padded/lined or malleolus pad
* L2275   Addition to lower extremity, varus/valgus correction, plastic modification, padded/lined

* L2280   Addition to lower extremity, molded inner boot
* L2300   Addition to lower extremity, abduction bar (bilateral hip involvement), jointed, adjustable
* L2310   Addition to lower extremity, abduction bar, straight
* L2320   Addition to lower extremity, non-molded lacer, for custom fabricated orthosis only
* L2330   Addition to lower extremity, lacer molded to patient model, for custom fabricated orthosis only
* L2335   Addition to lower extremity, anterior swing band
* L2340   Addition to lower extremity, pre-tibial shell, molded to patient model
* L2350   Addition to lower extremity, prosthetic type, (BK) socket, molded to patient model, (used for PTB and AFO orthoses)
* L2360   Addition to lower extremity, extended steel shank
* L2370   Addition to lower extremity, Patten bottom
* L2375   Addition to lower extremity, torsion control, ankle joint and half solid stirrup
* L2380   Addition to lower extremity, torsion control, straight knee joint, each joint
* L2385   Addition to lower extremity, straight knee joint, heavy duty, each joint
▶ * L2387   Addition to lower extremity, polycentric knee joint, for custom fabricated knee ankle foot orthosis, each joint
* L2390   Addition to lower extremity, offset knee joint, each joint
* L2395   Addition to lower extremity, offset knee joint, heavy duty, each joint
* L2397   Addition to lower extremity orthosis, suspension sleeve

Additions to Straight Knee or Offset Knee Joints

⇒ * L2405   Addition to knee joint, drop lock, each
* L2415   Addition to knee lock with integrated release mechanism (bail, cable, or equal), any material, each joint
* L2425   Addition to knee joint, disc or dial lock for adjustable knee flexion, each joint
* L2430   Addition to knee joint, ratchet lock for active and progressive knee extension, each joint
* L2492   Addition to knee joint, lift loop for drop lock ring

Additions to Thigh/Weight Bearing

Gluteal/Ischial Weight Bearing

* L2500   Addition to lower extremity, thigh/weight bearing, gluteal/ischial weight bearing, ring

* L2510   Addition to lower extremity, thigh/weight bearing, quadri-lateral brim, molded to patient model

* L2520   Addition to lower extremity, thigh/weight bearing, quadri-lateral brim, custom fitted

* L2525   Addition to lower extremity, thigh/weight bearing, ischial containment/narrow M-L brim molded to patient model

* L2526   Addition to lower extremity, thigh/weight bearing, ischial containment/narrow M-L brim, custom fitted

* L2530   Addition to lower extremity, thigh-weight bearing, lacer, non-molded

* L2540   Addition to lower extremity, thigh/weight bearing, lacer, molded to patient model

* L2550   Addition to lower extremity, thigh/weight bearing, high roll cuff

Additions to Pelvic and Thoracic Control

* L2570   Addition to lower extremity, pelvic control, hip joint, Clevis type two position joint, each

* L2580   Addition to lower extremity, pelvic control, pelvic sling

* L2600   Addition to lower extremity, pelvic control, hip joint, Clevis type, or thrust bearing, free, each

* L2610   Addition to lower extremity, pelvic control, hip joint, Clevis or thrust bearing, lock, each

* L2620   Addition to lower extremity, pelvic control, hip joint, heavy duty, each

* L2622   Addition to lower extremity, pelvic control, hip joint, adjustable flexion, each

* L2624   Addition to lower extremity, pelvic control, hip joint, adjustable flexion, extension, abduction control, each

* L2627   Addition to lower extremity, pelvic control, plastic, molded to patient model, reciprocating hip joint and cables

* L2628   Addition to lower extremity, pelvic control, metal frame, reciprocating hip joint and cables

* L2630   Addition to lower extremity, pelvic control, band and belt, unilateral

* L2640   Addition to lower extremity, pelvic control, band and belt, bilateral

* L2650   Addition to lower extremity, pelvic and thoracic control, gluteal pad, each

* L2660   Addition to lower extremity, thoracic control, thoracic band

* L2670   Addition to lower extremity, thoracic control, paraspinal uprights

* L2680   Addition to lower extremity, thoracic control, lateral support uprights

General Additions

* L2750   Addition to lower extremity orthosis, plating chrome or nickel, per bar

* L2755   Addition to lower extremity orthosis, high strength, lightweight material, all hybrid lamination/prepreg composite, per segment, for custom fabricated orthosis only

* L2760   Addition to lower extremity orthosis, extension, per extension, per bar (for lineal adjustment for growth)

* L2768   Orthotic side bar disconnect device, per bar

* L2770   Addition to lower extremity orthosis, any material—per bar or joint

* L2780   Addition to lower extremity orthosis, non-corrosive finish, per bar

* L2785   Addition to lower extremity orthosis, drop lock retainer, each

* L2795   Addition to lower extremity orthosis, knee control, full kneecap

* L2800   Addition to lower extremity orthosis, knee control, knee cap, medial or lateral pull, for use with custom fabricated orthosis only

* L2810   Addition to lower extremity orthosis, knee control, condylar pad

* L2820   Addition to lower extremity orthosis, soft interface for molded plastic, below knee section

* L2830   Addition to lower extremity orthosis, soft interface for molded plastic, above knee section

* L2840   Addition to lower extremity orthosis, tibial length sock, fracture or equal, each

* L2850   Addition to lower extremity orthosis, femoral length sock, fracture or equal, each

* L2860   Addition to lower extremity joint, knee or ankle, concentric adjustable torsion style mechanism, each

* L2999   Lower extremity orthoses, not otherwise specified

Foot (Orthopedic Shoes)

Insert, Removable, Molded to Patient Model

⊙ L3000   Foot, insert, removable, molded to patient model, UCB type, Berkeley shell, each
MCM 2323

⊙ L3001   Foot, insert, removable, molded to patient model, Spenco, each
MCM 2323

⊙ L3002   Foot, insert, removable, molded to patient model, Plastazote or equal, each
MCM 2323

⊛ L3003　Foot, insert, removable, molded to patient model, silicone gel, each
　　　　　MCM 2323

⊛ L3010　Foot, insert, removable, molded to patient model, longitudinal arch support, each
　　　　　MCM 2323

⊛ L3020　Foot, insert, removable, molded to patient model, longitudinal/metatarsal support, each
　　　　　MCM 2323

⊛ L3030　Foot, insert, removable, formed to patient foot, each
　　　　　MCM 2323

⇛ ✳ L3031　Foot, insert/plate, removable, addition to lower extremity orthosis, high strength, lightweight material, all hybrid lamination/prepreg composite, each

Arch Support, Removable, Premolded

⊛ L3040　Foot, arch support, removable, premolded, longitudinal, each
　　　　　MCM 2323

⊛ L3050　Foot, arch support, removable, premolded, metatarsal, each
　　　　　MCM 2323

⊛ L3060　Foot, arch support, removable, premolded, longitudinal/metatarsal, each
　　　　　MCM 2323

Arch Support, Non-removable, Attached to Shoe

⊛ L3070　Foot, arch support, non-removable attached to shoe, longitudinal, each
　　　　　MCM 2323

⊛ L3080　Foot, arch support, non-removable attached to shoe, metatarsal, each
　　　　　MCM 2323

⊛ L3090　Foot, arch support, non-removable attached to shoe, longitudinal/metatarsal, each
　　　　　MCM 2323

⊛ L3100　Hallus-valgus night dynamic splint
　　　　　MCM 2323

Abduction and Rotation Bars

⊛ L3140　Foot, abduction rotation bar, including shoes
　　　　　MCM 2323

⊛ L3150　Foot, abduction rotation bar, without shoes
　　　　　MCM 2323

✳ L3160　Foot, adjustable shoe-styled positioning device

⇛ ⊛ L3170　Foot, plastic, silicone or equal, heel stabilizer, each
　　　　　MCM 2323

Orthopedic Footwear

⊛ L3201　Orthopedic shoe, oxford with supinator or pronator, infant
　　　　　MCM 2323

⊛ L3202　Orthopedic shoe, oxford with supinator or pronator, child
　　　　　MCM 2323

⊛ L3203　Orthopedic shoe, oxford with supinator or pronator, junior
　　　　　MCM 2323

⊛ L3204　Orthopedic shoe, hightop with supinator or pronator, infant
　　　　　MCM 2323

⊛ L3206　Orthopedic shoe, hightop with supinator or pronator, child
　　　　　MCM 2323

⊛ L3207　Orthopedic shoe, hightop with supinator or pronator, junior
　　　　　MCM 2323

⊛ L3208　Surgical boot, infant, each
　　　　　MCM 2079

⊛ L3209　Surgical boot, each, child
　　　　　MCM 2079

⊛ L3211　Surgical boot, each, junior
　　　　　MCM 2079

⊛ L3212　Benesch boot, pair, infant
　　　　　MCM 2079

⊛ L3213　Benesch boot, pair, child
　　　　　MCM 2079

⊛ L3214　Benesch boot, pair, junior
　　　　　MCM 2079

⇛ ◆ L3215　Orthopedic footwear, ladies' shoe, oxford, each
　　　　　Medicare Statute 1862A8

⇛ ◆ L3216　Orthopedic footwear, ladies' shoe, depth inlay, each
　　　　　Medicare Statute 1862A8

⇛ ◆ L3217　Orthopedic footwear, ladies' shoe, hightop, depth inlay, each
　　　　　Medicare Statute 1862A8

⇛ ◆ L3219　Orthopedic footwear, men's shoe, oxford, each
　　　　　Medicare Statute 1862A8

⇛ ◆ L3221　Orthopedic footwear, men's shoe, depth inlay, each
　　　　　Medicare Statute 1862A8

⇛ ◆ L3222　Orthopedic footwear, men's shoe, hightop, depth inlay, each
　　　　　Medicare Statute 1862A8

⊛ L3224　Orthopedic footwear, ladies' shoe, oxford, used as an integral part of a brace (orthosis)
　　　　　MCM 2323D

⊛ L3225　Orthopedic footwear, men's shoe, oxford, used as an integral part of a brace (orthosis)
　　　　　MCM 2323D

⇛ ⊛ L3230　Orthopedic footwear, custom shoe, depth inlay, each
　　　　　MCM 2323

⊙ L3250 Orthopedic footwear, custom molded shoe, removable inner mold, prosthetic shoe, each
MCM 2323

⊙ L3251 Foot, shoe molded to patient model, silicone shoe, each
MCM 2323

⊙ L3252 Foot, shoe molded to patient model, Plastazote (or similar), custom fabricated, each
MCM 2323

⊙ L3253 Foot, molded shoe Plastazote (or similar), custom fitted, each
MCM 2323

⊙ L3254 Non-standard size or width
MCM 2323

⊙ L3255 Non-standard size or length
MCM 2323

⊙ L3257 Orthopedic footwear, additional charge for split size
MCM 2323

⊙ L3260 Surgical boot/shoe, each
MCM 2079

∗ L3265 Plastazote sandal, each

Shoe Modifications

Lifts

⊙ L3300 Lift, elevation, heel, tapered to metatarsals, per inch
MCM 2323

⊙ L3310 Lift, elevation, heel and sole, Neoprene, per inch
MCM 2323

⊙ L3320 Lift, elevation, heel and sole, cork, per inch
MCM 2323

⊙ L3330 Lift, elevation, metal extension (skate)
MCM 2323

⊙ L3332 Lift, elevation, inside shoe, tapered, up to 0.5 in
MCM 2323

⊙ L3334 Lift, elevation, heel, per inch
MCM 2323

Wedges

⊙ L3340 Heel wedge, SACH
MCM 2323

⊙ L3350 Heel wedge
MCM 2323

⊙ L3360 Sole wedge, outside sole
MCM 2323

⊙ L3370 Sole wedge, between sole
MCM 2323

⊙ L3380 Clubfoot wedge
MCM 2323

⊙ L3390 Outflare wedge
MCM 2323

⊙ L3400 Metatarsal bar wedge, rocker
MCM 2323

⊙ L3410 Metatarsal bar wedge, between sole
MCM 2323

⊙ L3420 Full sole and heel wedge, between sole
MCM 2323

Heels

⊙ L3430 Heel, counter, plastic reinforced
MCM 2323

⊙ L3440 Heel, counter, leather reinforced
MCM 2323

⊙ L3450 Heel, SACH cushion type
MCM 2323

⊙ L3455 Heel, new leather, standard
MCM 2323

⊙ L3460 Heel, new rubber, standard
MCM 2323

⊙ L3465 Heel, Thomas with wedge
MCM 2323

⊙ L3470 Heel, Thomas extended to ball
MCM 2323

⊙ L3480 Heel, pad and depression for spur
MCM 2323

⊙ L3485 Heel, pad, removable for spur
MCM 2323

Additions to Orthopedic Shoes

⊙ L3500 Orthopedic shoe addition, insole, leather
MCM 2323

⊙ L3510 Orthopedic shoe addition, insole, rubber
MCM 2323

⊙ L3520 Orthopedic shoe addition, insole, felt covered with leather
MCM 2323

⊙ L3530 Orthopedic shoe addition, sole, half
MCM 2323

⊙ L3540 Orthopedic shoe addition, sole, full
MCM 2323

⊙ L3550 Orthopedic shoe addition, toe tap, standard
MCM 2323

⊙ L3560 Orthopedic shoe addition, toe tap, horseshoe
MCM 2323

⊙ L3570 Orthopedic shoe addition, special extension to instep (leather with eyelets)
MCM 2323

⊙ L3580 Orthopedic shoe addition, convert instep to Velcro closure
MCM 2323

⊙ L3590 Orthopedic shoe addition, convert firm shoe counter to soft counter
MCM 2323

⊙ L3595 Orthopedic shoe addition, March bar
MCM 2323

Transfer or Replacement

☺ L3600   Transfer of an orthosis from one shoe to another, caliper plate, existing
     MCM 2323

☺ L3610   Transfer of an orthosis from one shoe to another, caliper plate, new
     MCM 2323

☺ L3620   Transfer of an orthosis from one shoe to another, solid stirrup, existing
     MCM 2323

☺ L3630   Transfer of an orthosis from one shoe to another, solid stirrup, new
     MCM 2323

☺ L3640   Transfer of an orthosis from one shoe to another, Dennis Browne splint (Riveton), both shoes
     MCM 2323

☺ L3649   Orthopedic shoe, modification, addition or transfer, not otherwise specified
     MCM 2323

Orthotic Devices: Upper Limb

NOTE: The procedures in this section are considered as *base* or *basic procedures* and may be modified by listing procedures from the Additions section and adding them to the base procedure.

Shoulder

* L3650   Shoulder orthosis, (SO), figure of eight (8) design abduction restrainer, prefabricated, includes fitting and adjustment

* L3651   Shoulder orthosis, single shoulder, elastic, prefabricated, includes fitting and adjustment (e.g. neoprene, Lycra)

* L3652   Shoulder orthosis, double shoulder, elastic, prefabricated, includes fitting and adjustment (e.g. neoprene, Lycra)

* L3660   SO, figure of eight (8) design abduction restrainer, canvas and webbing, prefabricated, includes fitting and adjustment

* L3670   SO, acromio/clavicular (canvas and webbing type), prefabricated, includes fitting and adjustment

▶* L3671   Shoulder orthosis, shoulder cap design, without joints, may include soft interface, straps, custom fabricated, includes fitting and adjustment

▶* L3672   Shoulder orthosis, abduction positioning (airplane design), thoracic component and support bar, without joints, may include soft interface, straps, custom fabricated, includes fitting and adjustment

▶* L3673   Shoulder orthosis, abduction positioning (airplane design), thoracic component and support bar, includes nontorsion joint/turnbuckle, may include soft interface, straps, custom fabricated, includes fitting and adjustment

* L3675   SO, vest type abduction restrainer, canvas webbing type, or equal, prefabricated, includes fitting and adjustment

☺ L3677   SO, hard plastic, shoulder stabilizer, pre-fabricated, includes fitting and adjustment
     MCM 2130

Elbow

* L3700   Elbow orthosis (EO), elastic with stays, prefabricated, includes fitting and adjustment

* L3701   Elbow orthosis, elastic, prefabricated, includes fitting and adjustment (e.g. neoprene, Lycra)

▶* L3702   Elbow orthosis, without joints, may include soft interface, straps, custom fabricated, includes fitting and adjustment

* L3710   EO, elastic with metal joints, prefabricated, includes fitting and adjustment

* L3720   EO, double upright with forearm/arm cuffs, free motion, custom fabrication

* L3730   EO, double upright with forearm/arm cuffs, extension/flexion assist, custom fabrication

* L3740   EO, double upright with forearm/arm cuffs, adjustable position lock with active control, custom fabrication

* L3760   Elbow orthosis, with adjustable position locking joint(s), prefabricated, includes fitting and adjustments, any type

* L3762   Elbow orthosis, rigid, without joints, includes soft interface material, prefabricated, includes fitting and adjustment

▶* L3763   Elbow wrist hand orthosis, rigid, without joints, may include soft interface, straps, custom fabricated, includes fitting and adjustment

▶* L3764   Elbow wrist hand orthosis, includes one or more nontorsion joints, elastic bands, turnbuckles, may include soft interface, straps, custom fabricated, includes fitting and adjustment

▶* L3765   Elbow wrist hand finger orthosis, rigid, without joints, may include soft interface, straps, custom fabricated, includes fitting and adjustment

▶* L3766   Elbow wrist hand finger orthosis, includes one or more nontorsion joints, elastic bands, turnbuckles, may include soft interface, straps, custom fabricated, includes fitting and adjustment

Wrist-Hand-Finger Orthosis (WHFO)

* L3800   Wrist-hand-finger orthosis (WHFO), short opponens, no attachments, custom fabrication
* L3805   Wrist-hand-finger orthosis (WHFO), long opponens, no attachment, custom fabrication
* L3807   Wrist-hand-finger orthosis (WHFO), without joint(s), prefabricated, includes fitting and adjustments, any type

Additions and Extensions

* L3810   Wrist-hand-finger orthosis (WHFO), addition to short and long opponens, thumb abduction (C) bar
* L3815   Wrist-hand-finger orthosis (WHFO), addition to short and long opponens, second MP abduction assist
* L3820   Wrist-hand-finger orthosis (WHFO), addition to short and long opponens, IP extension assist, with MP extension stop
* L3825   Wrist-hand-finger orthosis (WHFO), addition to short and long opponens, MP extension stop
* L3830   Wrist-hand-finger orthosis (WHFO), addition to short and long opponens, MP extension assist
* L3835   Wrist-hand-finger orthosis (WHFO), addition to short and long opponens, MP spring extension assist
* L3840   Wrist-hand-finger orthosis (WHFO), addition to short and long opponens, spring swivel thumb
* L3845   Wrist-hand-finger orthosis (WHFO), addition to short and long opponens, thumb IP extension assist, with MP stop
* L3850   WHO, addition to short and long opponens, action wrist, with dorsiflexion assist
* L3855   Wrist-hand-finger orthosis (WHFO), addition to short and long opponens, adjustable MP flexion control
* L3860   Wrist-hand-finger orthosis (WHFO), addition to short and long opponens, adjustable MP flexion control and IP
* L3890   Addition to upper extremity joint, wrist or elbow, concentric adjustable torsion style mechanism, each
* L3900   Wrist-hand-finger orthosis (WHFO), dynamic flexor hinge, reciprocal wrist extension/flexion, finger flexion/extension, wrist or finger driven, custom fabrication
* L3901   Wrist-hand-finger orthosis (WHFO), dynamic flexor hinge, reciprocal wrist extension/flexion, finger flexion/extension, cable driven, custom fabrication

External Power

◆ L3902   Wrist-hand-finger orthosis (WHFO), external powered, compressed gas, custom fabrication
* L3904   Wrist-hand-finger orthosis (WHFO), external powered, electric, custom fabrication
▶ * L3905   Wrist hand orthosis, includes one or more nontorsion joints, elastic bands, turnbuckles, may include soft interface, straps, custom fabricated, includes fitting and adjustment

Other Wrist-Hand-Finger Orthoses: Custom Fitted

⇒ * L3906   Wrist hand orthosis, without joints, may include soft interface, straps, custom fabricated, includes fitting and adjustment
* L3907   Wrist-hand-finger orthosis (WHFO), wrist gauntlet with thumb spica, molded to patient model, custom fabrication
* L3908   WHO, wrist extension control cock-up, non-molded, prefabricated, includes fitting and adjustment
* L3909   Wrist orthosis, elastic, prefabricated, includes fitting and adjustment (e.g. neoprene, Lycra)
* L3910   Wrist-hand-finger orthosis (WHFO), Swanson design, prefabricated, includes fitting and adjustment
* L3911   Wrist hand finger orthosis, elastic, prefabricated, includes fitting and adjustment (e.g. neoprene, Lycra)
* L3912   HFO, flexion glove with elastic finger control, prefabricated, includes fitting and adjustment
▶ * L3913   Hand finger orthosis, without joints, may include soft interface, straps, custom fabricated, includes fitting and adjustment
* L3914   WHO, wrist extension cock-up, prefabricated, includes fitting and adjustment
* L3916   Wrist-hand-finger orthosis (WHFO), wrist extension cock-up, with outrigger, prefabricated, includes fitting and adjustment
* L3917   Hand orthosis, metacarpal fracture orthosis, prefabricated, includes fitting and adjustment
* L3918   HFO, knuckle bender, prefabricated, includes fitting and adjustment
▶ * L3919   Hand orthosis, without joints, may include soft interface, straps, custom fabricated, includes fitting and adjustment
* L3920   HFO, knuckle bender, with outrigger, prefabricated, includes fitting and adjustment

▶ ✳ L3921 Hand finger orthosis, includes one or more nontorsion joints, elastic bands, turnbuckles, may include soft interface, straps, custom fabricated, includes fitting and adjustment

✳ L3922 HFO, knuckle bender, two segment to flex joints, prefabricated, includes fitting and adjustment

⇒ ✳ L3923 Hand finger orthosis, without joints, may include soft interface, straps, prefabricated, includes fitting and adjustments

✳ L3924 Wrist-hand-finger orthosis (WHFO), Oppenheimer, prefabricated, includes fitting and adjustment

✳ L3926 Wrist-hand-finger orthosis (WHFO), Thomas suspension, prefabricated, includes fitting and adjustment

✳ L3928 HFO, finger extension, with clock spring, prefabricated, includes fitting and adjustment

✳ L3930 Wrist-hand-finger orthosis (WHFO), finger extension, with wrist support, prefabricated, includes fitting and adjustment

✳ L3932 FO, safety pin, spring wire, prefabricated, includes fitting and adjustment

▶ ✳ L3933 Finger orthosis, without joints, may include soft interface, custom fabricated, includes fitting and adjustment

✳ L3934 FO, safety pin, modified, prefabricated, includes fitting and adjustment

▶ ✳ L3935 Finger orthosis, nontorsion joint, may include soft interface, custom fabricated, includes fitting and adjustment

✳ L3936 Wrist-hand-finger orthosis (WHFO), palmar, prefabricated, includes fitting and adjustment

✳ L3938 Wrist-hand-finger orthosis (WHFO), dorsal wrist, prefabricated, includes fitting and adjustment

✳ L3940 Wrist-hand-finger orthosis (WHFO), dorsal wrist, with outrigger attachment, prefabricated, includes fitting and adjustment

✳ L3942 HFO, reverse knuckle bender, prefabricated, includes fitting and adjustment

✳ L3944 HFO, reverse knuckle bender, with outrigger, prefabricated, includes fitting and adjustment

✳ L3946 HFO, composite elastic, prefabricated, includes fitting and adjustment

✳ L3948 FO, finger knuckle bender, prefabricated, includes fitting and adjustment

✳ L3950 Wrist-hand-finger orthosis (WHFO), combination Oppenheimer, with knuckle bender and two attachments, prefabricated, includes fitting and adjustment

✳ L3952 Wrist-hand-finger orthosis (WHFO), combination Oppenheimer, with reverse knuckle and two attachments, prefabricated, includes fitting and adjustment

✳ L3954 HFO, spreading hand, prefabricated, includes fitting and adjustment

✳ L3956 Addition of joint to upper extremity orthosis, any material, per joint

Shoulder-Elbow-Wrist-Hand Orthosis (SEWHO)

Abduction Positioning: Custom Fitted

✳ L3960 Shoulder-elbow-wrist-hand orthosis, (SEWHO), abduction positioning, airplane design, prefabricated, includes fitting and adjustment

▶ ✳ L3961 Shoulder elbow wrist hand orthosis, shoulder cap design, without joints, may include soft interface, straps, custom fabricated, includes fitting and adjustment

✳ L3962 SEWHO, abduction positioning, Erb's palsy design, prefabricated, includes fitting and adjustment

L3963 Deleted 12/31/05

✳ L3964 SEO, mobile arm support attached to wheelchair, balanced, adjustable, prefabricated, includes fitting and adjustment

✳ L3965 SEO, mobile arm support attached to wheelchair, balanced, adjustable Rancho type, prefabricated, includes fitting and adjustment

✳ L3966 SEO, mobile arm support attached to wheelchair, balanced, reclining, prefabricated, includes fitting and adjustment

▶ ✳ L3967 Shoulder elbow wrist hand orthosis, abduction positioning (airplane design), thoracic component and support bar, without joints, may include soft interface, straps, custom fabricated, includes fitting and adjustment

✳ L3968 SEO, mobile arm support attached to wheelchair, balanced, friction arm support (friction dampening to proximal and distal joints), prefabricated, includes fitting and adjustment

✳ L3969 SEO, mobile arm support, monosuspension arm and hand support, overhead elbow forearm hand sling support, yoke type arm suspension support, prefabricated, includes fitting and adjustment

Additions to Mobile Arm Supports and SEWHO

* L3970   SEO, addition to mobile arm support, elevating proximal arm

▶ * L3971   Shoulder elbow wrist hand orthosis, shoulder cap design, includes one or more nontorsion joints, elastic bands, turnbuckles, may include soft interface, straps, custom fabricated, includes fitting and adjustment

* L3972   SEO, addition to mobile arm support, offset or lateral rocker arm with elastic balance control

▶ * L3973   Shoulder elbow wrist hand orthosis, abduction positioning (airplane design), thoracic component and support bar, includes one or more nontorsion joints, elastic bands, turnbuckles, may include soft interface, straps, custom fabricated, includes fitting and adjustment

* L3974   SEO, addition to mobile arm support, supinator

▶ * L3975   Shoulder elbow wrist hand finger orthosis, shoulder cap design, without joints, may include soft interface, straps, custom fabricated, includes fitting and adjustment

▶ * L3976   Shoulder elbow wrist hand finger orthosis, abduction positioning (airplane design), thoracic component and support bar, without joints, may include soft interface, straps, custom fabricated, includes fitting and adjustment

▶ * L3977   Shoulder elbow wrist hand finger orthosis, shoulder cap design, includes one or more nontorsion joints, elastic bands, turnbuckles, may include soft interface, straps, custom fabricated, includes fitting and adjustment

▶ * L3978   Shoulder elbow wrist hand finger orthosis, abduction positioning (airplane design), thoracic component and support bar, includes one or more nontorsion joints, elastic bands, turnbuckles, may include soft interface, straps, custom fabricated, includes fitting and adjustment

Fracture Orthoses

* L3980   Upper extremity fracture orthosis, humeral, prefabricated, includes fitting and adjustment

* L3982   Upper extremity fracture orthosis, radius/ulnar, prefabricated, includes fitting and adjustment

* L3984   Upper extremity fracture orthosis, wrist, prefabricated, includes fitting and adjustment

* L3985   Upper extremity fracture orthosis, forearm, hand with wrist hinge, custom fabrication

* L3986   Upper extremity fracture orthosis, combination of humeral, radius/ulnar, wrist, (e.g., Colles' fracture), custom fabrication

* L3995   Addition to upper extremity orthosis, sock, fracture or equal, each

* L3999   Upper limb orthosis, not otherwise specified

Specific Repair

* L4000   Replace girdle for spinal orthosis (CTLSO or SO)

* L4002   Replacement strap, any orthosis; includes all components, any length, any type

* L4010   Replace trilateral socket brim

* L4020   Replace quadrilateral socket brim, molded to patient model

* L4030   Replace quadrilateral socket brim, custom fitted

* L4040   Replace molded thigh lacer, for custom fabricated orthosis only

* L4045   Replace non-molded thigh lacer, for custom fabricated orthosis only

* L4050   Replace molded calf lacer, for custom fabricated orthosis only

* L4055   Replace non-molded calf lacer, for custom fabricated orthosis only

* L4060   Replace high roll cuff

* L4070   Replace proximal and distal upright for KAFO

* L4080   Replace metal bands, KAFO, proximal thigh

* L4090   Replace metal bands, KAFO-AFO, calf or distal thigh

* L4100   Replace leather cuff, KAFO, proximal thigh

* L4110   Replace leather cuff, KAFO-AFO, calf or distal thigh

* L4130   Replace pretibial shell

Repairs

⊙ L4205   Repair of orthotic device, labor component, per 15 minutes
MCM 2100.4

⊙ L4210   Repair of orthotic device, repair or replace minor parts
MCM 2100.4, MCM 2130D, MCM 2133

Ancillary Orthotic Services

* L4350   Ankle control orthosis, stirrup style, rigid, includes any type interface (e.g., pneumatic, gel), prefabricated, includes fitting and adjustment

* L4360   Walking boot, pneumatic, with or without joints, with or without interface material, prefabricated, includes fitting and adjustment
* L4370   Pneumatic full leg splint, prefabricated, includes fitting and adjustment
* L4380   Pneumatic knee splint, prefabricated, includes fitting and adjustment
* L4386   Walking boot, non-pneumatic, with or without joints, with or without interface material, prefabricated, includes fitting and adjustment
* L4392   Replace soft interface material, static AFO
* L4394   Replace soft interface material, foot drop splint
* L4396   Static AFO, including soft interface material, adjustable for fit, for positioning, pressure reduction, may be used for minimal ambulation, prefabricated, includes fitting and adjustment
* L4398   Foot drop splint, recumbent positioning device, prefabricated, includes fitting and adjustment

PROSTHETIC PROCEDURES (L5000-L9999)

Lower Limb (L5000-L5999)

NOTE: The procedures in this sections are considered as *base* or *basic procedures* and may be modified by listing items/procedures or special materials from the Additions section and adding them to the base procedure.

Partial Foot

* ⊛ L5000   Partial foot, shoe insert with longitudinal arch, toe filler
  MCM 2323
* ⊛ L5010   Partial foot, molded socket, ankle height, with toe filler
  MCM 2323
* ⊛ L5020   Partial foot, molded socket, tibial tubercle height, with toe filler
  MCM 2323

Ankle

* L5050   Ankle, Symes, molded socket, SACH (solid ankle cushion heel) foot
* L5060   Ankle, Symes, metal frame, molded leather socket, articulated ankle/foot

Below Knee

* L5100   Below knee, molded socket, shin, SACH (solid ankle cushion heel) foot

* L5105   Below knee, plastic socket, joints and thigh lacer, SACH (solid ankle cushion heel) foot

Knee Disarticulation

* L5150   Knee disarticulation (or through knee), molded socket, external knee joints, shin, SACH (solid ankle cushion heel) foot
* L5160   Knee disarticulation (or through knee), molded socket, bent knee configuration, external knee joints, shin, SACH (solid ankle cushion heel) foot

Above Knee

* L5200   Above knee, molded socket, single axis constant friction knee, shin, SACH (solid ankle cushion heel) foot
* L5210   Above knee, short prosthesis, no knee joint ('stubbies'), with foot blocks, no ankle joints, each
* L5220   Above knee, short prosthesis, no knee joint ('stubbies'), with articulated ankle/foot, dynamically aligned, each
* L5230   Above knee, for proximal femoral focal deficiency, constant friction knee, shin, SACH (solid ankle cushion heel) foot

Hip Disarticulation

* L5250   Hip disarticulation, Canadian type; molded socket, hip joint, single axis constant friction knee, shin, SACH (solid ankle cushion heel) foot
* L5270   Hip disarticulation, tilt table type; molded socket, locking hip joint, single axis constant friction knee, shin, SACH (solid ankle cushion heel) foot

Hemipelvectomy

* L5280   Hemipelvectomy, Canadian type; molded socket, hip joint, single axis constant friction knee, shin, SACH (solid ankle cushion heel) foot

Endoskeleton: Below Knee

* L5301   Below knee, molded socket, shin, SACH (solid ankle cushion heel) foot, endoskeletal system

Endoskeletal: Knee Disarticulation

* L5311   Knee disarticulation (or through knee), molded socket, external knee joints, shin, SACH (solid ankle cushion heel) foot, endoskeletal system

Endoskeletal: Above Knee

* L5321   Above knee, molded socket, open end, SACH (solid ankle cushion heel) foot, endoskeletal system, single axis knee

Endoskeletal: Hip Disarticulation

* L5331   Hip disarticulation, Canadian type, molded socket, endoskeletal system, hip joint, single axis knee, SACH (solid ankle cushion heel) foot

Endoskeletal: Hemipelvectomy

* L5341   Hemipelvectomy, Canadian type, molded socket, endoskeletal system, hip joint, single axis knee, SACH (solid ankle cushion heel) foot

Immediate Postsurgical or Early Fitting Procedures

* L5400   Immediate postsurgical or early fitting, application of initial rigid dressing, including fitting, alignment, suspension, and one cast change, below knee

* L5410   Immediate post surgical or early fitting, application of initial rigid dressing, including fitting, alignment and suspension, below knee, each additional cast change and realignment

* L5420   Immediate postsurgical or early fitting, application of initial rigid dressing, including fitting, alignment and suspension and one cast change AK or knee disarticulation

* L5430   Immediate postsurgical or early fitting, application of initial rigid dressing, including fitting, alignment and suspension, AK or knee disarticulation, each additional cast change and realignment

* L5450   Immediate postsurgical or early fitting, application of non-weight bearing rigid dressing, below knee

* L5460   Immediate postsurgical or early fitting, application of non-weight bearing rigid dressing, above knee

Initial Prosthesis

* L5500   Initial, below knee PTB type socket, non-alignable system, pylon, no cover, SACH (solid ankle cushion heel) foot, plaster socket, direct formed

* L5505   Initial, above knee–knee disarticulation, ischial level socket, non-alignable system, pylon, no cover, SACH (solid ankle cushion heel) foot, plaster socket, direct formed

Preparatory Prosthesis

* L5510   Preparatory, below knee PTB type socket, non-alignable system, pylon, no cover, SACH (solid ankle cushion heel) foot, plaster socket, molded to model

* L5520   Preparatory, below knee PTB type socket, non-alignable system, pylon, no cover, SACH (solid ankle cushion heel) foot, thermoplastic or equal, direct formed

* L5530   Preparatory, below knee PTB type socket, non-alignable system, pylon, no cover, SACH (solid ankle cushion heel) foot, thermoplastic or equal, molded to model

* L5535   Preparatory, below knee PTB type socket, non-alignable system, no cover, SACH (solid ankle cushion heel) foot, prefabricated, adjustable open end socket

* L5540   Preparatory, below knee PTB type socket, non-alignable system, pylon, no cover, SACH (solid ankle cushion heel) foot, laminated socket, molded to model

* L5560   Preparatory, above knee-knee disarticulation, ischial level socket, non-alignable system, pylon, no cover, SACH (solid ankle cushion heel) foot, plaster socket, molded to model

* L5570   Preparatory, above knee-knee disarticulation, ischial level socket, non-alignable system, pylon, no cover, SACH (solid ankle cushion heel) foot, thermoplastic or equal, direct formed

* L5580   Preparatory, above knee-knee disarticulation, ischial level socket, non-alignable system, pylon, no cover, SACH (solid ankle cushion heel) foot, thermoplastic or equal, molded to model

* L5585   Preparatory, above knee-knee disarticulation, ischial level socket, non-alignable system, pylon, no cover, SACH (solid ankle cushion heel) foot, prefabricated adjustable open end socket

* L5590   Preparatory, above knee-knee disarticulation, ischial level socket, non-alignable system, pylon, no cover, SACH (solid ankle cushion heel) foot, laminated socket, molded to model
* L5595   Preparatory, hip disarticulation-hemipelvectomy, pylon, no cover, SACH (solid ankle cushion heel) foot, thermoplastic or equal, molded to patient model
* L5600   Preparatory, hip disarticulation-hemipelvectomy, pylon, no cover, SACH (solid ankle cushion heel) foot, laminated socket, molded to patient model

Additions to Lower Extremity

* L5610   Addition to lower extremity, endoskeletal system, above knee, hydracadence system
* L5611   Addition to lower extremity, endoskeletal system, above knee-knee disarticulation, 4-bar link-age, with friction wing phase control
* L5613   Addition to lower extremity, endoskeletal system, above knee-knee disarticulation, 4-bar linkage, with hydraulic swing phase control
* L5614   Addition to lower extremity, exoskeletal system, above knee-knee disarticulation, 4-bar linkage, with pneumatic swing phase control
* L5616   Addition to lower extremity, endoskeletal system, above knee, universal multiplex system, friction swing phase control
* L5617   Addition to lower extremity, quick change self-aligning unit, above knee or below knee, each

Additions to Test Sockets

* L5618   Addition to lower extremity, test socket, Symes
* L5620   Addition to lower extremity, test socket, below knee
* L5622   Addition to lower extremity, test socket, knee disarticulation
* L5624   Addition to lower extremity, test socket, above knee
* L5626   Addition to lower extremity, test socket, hip disarticulation
* L5628   Addition to lower extremity, test socket, hemipelvectomy
* L5629   Addition to lower extremity, below knee, acrylic socket

Additions to Socket Variations

* L5630   Addition to lower extremity, Symes type, expandable wall socket
* L5631   Addition to lower extremity, above knee or knee disarticulation, acrylic socket
* L5632   Addition to lower extremity, Symes type, PTB brim design socket
* L5634   Addition to lower extremity, Symes type, posterior opening (Canadian) socket
* L5636   Addition to lower extremity, Symes type, medial opening socket
* L5637   Addition to lower extremity, below knee, total contact
* L5638   Addition to lower extremity, below knee, leather socket
* L5639   Addition to lower extremity, below knee, wood socket
* L5640   Addition to lower extremity, knee disarticulation, leather socket
* L5642   Addition to lower extremity, above knee, leather socket
* L5643   Addition to lower extremity, hip disarticulation, flexible inner socket, external frame
* L5644   Addition to lower extremity, above knee, wood socket
* L5645   Addition to lower extremity, below knee, flexible inner socket, external frame
* L5646   Addition to lower extremity, below knee, air, fluid, gel or equal, cushion socket
* L5647   Addition to lower extremity, below knee, suction socket
* L5648   Addition to lower extremity, above knee, air, fluid, gel or equal, cushion socket
* L5649   Addition to lower extremity, ischial containment/narrow M-L socket
* L5650   Additions to lower extremity, total contact, above knee or knee disarticulation socket
* L5651   Addition to lower extremity, above knee, flexible inner socket, external frame
* L5652   Addition to lower extremity, suction suspension, above knee or knee disarticulation socket
* L5653   Addition to lower extremity, knee disarticulation, expandable wall socket

Additions to Socket Insert and Suspension

* L5654   Addition to lower extremity, socket insert, Symes, (Kemblo, Pelite, Aliplast, Plastazote or equal)

* L5655 Addition to lower extremity, socket insert, below knee (Kemblo, Pelite, Aliplast, Plastazote or equal)

* L5656 Addition to lower extremity, socket insert, knee disarticulation (Kemblo, Pelite, Aliplast, Plastazote or equal)

* L5658 Addition to lower extremity, socket insert, above knee (Kemblo, Pelite, Aliplast, Plastazote or equal)

* L5661 Addition to lower extremity, socket insert, multi-durometer Symes

* L5665 Addition to lower extremity, socket insert, multi-durometer, below knee

* L5666 Addition to lower extremity, below knee, cuff suspension

* L5668 Addition to lower extremity, below knee, molded distal cushion

* L5670 Addition to lower extremity, below knee, molded supracondylar suspension (PTS or similar)

* L5671 Addition to lower extremity, below knee/above knee suspension locking mechanism (shuttle, lanyard or equal), excludes socket insert

* L5672 Addition to lower extremity, below knee, removable medial brim suspension

* L5673 Addition to lower extremity, below knee/above knee, custom fabricated from existing mold or prefabricated, socket insert, silicone gel, elastomeric or equal, for use with locking mechanism

* L5676 Addition to lower extremity, below knee, knee joints, single axis, pair

* L5677 Addition to lower extremity, below knee, knee joints, polycentric, pair

* L5678 Addition to lower extremity, below knee, joint covers, pair

* L5679 Addition to lower extremity, below knee/above knee, custom fabricated from existing mold or prefabricated, socket insert, silicone gel, elastomeric or equal, not for use with locking mechanism

* L5680 Addition to lower extremity, below knee, thigh lacer, non-molded

* L5681 Addition to lower extremity, below knee/above knee, custom fabricated socket insert for congenital or atypical traumatic amputee, silicone gel, elastomeric or equal, for use with or without locking mechanism, initial only (for other than initial, use code L5673 or L5679)

* L5682 Addition to lower extremity, below knee, thigh lacer, gluteal/ischial, molded

* L5683 Addition to lower extremity, below knee/above knee, custom fabricated socket insert for other than congenital or atypical traumatic amputee, silicone gel, elastomeric or equal, for use with or without locking mechanism, initial only (for other than initial, use code L5673 or L5679)

* L5684 Addition to lower extremity, below knee, fork strap

* L5685 Addition to lower extremity prosthesis, below knee, suspension/sealing sleeve, with or without valve, any material, each

* L5686 Addition to lower extremity, below knee, back check (extension control)

* L5688 Addition to lower extremity, below knee, waist belt, webbing

* L5690 Addition to lower extremity, below knee, waist belt, padded and lined

* L5692 Addition to lower extremity, above knee, pelvic control belt, light

* L5694 Addition to lower extremity, above knee, pelvic control belt, padded and lined

* L5695 Addition to lower extremity, above knee, pelvic control, sleeve suspension, neoprene or equal, each

* L5696 Addition to lower extremity, above knee or knee disarticulation, pelvic joint

* L5697 Addition to lower extremity, above knee or knee disarticulation, pelvic band

* L5698 Addition to lower extremity, above knee or knee disarticulation, Silesian bandage

* L5699 All lower extremity prostheses, shoulder harness

Additions to Feet-Ankle Units

* L5700 Replacement, socket, below knee, molded to patient model

* L5701 Replacement, socket, above knee-knee disarticulation, including attachment plate, molded to patient model

* L5702 Replacement, socket, hip disarticulation, including hip joint, molded to patient model

▶ * L5703 Ankle, Symes, molded to patient model, socket without solid ankle cushion heel (Sach) foot, replacement only

* L5704 Custom shaped protective cover, below knee

* L5705 Custom shaped protective cover, above knee

* L5706 Custom shaped protective cover, knee disarticulation

* L5707 Custom shaped protective cover, hip disarticulation

Additions to Exoskeletal—Knee-Shin System

∗ L5710   Addition, exoskeletal knee-shin system, single axis, manual lock

∗ L5711   Addition, exoskeletal knee-shin system, single axis, manual lock, ultralight material

∗ L5712   Addition, exoskeletal knee-shin system, single axis, friction swing and stance phase control (safety knee)

∗ L5714   Addition, exoskeletal knee-shin system, single axis, variable friction swing phase control

∗ L5716   Addition, exoskeletal knee-shin system, polycentric, mechanical stance phase lock

∗ L5718   Addition, exoskeletal knee-shin system, polycentric, friction swing and stance phase control

∗ L5722   Addition, exoskeletal knee-shin system, single axis, pneumatic swing, friction stance phase control

∗ L5724   Addition, exoskeletal knee-shin system, single axis, fluid swing phase control

∗ L5726   Addition, exoskeletal knee-shin system, single axis, external joints, fluid swing phase control

∗ L5728   Addition, exoskeletal knee-shin system, single axis, fluid swing and stance phase control

∗ L5780   Addition, exoskeletal knee-shin system, single axis, pneumatic/hydra pneumatic swing phase control

∗ L5781   Addition to lower limb prosthesis, vacuum pump, residual limb volume management and moisture evacuation system

∗ L5782   Addition to lower limb prosthesis, vacuum pump, residual limb volume management and moisture evacuation system, heavy duty

Component Modification

∗ L5785   Addition, exoskeletal system, below knee, ultra-light material (titanium, carbon fiber or equal)

∗ L5790   Addition, exoskeletal system, above knee, ultra-light material (titanium, carbon fiber or equal)

∗ L5795   Addition, exoskeletal system, hip disarticulation, ultra-light material (titanium, carbon fiber or equal)

Endoskeletal

∗ L5810   Addition, endoskeletal knee-shin system, single axis, manual lock

∗ L5811   Addition, endoskeletal knee-shin system, single axis, manual lock, ultra light material

∗ L5812   Addition, endoskeletal knee-shin system, single axis, friction swing and stance phase control (safety knee)

∗ L5814   Addition, endoskeletal knee-shin system, polycentric, hydraulic swing phase control, mechanical stance phase lock

∗ L5816   Addition, endoskeletal knee-shin system, polycentric, mechanical stance phase lock

∗ L5818   Addition, endoskeletal knee-shin system, polycentric, friction swing, and stance phase control

∗ L5822   Addition, endoskeletal knee-shin system, single axis, pneumatic swing, friction stance phase control

∗ L5824   Addition, endoskeletal knee-shin system, single axis, fluid swing phase control

∗ L5826   Addition, endoskeletal knee-shin system, single axis, hydraulic swing phase control, with miniature high activity frame

∗ L5828   Addition, endoskeletal knee-shin system, single axis, fluid swing and stance phase control

∗ L5830   Addition, endoskeletal knee-shin system, single axis, pneumatic/ swing phase control

∗ L5840   Addition, endoskeletal knee-shin system, four-bar linkage or multiaxial, pneumatic swing phase control

∗ L5845   Addition, endoskeletal, knee-shin system, stance flexion feature, adjustable

∗ L5848   Addition to endoskeletal, knee-shin system, hydraulic stance extension, dampening feature, with or without adjustability

∗ L5850   Addition, endoskeletal system, above knee or hip disarticulation, knee extension assist

∗ L5855   Addition, endoskeletal system, hip disarticulation, mechanical hip extension assist

∗ L5856   Addition to lower extremity prosthesis, endoskeletal knee-shin system, microprocessor control feature, swing and stance phase; includes electronic sensor(s), any type

∗ L5857   Addition to lower extremity prosthesis, endoskeletal knee-shin system, microprocessor control feature, swing phase only; includes electronic sensor(s), any type

▶ ∗ L5858   Addition to lower extremity prosthesis, endoskeletal knee shin system, microprocessor control feature, stance phase only, includes electronic sensor(s), any type

* L5910 Addition, endoskeletal system, below knee, alignable system
* L5920 Addition, endoskeletal system, above knee or hip disarticulation, alignable system
* L5925 Addition, endoskeletal system, above knee, knee disarticulation or hip disarticulation, manual lock
* L5930 Addition, endoskeletal system, high activity knee control frame
* L5940 Addition, endoskeletal system, below knee, ultra light material (titanium, carbon fiber or equal)
* L5950 Addition, endoskeletal system, above knee, ultra light material (titanium, carbon fiber or equal)
* L5960 Addition, endoskeletal system, hip disarticulation, ultra light material (titanium, carbon fiber or equal)
* L5962 Addition, endoskeletal system, below knee, flexible protective outer surface covering system
* L5964 Addition, endoskeletal system, above knee, flexible protective outer surface covering system
* L5966 Addition, endoskeletal system, hip disarticulation, flexible protective outer surface covering system
* L5968 Addition to lower limb prosthesis, multiaxial ankle with swing phase active dorsiflexion feature
* L5970 All lower extremity prostheses, foot, external heel, SACH foot
▶* L5971 All lower extremity prosthesis, solid ankle cushion heel (SACH) foot, replacement only
* L5972 All lower extremity prostheses, flexible heel foot (Safe, Sten, Bock Dynamic or equal)
* L5974 All lower extremity prostheses, foot, single axis ankle/foot
* L5975 All lower extremity prostheses, combination single axis ankle and flexible keel foot
* L5976 All lower extremity prostheses, energy storing foot (Seattle Carbon Copy II or equal)
* L5978 All lower extremity prostheses, foot, multiaxial ankle/foot
* L5979 All lower extremity prostheses, multiaxial ankle, dynamic response foot, one piece system
* L5980 All lower extremity prostheses, flex foot system
* L5981 All lower extremity prostheses, flex-walk system or equal
* L5982 All exoskeletal lower extremity prostheses, axial rotation unit
* L5984 All endoskeletal lower extremity prostheses, axial rotation unit, with or without adjustability

* L5985 All endoskeletal lower extremity prostheses, dynamic prosthetic pylon
* L5986 All lower extremity prostheses, multiaxial rotation unit (MCP or equal)
* L5987 All lower extremity prostheses, shank foot system with vertical loading pylon
* L5988 Addition to lower limb prosthesis, vertical shock reducing pylon feature
* L5990 Addition to lower extremity prosthesis, user adjustable heel height
* L5995 Addition to lower extremity prosthesis, heavy duty feature (for patient weight > 300 lbs)
* L5999 Lower extremity prosthesis, not otherwise specified

Upper Limb

NOTE: The procedures in L6000-L6599 are considered as base or basic procedures and may be modified by listing procedures from the additions sections. The base procedures include only standard friction wrist and control cable system unless otherwise specified.

Partial Hand

* L6000 Partial hand, Robin-Aids, thumb remaining (or equal)
* L6010 Partial hand, Robin-Aids, little and/or ring finger remaining (or equal)
* L6020 Partial hand, Robin-Aids, no finger remaining (or equal)
* L6025 Transcarpal/metacarpal or partial hand disarticulation prosthesis, external power, self-suspended, inner socket with removable forearm section, electrodes and cables, two batteries, charger, myoelectric control of terminal device

Wrist Disarticulation

* L6050 Wrist disarticulation, molded socket, flexible elbow hinges, triceps pad
* L6055 Wrist disarticulation, molded socket with expandable interface, flexible elbow hinges, triceps pad

Below Elbow

* L6100 Below elbow, molded socket, flexible elbow hinge, triceps pad
* L6110 Below elbow, molded socket, (Muenster or Northwestern suspension types)
* L6120 Below elbow, molded double wall split socket, step-up hinges, half cuff

⊙ Special coverage instructions   ◆ Not covered by or valid for Medicare   * Carrier discretion   ◀▶ New   ⬛▶ Revised

* L6130   Below elbow, molded double wall split socket, stump activated locking hinge, half cuff

Elbow Disarticulation

* L6200   Elbow disarticulation, molded socket, outside locking hinge, forearm
* L6205   Elbow disarticulation, molded socket with expandable interface, outside locking hinges, forearm

Above Elbow

* L6250   Above elbow, molded double wall socket, internal locking elbow, forearm

Shoulder Disarticulation

* L6300   Shoulder disarticulation, molded socket, shoulder bulkhead, humeral section, internal locking elbow, forearm
* L6310   Shoulder disarticulation, passive restoration (complete prosthesis)
* L6320   Shoulder disarticulation, passive restoration (shoulder cap only)

Interscapular Thoracic

* L6350   Interscapular thoracic, molded socket, shoulder bulkhead, humeral section, internal locking elbow, forearm
* L6360   Interscapular thoracic, passive restoration (complete prosthesis)
* L6370   Interscapular thoracic, passive restoration (shoulder cap only)

Immediate and Early Postsurgical Procedures

* L6380   Immediate postsurgical or early fitting, application of initial rigid dressing, including fitting alignment and suspension of components, and one cast change, wrist disarticulation or below elbow
* L6382   Immediate postsurgical or early fitting, application of initial rigid dressing including fitting alignment and suspension of components, and one cast change, elbow disarticulation or above elbow
* L6384   Immediate postsurgical or early fitting, application of initial rigid dressing including fitting alignment and suspension of components, and one cast change, shoulder disarticulation or interscapular thoracic

* L6386   Immediate postsurgical or early fitting, each additional cast change and re-alignment
* L6388   Immediate postsurgical or early fitting, application of rigid dressing only

Endoskeletal: Below Elbow

* L6400   Below elbow, molded socket, endoskeletal system, including soft prosthetic tissue shaping

Endoskeletal: Elbow Disarticulation

* L6450   Elbow disarticulation, molded socket, endoskeletal system, including soft prosthetic tissue shaping

Endoskeletal: Above Elbow

* L6500   Above elbow, molded socket, endoskeletal system, including soft prosthetic tissue shaping

Endoskeletal: Shoulder Disarticulation

* L6550   Shoulder disarticulation, molded socket, endoskeletal system, including soft prosthetic tissue shaping

Endoskeletal: Interscapular Thoracic

* L6570   Interscapular thoracic, molded socket, endoskeletal system, including soft prosthetic tissue shaping
* L6580   Preparatory, wrist disarticulation or below elbow, single wall plastic socket, friction wrist, flexible elbow hinges, figure of eight harness, humeral cuff, Bowden cable control, USMC or equal pylon, no cover, molded to patient model
* L6582   Preparatory, wrist disarticulation or below elbow, single wall socket, friction wrist, flexible elbow hinges, figure of eight harness, humeral cuff, Bowden cable control, USMC or equal pylon, no cover, direct formed
* L6584   Preparatory, elbow disarticulation or above elbow, single wall plastic socket, friction wrist, locking elbow, figure of eight harness, fair lead cable control, USMC or equal pylon, no cover, molded to patient model

* L6586　Preparatory, elbow disarticulation or above elbow, single wall socket, friction wrist, locking elbow, figure of eight harness, fair lead cable control, USMC or equal pylon, no cover, direct formed

* L6588　Preparatory, shoulder disarticulation or interscapular thoracic, single wall plastic socket, shoulder joint, locking elbow, friction wrist, chest strap, fair lead cable control, USMC or equal pylon, no cover, molded to patient model

* L6590　Preparatory, shoulder disarticulation or interscapular thoracic, single wall socket, shoulder joint, locking elbow, friction wrist, chest strap, fair lead cable control, USMC or equal pylon, no cover, direct formed

Additions to Upper Limb

NOTE: The following procedures/modifications/ components may be added to other base procedures. The items in this section should reflect the additional complexity of each modification procedure, in addition to base procedure, at the time of the original order.

* L6600　Upper extremity addition, polycentric hinge, pair

* L6605　Upper extremity addition, single pivot hinge, pair

* L6610　Upper extremity addition, flexible metal hinge, pair

* L6615　Upper extremity addition, disconnect locking wrist unit

* L6616　Upper extremity addition, additional disconnect insert for locking wrist unit, each

* L6620　Upper extremity addition, flexion-friction wrist unit, with or without friction

▶ * L6621　Upper extremity prosthesis addition, flexion/extension wrist with or without friction, for use with external powered terminal device

* L6623　Upper extremity addition, spring assisted rotational wrist unit with latch release

* L6625　Upper extremity addition, rotation wrist unit with cable lock

* L6628　Upper extremity addition, quick disconnect hook adapter, Otto Bock or equal

* L6629　Upper extremity addition, quick disconnect lamination collar with coupling piece, Otto Bock or equal

* L6630　Upper extremity addition, stainless steel, any wrist

* L6632　Upper extremity addition, latex suspension sleeve, each

* L6635　Upper extremity addition, lift assist for elbow

* L6637　Upper extremity addition, nudge control elbow lock

* L6638　Upper extremity addition to prosthesis, electric locking feature, only for use with manually powered elbow

* L6640　Upper extremity additions, shoulder abduction joint, pair

* L6641　Upper extremity addition, excursion amplifier, pulley type

* L6642　Upper extremity addition, excursion amplifier, lever type

* L6645　Upper extremity addition, shoulder flexion-abduction joint, each

* L6646　Upper extremity addition, shoulder joint, multipositional locking, flexion, adjustable abduction friction control, for use with body powered or external powered system

* L6647　Upper extremity addition, shoulder lock mechanism, body powered actuator

* L6648　Upper extremity addition, shoulder lock mechanism, external powered actuator

* L6650　Upper extremity addition, shoulder universal joint, each

* L6655　Upper extremity addition, standard control cable, extra

* L6660　Upper extremity addition, heavy duty control cable

* L6665　Upper extremity addition, Teflon, or equal, cable lining

* L6670　Upper extremity addition, hook to hand, cable adapter

* L6672　Upper extremity addition, harness, chest or shoulder, saddle type

* L6675　Upper extremity addition, harness, (e.g. figure of eight type), single cable design

* L6676　Upper extremity addition, harness, (e.g. figure of eight type), dual cable design

▶ * L6677　Upper extremity addition, harness, triple control, simultaneous operation of terminal device and elbow

* L6680　Upper extremity addition, test socket, wrist disarticulation or below elbow

* L6682　Upper extremity addition, test socket, elbow disarticulation or above elbow

* L6684　Upper extremity addition, test socket, shoulder disarticulation or interscapular thoracic

* L6686　Upper extremity addition, suction socket

* L6687　Upper extremity addition, frame type socket, below elbow or wrist disarticulation

* L6688　Upper extremity addition, frame type socket, above elbow or elbow disarticulation

* L6689　Upper extremity addition, frame type socket, shoulder disarticulation

　☺ Special coverage instructions　◆ Not covered by or valid for Medicare　✳ Carrier discretion　◀▶ New　◀▥▥▶ Revised

✳ L6690   Upper extremity addition, frame type socket, interscapular-thoracic

✳ L6691   Upper extremity addition, removable insert, each

✳ L6692   Upper extremity addition, silicone gel insert or equal, each

✳ L6693   Upper extremity addition, locking elbow, forearm counterbalance

✳ L6694   Addition to upper extremity prosthesis, below elbow/above elbow, custom fabricated from existing mold or prefabricated, socket insert, silicone gel, elastomeric or equal, for use with locking mechanism

✳ L6695   Addition to upper extremity prosthesis, below elbow/above elbow, custom fabricated from existing mold or prefabricated, socket insert, silicone gel, elastomeric or equal, not for use with locking mechanism

✳ L6696   Addition to upper extremity prosthesis, below elbow/above elbow, custom fabricated socket insert for congenital or atypical traumatic amputee, silicone gel, elastomeric or equal, for use with or without locking mechanism, initial only (for other than initial, use code L6694 or L6695)

✳ L6697   Addition to upper extremity prosthesis, below elbow/above elbow, custom fabricated socket insert for other than congenital or atypical traumatic amputee, silicone gel, elastomeric or equal, for use with or without locking mechanism, initial only (for other than initial, use code L6694 or L6695)

✳ L6698   Addition to upper extremity prosthesis, below elbow/above elbow, lock mechanism, excludes socket insert

Terminal Devices

Hooks

⊗ L6700   Terminal device, hook, Dorrance, or equal, model #3
        MCM 2133

⊗ L6705   Terminal device, hook, Dorrance, or equal, model #5
        MCM 2133

⊗ L6710   Terminal device, hook, Dorrance, or equal, model #5X
        MCM 2133

⊗ L6715   Terminal device, hook, Dorrance, or equal, model #5XA
        MCM 2133

⊗ L6720   Terminal device, hook, Dorrance, or equal, model #6
        MCM 2133

⊗ L6725   Terminal device, hook, Dorrance, or equal, model #7
        MCM 2133

⊗ L6730   Terminal device, hook, Dorrance, or equal, model #7LO
        MCM 2133

⊗ L6735   Terminal device, hook, Dorrance, or equal, model #8
        MCM 2133

⊗ L6740   Terminal device, hook, Dorrance, or equal, model #8X
        MCM 2133

⊗ L6745   Terminal device, hook, Dorrance, or equal, model #88X
        MCM 2133

⊗ L6750   Terminal device, hook, Dorrance, or equal, model #10P
        MCM 2133

⊗ L6755   Terminal device, hook, Dorrance, or equal, model #10X
        MCM 2133

⊗ L6765   Terminal device, hook, Dorrance, or equal, model #12P
        MCM 2133

⊗ L6770   Terminal device, hook, Dorrance, or equal, model #99X
        MCM 2133

⊗ L6775   Terminal device, hook, Dorrance, or equal, model #555
        MCM 2133

⊗ L6780   Terminal device, hook, Dorrance, or equal, model #SS555
        MCM 2133

⊗ L6790   Terminal device, hook, Accu hook, or equal
        MCM 2133

⊗ L6795   Terminal device, hook, 2 load, or equal
        MCM 2133

⊗ L6800   Terminal device, hook, APRL VC, or equal
        MCM 2133

⊗ L6805   Terminal device, modifier wrist flexion unit
        MCM 2133

⊗ L6806   Terminal device, hook, TRS Grip, Grip III, VC, or equal
        MCM 2133

⊗ L6807   Terminal device, hook, Grip I, Grip II, VC, or equal
        MCM 2133

⊗ L6808   Terminal device, hook, TRS Adept, infant or child, VC, or equal
        MCM 2133

⊗ L6809   Terminal device, hook, TRS Super Sport, passive
        MCM 2133

⊗ L6810   Terminal device, pincher tool, Otto Bock or equal
        MCM 2133

Hands

- ✪ L6825 Terminal device, hand, Dorrance, VO
MCM 2133
- ✪ L6830 Terminal device, hand, APRL, VC
MCM 2133
- ✪ L6835 Terminal device, hand, Sierra, VO
MCM 2133
- ✪ L6840 Terminal device, hand, Becker Imperial
MCM 2133
- ✪ L6845 Terminal device, hand, Becker Lock Grip
MCM 2133
- ✪ L6850 Terminal device, hand, Becker Plylite
MCM 2133
- ✪ L6855 Terminal device, hand, Robin-Aids, VO
MCM 2133
- ✪ L6860 Terminal device, hand, Robin-Aids, VO soft
MCM 2133
- ✪ L6865 Terminal device, hand, passive hand
MCM 2133
- ✪ L6867 Terminal device, hand, Detroit infant hand (mechanical)
MCM 2133
- ✪ L6868 Terminal device, hand, passive infant hand, (Steeper, Hosmer or equal)
MCM 2133
- ✪ L6870 Terminal device, hand, child MITT
MCM 2133
- ✪ L6872 Terminal device, hand, NYU child hand
MCM 2133
- ✪ L6873 Terminal device, hand, mechanical infant hand, Steeper or equal
MCM 2133
- ✪ L6875 Terminal device, hand, Bock, VC
MCM 2133
- ✪ L6880 Terminal device, hand, Bock, VO
MCM 2133
- ✳ L6881 Automatic grasp feature, addition to upper limb prosthetic terminal device
- ✪ L6882 Microprocessor control feature, addition to upper limb prosthetic terminal device
MCM 2133

Replacement Sockets

- ▶ ✳ L6883 Replacement socket, below elbow/wrist disarticulation, molded to patient model, for use with or without external power
- ▶ ✳ L6884 Replacement socket, above elbow disarticulation, molded to patient model, for use with or without external power
- ▶ ✳ L6885 Replacement socket, shoulder disarticulation/interscapular thoracic, molded to patient model, for use with or without external power

Gloves for Above Hands

- L6890 Addition to upper extremity prosthesis, glove for terminal device, any material, prefabricated, includes fitting and adjustment
- L6895 Addition to upper extremity prosthesis, glove for terminal device, any material, custom fabricated

Hand Restoration

- ✳ L6900 Hand restoration (casts, shading and measurements included), partial hand, with glove, thumb or one finger remaining
- ✳ L6905 Hand restoration (casts, shading and measurements included), partial hand, with glove, multiple fingers remaining
- ✳ L6910 Hand restoration (casts, shading and measurements included), partial hand, with glove, no fingers remaining
- ✳ L6915 Hand restoration (shading, and measurements included), replacement glove for above

External Power

Base Devices

- ✳ L6920 Wrist disarticulation, external power, self-suspended inner socket, removable forearm shell, Otto Bock or equal, switch, cables, two batteries and one charger, switch control of terminal device
- ✳ L6925 Wrist disarticulation, external power, self-suspended inner socket, removable forearm shell, Otto Bock or equal, electrodes, cables, two batteries and one charger, myoelectronic control of terminal device
- ✳ L6930 Below elbow, external power, self-suspended inner socket, removable forearm shell, Otto Bock or equal, switch, cables, two batteries and one charger, switch control of terminal device
- ✳ L6935 Below elbow, external power, self-suspended inner socket, removable forearm shell, Otto Bock or equal, electrodes, cables, two batteries and one charger, myoelectronic control of terminal device
- ✳ L6940 Elbow disarticulation, external power, molded inner socket, removable humeral shell, outside locking hinges, forearm, Otto Bock or equal, switch, cables, two batteries and one charger, switch control of terminal device

* L6945   Elbow disarticulation, external power, molded inner socket, removable humeral shell, outside locking hinges, forearm, Otto Bock or equal, electrodes, cables, two batteries and one charger, myoelectronic control of terminal device

* L6950   Above elbow, external power, molded inner socket, removable humeral shell, internal locking elbow, forearm, Otto Bock or equal, switch, cables, two batteries and one charger, switch control of terminal device

* L6955   Above elbow, external power, molded inner socket, removable humeral shell, internal locking elbow, forearm, Otto Bock or equal, electrodes, cables, two batteries and one charger, myoelectronic control of terminal device

* L6960   Shoulder disarticulation, external power, molded inner socket, removable shoulder shell, shoulder bulkhead, humeral section, mechanical elbow, forearm, Otto Bock or equal, switch, cables, two batteries and one charger, switch control of terminal device

* L6965   Shoulder disarticulation, external power, molded inner socket, removable shoulder shell, shoulder bulkhead, humeral section, mechanical elbow, forearm, Otto Bock or equal, electrodes, cables, two batteries and one charger, myoelectronic control of terminal device

* L6970   Interscapular-thoracic, external power, molded inner socket, removable shoulder shell, shoulder bulkhead, humeral section, mechanical elbow, forearm, Otto Bock or equal, switch, cables, two batteries and one charger, switch control of terminal device

* L6975   Interscapular-thoracic, external power, molded inner socket, removable shoulder shell, shoulder bulkhead, humeral section, mechanical elbow, forearm, Otto Bock or equal, electrodes, cables, two batteries and one charger, myoelectronic control of terminal device

Terminal Devices

* L7010   Electronic hand, Otto Bock, Steeper or equal, switch controlled

* L7015   Electronic hand, System Teknik, Variety Village or equal, switch controlled

* L7020   Electronic Greifer, Otto Bock or equal, switch controlled

* L7025   Electronic hand, Otto Bock or equal, myoelectronically controlled

* L7030   Electronic hand, System Teknik, Variety Village or equal, myoelectronically controlled

* L7035   Electronic Greifer, Otto Bock or equal, myoelectronically controlled

* L7040   Prehensile actuator, Hosmer or equal, switch controlled

* L7045   Electronic hook, child, Michigan or equal, switch controlled

Elbow

* L7170   Electronic elbow, Hosmer or equal, switch controlled

* L7180   Electronic elbow, microprocessor sequential control of elbow and terminal device

* L7181   Electronic elbow, microprocessor simultaneous control of elbow and terminal device

* L7185   Electronic elbow, adolescent, Variety Village or equal, switch controlled

* L7186   Electronic elbow, child, Variety Village or equal, switch controlled

* L7190   Electronic elbow, adolescent, Variety Village or equal, myoelectronically controlled

* L7191   Electronic elbow, child, Variety Village or equal, myoelectronically controlled

* L7260   Electronic wrist rotator, Otto Bock or equal

* L7261   Electronic wrist rotator, for Utah arm

* L7266   Servo control, Steeper or equal

* L7272   Analogue control, UNB or equal

* L7274   Proportional control, 6-12 volt, Liberty, Utah or equal

Battery Components

* L7360   Six-volt battery, Otto Bock or equal, each

* L7362   Battery charger, 6 volt, Otto Bock or equal

* L7364   Twelve volt battery, Utah or equal, each

* L7366   Battery charger, 12 volt, Utah or equal

* L7367   Lithium ion battery, replacement

* L7368   Lithium ion battery charger

Other

▶ * L7400   Addition to upper extremity prosthesis, below elbow/wrist disarticulation, ultralight material (titanium, carbon fiber or equal)

▶ * L7401   Addition to upper extremity prosthesis, above elbow disarticulation, ultralight material (titanium, carbon fiber or equal)

▶ * L7402   Addition to upper extremity prosthesis, shoulder disarticulation/interscapular thoracic, ultralight material (titanium, carbon fiber or equal)

▶ * L7403   Addition to upper extremity prosthesis, below elbow/wrist disarticulation, acrylic material

▶ * L7404   Addition to upper extremity prosthesis, above elbow disarticulation, acrylic material

▶ * L7405   Addition to upper extremity prosthesis, shoulder disarticulation/interscapular thoracic, acrylic material

* L7499   Upper extremity prosthesis, not otherwise specified

☉ L7500   Repair of prosthetic device, hourly rate (excludes V5335 repair of oral or laryngeal prosthesis or artificial larynx)
MCM 2100.4, MCM 2130D, MCM 2133

☉ L7510   Repair of prosthetic device, repair or replace minor parts
MCM 2100.4, MCM 2130D, MCM 2133

* L7520   Repair prosthetic device, labor component, per 15 minutes

▶ * L7600   Prosthetic donning sleeve, any material, each

* L7900   Male vacuum erection system

Breast Prostheses

☉ L8000   Breast prosthesis, mastectomy bra
MCM 2130A

☉ L8001   Breast prosthesis, mastectomy bra, with integrated breast prosthesis form, unilateral
MCM 2130A

☉ L8002   Breast prosthesis, mastectomy bra, with integrated breast prosthesis form, bilateral
MCM 2130A

⇒ ☉ L8010   Breast prosthesis, mastectomy sleeve
MCM 2130A

☉ L8015   External breast prosthesis garment, with mastectomy form, post mastectomy
MCM 2130

☉ L8020   Breast prosthesis, mastectomy form
MCM 2130A

☉ L8030   Breast prosthesis, silicone or equal
MCM 2130A

☉ L8035   Custom breast prosthesis, post mastectomy, molded to patient mode
IMCM 2130

* L8039   Breast prosthesis, not otherwise specified

Nasal, Orbital, Auricular Prosthesis

* L8040   Nasal prosthesis, provided by a non-physician

* L8041   Midfacial prosthesis, provided by a non-physician

* L8042   Orbital prosthesis, provided by a non-physician

* L8043   Upper facial prosthesis, provided by a non-physician

* L8044   Hemi-facial prosthesis, provided by a non-physician

* L8045   Auricular prosthesis, provided by a non-physician

* L8046   Partial facial prosthesis, provided by a non-physician

* L8047   Nasal septal prosthesis, provided by a non-physician

* L8048   Unspecified maxillofacial prosthesis, by report, provided by a non-physician

* L8049   Repair or modification of maxillofacial prosthesis, labor component, 15-minute increments, provided by a non-physician

Elastic Supports

L8100   Deleted 12/31/05
L8110   Deleted 12/31/05
L8120   Deleted 12/31/05
L8130   Deleted 12/31/05
L8140   Deleted 12/31/05
L8150   Deleted 12/31/05
L8160   Deleted 12/31/05
L8170   Deleted 12/31/05
L8180   Deleted 12/31/05
L8190   Deleted 12/31/05
L8195   Deleted 12/31/05
L8200   Deleted 12/31/05
L8210   Deleted 12/31/05
L8220   Deleted 12/31/05
L8230   Deleted 12/31/05
L8239   Deleted 12/31/05

Trusses

☉ L8300   Truss, single with standard pad
MCM 2133, CIM 70-1, CIM 70-2

☉ L8310   Truss, double with standard pads
MCM 2133, CIM 70-1, CIM 70-2

☉ L8320   Truss, addition to standard pad, water pad
MCM 2133, CIM 70-1, CIM 70-2

☉ L8330   Truss, addition to standard pad, scrotal pad
MCM 2133, CIM 70-1, CIM 70-2

Prosthetic Socks

☉ L8400   Prosthetic sheath, below knee, each
MCM 2133

☉ L8410   Prosthetic sheath, above knee, each
MCM 2133

⊛ L8415 Prosthetic sheath, upper limb, each
MCM 2133

✳ L8417 Prosthetic sheath/sock, including a gel cushion layer, below knee or above knee, each

⊛ L8420 Prosthetic sock, multiple ply, below knee, each
MCM 2133

⊛ L8430 Prosthetic sock, multiple ply, above knee, each
MCM 2133

⊛ L8435 Prosthetic sock, multiple ply, upper limb, each
MCM 2133

⊛ L8440 Prosthetic shrinker, below knee, each
MCM 2133

⊛ L8460 Prosthetic shrinker, above knee, each
MCM 2133

⊛ L8465 Prosthetic shrinker, upper limb, each
MCM 2133

⊛ L8470 Prosthetic sock, single ply, fitting, below knee, each
MCM 2133

⊛ L8480 Prosthetic sock, single ply, fitting, above knee, each
MCM 2133

⊛ L8485 Prosthetic sock, single ply, fitting, upper limb, each
MCM 2133

L8490 Deleted 1/1/05

✳ L8499 Unlisted procedure for miscellaneous prosthetic services

Prosthetic Implants

Integumentary System

⊛ L8500 Artificial larynx, any type
MCM 2130, CIM 65-5

⊛ L8501 Tracheostomy speaking valve
CIM 65-16

✳ L8505 Artificial larynx replacement battery/accessory, any type

✳ L8507 Tracheo-esophageal voice prosthesis, patient inserted, any type, each

✳ L8509 Tracheo-esophageal voice prosthesis, inserted by licensed health car provider, any type

⊛ L8510 Voice amplifier
CIM 65-5

✳ L8511 Insert for indwelling tracheoesophageal prosthesis, with or without valve, replacement only, each

✳ L8512 Gelatin capsules or equivalent, for use with tracheoesophageal voice prosthesis, replacement only, per 10

✳ L8513 Cleaning device used with tracheo-esophageal voice prosthesis, pipet, brush, or equal, replacement only, each

✳ L8514 Tracheoesophageal puncture dilator, replacement only, each

✳ L8515 Gelatin capsule, application device for use with tracheoesophageal voice prosthesis, each

⊛ L8600 Implantable breast prosthesis, silicone or equal
MCM 2130, CIM 35-47

Urinary System

⊛ L8603 Injectable bulking agent, collagen implant, urinary tract, per 2.5 ml syringe, includes shipping and necessary supplies
CIM 65-9

⊛ L8606 Injectable bulking agent, synthetic implant, urinary tract, 1 ml syringe, includes shipping and necessary supplies
CIM 65.9

Head (Skull, Facial Bones, and Temporomandibular Joint)

▶ ✳ L8609 Artificial cornea

⊛ L8610 Ocular implant
MCM 2130

⊛ L8612 Aqueous shunt
MCM 2130, Cross Reference Q0074

⊛ L8613 Ossicula implant
MCM 2130

⊛ L8614 Cochlear device/system
MCM 2130, CIM 65-14

⊛ L8615 Headset/headpiece for use with cochlear implant device, replacement

⊛ L8616 Microphone for use with cochlear implant device, replacement

⊛ L8617 Transmitting coil for use with cochlear implant device, replacement

⊛ L8618 Transmitter cable for use with cochlear implant device, replacement

⊛ L8619 Cochlear implant external speech processor, replacement
CIM 65-14

L8620 Deleted 12/31/05

✳ L8621 Zinc air battery for use with cochlear implant device, replacement, each

✳ L8622 Alkaline battery for use with cochlear implant device, any size, replacement, each

▶ ✳ L8623 Lithium ion battery for use with cochlear implant device speech processor, other than ear level, replacement, each

▶ ✳ L8624 Lithium ion battery for use with cochlear implant device speech processor, ear level, replacement, each

Upper Extremity

⊛ L8630 Metacarpophalangeal joint implant
MCM 2130

⊛ L8631 Metacarpal phalangeal joint replacement, two or more pieces, metal (e.g., stainless steel or cobalt chrome), ceramic-like material (e.g., pyrocarbon), for surgical implantation (all sizes, includes entire system)
MCM 2130

Lower Extremity (Joint: Knee, Ankle, Toe)

⊛ L8641 Metatarsal joint implant
MCM 2130

⊛ L8642 Hallux implant
MCM 2130, Cross Reference Q0073

Miscellaneous Muscular-Skeletal

⊛ L8658 Interphalangeal joint spacer, silicone or equal, each
MCM 2130

⊛ L8659 Interphalangeal finger joint replacement, 2 or more pieces, metal (e.g., stainless steel or cobalt chrome), ceramic-like material (e.g., pyrocarbon) for surgical implantation, any size
MCM 2130

Cardiovascular System

⊛ L8670 Vascular graft material, synthetic, implant
MCM 2130

Neurostimulator

▶⊛ L8680 Implantable neurostimulator electrode, each
CIM 65-8

▶⊛ L8681 Patient programmer (external) for use with implantable programmable neurostimulator pulse generator
CIM 65-8

▶⊛ L8682 Implantable neurostimulator radiofrequency receiver
CIM 65-8

▶⊛ L8683 Radiofrequency transmitter (external) for use with implantable neurostimulator radiofrequency receiver
CIM 65-8

▶⊛ L8684 Radiofrequency transmitter (external) for use with implantable sacral root neurostimulator receiver for bowel and bladder management, replacement
CIM 65-8

▶⊛ L8685 Implantable neurostimulator pulse generator, single array, rechargeable, includes extension
CIM 65-8

▶⊛ L8686 Implantable neurostimulator pulse generator, single array, non-rechargeable, includes extension
CIM 65-8

▶⊛ L8687 Implantable neurostimulator pulse generator, dual array, rechargeable, includes extension
CIM 65-8

▶⊛ L8688 Implantable neurostimulator pulse generator, dual array, non-rechargeable, includes extension
CIM 65-8

▶⊛ L8689 External recharging system for implanted neurostimulator, replacement only
CIM 65-8

Genital

✳ L8699 Prosthetic implant, not otherwise specified

✳ L9900 Orthotic and prosthetic supply, accessory, and/or service component of another HCPCS L code

MEDICAL SERVICES (M0000-M0399)

Other Medical Services

⊛ M0064 Brief office visit for the sole purpose of monitoring or changing drug prescriptions used in the treatment of mental psychoneurotic and personality disorders
MCM 2476.3

◆ M0075 Cellular therapy
CIM 35-5

◆ M0076 Prolotherapy
CIM 35-13

◆ M0100 Intragastric hypothermia using gastric freezing
CIM 35-65

◆ M0300 IV chelation therapy (chemical endarterectomy)
CIM 35-64

◆ M0301 Fabric wrapping of abdominal aneurysm
CIM 35-34

PATHOLOGY AND LABORATORY TESTS (P0000-P2999)

Chemistry and Toxicology Tests

⊛ P2028 Cephalin flocculation, blood
CIM 50-34

⊚ P2029   Congo red, blood
         CIM 50-34
◆ P2031   Hair analysis (excluding arsenic)
         CIM 50-24
⊚ P2033   Thymol turbidity, blood
         CIM 50-34
⊚ P2038   Mucoprotein, blood (seromucoid) (medical necessity procedure)
         CIM 50-34

Pathology Screening Tests

⊚ P3000   Screening Papanicolaou smear, cervical or vaginal, up to three smears, by technician under physician supervision
         CIM 50-20, Laboratory Certification: cytology
⊚ P3001   Screening Papanicolaou smear, cervical or vaginal, up to three smears, requiring interpretation by physician
         CIM 50-20, Laboratory Certification: cytology

Microbiology Tests

◆ P7001   Culture, bacterial, urine; quantitative, sensitivity study
         Cross Reference CPT, Laboratory Certification: bacteriology

Miscellaneous Pathology

⊚ P9010   Blood (whole), for transfusion, per unit
         MCM 2455A
⊚ P9011   Blood (split unit), specify amount
         MCM 2455A
⊚ P9012   Cryoprecipitate, each unit
         MCM 2455B
⊚ P9016   Red blood cells, leukocytes reduced, each unit
         MCM 2455B
⊚ P9017   Fresh frozen plasma (single donor), frozen within 8 hours of collection, each unit
         MCM 2455B
    P9018   Deleted 01/01/01
⊚ P9019   Platelets, each unit
         MCM 2455B
⊚ P9020   Platelet rich plasma, each unit
         MCM 2455B
⊚ P9021   Red blood cells, each unit
         MCM 2455A
⊚ P9022   Red blood cells, washed, each unit
         MCM 2455A

⊚ P9023   Plasma, pooled multiple donor, solvent/detergent treated, frozen, each unit
         MCM 2455B
⊚ P9031   Platelets, leukocytes reduced, each unit
         MCM 2455
⊚ P9032   Platelets, irradiated, each unit
         MCM 2455
⊚ P9033   Platelets, leukocytes reduced, irradiated, each unit
         MCM 2455
⊚ P9034   Platelets, pheresis, each unit
         MCM 2455
⊚ P9035   Platelets, pheresis, leukocytes reduced, each unit
         MCM 2455
⊚ P9036   Platelets, pheresis, irradiated, each unit
         MCM 2455
⊚ P9037   Platelets, pheresis, leukocytes reduced, irradiated, each unit
         MCM 2455
⊚ P9038   Red blood cells, irradiated, each unit
         MCM 2455
⊚ P9039   Red blood cells, deglycerolized, each unit
         MCM 2455
⊚ P9040   Red blood cells, leukocytes reduced, irradiated, each unit
         MCM 2455
∗ P9041   Infusion, albumin (human), 5%, 50 ml
⊚ P9043   Infusion, plasma protein fraction (human), 5%, 50 ml
         MCM 2455B
⊚ P9044   Plasma, cryoprecipitate reduced, each unit
         MCM 2455B
∗ P9045   Infusion, albumin (human), 5%, 250 ml
∗ P9046   Infusion, albumin (human), 25%, 20 ml
∗ P9047   Infusion, albumin (human), 25%, 50 ml
∗ P9048   Infusion, plasma protein fraction (human), 5%, 250 ml
∗ P9050   Granulocytes, pheresis, each unit
⊚ P9051   Whole blood or red blood cells, leukocytes reduced, CMV-negative, each unit
         Medicare Statute 1833(t)
⊚ P9052   Platelets, HLA-matched leukocytes reduced, apheresis/pheresis, each unit
         Medicare Statute 1833(t)
⊚ P9053   Platelets, pheresis, leukocytes reduced, CMV-negative, irradiated, each unit
         Medicare Statute 1833(t)
⊚ P9054   Whole blood or red blood cells, leukocytes reduced, frozen, deglycerol, washed, each unit
         Medicare Statute 1833(t)
⊚ P9055   Platelets, leukocytes reduced, CMV-negative, apheresis/pheresis, each unit
         Medicare Statute 1833(t)
⊚ P9056   Whole blood, leukocytes reduced, irradiated, each unit
         Medicare Statute 1833(t)

☺ P9057 Red blood cells, frozen/deglycerolized/washed, leukocytes reduced, irradiated, each unit
Medicare Statute 1833(t)

☺ P9058 Red blood cells, leukocytes reduced, CMV-negative, irradiated, each unit
Medicare Statute 1833(t)

☺ P9059 Fresh frozen plasma between 8-24 hours of collection, each unit
Medicare Statute 1833(t)

☺ P9060 Fresh frozen plasma, donor retested, each unit
Medicare Statute 1833(t)

☺ P9603 Travel allowance one way in connection with medically necessary laboratory specimen collection drawn from home bound or nursing home bound patient; prorated miles actually traveled.
MCM 5114.1K

☺ P9604 Travel allowance one way in connection with medically necessary laboratory specimen collection drawn from home bound or nursing home bound patient; prorated trip charge
MCM 5114.1K

☺ P9612 Catheterization for collection of specimen, single patient, all places of service
MCM 5114.1D

☺ P9615 Catheterization for collection of specimen(s) (multiple patients)
MCM 5114.1D

Q CODES: TEMPORARY CODES (Q0000-Q9999)

☺ Q0035 Cardiokymography
CIM 50-50

☺ Q0081 Infusion therapy, using other than chemotherapy drugs, per visit
CIM 60-14

✻ Q0083 Chemotherapy administration by other than infusion technique only (e.g., subcutaneous, intramuscular, push), per visit

☺ Q0084 Chemotherapy administration by infusion technique only, per visit
CIM 60-14

✻ Q0085 Chemotherapy administration by both infusion technique and other technique(s) (e.g., subcutaneous, intramuscular, push), per visit

☺ Q0091 Screening Papanicolaou smear; obtaining, preparing and conveyance of cervical or vaginal smear to laboratory
CIM 50-20

☺ Q0092 Setup portable x-ray equipment
MCM 2070.4

✻ Q0111 Wet mounts, including preparations of vaginal, cervical or skin specimens; Laboratory Certification: bacteriology, mycology, parasitology

✻ Q0112 All potassium hydroxide (KOH) preparations; Laboratory Certification: mycology

✻ Q0113 Pinworm examinations; Laboratory Certification: parasitology

✻ Q0114 Fern test; Laboratory certification: routine chemistry

✻ Q0115 Post-coital direct, qualitative examinations of vaginal or cervical mucus; Laboratory Certification: hematology

Q0136 Deleted 12/31/05

Q0137 Deleted 12/31/05

◆ Q0144 Azithromycin dihydrate, oral, capsules/powder, 1 gm

☺ Q0163 Diphenhydramine HCl, 50 mg, oral, FDA-approved prescription antiemetic, for use as a complete therapeutic substitute for an IV antiemetic at time of chemotherapy treatment not to exceed a 48-hour dosage regimen
Medicare Statute 4557

☺ Q0164 Prochlorperazine maleate, 5 mg, oral, FDA-approved prescription antiemetic, for use as a complete therapeutic substitute for an IV antiemetic at the time of chemotherapy treatment, not to exceed a 48-hour dosage regimen
Medicare Statute 4557

☺ Q0165 Prochlorperazine maleate, 10 mg, oral, FDA-approved prescription antiemetic, for use as a complete therapeutic substitute for an IV antiemetic at the time of chemotherapy treatment, not to exceed a 48-hour dosage regimen
Medicare Statute 4557

☺ Q0166 Granisetron HCl, 1 mg, oral, FDA-approved prescription antiemetic, for use as a complete therapeutic substitute for an IV antiemetic at the time of chemotherapy treatment, not to exceed a 24-hour dosage regimen
Medicare Statute 4557

☺ Q0167 Dronabinol, 2.5 mg, oral, FDA-approved prescription antiemetic, for use as a complete therapeutic substitute for an IV antiemetic at the time of chemotherapy treatment, not to exceed a 48-hour dosage regimen
Medicare Statute 4557

☺ Q0168 Dronabinol, 5 mg, oral, FDA-approved prescription antiemetic, for use as a complete therapeutic substitute for an IV antiemetic at the time of chemotherapy treatment, not to exceed a 48-hour dosage regimen
Medicare Statute 4557

⊛ Q0169 Promethazine HCl, 12.5 mg, oral, FDA-approved prescription antiemetic, for use as a complete therapeutic substitute for an IV antiemetic at the time of chemotherapy treatment, not to exceed a 48-hour dosage regimen
Medicare Statute 4557

⊛ Q0170 Promethazine HCl, 25 mg, oral, FDA-approved prescription antiemetic, for use as a complete therapeutic substitute for an IV antiemetic at the time of chemotherapy treatment, not to exceed a 48-hour dosage regimen
Medicare Statute 4557

⊛ Q0171 Chlorpromazine HCl, 10 mg, oral, FDA-approved prescription antiemetic, for use as a complete therapeutic substitute for an IV antiemetic at the time of chemotherapy treatment, not to exceed a 48-hour dosage regimen
Medicare Statute 4557

⊛ Q0172 Chlorpromazine HCl, 25 mg, oral, FDA-approved prescription antiemetic, for use as a complete therapeutic substitute for an IV antiemetic at the time of chemotherapy treatment, not to exceed a 48-hour dosage regimen
Medicare Statute 4557

⊛ Q0173 Trimethobenzamide HCl, 250 mg, oral, FDA-approved prescription antiemetic, for use as a complete therapeutic substitute for an IV antiemetic at the time of chemotherapy treatment, not to exceed a 48-hour dosage regimen
Medicare Statute 4557

⊛ Q0174 Thiethylperazine maleate, 10 mg, oral, FDA-approved prescription antiemetic, for use as a complete therapeutic substitute for an IV antiemetic at the time of chemotherapy treatment, not to exceed a 48-hour dosage regimen
Medicare Statute 4557

⊛ Q0175 Perphenazine, 4 mg, oral, FDA-approved prescription antiemetic, for use as a complete therapeutic substitute for an IV antiemetic at the time of chemotherapy treatment, not to exceed a 48-hour dosage regimen
Medicare Statute 4557

⊛ Q0176 Perphenazine, 8 mg, oral, FDA-approved prescription antiemetic, for use as a complete therapeutic substitute for an IV antiemetic at the time of chemotherapy treatment, not to exceed a 48-hour dosage regimen
Medicare Statute 4557

⊛ Q0177 Hydroxyzine pamoate, 25 mg, oral, FDA-approved prescription antiemetic, for use as a complete therapeutic substitute for an IV antiemetic at the time of chemotherapy treatment, not to exceed a 48-hour dosage regimen
Medicare Statute 4557

⊛ Q0178 Hydroxyzine pamoate, 50 mg, oral, FDA-approved prescription antiemetic, for use as a complete therapeutic substitute for an IV antiemetic at the time of chemotherapy treatment, not to exceed a 48-hour dosage regimen
Medicare Statute 4557

⊛ Q0179 Ondansetron HCl, 8 mg, oral, FDA-approved prescription antiemetic, for use as a complete therapeutic substitute for an IV antiemetic at the time of chemotherapy treatment, not to exceed a 48-hour dosage regimen
Medicare Statute 4557

⊛ Q0180 Dolasetron mesylate, 100 mg, oral, FDA-approved prescription antiemetic, for use as a complete therapeutic substitute for an IV antiemetic at the time of chemotherapy treatment, not to exceed a 24-hour dosage regimen
Medicare Statute 4557

⊛ Q0181 Unspecified oral dosage form, FDA-approved prescription antiemetic, for use as a complete therapeutic substitute for a IV antiemetic at the time of chemotherapy treatment, not to exceed a 48-hour dosage regimen
Medicare Statute 4557

Q0187 Deleted 12/31/05

▶ ⊛ Q0480 Driver for use with pneumatic ventricular assist device, replacement only

▶ ⊛ Q0481 Microprocessor control unit for use with electric ventricular assist device, replacement only

▶ ⊛ Q0482 Microprocessor control unit for use with electric/pneumatic combination ventricular assist device, replacement only

▶ ⊛ Q0483 Monitor/display module for use with electric ventricular assist device, replacement only

▶ ⊛ Q0484 Monitor/display module for use with electric or electric/pneumatic ventricular assist device, replacement only

▶ ⊛ Q0485 Monitor control cable for use with electric ventricular assist device, replacement only

▶ ⊛ Q0486 Monitor control cable for use with electric/pneumatic ventricular assist device, replacement only

▶ ⊛ Q0487 Leads (pneumatic/electrical) for use with any type electric/pneumatic ventricular assist device, replacement only

▶ ☺ Q0488   Power pack base for use with electric ventricular assist device, replacement only

▶ ☺ Q0489   Power pack base for use with electric/pneumatic ventricular assist device, replacement only

▶ ☺ Q0490   Emergency power source for use with electric ventricular assist device, replacement only

▶ ☺ Q0491   Emergency power source for use with electric/pneumatic ventricular assist device, replacement only

▶ ☺ Q0492   Emergency power supply cable for use with electric ventricular assist device, replacement only

▶ ☺ Q0493   Emergency power supply cable for use with electric/pneumatic ventricular assist device, replacement only

▶ ☺ Q0494   Emergency hand pump for use with electric or electric/pneumatic ventricular assist device, replacement only

▶ ☺ Q0495   Battery/power pack charger for use with electric or electric/pneumatic ventricular assist device, replacement only

▶ ☺ Q0496   Battery for use with electric or electric/pneumatic ventricular assist device, replacement only

▶ ☺ Q0497   Battery clips for use with electric or electric/pneumatic ventricular assist device, replacement only

▶ ☺ Q0498   Holster for use with electric or electric/pneumatic ventricular assist device, replacement only

▶ ☺ Q0499   Belt/vest for use with electric or electric/pneumatic ventricular assist device, replacement only

▶ ☺ Q0500   Filters for use with electric or electric/pneumatic ventricular assist device, replacement only

▶ ☺ Q0501   Shower cover for use with electric or electric/pneumatic ventricular assist device, replacement only

▶ ☺ Q0502   Mobility cart for pneumatic ventricular assist device, replacement only

▶ ☺ Q0503   Battery for pneumatic ventricular assist device, replacement only, each

▶ ☺ Q0504   Power adapter for pneumatic ventricular assist device, replacement only, vehicle type

▶ ☺ Q0505   Miscellaneous supply or accessory for use with ventricular assist device

▶ ☺ Q0510   Pharmacy supply fee for initial immunosuppressive drug(s), first month following implant

▶ ☺ Q0511   Pharmacy supply fee for oral anti-cancer, oral anti-emetic or immunosuppressive

▶   Q0511   Drug(s); for the first prescription in a 30-day period

▶ ☺ Q0512   Pharmacy supply fee for oral anti-cancer, oral anti-emetic or immunosuppressive drug(s); for a subsequent prescription in a 30-day period

▶ ☺ Q0513   Pharmacy dispensing fee for inhalation drug(s); per 30 days

▶ ☺ Q0514   Pharmacy dispensing fee for inhalation drug(s); per 90 days

▶ ☺ Q0515   Injection, sermorelin acetate, 1 µg
MCM 2049

  Q1001   Deleted 06/30/05
  Q1002   Deleted 06/30/05

☺ Q1003   New technology intraocular lens category 3 as defined in Federal Register notice

☺ Q1004   New technology intraocular lens category 4 as defined in Federal Register notice

☺ Q1005   New technology intraocular lens category 5 as defined in Federal Register notice

  Q2001   Deleted 12/31/05
  Q2002   Deleted 12/31/05
  Q2003   Deleted 12/31/05

☺ Q2004   Irrigation solution for treatment of bladder calculi, for example renacidin, per 500 ml
MCM 2049, Medicare Statute 1861S2B

  Q2005   Deleted 12/31/05
  Q2006   Deleted 12/31/05
  Q2007   Deleted 12/31/05
  Q2008   Deleted 12/31/05

☺ Q2009   Injection, fosphenytoin, 50 mg
MCM 2049, Medicare Statute 1861S2B

  Q2011   Deleted 12/31/05
  Q2012   Deleted 12/31/05
  Q2013   Deleted 12/31/05
  Q2014   Deleted 12/31/05

☺ Q2017   Injection, teniposide, 50 mg
MCM 2049, Medicare Statute 1861S2B

  Q2018   Deleted 12/31/05
  Q2019   Deleted 12/31/05
  Q2020   Deleted 12/31/05
  Q2021   Deleted 12/31/05
  Q2022   Deleted 12/31/05
  Q3000   Deleted 12/31/05

⇒ ☺ Q3001   Radioelements for brachytherapy, any type, each
MCM 15022

  Q3002   Deleted 12/31/05
  Q3003   Deleted 12/31/05
  Q3004   Deleted 12/31/05
  Q3005   Deleted 12/31/05
  Q3006   Deleted 12/31/05
  Q3007   Deleted 12/31/05
  Q3008   Deleted 12/31/05
  Q3009   Deleted 12/31/05
  Q3010   Deleted 12/31/05
  Q3011   Deleted 12/31/05
  Q3012   Deleted 12/31/05

✳ Q3014   Telehealth originating site facility fee

✳ Q3019   ALS vehicle used, emergency transport, no ALS level services furnished.

✳ Q3020   ALS vehicle used, non-emergency transport, no ALS level service furnished

⊙ Q3025   Injection, interferon beta-1a, 11 mcg for intramuscular use
MCM 2049

◆ Q3026   Injection, interferon beta-1a, 11 mcg for subcutaneous use

⊙ Q3031   Collagen skin test
CIM 65-9

✳ Q4001   Casting supplies, body cast adult, with or without head, plaster

✳ Q4002   Cast supplies, body cast adult, with or without head, fiberglass

✳ Q4003   Cast supplies, shoulder cast, adult (11 years +), plaster

✳ Q4004   Cast supplies, shoulder cast, adult (11 years +), fiberglass

✳ Q4005   Cast supplies, long arm cast, adult (11 years +), plaster

✳ Q4006   Cast supplies, long arm cast, adult (11 years +), fiberglass

✳ Q4007   Cast supplies, long arm cast, pediatric (0-10 years), plaster

✳ Q4008   Cast supplies, long arm cast, pediatric (0-10 years), fiberglass

✳ Q4009   Cast supplies, short arm cast, adult (11 years +), plaster

✳ Q4010   Cast supplies, short arm cast, adult (11 years +), fiberglass

✳ Q4011   Cast supplies, short arm cast, pediatric (0-10 years), plaster

✳ Q4012   Cast supplies, short arm cast, pediatric (0-10 years), fiberglass

✳ Q4013   Cast supplies, gauntlet cast (includes lower forearm and hand), adult (11 years +), plaster

✳ Q4014   Cast supplies, gauntlet cast (includes lower forearm and hand), adult (11 years +), fiberglass

✳ Q4015   Cast supplies, gauntlet cast (includes lower forearm and hand), pediatric (0-10 years), plaster

✳ Q4016   Cast supplies, gauntlet cast (includes lower forearm and hand), pediatric (0-10 years), fiberglass

✳ Q4017   Cast supplies, long arm splint, adult (11 years +), plaster

✳ Q4018   Cast supplies, long arm splint, adult (11 years +), fiberglass

✳ Q4019   Cast supplies, long arm splint, pediatric (0-10 years), plaster

✳ Q4020   Cast supplies, long arm splint, pediatric (0-10 years), fiberglass

✳ Q4021   Cast supplies, short arm splint, adult (11 years +), plaster

✳ Q4022   Cast supplies, short arm splint, adult (11 years +), fiberglass

✳ Q4023   Cast supplies, short arm splint, pediatric (0-10 years), plaster

✳ Q4024   Cast supplies, short arm splint, pediatric (0-10 years), fiberglass

✳ Q4025   Cast supplies, hip spica (one or both legs), adult (11 years +), plaster

✳ Q4026   Cast supplies, hip spica (one or both legs), adult (11 years +), fiberglass

✳ Q4027   Cast supplies, hip spica (one or both legs), pediatric (0-10 years), plaster

✳ Q4028   Cast supplies, hip spica (one or both legs), pediatric (0-10 years), fiberglass

✳ Q4029   Cast supplies, long leg cast, adult (11 years +), plaster

✳ Q4030   Cast supplies, long leg cast, adult (11 years +), fiberglass

✳ Q4031   Cast supplies, long leg cast, pediatric (0-10 years), plaster

✳ Q4032   Cast supplies, long leg cast, pediatric (0-10 years), fiberglass

✳ Q4033   Cast supplies, long leg cylinder cast, adult (11 years +), plaster

✳ Q4034   Cast supplies, long leg cylinder cast, adult (11 years +), fiberglass

✳ Q4035   Cast supplies, long leg cylinder cast, pediatric (0-10 years), plaster

✳ Q4036   Cast supplies, long leg cylinder cast, pediatric (0-10 years), fiberglass

✳ Q4037   Cast supplies, short leg cast, adult (11 years +), plaster

✳ Q4038   Cast supplies, short leg cast, adult (11 years +), fiberglass

✳ Q4039   Cast supplies, short leg cast, pediatric (0-10 years), plaster

✳ Q4040   Cast supplies, short leg cast, pediatric (0-10 years), fiberglass

✳ Q4041   Cast supplies, long leg splint, adult (11 years +), plaster

✳ Q4042   Cast supplies, long leg splint, adult (11 years +), fiberglass

✳ Q4043   Cast supplies, long leg splint, pediatric (0-10 years), plaster

✳ Q4044   Cast supplies, long leg splint, pediatric (0-10 years), fiberglass

✳ Q4045   Cast supplies, short leg splint, adult (11 years +), plaster

✳ Q4046   Cast supplies, short leg splint, adult (11 years +), fiberglass

✳ Q4047   Cast supplies, short leg splint, pediatric (0-10 years), plaster

✳ Q4048   Cast supplies, short leg splint, pediatric (0-10 years), fiberglass

✳ Q4049   Finger splint, static

✳ Q4050   Cast supplies, for unlisted types and materials of casts

✳ Q4051   Splint supplies, miscellaneous (includes thermoplastics, strapping, fasteners, padding and other supplies)

Q4054   Deleted 12/31/05

Q4055   Deleted 12/31/05

Q4075   Deleted 12/31/05

Q4076   Deleted 12/31/05
Q4077   Deleted 12/31/05
▶✳ Q4079   Injection, natalizumab, 1 mg
▶✳ Q4080   Iloprost, inhalation solution, adminis-tered through DME, 20 μg

Injection Codes for Epoetin Alfa

Q9941   Deleted 12/31/05
Q9942   Deleted 12/31/05
Q9943   Deleted 12/31/05
Q9944   Deleted 12/31/05

Contrast

▶✪ Q9945   Low osmolar contrast material, up to 149 mg/ml iodine concentration, per ml
MCM 15022

▶✪ Q9946   Low osmolar contrast material, 150–199 mg/ml iodine concentration, per ml
MCM 15022

▶✪ Q9947   Low osmolar contrast material, 200–249 mg/ml iodine concentration, per ml
MCM 15022

▶✪ Q9948   Low osmolar contrast material, 250–299 mg/ml iodine concentration, per ml
MCM 15022

▶✪ Q9949   Low osmolar contrast material, 300–349 mg/ml iodine concentration, per ml
MCM 15022

▶✪ Q9950   Low osmolar contrast material, 350–399 mg/ml iodine concentration, per ml
MCM 15022

▶✪ Q9951   Low osmolar contrast material, 400 or greater mg/ml iodine concentration, per ml
MCM 15022

▶✪ Q9952   Injection, gadolinium-based magnetic resonance contrast agent, per ml
MCM 15022

▶✪ Q9953   Injection, iron-based magnetic reso-nance contrast agent, per ml
MCM 15022

▶✪ Q9954   Oral magnetic resonance contrast agent, per 100 ml
MCM 15022

▶✳ Q9955   Injection, perflexane lipid microspheres, per ml

▶✳ Q9956   Injection, octafluoropropane micro-spheres, per ml

▶✳ Q9957   Injection, perflutren lipid microspheres, per ml

▶✪ Q9958   High osmolar contrast material, up to 149 mg/ml iodine concentration, per ml
MCM 15022

▶✪ Q9959   High osmolar contrast material, 150–199 mg/ml iodine concentration, per ml
MCM 15022

▶✪ Q9960   High osmolar contrast material, 200–249 mg/ml iodine concentration, per ml
MCM 15022

▶✪ Q9961   High osmolar contrast material, 250–299 mg/ml iodine concentration, per ml
MCM 15022

▶✪ Q9962   High osmolar contrast material, 300–349 mg/ml iodine concentration, per ml
MCM 15022

▶✪ Q9963   High osmolar contrast material, 350–399 mg/ml iodine concentration, per ml
MCM 15022

▶✪ Q9964   High osmolar contrast material, 400 or greater mg/ml iodine concentration, per ml
MCM 15022

DOMESTIC RADIOLOGY SERVICES (R0000-R5999)
Transportation/Setup of Portable X-Ray Equipment

✪ R0070   Transportation of portable x-ray equip-ment and personnel to home or nursing home, per trip to facility or location, one patient seen
MCM 2070.4, MCM 5244B

✪ R0075   Transportation of portable x-ray equip-ment and personnel to home or nursing home, per trip to facility or location, more than one patient seen, per patient
MCM 2070.4, MCM 5244B

✪ R0076   Transportation of portable ECG to facil-ity or location, per patient
MCM 2070.1, MCM 2070.4, CIM 50-15

TEMPORARY NATIONAL CODES (S0009-S9999)

◆ S0012   Butorphanol tartrate, nasal spray, 25 mg
◆ S0014   Tacrine HCl, 10 mg
S0016   Deleted 03/31/05
◆ S0017   Injection, aminocaproic acid, 5 gm
◆ S0020   Injection, bupivacaine HCl, 30 ml
◆ S0021   Injection, cefoperazone sodium, 1 gm
◆ S0023   Injection, cimetidine HCl, 300 mg
◆ S0028   Injection, famotidine, 20 mg
◆ S0030   Injection, metronidazole, 500 mg
◆ S0032   Injection, nafcillin sodium, 2 gm

◆ S0034   Injection, ofloxacin, 400 mg

◆ S0039   Injection, sulfamethoxazole and trimethoprim, 10 ml

◆ S0040   Injection, ticarcillin disodium and clavulanate potassium, 3.1 gm

S0071   Deleted 12/31/05

S0072   Deleted 12/31/05

◆ S0073   Injection, aztreonam, 500 mg

◆ S0074   Injection, cefotetan disodium, 500 mg

◆ S0077   Injection, clindamycin phosphate, 300 mg

◆ S0078   Injection, fosphenytoin sodium, 750 mg

◆ S0080   Injection, pentamidine isethionate, 300 mg

◆ S0081   Injection, piperacillin sodium, 500 mg

◆ S0088   Imatinib, 100 mg

◆ S0090   Sildenafil citrate, 25 mg

◆ S0091   Granisetron hydrochloride, 1 mg (for circumstances falling under the Medicare statute, use Q0166)

◆ S0092   Injection, hydromorphone hydrochloride, 250 mg (loading dose for infusion pump)

◆ S0093   Injection, morphine sulfate, 500 mg (loading dose for infusion pump)

◆ S0104   Zidovudine, oral, 100 mg

◆ S0106   Bupropion HCl sustained release tablet, 150 mg, per bottle of 60 tablets

S0107   Deleted 03/31/05

◆ S0108   Mercaptopurine, oral, 50 mg

◆ S0109   Methadone, oral, 5 mg

S0114   Deleted 12/31/05

◆ S0116   Bevacizumab, 100 mg

◆ S0117   Tretinoin, topical, 5 grams

S0118   Deleted 12/31/05

◆ S0122   Injection, menotropins, 75 IU

◆ S0126   Injection, follitropin alfa, 75 IU

◆ S0128   Injection, follitropin beta, 75 IU

◆ S0132   Injection, ganirelix acetate, 250 mcg

▶◆ S0133   Histrelin, implant, 50 mg

◆ S0136   Clozapine, 25 mg

◆ S0137   Didanosine (DDI), 25 mg

◆ S0138   Finasteride, 5 mg

◆ S0139   Minoxidil, 10 mg

◆ S0140   Saquinavir, 200 mg

◆ S0141   Zalcitabine (DDC), 0.375 mg

▶◆ S0142   Colistimethate sodium, inhalation solution administered through DME, concentrated form, per mg

▶◆ S0143   Aztreonam, inhalation solution administered through DME, concentrated form, per gram

▶◆ S0145   Injection, pegylated interferon alfa-2a, 180 mcg per ml

▶◆ S0146   Injection, pegylated interferon alfa-2b, 10 mcg per 0.5 ml

◆ S0155   Sterile dilatant for epoprostenol, 50 ml

◆ S0156   Exemestane, 25 mg

◆ S0157   Becaplermin gel 0.01%, 0.5 gm

S0158   Deleted 03/31/05

S0159   Deleted 03/31/05

◆ S0160   Dextroamphetamine sulfate, 5 mg

◆ S0161   Calcitrol, 0.25 mcg

◆ S0162   Injection, efalizumab, 125 mg

◆ S0164   Injection, pantoprazole sodium, 40 mg

◆ S0166   Injection, olanzapine, 2.5 mg

◆ S0167   Injection, apomorphine hydrochloride, 1 mg

S0168   Deleted 12/31/05

◆ S0170   Anastrozole, oral, 1 mg

◆ S0171   Injection, bumetanide, 0.5 mg

◆ S0172   Chlorambucil, oral, 2 mg

S0173   Deleted 12/31/05

◆ S0174   Dolasetron mesylate, oral 50 mg (for circumstances falling under the Medicare statute, use Q0180)

◆ S0175   Flutamide, oral, 125 mg

◆ S0176   Hydroxyurea, oral, 500 mg

◆ S0177   Levamisole HCl, oral, 50 mg

◆ S0178   Lomustine, oral, 10 mg

◆ S0179   Megestrol acetate, oral, 20 mg

◆ S0181   Ondansetron HCl, oral, 4 mg (for circumstances falling under the Medicare statute, use Q0179)

◆ S0182   Procarbazine HCl, oral, 50 mg

◆ S0183   Prochlorperazine maleate, oral, 5 mg (for circumstances falling under the Medicare statute, use Q0164-Q0165)

◆ S0187   Tamoxifen citrate, oral, 10 mg

◆ S0189   Testosterone pellet, 75 mg

◆ S0190   Mifepristone, oral, 200 mg

◆ S0191   Misoprostol, oral 200 mcg

◆ S0194   Dialysis/stress vitamin supplement, oral, 100 capsules

◆ S0195   Pneumococcal conjugate vaccine, polyvalent, intramuscular, for children from five years to nine years of age who have not previously received the vaccine

◆ S0196   Injectable poly-l-lactic acid, restorative implant, 1 ml, face (deep dermis, subcutaneous layers)

▶ S0197   Prenatal vitamins, 30-day supply

▶◆ S0198   Injection, pegaptanib sodium, 0.3 mg

◆ S0199   Medically induced abortion by oral ingestion of medication including all associated services and supplies (e.g., patient counseling, office visits, confirmation of pregnancy by HCG, ultrasound to confirm duration of pregnancy, ultrasound to confirm completion of abortion), except drugs

◆ S0201   Partial hospitalization services, less than 24 hours, per diem

◆ S0207   Paramedic intercept, non-hospital based ALS service (non-voluntary), non-transport

◆ S0208   Paramedic intercept, hospital-based ALS service (non-voluntary), non-transport

◆ S0209   Wheelchair van, mileage, per mile

◆ S0215   Non-emergency transportation; mileage per mile

◆ S0220 Medical conference by a physician with interdisciplinary team of health professionals or representatives of community agencies to coordinate activities of patient care (patient is present); approximately 30 minutes

◆ S0221 Medical conference by a physician with interdisciplinary team of health professionals or representatives of community agencies to coordinate activities of patient care (patient is present); approximately 60 minutes

◆ S0250 Comprehensive geriatric assessment and treatment planning performed by assessment team

◆ S0255 Hospice referral visit (advising patient and family of care options) performed by nurse, social worker, or other designated staff

◆ S0257 Counseling and discussion regarding advance directives or end of life care planning and decisions, with patient and/or surrogate (list separately in addition to code for appropriate evaluation and management service)

◆ S0260 History and physical (outpatient or office) related to surgical procedure (list separately in addition to code for appropriate evaluation and management service)

▶ ◆ S0265 Genetic counseling, under physician supervision, each 15 minutes

◆ S0302 Completed EPSDT service (list in addition to code for appropriate evaluation and management service)

◆ S0310 Hospitalist services (list separately in addition to code for appropriate evaluation and management service)

◆ S0315 Disease management program; initial assessment and initiation of the program

◆ S0316 Follow-up/assessment

◆ S0317 Disease management program; per diem

◆ S0320 Telephone calls by a registered nurse to a disease management program member for monitoring purposes; per month

◆ S0340 Lifestyle modification program for management of coronary artery disease, including all supportive services; first quarter/stage

◆ S0341 Lifestyle modification program for management of coronary artery disease, including all supportive services; second or third quarter/stage

◆ S0342 Lifestyle modification program for management of coronary artery disease, including all supportive services; fourth quarter/stage

◆ S0390 Routine foot care; removal and/or trimming of corns, calluses and/or nails and preventive maintenance in specific medical conditions (e.g., diabetes), per visit

◆ S0395 Impression casting of a foot performed by a practitioner other than the manufacturer of the orthotic

◆ S0400 Global fee for extracorporeal shock wave lithotripsy treatment of kidney stone(s)

◆ S0500 Disposable contact lens, per lens

◆ S0504 Single vision prescription lens (safety, athletic, or sunglass), per lens

◆ S0506 Bifocal vision prescription lens (safety, athletic, or sunglass), per lens

◆ S0508 Trifocal vision prescription lens (safety, athletic, or sunglass), per lens

◆ S0510 Non-prescription lens (safety, athletic, or sunglass), per lens

◆ S0512 Daily wear specialty contact lens, per lens

◆ S0514 Color contact lens, per lens

◆ S0515 Scleral lens, liquid bandage device, per lens

◆ S0516 Safety eyeglass frames

◆ S0518 Sunglasses frames

◆ S0580 Polycarbonate lens (list this code in addition to the basic code for the lens)

◆ S0581 Nonstandard lens (list this code in addition to the basic code for the lens)

◆ S0590 Integral lens service, miscellaneous services reported separately

◆ S0592 Comprehensive contact lens evaluation

▶ ◆ S0595 Dispensing new spectacle lenses for patient supplied frame

◆ S0601 Screening proctoscopy

◆ S0605 Digital rectal examination, annual

◆ S0610 Annual gynecological examination, new patient

◆ S0612 Annual gynecological examination, established patient

▶ ◆ S0613 Annual gynecological examination; clinical breast examination without pelvic evaluation

◆ S0618 Audiometry for hearing aid evaluation to determine the level and degree of hearing loss

◆ S0620 Routine ophthalmological examination including refraction; new patient

◆ S0621 Routine ophthalmological examination including refraction; established patient

◆ S0622 Physical exam for college, new or established patient (list separately) in addition to appropriate evaluation and management code)

▶ S0625 Retinal telescreening by digital imaging of multiple different fundus areas to screen for vision-threatening conditions, including imaging, interpretation and report

◆ S0630   Removal of sutures; by a physician other than the physician who originally closed the wound

◆ S0800   Laser in situ keratomileusis (LASIK)

◆ S0810   Photorefractive keratectomy (PRK)

◆ S0812   Phototherapeutic keratectomy (PTK)

◆ S0820   Computerized corneal topography, unilateral

◆ S1001   Deluxe item, patient aware (list in addition to code for basic item)

◆ S1002   Customized item (list in addition to code for basic item)

◆ S1015   IV tubing extension set

◆ S1016   Non–polyvinyl chloride (PVC) IV administration set, for use with drugs that are not stable in PVC (e.g., paclitaxel)

◆ S1025   Inhaled nitric oxide for the treatment of hypoxic respiratory failure in the neonate; per diem

◆ S1030   Continuous noninvasive glucose monitoring device, purchase (for physician interpretation of data, use CPT code)

◆ S1031   Continuous noninvasive glucose monitoring device, rental, including sensor, sensor replacement, and download to monitor (for physician interpretation of data, use CPT code)

◆ S1040   Cranial remolding orthosis, rigid, with soft interface material, custom fabricated, includes fitting and adjustment(s)

◆ S2053   Transplantation of small intestine and liver allografts

◆ S2054   Transplantation of multivisceral organs

◆ S2055   Harvesting of donor multivisceral organs, with preparation and maintenance of allografts; from cadaver donor

◆ S2060   Lobar lung transplantation

◆ S2061   Donor lobectomy (lung) for transplantation, living donor

◆ S2065   Simultaneous pancreas kidney transplantation

▶◆ S2068   Breast reconstruction with deep inferior epigastric perforator (DIEP) flap, including microvascular anastomosis and closure of donor site, unilateral

◆ S2070   Cystourethroscopy, with ureteroscopy and/or pyeloscopy; with endoscopic laser treatment of ureteral calculi (includes ureteral catheterization)

▶◆ S2075   Laparoscopy, surgical; repair incisional or ventral hernia laparoscopy, surgical; repair umbilical hernia

▶◆ S2076   Laparoscopy, surgical; repair umbilical hernia

▶◆ S2077   Laparoscopy, surgical; implantation of mesh or other prosthesis for incisional or ventral hernia repair (list separately in addition to code for incisional or ventral hernia repair)

▶◆ S2078   Laparoscopic supracervical hysterectomy (subtotal hysterectomy), with or without removal of tube(s), with or without removal of ovary(s)

▶◆ S2079   Laparoscopic esophagomyotomy (Heller type)

◆ S2080   Laser-assisted uvulopalatoplasty (LAUP)

   S2082   Deleted 12/31/05

◆ S2083   Adjustment of gastric band diameter via subcutaneous port by injection or aspiration of saline

   S2090   Deleted 12/31/05

   S2091   Deleted 12/31/05

◆ S2095   Transcatheter occlusion or embolization for tumor destruction, percutaneous, any method, using yttrium-90 microspheres

◆ S2102   Islet cell tissue transplant from pancreas allogeneic

◆ S2103   Adrenal tissue transplant to brain

◆ S2107   Adoptive immunotherapy i.e. development of specific anti-tumor reactivity (e.g. tumor-infiltrating lymphocyte therapy) per course of treatment

◆ S2112   Arthroscopy, knee, surgical for harvesting of cartilage (chondrocyte cells)

▶◆ S2114   Arthroscopy, shoulder, surgical; tenodesis of biceps

   S2115   Deleted 12/31/05

▶◆ S2117   Arthroereisis, subtalar

◆ S2120   Low-density lipoprotein (LDL) apheresis using heparin-induced extracorporeal LDL precipitation

◆ S2135   Neurolysis, by injection, of metatarsal neuroma/interdigital neuritis, any interspace of the foot

◆ S2140   Cord blood harvesting for transplantation, allogeneic

◆ S2142   Cord blood–derived stem cell transplantation, allogeneic

◆ S2150   Bone marrow or blood-derived stem cells (peripheral or umbilical), allogeneic or autologous, harvesting, transplantation, and related complications; including: pheresis and cell preparation/storage; marrow ablative therapy; drugs; supplies; hospitalization with outpatient follow-up; medical/surgical, diagnostic, emergency, and rehabilitative services; and the number of days of pre- and post-transplant care in the global definition

◆ S2152   Solid organ(s), complete or segmental, single organ or combination of organs; deceased or living donor(s), procurement, transplantation, and related complications; including: drugs; supplies; hospitalization with outpatient follow-up; medical/surgical, diagnostic, emergency, and rehabilitative services; and the number of days of pre- and post-transplant care in the global definition

◆ S2202 Echosclerotherapy

◆ S2205 Minimally invasive direct coronary artery bypass surgery involving mini-thoracotomy or mini-sternotomy surgery, performed under direct vision; using arterial graft(s), single coronary arterial graft

◆ S2206 Minimally invasive direct coronary artery bypass surgery involving mini-thoracotomy or mini-sternotomy surgery, performed under direct vision; using arterial graft(s), two coronary arterial grafts

◆ S2207 Minimally invasive direct coronary artery bypass surgery involving mini-thoracotomy or mini-sternotomy surgery, performed under direct vision; using venous graft only, single coronary venous graft

◆ S2208 Minimally invasive direct coronary artery bypass surgery involving mini-thoracotomy or mini-sternotomy surgery, performed under direct vision; using single arterial and venous graft(s), single venous graft

◆ S2209 Minimally invasive direct coronary artery bypass surgery involving mini-thoracotomy or mini-sternotomy surgery, performed under direct vision; using two arterial grafts and single venous graft

◆ S2213 Implantation of gastric electrical stimulation device

S2215 Deleted 12/31/05

◆ S2225 Myringotomy, laser-assisted

◆ S2230 Implantation of magnetic component of semi-implantable hearing device on ossicles in middle ear

◆ S2235 Implantation of auditory brain stem implant

◆ S2250 Uterine artery embolization for uterine fibroids

◆ S2260 Induced abortion, 17-24 weeks, any surgical method

◆ S2262 Abortion for maternal indications, 25 weeks or greater

◆ S2265 Abortion for fetal indications, 25-28 weeks

◆ S2266 Abortion for fetal indication, 29-31 weeks

◆ S2267 Abortion for fetal indication, 32 weeks or greater

◆ S2300 Arthroscopy, shoulder, surgical; with thermally induced capsulorrhaphy

◆ S2340 Chemodenervation of abductor muscle(s) of vocal cord

◆ S2341 Chemodenervation of adductor muscle(s) of vocal cord

◆ S2342 Nasal endoscopy for post-operative debridement following functional endoscopic sinus surgery, nasal and/or sinus cavity(s), unilateral or bilateral

◆ S2348 Decompression procedure, percutaneous, or nucleus pulpous of intervertebral disc, using radiofrequency energy, single or multiple levels, lumbar

◆ S2350 Diskectomy, anterior, with decompression of spinal cord and/or nerve root(s) including osteophytectomy; lumbar, single interspace

◆ S2351 Diskectomy, anterior, with decompression of spinal cord and/or nerve root(s) including osteophytectomy; lumbar, each additional interspace (list separately in addition to code for primary procedure)

◆ S2360 Percutaneous vertebroplasty, one vertebral body, unilateral or bilateral injection; cervical

◆ S2361 Each additional cervical vertebral body (list separately in addition to code for primary procedure)

◆ S2362 Kyphoplasty, one vertebral body, unilateral or bilateral injection

◆ S2363 Kyphoplasty, one vertebral body, unilateral or bilateral injection; each additional vertebral body (list separately in addition to code for primary procedure)

◆ S2400 Repair, congenital diaphragmatic hernia in the fetus using temporary tracheal occlusion, procedure performed in utero

◆ S2401 Repair, urinary tract obstruction in the fetus, procedure performed in utero

◆ S2402 Repair, congenital cystic adenomatoid malformation in the fetus, procedure performed in utero

◆ S2403 Repair, extralobar pulmonary sequestration in the fetus, procedure performed in utero

◆ S2404 Repair, myelomeningocele in the fetus, procedure performed in utero

◆ S2405 Repair of sacrococcygeal teratoma in the fetus, procedure performed in utero

◆ S2409 Repair, congenital malformation of fetus, procedure performed in utero, not otherwise classified

◆ S2411 Fetoscopic laser therapy for treatment of twin-to-twin transfusion syndrome (TTTS)

▶◆ S2900 Surgical techniques requiring use of robotic surgical system (list separately In addition to code for primary procedure)

◆ S3000 Diabetic indicator; retinal eye exam, dilated, bilateral

▶◆ S3005 Performance measurement, evaluation of patient self assessment, depression

☺ Special coverage instructions ◆ Not covered by or valid for Medicare ✳ Carrier discretion ◀▶ New ◀▥▥▶ Revised

◆ S3600 STAT laboratory request (situations other than S3601)

◆ S3601 Emergency STAT laboratory charge for patient who is homebound or residing in a nursing facility

☺ S3620 Newborn metabolic screening panel, includes test kit, postage, and the laboratory tests specified by the sate for inclusion in this panel (e.g., galactose, hemoglobin; electrophoresis; hydroxy-progesterone; 17-D; phenylalanine (PKU); and thyroxine, total)

◆ S3625 Maternal serum triple marker screen including alpha-fetoprotein (AFP), estriol, and human chorionic gonadotropin (hcG)

▶◆ S3626 Maternal serum quadruple marker screen including alpha-fetoprotein (AFP), estriol, human chorionic gonadotropin (HCG) and inhibin a

◆ S3630 Eosinophil count, blood, direct

◆ S3645 Human immunodeficiency virus-1 (HIV-1) antibody testing of oral mucosal transudate

◆ S3650 Saliva test, hormone level; during menopause

◆ S3652 Saliva test, hormone level; to assess preterm labor risk

◆ S3655 Antisperm antibodies test (immunobead)

◆ S3701 Immunoassay for nuclear matrix protein 22 (NMP-22), quantitative

◆ S3708 Gastrointestinal fat absorption study

◆ S3818 Complete gene sequence analysis; BRCA1 gene

◆ S3819 Complete gene sequence analysis; BRCA2 gene

◆ S3820 Complete BRAL1 and BRCA2 gene sequence analysis for susceptibility to breast and ovarian cancer

◆ S3822 Single mutation analysis (in individual with a known BRCA1 or BRCA2 mutation in the family) for susceptibility to breast and ovarian cancer

◆ S3823 Three-mutation BRCA1 and BRCA2 analysis for susceptibility to breast and ovarian cancer in Ashkenazi individuals

◆ S3828 Complete gene sequence analysis; MLH1 gene

◆ S3829 Complete gene sequence analysis; MLH2 gene

◆ S3830 Complete MLH and MLH gene sequence analysis for hereditary nonpolyposis colorectal cancer (HNPCC) genetic testing

◆ S3831 Single-mutation analysis (in individual with a known MLH and MLH mutation in the family) for hereditary nonpolyposis colorectal cancer (HNPCC) genetic testing

◆ S3833 Complete APC gene sequence analysis for susceptibility to familial adenomatous polyposis (FAP) and attenuated FAP

◆ S3834 Single-mutation analysis (in individual with a known APC mutation in the family) for susceptibility to familial adenomatous polyposis (FAP) and attenuated FAP

◆ S3835 Complete gene sequence analysis for cystic fibrosis genetic testing

◆ S3837 Complete gene sequence analysis for hemochromatosis genetic testing

◆ S3840 DNA analysis for germline mutations of the ret proto-oncogene for susceptibility to multiple endocrine neoplasia type 2

◆ S3841 Genetic testing for retinoblastoma

◆ S3842 Genetic testing for von Hippel-Lindau disease

◆ S3843 DNA analysis of the F5 gene for susceptibility to Factor V Leiden thrombophilia

◆ S3844 DNA analysis of the connexin 26 gene (GJB2) for susceptibility to congenital, profound deafness

◆ S3845 Genetic testing for alpha-thalassemia

◆ S3846 Genetic testing for hemoglobin E beta-thalassemia

◆ S3847 Genetic testing for Tay-Sachs disease

◆ S3848 Genetic testing for Gaucher disease

◆ S3849 Genetic testing for Niemann-Pick disease

◆ S3850 Genetic testing for sickle cell anemia

◆ S3851 Genetic testing for Canavan disease

◆ S3852 DNA analysis for APOE epilson 4 allele for susceptibility to Alzheimer's disease

◆ S3853 Genetic testing for myotonic muscular dystrophy

▶◆ S3854 Gene expression profiling panel for use in the management of breast cancer treatment

◆ S3890 DNA analysis, fecal, for colorectal cancer screening

◆ S3900 Surface electromyography (EMG)

◆ S3902 Ballistrocardiogram

◆ S3904 Masters two step

◆ S4005 Interim labor facility global (labor occurring but not resulting in delivery)

◆ S4011 In vitro fertilization (IVF); including but not limited to identification and incubation of mature oocytes, fertilization with sperm, incubation of embryo(s), and subsequent visualization for determination of development

◆ S4013 Complete cycle, gamete intrafallopian transfer (GIFT), case rate

◆ S4014 Complete cycle, zygote intrafallopian transfer (ZIFT), case rate

◆ S4015 Complete in vitro fertilization cycle, not otherwise specified, case rate

◆ S4016 Frozen in vitro fertilization cycle, case rate

◆ S4017 Incomplete cycle, treatment canceled prior to stimulation, case rate

◆ S4018 Frozen embryo transfer procedure cancelled before transfer, case rate

◆ S4020 In vitro fertilization procedure cancelled before aspiration, case rate

◆ S4021 In vitro fertilization procedure cancelled after aspiration, case rate

◆ S4022 Assisted oocyte fertilization, case rate

◆ S4023 Donor egg cycle, incomplete, case rate

◆ S4025 Donor services for in vitro fertilization (sperm or embryo), case rate

◆ S4026 Procurement of donor sperm from sperm bank

◆ S4027 Storage of previously frozen embryos

◆ S4028 Microsurgical epididymal sperm aspiration (MESA)

◆ S4030 Sperm procurement and cryopreservation services; initial visit

◆ S4031 Sperm procurement and cryopreservation services; subsequent visit

◆ S4035 Stimulated intrauterine insemination (IUI), case rate

◆ S4036 Intravaginal culture (IVC), case rate

◆ S4037 Cryopreserved embryo transfer, case rate

◆ S4040 Monitoring and storage of cryopreserved embryos, per 30 days

◆ S4042 Management of ovulation induction (interpretation of diagnostic tests and studies, non–face-to-face medical management of the patient), per cycle

◆ S4981 Insertion of levonorgestrel-releasing intrauterine system

◆ S4989 Contraceptive intrauterine device (IUD) (e.g. Progestasert), including implants and supplies

◆ S4990 Nicotine patches, legend

◆ S4991 Nicotine patches, non-legend

◆ S4993 Contraceptive pills for birth control

◆ S4995 Smoking cessation gum

◆ S5000 Prescription drug, generic

◆ S5001 Prescription drug, brand name

S5002 Deleted 01/01/02

◆ S5010 5% dextrose and 45% normal saline, 1000 ml

◆ S5011 5% dextrose in lactated Ringer's, 1000 ml

◆ S5012 5% dextrose with potassium chloride, 1000 ml

◆ S5013 5% dextrose/45% normal saline with potassium chloride and magnesium sulfate, 1000 ml

◆ S5014 5% dextrose/45% normal saline with potassium chloride and magnesium sulfate, 1500 ml

◆ S5035 Home infusion therapy, routine service of infusion device (e.g., pump maintenance)

◆ S5036 Home infusion therapy, repair of infusion device (e.g., pump repair)

◆ S5100 Day care services, adult; per 15 minutes

◆ S5101 Day care services, adult; per half day

◆ S5102 Day care services, adult; per diem

◆ S5105 Day care services, center-based; services not included in program fee, per diem

◆ S5108 Home care training to home care client, per 15 minutes

◆ S5109 Home care training to home care client, per session

◆ S5110 Home care training, family; per 15 minutes

◆ S5111 Home care training, family; per session

◆ S5115 Home care training, non-family; per 15 minutes

◆ S5116 Home care training, non-family; per session

◆ S5120 Chore services; per 15 minutes

◆ S5121 Chore services; per diem

◆ S5125 Attendant care services; per 15 minutes

◆ S5126 Attendant care services; per diem

◆ S5130 Homemaker service, NOS; per 15 minutes

◆ S5131 Homemaker service, NOS; per diem

◆ S5135 Companion care, adult (e.g., IADL/ADL); per 15 minutes

◆ S5136 Companion care, adult (e.g., IADL/ADL); per diem

◆ S5140 Foster care, adult; per diem

◆ S5141 Foster care, adult; per month

◆ S5145 Foster care, therapeutic, child; per diem

◆ S5146 Foster care, therapeutic, child; per month

◆ S5150 Unskilled respite care, not hospice; per 15 minutes

◆ S5151 Unskilled respite care, not hospice; per diem

◆ S5160 Emergency response system; installation and testing

◆ S5161 Emergency response system; service fee, per month (excludes installation and testing)

◆ S5162 Emergency response system; purchase only

◆ S5165 Home modifications; per service

◆ S5170 Home delivered meals, including preparation; per meal

◆ S5175 Laundry service, external, professional; per order

◆ S5180 Home health respiratory therapy, initial evaluation

◆ S5181 Home health respiratory therapy, NOS, per diem

◆ S5185 Medication reminder service, non-face-to-face; per month

◆ S5190 Wellness assessment, performed by non-physician

◆ S5199 Personal care item, NOS, each

☺ **Special coverage instructions**   ◆ **Not covered by or valid for Medicare**   ✳ **Carrier discretion**   ◀▶ **New**   ⬸⬗ **Revised**

◆ S5497 Home infusion therapy, catheter care/ maintenance, not otherwise classified; includes administration services, professional pharmacy services, care coordination, and all necessary supplies and equipment (drugs and nursing visits coded separately), per diem

◆ S5498 Home infusion therapy, catheter care/ maintenance, simple (single lumen), includes administrative services, professional pharmacy services, care coordination and all necessary supplies and equipment, (drugs and nursing visits coded separately), per diem

◆ S5501 Home infusion therapy, catheter care/ maintenance, complex (more than one lumen), includes administrative services, professional pharmacy services, care coordination, and all necessary supplies and equipment (drugs and nursing visits coded separately), per diem

◆ S5502 Home infusion therapy, catheter care/ maintenance, implanted access device, includes administrative services, professional pharmacy services, care coordination and all necessary supplies and equipment, (drugs and nursing visits coded separately), per diem (use this code for interim maintenance of vascular access not currently in use)

◆ S5517 Home infusion therapy, all supplies necessary for restoration of catheter patency or declotting

◆ S5518 Home infusion therapy, all supplies necessary for catheter repair

◆ S5520 Home infusion therapy, all supplies (including catheter) necessary for a peripherally inserted central venous catheter (PICC) line insertion

◆ S5521 Home infusion therapy, all supplies (including catheter) necessary for a midline catheter insertion

◆ S5522 Home infusion therapy, insertion of PICC, nursing services only (no supplies or catheter included)

◆ S5523 Home infusion therapy, insertion of midline central venous catheter, nursing services only (no supplies or catheter included)

◆ S5550 Insulin, rapid onset, 5 units

◆ S5551 Insulin, most rapid onset (Lispro or Aspart); 5 units

◆ S5552 Insulin, intermediate acting (NPH or Lente); 5 units

◆ S5553 Insulin, long acting; 5 units

◆ S5560 Insulin delivery device, reusable pen; 1.5 ml size

◆ S5561 Insulin delivery device, reusable pen; 3 ml size

◆ S5565 Insulin cartridge for use in insulin delivery device other than pump; 150 units

◆ S5566 Insulin cartridge for use in insulin delivery device other than pump; 300 units

◆ S5570 Insulin delivery device, disposable pen (including insulin); 1.5 ml size

◆ S5571 Insulin delivery device, disposable pen (including insulin); 3 ml size

S8004 Deleted 03/31/05

◆ S8030 Scleral application of tantalum ring(s) for localization of lesions for proton beam therapy

◆ S8035 Magnetic source imaging

◆ S8037 Magnetic resonance cholangiopancreatography (MRCP)

◆ S8040 Topographic brain mapping

◆ S8042 Magnetic resonance imaging (MRI), low-field

◆ S8049 Intraoperative radiation therapy (single administration)

◆ S8055 Ultrasound guidance for multifetal pregnancy reduction(s), technical component (only to be used when the physician doing the reduction procedure does not perform the ultrasound, guidance is included in the CPT code for multifetal pregnancy reduction-59866*)

◆ S8075 Computer analysis of full-field digital mammogram and further physician review for interpretation, mammography (list separately in addition to code for primary procedure)

◆ S8080 Scintimammography (radioimmunoscintigraphy of the breast), unilateral, including supply of radiopharmaceutical

◆ S8085 Fluorine-18 fluorodeoxyglucose (F-18 FDG) imaging using dual-head coincidence detection system (non-dedicated postiron emission test [PET] scan)

◆ S8092 Electron beam computed tomography (also known as ultrafast CT, cine CT)

◆ S8093 Computed tomographic angiography, coronary arteries, with contrast material(s)

S8095 Deleted 12/31/05

◆ S8096 Portable peak flow meter

◆ S8097 Asthma kit (including but not limited to portable peak expiratory flow meter, instructional video, brochure, and/or spacer)

◆ S8100 Holding chamber or spacer for use with an inhaler or nebulizer; without mask

◆ S8101 Holding chamber or spacer for use with an inhaler or nebulizer; with mask

◆ S8110 Peak expiratory flow rate (physician services)

*CPT only © 2005. Current Procedural Terminology, 2006, Professional Edition, American Medical Association. All Rights Reserved.

- ◆ S8120 Oxygen contents, gaseous, 1 unit equals 1 cubic foot
- ◆ S8121 Oxygen contents, liquid, 1 unit equals 1 pound
- ◆ S8185 Flutter device
- ◆ S8186 Swivel adaptor
- ◆ S8189 Tracheostomy supply, not otherwise classified
- ◆ S8190 Electronic spirometer (or micro spirometer)
- ◆ S8210 Mucus trap
- ◆ S8260 Oral orthotic for treatment of sleep apnea, includes fitting, fabrication, and materials
- ◆ S8262 Mandibular orthopedic repositioning device, each
- ◆ S8265 Haberman Feeder for cleft lip/palate
- ▶◆ S8270 Enuresis alarm, using auditory buzzer and/or vibration device
- ◆ S8301 Infection control supplies, not otherwise specified
- ◆ S8415 Supplies for home delivery of infant
- ◆ S8420 Gradient pressure aid (sleeve and glove combination), custom made
- ◆ S8421 Gradient pressure aid (sleeve and glove combination), ready made
- ◆ S8422 Gradient pressure aid (sleeve), custom made, medium weight
- ◆ S8423 Gradient pressure aid (sleeve), custom made, heavy weight
- ◆ S8424 Gradient pressure aid (sleeve), ready made
- ◆ S8425 Gradient pressure aid (glove), custom made, medium weight
- ◆ S8426 Gradient pressure aid (glove), custom made, heavy weight
- ◆ S8427 Gradient pressure aid (glove), ready made
- ◆ S8428 Gradient pressure aid (gauntlet), ready made
- ◆ S8429 Gradient pressure exterior wrap
- ◆ S8430 Padding for compression bandage, roll
- ◆ S8431 Compression bandage, roll
- S8434 Deleted 12/31/05
- ◆ S8450 Splint, prefabricated, digit (specify digit by use of modifier)
- ◆ S8451 Splint, prefabricated, wrist or ankle
- ◆ S8452 Splint, prefabricated, elbow
- ◆ S8460 Camisole, post-mastectomy
- ◆ S8490 Insulin syringes (100 syringes, any size)
- ▶◆ S8940 Equestrian/Hippotherapy, per session
- ◆ S8948 Application of a modality (requiring constant provider attendance) to one or more areas; low-level laser; each 15 minutes
- ◆ S8950 Complex lymphedema therapy, each 15 minutes
- ◆ S8990 Physical or manipulative therapy performed for maintenance rather than restoration

- ◆ S8999 Resuscitation bag (for use by patient on artificial respiration during power failure or other catastrophic event)
- ◆ S9001 Home uterine monitor with or without associated nursing services
- ◆ S9007 Ultrafiltration monitor
- ◆ S9015 Automated electroencephalogram (EEG) monitoring
- ◆ S9022 Digital subtraction angiography (use in addition to CPT code for the procedure for further identification)
- ◆ S9024 Paranasal sinus ultrasound
- ◆ S9025 Omnicardiogram/cardiointegram
- ◆ S9034 Extracorporeal shockwave lithotripsy for gall stones (if performed with ERCP, use 43265*)
- ◆ S9055 Procuren or other growth factor preparation to promote wound healing
- ◆ S9056 Coma stimulation per diem
- ◆ S9061 Home administration of aerosolized drug therapy (e.g., pentamidine); administrative services, professional pharmacy services, care coordination, all necessary supplies and equipment (drugs and nursing visits coded separately), per diem
- ◆ S9075 Smoking cessation treatment
- ◆ S9083 Global fee urgent care centers
- ◆ S9088 Services provided in an urgent care center (list in addition to code for service)
- ◆ S9090 Vertebral axial decompression, per session
- ◆ S9092 Canolith repositioning, per visit
- ◆ S9097 Home visit for wound care
- ◆ S9098 Home visit, phototherapy services (e.g. Bili-Lite), including equipment rental, nursing services, blood draw, supplies, and other services, per diem
- ◆ S9109 Congestive heart failure telemonitoring, equipment rental, including telescale, computer system and software, telephone connections, and maintenance, per month
- ◆ S9117 Back school, per visit
- ◆ S9122 Home health aide or certified nurse assistant, providing care in the home; per hour
- ◆ S9123 Nursing care, in the home; by registered nurse, per hour (use for general nursing care only, not to be used when CPT codes 99500-99602* can be used)
- ◆ S9124 Nursing care, in the home; by licensed practical nurse, per hour
- ◆ S9125 Respite care, in the home, per diem
- ◆ S9126 Hospice care, in the home, per diem
- ◆ S9127 Social work visit, in the home, per diem

- S9128   Speech therapy, in the home, per diem
- S9129   Occupational therapy, in the home, per diem
- S9131   Physical therapy; in the home, per diem
- S9140   Diabetic management program, follow-up visit to non-physician provider
- S9141   Diabetic management program, follow-up visit to physcian provider
- S9145   Insulin pump initiation, instruction in initial use of pump (pump not included)
- S9150   Evaluation by ocularist
- S9208   Home management of preterm labor, including administrative services, professional pharmacy services, care coordination, and all necessary supplies or equipment (drugs and nursing visits coded separately), per diem (do not use this code with any home infusion per diem code)
- S9209   Home management of preterm premature rupture of membranes (PPROM), including administrative services, professional pharmacy services, care coordination, and all necessary supplies or equipment (drugs and nursing visits coded separately), per diem (do not use this code with any home infusion per diem code)
- S9211   Home management of gestational hypertension, includes administrative services, professional pharmacy services, care coordination and all necessary supplies and equipment (drugs and nursing visits coded separately); per diem (do not use this code with any home infusion per diem code)
- S9212   Home management of postpartum hypertension, includes administrative services, professional pharmacy services, care coordination, and all necessary supplies and equipment (drugs and nursing visits coded separately), per diem (do not use this code with any home infusion per diem code)
- S9213   Home management of preeclampsia, includes administrative services, professional pharmacy services, care coordination, and all necessary supplies and equipment (drugs and nursing services coded separately); per diem (do not use this code with any home infusion per diem code)
- S9214   Home management of gestational diabetes, includes administrative services, professional pharmacy services, care coordination, and all necessary supplies and equipment (drugs and nursing visits coded separately); per diem (do not use this code with any home infusion per diem code)
- S9325   Home infusion therapy, pain management infusion; administrative services, professional pharmacy services, care coordination, and all necessary supplies and equipment, (drugs and nursing visits coded separately), per diem (do not use this code with S9326, S9327 or S9328)
- S9326   Home infusion therapy, continuous (twenty-four hours or more) pain management infusion; administrative services, professional pharmacy services, care coordination and all necessary supplies and equipment (drugs and nursing visits coded separately), per diem
- S9327   Home infusion therapy, intermittent (less than twenty-four hours) pain management infusion; administrative services, professional pharmacy services, care coordination, and all necessary supplies and equipment (drugs and nursing visits coded separately), per diem
- S9328   Home infusion therapy, implanted pump pain management infusion; administrative services, professional pharmacy services, care coordination, and all necessary supplies and equipment (drugs and nursing visits coded separately), per diem
- S9329   Home infusion therapy, chemotherapy infusion; administrative services, professional pharmacy services, care coordination, and all necessary supplies and equipment (drugs and nursing visits coded separately), per diem (do not use this code with S9330 or S9331)
- S9330   Home infusion therapy, continuous (twenty-four hours or more) chemotherapy infusion; administrative services, professional pharmacy services, care coordination, and all necessary supplies and equipment (drugs and nursing visits coded separately), per diem
- S9331   Home infusion therapy, intermittent (less than twenty-four hours) chemotherapy infusion; administrative services, professional pharmacy services, care coordination, and all necessary supplies and equipment (drugs and nursing visits coded separately), per diem
- S9335   Home therapy, hemodialysis; administrative services, professional pharmacy services, care coordination, and all necessary supplies and equipment (drugs and nursing services coded separately), per diem

◆ S9336   Home infusion therapy, continuous anticoagulant infusion therapy (e.g. heparin), administrative services, professional pharmacy services, care coordination and all necessary supplies and equipment (drugs and nursing visits coded separately), per diem

◆ S9338   Home infusion therapy, immunotherapy therapy; (e.g., intravenous immunoglobulin, interferon); administrative services, professional pharmacy services, care coordination, and all necessary supplies and equipment (drug and nursing visits coded separately), per diem

◆ S9339   Home therapy; peritoneal dialysis, administrative services, professional pharmacy services, care coordination and all necessary supplies and equipment (drugs and nursing visits coded separately), per diem

◆ S9340   Home therapy; enteral nutrition; administrative services, professional pharmacy services, care coordination, and all necessary supplies and equipment (enteral formula and nursing visits coded separately), per diem

◆ S9341   Home therapy; enteral nutrition via gravity; administrative services, professional pharmacy services, care coordination, and all necessary supplies and equipment (enteral formula and nursing visits coded separately), per diem

◆ S9342   Home therapy; enteral nutrition via pump; administrative services, professional pharmacy services, care coordination, and all necessary supplies and equipment (enteral formula and nursing visits coded separately), per diem

◆ S9343   Home therapy; enteral nutrition via bolus; administrative services, professional pharmacy services, care coordination, and all necessary supplies and equipment (enteral formula and nursing visits coded separately), per diem

◆ S9345   Home infusion therapy, anti-hemophilic agent infusion therapy (e.g. Factor VIII); administrative services, professional pharmacy services, care coordination, and all necessary supplies and equipment (drugs and nursing visits coded separately), per diem

◆ S9346   Home infusion therapy, alpha-1-proteinase inhibitor (e.g., Prolastin); administrative services, professional pharmacy services, care coordination, and all necessary supplies and equipment (drugs and nursing visits coded separately), per diem

◆ S9347   Home infusion therapy, uninterrupted, long-term, controlled rate IV or subcutaneous infusion therapy (e.g. Epoprostenol); administrative services, professional pharmacy services, care coordination, and all necessary supplies and equipment (drugs and nursing visits coded separately), per diem

◆ S9348   Home infusion therapy, sympathomimetic/inotropic agent infusion therapy (e.g., Dobutamine); administrative services, professional pharmacy services, care coordination, all necessary supplies and equipment (drugs and nursing visits coded separately), per diem

◆ S9349   Home infusion therapy, tocolytic infusion therapy; administrative services, professional pharmacy services, care coordination, and all necessary supplies and equipment (drugs and nursing visits coded separately), per diem

◆ S9351   Home infusion therapy, continuous antiemetic infusion therapy; administrative services, professional pharmacy services, care coordination, all necessary supplies and equipment (drugs and nursing visits coded separately), per diem

◆ S9353   Home infusion therapy, continuous insulin infusion therapy; administrative services, professional pharmacy services, care coordination, and all necessary supplies and equipment (drugs and nursing visits coded separately), per diem

◆ S9355   Home infusion therapy, chelation therapy; administrative services, professional pharmacy services, care coordination, and all necessary supplies and equipment (drugs and nursing visits coded separately), per diem

◆ S9357   Home infusion therapy, enzyme replacement IV therapy; (e.g. Imiglucerase); administrative services, professional pharmacy services, care coordination, and all necessary supplies and equipment (drugs and nursing visits coded separately), per diem

◆ S9359   Home infusion therapy, anti-tumor necrosis factor IV therapy; (e.g. Infliximab); administrative services, professional pharmacy services, care coordination, and all necessary supplies and equipment (drugs and nursing visits coded separately), per diem

◆ S9361   Home infusion therapy, diuretic IV therapy; administrative services, professional pharmacy services, care coordination, and all necessary supplies and equipment (drugs and nursing visits coded separately), per diem

◆ S9363   Home infusion therapy, anti-spasmotic therapy; administrative services, professional pharmacy services, care coordination, and all necessary supplies and equipment (drugs and nursing visits coded separately), per diem

◆ S9364   Home infusion therapy, total parenteral nutrition (TPN); administrative services, professional pharmacy services, care co-ordination, and all necessary supplies and equipment including standard TPN formula (lipids, specialty amino acid formulas, drugs other than in standard formula and nursing visits coded separately) per diem (do not use with home infusion codes S9365-S9368 using daily volume scales)

◆ S9365   Home infusion therapy, total parenteral nutrition (TPN); one liter per day, administrative services, professional pharmacy services, care coordination, and all necessary supplies and equipment including standard TPN formula (lipids, specialty amino acid formulas, drugs other than in standard formula and nursing visits coded separately), per diem

◆ S9366   Home infusion therapy, total parenteral nutrition (TPN); more than one liter but no more than two liters per day, administrative services, professional pharmacy services, care coordination, and all necessary supplies and equipment including standard TPN formula; (lipids, specialty amino acid formulas, drugs other than in standard formula and nursing visits coded separately), per diem

◆ S9367   Home infusion therapy, total parenteral nutrition (TPN); more than two liters but no more than three liters per day, administrative services, professional pharmacy services, care coordination, and all necessary supplies and equipment including standard TPN formula; (lipids, specialty amino acid formulas, drugs other than in standard formula and nursing visits coded separately), per diem

◆ S9368   Home infusion therapy, total parenteral nutrition (TPN); more than three liters per day, administrative services, professional pharmacy services, care coordination, and all necessary supplies and equipment (includes standard TPN formula; (lipids, specialty amino acid formulas, drugs other than in standard formula and nursing visits coded separately), per diem

◆ S9370   Home therapy, intermittent antiemetic injection therapy; administrative services, professional pharmacy services, care coordination, and all necessary supplies and equipment (drugs and nursing visits coded separately), per diem

◆ S9372   Home therapy; intermittent anti-coagulant injection therapy (e.g. heparin); administrative services, professional pharmacy services, care coordination, and all necessary supplies and equipment (drugs and nursing visits coded separately), per diem (do not use this code for flushing of infusion devices with heparin to maintain patency)

◆ S9373   Home infusion therapy, hydration therapy; administrative services, professional pharmacy services, care coordination, and all necessary supplies and equipment (drugs and nursing visits coded separately), per diem (do not use with hydration therapy codes S9374-S9377 using daily volume scales)

◆ S9374   Home infusion therapy, hydration therapy; one liter per day, administrative services, professional pharmacy services, care coordination, and all necessary supplies and equipment (drugs and nursing visits coded separately), per diem

◆ S9375   Home infusion therapy, hydration therapy; more than one liter but no more than two liters per day, administrative services, professional pharmacy services, care coordination, and all necessary supplies and equipment (drugs and nursing visits coded separately), per diem

◆ S9376   Home infusion therapy, hydration therapy; more than two liters but no more than three liters per day, administrative services, professional pharmacy services, care coordination, and all necessary supplies and equipment (drugs and nursing visits coded separately), per diem

◆ S9377   Home infusion therapy, hydration therapy; more than three liters per day, administrative services, professional pharmacy services, care coordination, and all necessary supplies (drugs and nursing visits coded separately), per diem

◆ S9379   Home infusion therapy, infusion therapy, not otherwise classified; administrative services, professional pharmacy services, care coordination, and all necessary supplies and equipment (drugs and nursing visits coded separately), per diem

◆ S9381   Delivery or service to high risk areas requiring escort or extra protection, per visit

◆ S9401   Anti-coagulation clinic, inclusive of all services except laboratory tests, per session

◆ S9430   Pharmacy compounding and dispensing services

◆ S9434   Modified solid food supplements for inborn errors of metabolism

◆ S9435   Medical foods for inborn errors of metabolism

◆ S9436   Childbirth preparation/Lamaze classes, non-physician provider, per session

◆ S9437   Childbirth refresher classes, non-physician provider, per session

◆ S9438   Cesarean birth classes, non-physician provider, per session

◆ S9439   Vaginal birth after cesarean (VBAC) classes, non-physician provider, per session

◆ S9441   Asthma education, non-physician provider, per session

◆ S9442   Birthing classes, non-physician provider, per session

◆ S9443   Lactation classes, non-physician provider, per session

◆ S9444   Parenting classes, non-physician provider, per session

◆ S9445   Patient education, not otherwise classified, non-physician provider, individual, per session

◆ S9446   Patient education, not otherwise classified, non-physician provider, group, per session

◆ S9447   Infant safety (including cardiopulmonary resuscitation [CPR]) classes, non-physician provider, per session

◆ S9449   Weight management classes, non-physician provider, per session

◆ S9451   Exercise classes, non-physician provider, per session

◆ S9452   Nutrition classes, non-physician provider, per session

◆ S9453   Smoking cessation classes, non-physician provider, per session

◆ S9454   Stress management classes, non-physician provider, per session

◆ S9455   Diabetic management program, group session

◆ S9460   Diabetic management program, nurse visit

◆ S9465   Diabetic management program, dietitian visit

◆ S9470   Nutritional counseling, dietitian visit

◆ S9472   Cardiac rehabilitation program, non-physician provider, per diem

◆ S9473   Pulmonary rehabilitation program, non-physician provider, per diem

◆ S9474   Enterostomal therapy by a registered nurse certified in enterostomal therapy, per diem

◆ S9475   Ambulatory setting substance abuse treatment or detoxification services, per diem

◆ S9476   Vestibular rehabilitation program, non-physician provider, per diem

◆ S9480   Intensive outpatient psychiatric services, per diem

◆ S9482   Family stabilization services, per 15 minutes

◆ S9484   Crisis intervention mental health services, per hour

◆ S9485   Crisis intervention mental health services, per diem

◆ S9490   Home infusion therapy, corticosteroid infusion; administrative services, professional pharmacy services, care coordination, and all necessary supplies and equipment (drugs and nursing visits coded separately), per diem

◆ S9494   Home infusion therapy, antibiotic, antiviral, or anti-fungal therapy; administrative services, professional pharmacy services, care coordination, and all necessary supplies and equipment (drug and nursing visits coded separately, per diem), (do not use with home infusion codes for hourly dosing schedules S9497-S9504)

◆ S9497   Home infusion therapy, antibiotic, antiviral, or anti-fungal therapy; once every 3 hours; administrative services, professional pharmacy services, care coordination, and all necessary supplies and equipment (drugs and nursing visits coded separately), per diem

◆ S9500   Home infusion therapy, antibiotic, antiviral, or anti-fungal therapy; once every 24 hours; administrative services, professional pharmacy services, care coordination, and all necessary supplies and equipment (drugs and nursing visits coded separately), per diem

◆ S9501   Home infusion therapy, antibiotic, antiviral, or anti-fungal therapy; once every 12 hours; administrative services, professional pharmacy services, care coordination, and all necessary supplies and equipment (drugs and nursing visits coded separately), per diem

◆ S9502   Home infusion therapy, antibiotic, antiviral, or anti-fungal therapy; once every 8 hours, administrative services, professional pharmacy services, care coordination, and all necessary supplies and equipment (drugs and nursing visits coded separately), per diem

◆ S9503 Home infusion therapy, antibiotic, anti-viral, or anti-fungal; once every 6 hours; administrative services, professional pharmacy services, care coordination, and all necessary supplies and equipment (drugs and nursing visits coded separately), per diem

◆ S9504 Home infusion therapy, antibiotic, anti-viral, or anti-fungal; once every 4 hours; administrative services, professional pharmacy services, care coordination, and all necessary supplies and equipment (drugs and nursing visits coded separately), per diem

◆ S9529 Routine venipuncture for collection of specimen(s), single home bound, nursing home, or skilled nursing facility patient

◆ S9537 Home therapy; hematopoietic hormone injection therapy (e.g. erythropoietin, G-CSF, GM-CSF); administrative services, professional pharmacy services, care coordination, and all necessary supplies and equipment (drugs and nursing visits coded separately), per diem

◆ S9538 Home transfusion of blood product(s); administrative services, professional pharmacy services, care coordination and all necessary supplies and equipment (blood products, drugs, and nursing visits coded separately), per diem

◆ S9542 Home injectable therapy; not otherwise classified, including administrative services, professional pharmacy services, care coordination, and all necessary supplies and equipment (drugs and nursing visits coded separately), per diem

◆ S9558 Home infusion therapy; growth hormone, including administrative services, professional pharmacy services, care coordination, and all necessary supplies and equipment (drugs and nursing visits coded separately), per diem

◆ S9559 Home infusion therapy; interferon, including administrative services, professional pharmacy services, care coordination, and all necessary supplies and equipment (drugs and nursing visits coded separately), per diem

◆ S9560 Home injectable therapy; hormonal therapy (e.g.; Leuprolide, Goserelin), including administrative services, professional pharmacy services, care coordination, and all necessary supplies and equipment (drugs and nursing visits coded separately), per diem

◆ S9562 Home injectable therapy, palivizumab, including administrative services, professional pharmacy services, care coordination, and all necessary supplies and equipment (drugs and nursing visits coded separately), per diem

◆ S9590 Home therapy, irrigation therapy (e.g. sterile irrigation of an organ or anatomical cavity); including administrative services, professional pharmacy services, care coordination, and all necessary supplies and equipment (drugs and nursing visits coded separately), per diem

◆ S9810 Home therapy; professional pharmacy services for provision of infusion, specialty drug administration, and/or disease state management, not otherwise classified, per hour (do not use this code with any per diem code)

◆ S9900 Services by authorized Christian Science Practitioner for the process of healing, per diem; not to be used for rest or study; excludes in-patient services

◆ S9970 Health club membership, annual

◆ S9975 Transplant related lodging, meals and transportation, per diem

◆ S9976 Lodging, per diem, not otherwise specified

◆ S9977 Meals, per diem, not otherwise specified

◆ S9981 Medical records copying fee, administrative

◆ S9982 Medical records copying fee, per page

◆ S9986 Not medically necessary service (patient is aware that service not medically necessary)

◆ S9988 Services provided as part of phase I clinical trial

◆ S9989 Services provided outside of the United States of America (list in addition to code[s] for services[s])

◆ S9990 Services provided as part of a phase II clinical trial

◆ S9991 Services provided as part of a phase III clinical trial

◆ S9992 Transportation costs to and from trial location and local transportation costs (e.g., fares for taxicab or bus) for clinical trial participant and one caregiver/companion

◆ S9994 Lodging costs (e.g., hotel charges) for clinical trial participant and one caregiver/companion

◆ S9996 Meals for clinical trial participant and one caregiver/companion

◆ S9999 Sales tax

NATIONAL T CODES FOR STATE MEDICAID AGENCIES (T1000-T9999)

Not Valid For Medicare

◆ T1000 Private duty/independent nursing service(s), licensed, up to 15 minutes
◆ T1001 Nursing assessment/evaluation
◆ T1002 RN services, up to 15 minutes
◆ T1003 Licensed practical nurse/licensed nurse (LPN/LVN) services, up to 15 minutes
◆ T1004 Services of a qualified nursing aide, up to 15 minutes
◆ T1005 Respite care services, up to 15 minutes
◆ T1006 Alcohol and/or substance abuse services, family/couple counseling
◆ T1007 Alcohol and/or substance abuse services, treatment plan development and/or modification
◆ T1009 Child sitting services for children of the individual receiving alcohol and/or substance abuse services
◆ T1010 Meals for individuals receiving alcohol and/or substance abuse services (when meals not included in the program)
◆ T1012 Alcohol and/or substance abuse services, skills development
◆ T1013 Sign language or oral interpreter services, per 15 minutes
◆ T1014 Telehealth transmission, per minute, professional services bill separately
◆ T1015 Clinic visit/encounter, all-inclusive
◆ T1016 Case Management, each 15 minutes
◆ T1017 Targeted Case Management, each 15 minutes
◆ T1018 School-based IEP services, bundled
◆ T1019 Personal care services, per 15 minutes, not for an in-patient or resident of a hospital, nursing facility, ICF/MR or IMD, part of the individualized plan of treatment (code may not be used to identify services provided by home health aide or certified nurse assistant)
◆ T1020 Personal care services, per diem, not for an inpatient or resident of a hospital, nursing facility, ICF/MR or IMD, part of the individualized plan of treatment (code may not be used to identify services provided by home health aide or certified nurse assistant)
◆ T1021 Home health aide or certified nurse assistant, per visit
◆ T1022 Contracted home health agency services, all services provided under contract, per day
◆ T1023 Screening to determine the appropriateness of consideration of an individual for participation in a specified program, project or treatment protocol, per encounter

◆ T1024 Evaluation and treatment by an integrated, specialty team contracted to provide coordinated care to multiple or severely handicapped children, per encounter
◆ T1025 Intensive, extended multidisciplinary services provided in a clinic setting to children with complex medical, physical, mental and psychosocial impairments, per diem
◆ T1026 Intensive, extended multidisciplinary services provided in a clinic setting to children with complex medical, physical, medical and psychosocial impairments, per hour
◆ T1027 Family training and counseling for child development, per 15 minutes
◆ T1028 Assessment of home, physical and family environment, to determine suitability to meet patient's medical needs
◆ T1029 Comprehensive environmental lead investigation, not including laboratory analysis, per dwelling
◆ T1030 Nursing care, in the home, by registered nurse, per diem
◆ T1031 Nursing care, in the home, by licensed practical nurse, per diem
◆ T1502 Administration of oral, intramuscular and/or subcutaneous medication by health care agency/professional, per visit
◆ T1999 Miscellaneous therapeutic items and supplies, retail purchases, not otherwise classified; identify product in "remarks"
◆ T2001 Non-emergency transportation; patient attendant/escort
◆ T2002 Non-emergency transportation; per diem
◆ T2003 Non-emergency transportation; encounter/trip
◆ T2004 Non-emergency transport; commercial carrier, multi-pass
➡ ◆ T2005 Non-emergency transportation: stretcher van
  T2006 Deleted 12/31/05
◆ T2007 Transportation waiting time, air ambulance and non-emergency vehicle, one-half (1/2) hour increments
◆ T2010 Preadmission screening and resident review (PASRR) level I identification screening, per screen
◆ T2011 Preadmission screening and resident review (PASRR) level II evaluation, per evaluation
◆ T2012 Habilitation, educational; waiver, per diem
◆ T2013 Habilitation, educational, waiver; per hour
◆ T2014 Habilitation, prevocational, waiver; per diem

◆ T2015   Habilitation, prevocational, waiver; per hour

◆ T2016   Habilitation, residential, waiver; per diem

◆ T2017   Habilitation, residential, waiver; 15 minutes

◆ T2018   Habilitation, supported employment, waiver; per diem

◆ T2019   Habilitation, supported employment, waiver; per 15 minutes

◆ T2020   Day habilitation, waiver; per diem

◆ T2021   Day habilitation, waiver; per 15 minutes

◆ T2022   Case management, per month

◆ T2023   Targeted case management; per month

◆ T2024   Service assessment/plan of care development, waiver

◆ T2025   Waiver services; not otherwise specified (NOS)

◆ T2026   Specialized childcare, waiver; per diem

◆ T2027   Specialized childcare, waiver; per 15 minutes

◆ T2028   Specialized supply, not otherwise specified, waiver

◆ T2029   Specialized medical equipment, not otherwise specified, waiver

◆ T2030   Assisted living, waiver; per month

◆ T2031   Assisted living; waiver, per diem

◆ T2032   Residential care, not otherwise specified (NOS), waiver; per month

◆ T2033   Residential care, not otherwise specified (NOS), waiver; per diem

◆ T2034   Crisis intervention, waiver; per diem

◆ T2035   Utility services to support medical equipment and assistive technology/devices, waiver

◆ T2036   Therapeutic camping, overnight, waiver; each session

◆ T2037   Therapeutic camping, day, waiver; each session

◆ T2038   Community transition, waiver; per service

◆ T2039   Vehicle modifications, waiver; per service

◆ T2040   Financial management, self-directed, waiver; per 15 minutes

◆ T2041   Supports brokerage, self-directed, waiver; per 15 minutes

◆ T2042   Hospice routine home care; per diem

◆ T2043   Hospice continuous home care; per hour

◆ T2044   Hospice inpatient respite care; per diem

◆ T2045   Hospice general inpatient care; per diem

◆ T2046   Hospice long term care, room and board only; per diem

◆ T2048   Behavioral health; long-term care residential (non-acute care in a residential treatment program where stay is typically longer than 30 days), with room and board, per diem

◆ T2049   Non-emergency transportation; stretcher van, mileage; per mile

◆ T2101   Human breast milk processing, storage and distribution only

◆ T4521   Adult sized disposable incontinence product, brief/diaper, small, each
CIM 60-9

◆ T4522   Adult sized disposable incontinence product, brief/diaper, medium, each
CIM 60-9

◆ T4523   Adult sized disposable incontinence product, brief/diaper, large, each
CIM 60-9

◆ T4524   Adult sized disposable incontinence product, brief/diaper, extra large, each
CIM 60-9

◆ T4525   Adult sized disposable incontinence product, protective underwear/pull-on, small size, each
CIM 60-9

◆ T4526   Adult sized disposable incontinence product, protective underwear/pull-on, medium size, each
CIM 60-9

◆ T4527   Adult sized disposable incontinence product, protective underwear/pull-on, large size, each
CIM 60-9

◆ T4528   Adult sized disposable incontinence product, protective underwear/pull-on, extra large size, each
CIM 60-9

◆ T4529   Pediatric sized disposable incontinence product, brief/diaper, small/medium size, each
CIM 60-9

◆ T4530   Pediatric sized disposable incontinence product, brief/diaper, large size, each
CIM 60-9

◆ T4531   Pediatric sized disposable incontinence product, protective underwear/pull-on, small/medium size, each
CIM 60-9

◆ T4532   Pediatric sized disposable incontinence product, protective underwear/pull-on, large size, each
CIM 60-9

◆ T4533   Youth sized disposable incontinence product, brief/diaper, each
CIM 60-9

◆ T4534   Youth sized disposable incontinence product, protective underwear/pull-on, each
CIM 60-9

◆ T4535   Disposable liner/shield/guard/pad/undergarment, for incontinence, each
CIM 60-9

◆ T4536   Incontinence product, protective underwear/pull-on, reusable, any size, each
CIM 60-9

◆ T4537   Incontinence product, protective under-
          pad, reusable, bed size, each
          CIM 60-9
◆ T4538   Diaper service, reusable diaper, each di-
          aper
          CIM 60-9
◆ T4539   Incontinence product, diaper/brief, re-
          usable, any size, each
          CIM 60-9
◆ T4540   Incontinence product, protective under-
          pad, reusable, chair size, each
          CIM 60-9
◆ T4541   Incontinence product, disposable under-
          pad, large, each
◆ T4542   Incontinence product, disposable under-
          pad, small size, each
◆ T5001   Positioning seat for persons with spe-
          cial orthopedic needs, for use in vehi-
          cles
◆ T5999   Supply, not otherwise specified

VISION SERVICES (V0000-V2999)

Frames

◎ V2020   Frames, purchases
          MCM 2130
◆ V2025   Deluxe frame
          MCM 3045.4

Spectacle Lenses

NOTE: If a CPT procedure code for supply of spectacles or a permanent prosthesis is reported, recode
with the specific lens type listed below. For aphakic
temporary spectacle correction, see CPT.*

Single Vision, Glass or Plastic

∗ V2100   Sphere, single vision, plano to plus or
          minus 4.00, per lens
∗ V2101   Sphere, single vision, plus or minus
          4.12 to plus or minus 7.00d, per lens
∗ V2102   Sphere, single vision, plus or minus
          7.12 to plus or minus 20.00d, per lens
∗ V2103   Spherocylinder, single vision, plano to
          plus or minus 4.00d sphere, 0.12 to
          2.00d cylinder, per lens
∗ V2104   Spherocylinder, single vision, plano to
          plus or minus 4.00d sphere, 2.12 to
          4.00d cylinder, per lens
∗ V2105   Spherocylinder, single vision, plano to
          plus or minus 4.00d sphere, 4.25 to
          6.00d cylinder, per lens

∗ V2106   Spherocylinder, single vision, plano to
          plus or minus 4.00d sphere, over 6.00d
          cylinder, per lens
∗ V2107   Spherocylinder, single vision, plus or
          minus 4.25 to plus or minus 7.00
          sphere, 0.12 to 2.00d cylinder, per lens
∗ V2108   Spherocylinder, single vision, plus or
          minus 4.25d to plus or minus 7.00d
          sphere, 2.12 to 4.00d cylinder, per lens
∗ V2109   Spherocylinder, single vision, plus or
          minus 4.25 to plus or minus 7.00d
          sphere, 4.25 to 6.00d cylinder, per lens
∗ V2110   Sperocylinder, single vision, plus or mi-
          nus 4.25 to 7.00d sphere, over 6.00d
          cylinder, per lens
∗ V2111   Spherocylinder, single vision, plus or
          minus 7.25 to plus or minus 12.00d
          sphere, 0.25 to 2.25d cylinder, per lens
∗ V2112   Spherocylinder, single vision, plus or
          minus 7.25 to plus or minus 12.00d
          sphere, 2.25d to 4.00d cylinder, per lens
∗ V2113   Spherocylinder, single vision, plus or
          minus 7.25 to plus or minus 12.00d
          sphere, 4.25 to 6.00d cylinder, per lens
∗ V2114   Spherocylinder, single vision, sphere
          over plus or minus 12.00d, per lens
∗ V2115   Lenticular (myodisc), per lens, single
          vision
∗ V2118   Aniseikonic lens, single vision
◎ V2121   Lenticular lens, per lens, single
          MCM 2130B
∗ V2199   Not otherwise classified, single vision
          lens

Bifocal, Glass or Plastic

∗ V2200   Sphere, bifocal, plano to plus or minus
          4.00d, per lens
∗ V2201   Sphere, bifocal, plus or minus 4.12 to
          plus or minus 7.00d, per lens
∗ V2202   Sphere, bifocal, plus or minus 7.12 to
          plus or minus 20.00d, per lens
∗ V2203   Spherocylinder, bifocal, plano to plus
          or minus 4.00d sphere, 0.12 to 2.00d
          cylinder, per lens
∗ V2204   Spherocylinder, bifocal, plano to plus
          or minus 4.00d sphere, 2.12 to 4.00d
          cylinder, per lens
∗ V2205   Spherocylinder, bifocal, plano to plus
          or minus 4.00d sphere, 4.25 to 6.00d
          cylinder, per lens
∗ V2206   Spherocylinder, bifocal, plano to plus
          or minus 4.00d sphere, over 6.00d cyl-
          inder, per lens
∗ V2207   Spherocylinder, bifocal, plus or minus
          4.25 to plus or minus 7.00d sphere, 0.12
          to 2.00d cylinder, per lens
∗ V2208   Spherocylinder, bifocal, plus or minus
          4.25 to plus or minus 7.00d sphere, 2.12
          to 4.00d cylinder, per lens

---

* V2209 Spherocylinder, bifocal, plus or minus 4.25 to plus or minus 7.00d sphere, 4.25 to 6.00d cylinder, per lens
* V2210 Spherocylinder, bifocal, plus or minus 4.25 to plus or minus 7.00d sphere, over 6.00d cylinder, per lens
* V2211 Spherocylinder, bifocal, plus or minus 7.25 to plus or minus 12.00d sphere, 0.25 to 2.25d cylinder, per lens
* V2212 Spherocylinder, bifocal, plus or minus 7.25 to plus or minus 12.00d sphere, 2.25 to 4.00d cylinder, per lens
* V2213 Spherocylinder, bifocal, plus or minus 7.25 to plus or minus 12.00d sphere, 4.25 to 6.00d cylinder, per lens
* V2214 Spherocylinder, bifocal, sphere over plus or minus 12.00d, per lens
* V2215 Lenticular (myodisc), per lens, bifocal
* V2218 Aniseikonic, per lens, bifocal
* V2219 Bifocal seg width over 28 mm
* V2220 Bifocal add over 3.25d
⊚ V2221 Lenticular lens, per lens, bifocal
         MCM 2130B
* V2299 Specialty bifocal (by report)

Trifocal, Glass or Plastic

* V2300 Sphere, trifocal, plano to plus or minus 4.00d, per lens
* V2301 Sphere, trifocal, plus or minus 4.12 to plus or minus 7.00d per lens
* V2302 Sphere, trifocal, plus or minus 7.12 to plus or minus 20.00, per lens
* V2303 Spherocylinder, trifocal, plano to plus or minus 4.00d sphere, 0.12 to 2.00d cylinder, per lens
* V2304 Spherocylinder, trifocal, plano to plus or minus 4.00d sphere, 2.25 to 4.00d cylinder, per lens
* V2305 Spherocylinder, trifocal, plano to plus or minus 4.00d sphere, 4.25 to 6.00 cylinder, per lens
* V2306 Spherocylinder, trifocal, plano to plus or minus 4.00d sphere, over 6.00d cylinder, per lens
* V2307 Spherocylinder, trifocal, plus or minus 4.25 to plus or minus 7.00d sphere, 0.12 to 2.00d cylinder, per lens
* V2308 Spherocylinder, trifocal, plus or minus 4.25 to plus or minus 7.00d sphere, 2.12 to 4.00d cylinder, per lens
* V2309 Spherocylinder, trifocal, plus or minus 4.25 to plus or minus 7.00d sphere, 4.25 to 6.00d cylinder, per lens
* V2310 Spherocylinder, trifocal, plus or minus 4.25 to plus or minus 7.00d sphere, over 6.00d cylinder, per lens
* V2311 Spherocylinder, trifocal, plus or minus 7.25 to plus or minus 12.00d sphere, 0.25 to 2.25d cylinder, per lens

* V2312 Spherocylinder, trifocal, plus or minus 7.25 to plus or minus 12.00d sphere, 2.25 to 4.00d cylinder, per lens
* V2313 Spherocylinder, trifocal, plus or minus 7.25 to plus or minus 12.00d sphere, 4.25 to 6.00d cylinder, per lens
* V2314 Spherocylinder, trifocal, sphere over plus or minus 12.00d, per lens
* V2315 Lenticular (myodisc), per lens, trifocal
* V2318 Aniseikonic lens, trifocal
* V2319 Trifocal seg width over 28 mm
* V2320 Trifocal add over 3.25d
⊚ V2321 Lenticular lens, per lens, trifocal
         MCM 2130B
* V2399 Specialty trifocal (by report)

Variable Asphericity

* V2410 Variable asphericity lens, single vision, full field, glass or plastic, per lens
* V2430 Variable asphericity lens, bifocal, full field, glass or plastic, per lens
* V2499 Variable sphericity lens, other type

Contact Lenses

If a CPT procedure code for supply of contact lens is reported, recode with specific lens type listed below (per lens).

* V2500 Contact lens, PMMA, spherical, per lens
* V2501 Contact lens, PMMA, toric or prism ballast, per lens
* V2502 Contact lens PMMA, bifocal, per lens
* V2503 Contact lens PMMA, color vision deficiency, per lens
* V2510 Contact lens, gas permeable, spherical, per lens
* V2511 Contact lens, gas permeable, toric, prism ballast, per lens
* V2512 Contact lens, gas permeable, bifocal, per lens
* V2513 Contact lens, gas permeable, extended wear, per lens
⊚ V2520 Contact lens, hydrophilic, spherical, per lens
         CIM 45-7, CIM 65-1
⊚ V2521 Contact lens, hydrophilic, toric, or prism ballast, per lens
         CIM 45-7, CIM 65-1
⊚ V2522 Contact lens, hydrophilic, bifocal, per lens
         CIM 45-7, CIM 65-1
⊚ V2523 Contact lens, hydrophilic, extended wear, per lens
         CIM 45-7, CIM 65-1
* V2530 Contact lens, scleral, gas impermeable, per lens (for modification, see contact lens, 92325*)

⊚ **Special coverage instructions** ◆ **Not covered by or valid for Medicare** * **Carrier discretion** ◀▶ **New** ◀▥▶ **Revised**

⊙ V2531   Contact lens, scleral, gas permeable, per lens (for contact lens modification, see 92325*)
CIM 65-3

∗ V2599   Contact lens, other type

Low Vision Aids

If a CPT procedure code for supply of low vision aid is reported, recode with specific systems listed below.

∗ V2600   Hand-held low vision aids and other nonspectacle mounted aids

∗ V2610   Single lens spectacle mounted low vision aids

∗ V2615   Telescopic and other compound lens system, including distance vision telescopic, near vision telescopes and compound microscopic lens system

Prosthetic Eye

⊙ V2623   Prosthetic eye, plastic, custom
MCM 2133

∗ V2624   Polishing/resurfacing of ocular prosthesis

∗ V2625   Enlargement of ocular prosthesis

∗ V2626   Reduction of ocular prosthesis

⊙ V2627   Scleral cover shell
CIM 65-3

∗ V2628   Fabrication and fitting of ocular conformer

∗ V2629   Prosthetic eye, other type

Intraocular Lenses

⊙ V2630   Anterior chamber intraocular lens
MCM 2130

⊙ V2631   Iris supported intraocular lens
MCM 2130

⊙ V2632   Posterior chamber intraocular lens
MCM 2130

Miscellaneous

∗ V2700   Balance lens, per lens

◆ V2702   Deluxe lens feature
MCM 2130B

∗ V2710   Slab off prism, glass or plastic, per lens

∗ V2715   Prism, per lens

∗ V2718   Press-on lens, Fresnel prism, per lens

∗ V2730   Special base curve, glass or plastic, per lens

⊙ V2744   Tint, photochromatic, per lens
MCM 2130B

⊙ V2745   Addition to lens, tint, any color, solid, gradient or equal, excludes photochromatic, any lens material, per lens
MCM 2130B

⊙ V2750   Anti-reflective coating, per lens
MCM 2130B

⊙ V2755   U-V lens, per lens
MCM 2130B

◆ V2756   Eye glass case

∗ V2760   Scratch resistant coating, per lens

⊙ V2761   Mirror coating, any type, solid, gradient or equal, any lens material, per lens
MCM 2130B

⊙ V2762   Polarization, any lens material, per lens
MCM 2130B

∗ V2770   Occluder lens, per lens

∗ V2780   Oversize lens, per lens

∗ V2781   Progressive lens, per lens

⊙ V2782   Lens, index 1.54 to 1.65 plastic or 1.60 to 1.79 glass, excludes polycarbonate, per lens
MCM 2130B

⊙ V2783   Lens, index greater than or equal to 1.66 plastic or greater than or equal to 1.80 glass, excludes polycarbonate, per lens
MCM 2130B

⊙ V2784   Lens, polycarbonate or equal, any index, per lens
MCM 2130B

∗ V2785   Processing, preserving and transporting corneal tissue

⊙ V2786   Specialty occupational multifocal lens, per lens
MCM 2130B

▶◆ V2788   Presbyopia correcting function of intraocular lens
Medicare Statute 1862(a)(7)

∗ V2790   Amniotic membrane for surgical reconstruction, per procedure

∗ V2797   Vision supply, accessory and/or service component of another HCPCS vision code

∗ V2799   Vision service, miscellaneous

HEARING SERVICES (V5000-V5999)

NOTE: These codes are for non-physician services.

◆ V5008   Hearing screening
MCM 2320

◆ V5010   Assessment for hearing aid
Medicare Statute 1862A7

◆ V5011   Fitting/orientation/checking of hearing aid
Medicare Statute 1862A7

◆ V5014   Repair/modification of a hearing aid
Medicare Statute 1862A7

◆ V5020 Conformity evaluation
Medicare Statute 1862A7

◆ V5030 Hearing aid, monaural, body worn, air conduction
Medicare Statute 1862A7

◆ V5040 Hearing aid, monaural, body worn, bone conduction
Medicare Statute 1862A7

◆ V5050 Hearing aid, monaural, in the ear
Medicare Statute 1862A7

◆ V5060 Hearing aid, monaural, behind the ear
Medicare Statute 1862A7

◆ V5070 Glasses, air conduction
Medicare Statute 1862A7

◆ V5080 Glasses, bone conduction
Medicare Statute 1862A7

◆ V5090 Dispensing fee, unspecified hearing aid
Medicare Statute 1862A7

◆ V5095 Semi-implantable middle ear hearing prosthesis
Medicare Statute 1862a7

◆ V5100 Hearing aid, bilateral, body worn
Medicare Statute 1862A7

◆ V5110 Dispensing fee, bilateral
Medicare Statute 1862A7

◆ V5120 Binaural, body
Medicare Statute 1862A7

◆ V5130 Binaural, in the ear
Medicare Statute 1862A7

◆ V5140 Binaural, behind the ear
Medicare Statute 1862A7

◆ V5150 Binaural, glasses
Medicare Statute 1862A7

◆ V5160 Dispensing fee, binaural
Medicare Statute 1862A7

◆ V5170 Hearing aid, CROS, in the ear
Medicare Statute 1862A7

◆ V5180 Hearing aid, CROS, behind the ear
Medicare Statute 1862A7

◆ V5190 Hearing aid, CROS, glasses
Medicare Statute 1862A7

◆ V5200 Dispensing fee, CROS
Medicare Statute 1862A7

◆ V5210 Hearing aid, BICROS, in the ear
Medicare Statute 1862A7

◆ V5220 Hearing aid, BICROS, behind the ear
Medicare Statute 1862A7

◆ V5230 Hearing aid, BICROS, glasses
Medicare Statute 1862A7

◆ V5240 Dispensing fee, BICROS
Medicare Statute 1862A7

◆ V5241 Dispensing fee, monaural hearing aid, any type
Medicare Statute 1862A7

◆ V5242 Hearing aid, analog, monaural, completely in the ear canal (CIC)
Medicare Statute 1862A7

◆ V5243 Hearing aid, analog, monaural, in the canal (ITC)
Medicare Statute 1862A9

◆ V5244 Hearing aid, digitally programmable analog, monaural, CIC
Medicare Statute 1862A7

◆ V5245 Hearing aid, digitally programmable, analog, monaural, ITC
Medicare Statute 1862A7

◆ V5246 Hearing aid, digitally programmable analog, monaural, in the ear (ITE)
Medicare Statute 1862A7

◆ V5247 Hearing aid, digitally programmable analog, monaural, behind the ear (BTE)
Medicare Statute 1862A7

◆ V5248 Hearing aid, analog, binaural, CIC
Medicare Statute 1862A7

◆ V5249 Hearing aid, analog, binaural, ITC
Medicare Statute 1862A7

◆ V5250 Hearing aid, digitally programmable analog, binaural, CIC
Medicare Statute 1862A7

◆ V5251 Hearing aid, digitally programmable analog, binaural, ITC
Medicare Statute 1862A7

◆ V5252 Hearing aid, digitally programmable, binaural, ITE
Medicare Statute 1862A7

◆ V5253 Hearing aid, digitally programmable, binaural, BTE
Medicare Statute 1862A7

◆ V5254 Hearing aid, digital, monaural, CIC
Medicare Statute 1862A7

◆ V5255 Hearing aid, digital, monaural, ITC
Medicare Statute 1862A7

◆ V5256 Hearing aid, digital, monaural, ITE
Medicare Statute 1862A7

◆ V5257 Hearing aid, digital, monaural, BTE
Medicare Statute 1862A7

◆ V5258 Hearing aid, digital, binaural, CIC
Medicare Statute 1862A7

◆ V5259 Hearing aid, digital, binaural, ITC
Medicare Statute 1862A7

◆ V5260 Hearing aid, digital, binaural, ITE
Medicare Statute 1862A7

◆ V5261 Hearing aid, digital, binaural, BTE
Medicare Statute 1862A7

◆ V5262 Hearing aid, disposable, any type, monaural
Medicare Statute 1862A7

◆ V5263 Hearing aid, disposable, any type, binaural
Medicare Statute 1862A7

◆ V5264 Ear mold/insert, not disposable, any type
Medicare Statute 1862A7

◆ V5265 Ear mold/insert, disposable, any type
Medicare Statute 1862A7

◆ V5266 Battery for use in hearing device
Medicare Statute 1862A7

◆ V5267 Hearing aid supplies/accessories
Medicare Statute 1862A7

◆ V5268   Assistive listening device, telephone amplifier, any type
Medicare Statute 1862A7

◆ V5269   Assistive listening device, alerting, any type
Medicare Statute 1862A7

◆ V5270   Assistive listening device, television amplifier, any type
Medicare Statute 1862A7

◆ V5271   Assistive listening device, television caption decoder
Medicare Statute 1862A7

◆ V5272   Assistive listening device, TDD
Medicare Statute 1862A7

◆ V5273   Assistive listening device, for use with cochlear implant
Medicare Statute 1862A7

◆ V5274   Assistive listening device, not otherwise specified
Medicare Statute 1862A7

◆ V5275   Ear impression, each
Medicare Statute 1862A7

◆ V5298   Hearing aid, not otherwise classified
Medicare Statute 1862a7

⊙ V5299   Hearing service, miscellaneous
MCM 2320

Speech-Language Pathology Services

NOTE: These codes are for non-physician services.

◆ V5336   Repair/modification of augmentative communicative system or device (excludes adaptive hearing aid)
Medicare Statute 1862A7

◆ V5362   Speech screening
MCM 2320

◆ V5363   Language screening
MCM 2320

◆ V5364   Dysphagia screening
MCM 2320

2006 TABLE OF DRUGS

IA—Intra-arterial administration
IV—Intravenous administration
IM—Intramuscular administration
IT—Intrathecal
SC—Subcutaneous administration
INH—Administration by inhaled solution
VAR—Various routes of administration
OTH—Other routes of administration
ORAL—Administered orally

Intravenous administration includes all methods, such as gravity infusion, injections, and timed pushes. The "VAR" posting denotes various routes of administration and is used for drugs that are commonly administered into joints, cavities, tissues, or topical applications, in addition to other parenteral administrations. Listings posted with "OTH" indicate other administration methods, such as suppositories or catheter injections.

A

Abarelix	10 mg		J0128
Abbokinase, *see* Urokinase			
Abbokinase, Open Cath, *see* Urokinase			
Abciximab	10 mg	IV	J0130
Abelcet, *see* Amphotericin B lipid complex			
ABLC, *see* Amphotericin B			
Acetazolamide sodium	up to 500 mg	IM, IV	J1120
Acetylcysteine, injection	100 mg		J0132
Acetylcysteine, unit dose form	per gram	INH	J7608
Achromycin, *see* Tetracycline			
ACTH, *see* Corticotropin			
Acthar, *see* Corticotropin			
Actimmune, *see* Interferon gamma 1-B			
Activase, *see* Alteplase recombinant			
Acyclovir	5 mg		J0133
Adalimumab	20 mg		J0135
Adenocard, *see* Adenosine			
Adenoscan, *see* Adenosine			
Adenosine	6 mg	IV	J0150
Adenosine	30 mg	IV	J0152
Adrenalin Chloride, *see* Adrenalin, epinephrine			
Adrenalin, epinephrine	up to 1 ml ampule	SC, IM	J0170
Adriamycin PFS, *see* Doxorubicin HCl			
Adriamycin RDF, *see* Doxorubicin HCl			
Adrucil, *see* Fluorouracil			
Agalsidase beta	1 mg		J0180
Aggrastat, *see* Tirofiban hydrochloride			
A-hydroCort, *see* Hydrocortisone sodium phosphate			
Akineton, *see* Biperiden			
Alatrofloxacin mesylate, injection 100 mg		IV	J0200
Albuterol	0.5 mg	INH	J7620
Albuterol, concentrated form	per mg	INH	J7611
Albuterol, unit dose form	per mg	INH	J7613
Aldesleukin	per single use vial	IM, IV	J9015
Aldomet, *see* Methyldopate HCl			
Alefacept	0.5 mg		J0215
Alemtuzumab	10 mg		J9010

Alferon N, *see* Interferon alfa-n3			
Alglucerase	per 10 units	IV	J0205
Alkaban-AQ, *see* Vinblastine sulfate			
Alkeran, *see* Melphalan, oral			
Alpha-1-proteinase inhibitor, human	10 mg	IV	J0256
Alprostadil, injection	1.25 mcg	OTH injection	J0270
Alprostadil, urethral suppository		OTH	J0275
Alteplase recombinant	1 mg	IV	J2997
Alupent, *see* Metaproterenol sulfate or Metaproterenol, compounded			
Amcort, *see* Triamcinolone diacetate			
A-Methapred, *see* Methylprednisolone sodium succinate			
Amgen, *see* Interferon alpha-con-1			
Amifostine	500 mg	IV	J0207
Amikacin sulfate	100 mg		J0278
Aminolevalinic acid HCl	unit dose (354 mg)	OTH	J7308
Aminophylline/Aminophyllin	up to 250 mg	IV	J0280
Amiodarone HCl	30 mg	IV	J0282
Amitriptyline HCl	up to 20 mg	IM	J1320
Amobarbital	up to 125 mg	IM, IV	J0300
Amphocin, *see* Amphotericin B			
Amphotericin B	50 mg	IV	J0285
Amphotericin B lipid complex	10 mg	IV	J0287 J0289
Ampicillin sodium	up to 500 mg	IM, IV	J0290
Ampicillin sodium/sulbactam sodium	per 1.5 gm	IM, IV	J0295
Amygdalin, *see* Laetrile, Amygdalin, vitamin B-17			
Amytal, *see* Amobarbital			
Anabolin LA 100, *see* Nandrolone decanoate			
Ancef, *see* Cefazolin sodium			
Andrest 90-4, *see* Testosterone enanthate and estradiol valerate			
Andro-Cyp, *see* Testosterone cypionate			
Andro-Cyp 200, *see* Testosterone cypionate			
Andro L.A. 200, *see* Testosterone enanthate			
Andro-Estro 90-4, *see* Testosterone enanthate and estradiol valerate			
Andro/Fem, *see* Testosterone cypionate and estradiol cypionate			
Androgyn L.A., *see* Testosterone enanthate and estradiol valerate			
Androlone-50, *see* Nandrolone phenpropionate			
Androlone-D 100, *see* Nandrolone decanoate			
Andronaq-50, *see* Testosterone suspension			
Andronaq-LA, *see* Testosterone cypionate			

Andronate-200, *see* Testosterone cypionate
Andronate-100, *see* Testosterone cypionate
Andropository 100, *see* Testosterone enanthate
Andryl 200, *see* Testosterone enanthate
Anectine, *see* Succinylcholine chloride
Anergan 25, *see* Promethazine HCl
Anergan 50, *see* Promethazine HCl

Anistreplase	30 units	IV	J0350
Anti-Inhibitor	per IU	IV	J7198

Antispas, *see* Dicyclomine HCl

Antithrombin III (human)	per IU	IV	J7197

Anzemet, *see* Dolasetron mesylate injection
A.P.L., *see* Chorionic gonadotropin
Apresoline, *see* Hydralazine HCl

Aprotinin	10,000 KIU		J0365

AquaMEPHYTON, *see* Vitamin K
Aralen, *see* Chloroquine HCl
Aramine, *see* Metaraminol
Aranesp, *see* Darbepoietin Alfa

Arbutamine	1 mg	IV	J0395

Aredia, *see* Pamidronate disodium
Arfonad, *see* Trimethaphan camsylate
Aristocort Forte, *see* Triamcinolone diacetate
Aristocort Intralesional, *see* Triamcinolone diacetate
Aristospan Intra-Articular, *see* Triamcinolone hexacetonide
Aristospan Intralesional, *see* Triamcinolone hexacetonide
Arrestin, *see* Trimethobenzamide HCl

Arsenic trioxide	1 mg	IV	J9017
Asparaginase	10,000 units	IV, IM	J9020

Astramorph PF, *see* Morphine sulfate
Atgam, *see* Lymphocyte immune globulin
Ativan, *see* Lorazepam

Atropine, concentrated form	per mg	INH	J7635
Atropine, unit dose form	per mg	INH	J7636
Atropine sulfate	up to 0.3 mg	IV, IM, SC	J0460

Atrovent, *see* Ipratropium bromide

Aurothioglucose	up to 50 mg	IM	J2910
Autologous cultured chondrocytes implant			J7330

Autoplex T, *see* Hemophilia clotting factors
Avonex, *see* Interferon beta-1a

Azacitidine	1 mg		J9025
Azathioprine	50 mg	ORAL	J7500
Azathioprine, parenteral	100 mg	IV	J7501
Azithromycin, dihydrate	1 gm	ORAL	Q0144
Azithromycin, injection	500 mg	IV	J0456

B

Baclofen	10 mg	IT	J0475
Baclofen for intrathecal trial	50 mcg	OTH	J0476

Bactocill, *see* Oxacillin sodium
BAL in oil, *see* Dimercaprol
Banflex, *see* Orphenadrine citrate

Basiliximab	20 mg		J0480
BCG (Bacillus Calmette and Guérin), live	per vial instillation	IV	J9031
Beclomethasone inhalation solution, unit dose form	per mg	INH	J7622

Bena-D 10, *see* Diphenhydramine HCl
Bena-D 50, *see* Diphenhydramine HCl
Benadryl, *see* Diphenhydramine HCl
Benahist 10, *see* Diphenhydramine HCl
Benahist 50, *see* Diphenhydramine HCl
Ben-Allergin-50, *see* Diphenhydramine HCl
Benefix, *see* Factor IX, recombinant
Benoject-10, *see* Diphenhydramine HCl
Benoject-50, *see* Diphenhydramine HCl
Bentyl, *see* Dicyclomine

Benztropine mesylate	per 1 mg	IM, IV	J0515

Berubigen, *see* Vitamin B-12, cyanocobalamin
Betalin 12, *see* Vitamin B-12, cyanocobalamin
Betameth, *see* Betamethasone sodium phosphate

Betamethasone acetate & betamethasone sodium phosphate	3 mg of ea	IM	J0702
Betamethasone inhalation solution, unit dose form	per mg	INH	J7624
Betamethasone sodium phosphate	4 mg	IM, IV	J0704

Betaseron, *see* Interferon beta-1b

Bethanechol chloride	up to 5 mg	SC	J0520
Bevacizumab	10 mg		J9035

Bicillin L-A, *see* Penicillin G benzathine
Bicillin C-R 900/300, *see* Penicillin G procaine and penicillin G benzathine
Bicillin C-R, *see* Penicillin G benzathine and penicillin G procaine
BiCNU, *see* Carmustine

Biperiden lactate	per 5 mg	IM, IV	J0190
Bitolterol mesylate, concentrated form	per mg	INH	J7628
Bitolterol mesylate, unit dose form	per mg	INH	J7629
Bivalirudin	1 mg		J0583

Blenoxane, *see* Bleomycin sulfate

Bleomycin sulfate	15 units	IM, IV, SC	J9040
Bortezomib	0.1 mg		J9041
Botulinum toxin type A	per unit	IM	J0585
Botulinum toxin type B	per 100 units	IM	J0587

Brethine, *see* Terbutaline sulfate or Terbutaline, compounded
Bricanyl Subcutaneous, *see* Terbutaline sulfate

Brompheniramine maleate	per 10 mg	IM, SC, IV	J0945

Drug	Amount	Route	Code
Bronkephrine, *see* Ethylnore-pinephrine HCl			
Bronkosol, *see* Isoetharine HCl			
Budesonide inhalation solution, concentrated form	0.25 mg	INH	J7633
Budesonide inhalation solution, unit dose form	0.25 mg	INH	J7626, J7627
Buprenorphine Hydrochloride	0.1 mg		J0592
Busulfan	2 mg	ORAL	J8510
Butorphanol tartrate	2 mg		J0595
C			
Cabergoline	0.25 mg	ORAL	J8515
Cafcit, *see* Caffeine citrate			
Caffeine citrate	5 mg	IV	J0706
Caine-1, *see* Lidocaine HCl			
Caine-2, *see* Lidocaine HCl			
Calcijex, *see* Calcitriol			
Calcimar, *see* Calcitonin-salmon			
Calcitonin-salmon	up to 400 units	SC, IM	J0630
Calcitriol	0.1 mcg	IM	J0636
Calcium Disodium Versenate, *see* Edetate calcium disodium			
Calcium gluconate	per 10 ml	IV	J0610
Calcium glycerophosphate & calcium lactate	per 10 ml	IM, SC	J0620
Calphosan, *see* Calcium glycerophosphate & calcium lactate			
Camptosar, *see* Irinotecan			
Capecitabine	150 mg	ORAL	J8520
	500 mg	ORAL	J8521
Carbocaine with Neo-Cobefrin, *see* Mepivacaine			
Carbocaine, *see* Mepivacaine			
Carboplatin	50 mg	IV	J9045
Carmustine	100 mg	IV	J9050
Carnitor, *see* Levocarnitine			
Carticel, *see* Autologous cultured chondrocytes			
Caspofungin Acetate	5 mg	IV	J0637
Cefadyl, *see* Cephapirin sodium			
Cefazolin sodium	up to 500 mg	IV, IM	J0690
Cefepime hydrochloride	500 mg	IV	J0692
Cefizox, *see* Ceftizoxime sodium			
Cefotaxime sodium	per 1 g	IV, IM	J0698
Cefoxitin sodium	1 g	IV, IM	J0694
Ceftazidime	per 500 mg	IM, IV	J0713
Ceftizoxime sodium	per 500 mg	IV, IM	J0715
Ceftriaxone sodium	per 250 mg	IV, IM	J0696
Cefuroxime sodium, sterile	per 750 mg	IM, IV	J0697
Celestone Phosphate, *see* Betamethasone sodium phosphate			
Celestone Soluspan, *see* Betamethasone acetate and betamethasone sodium phosphate			
CellCept, *see* Mycophenolate mofetil			
Cel-U-Jec, *see* Betamethasone sodium phosphate			
Cenacort Forte, *see* Triamcinolone diacetate			
Cenacort A-40, *see* Triamcinolone acetonide			
Cephalothin sodium	up to 1 g	IM, IV	J1890
Cephapirin sodium	up to 1 g	IV, IM	J0710
Ceredase, *see* Alglucerase			
Cerezyme, *see* Imiglucerase			
Cerubidine, *see* Daunorubicin HCl			
Cetuximab	10 mg		J9055
Chealamide, *see* Endrate ethylenediamine-tetra-/acetic acid			
Chloramphenicol sodium succinate	up to 1 g	IV	J0720
Chlordiazepoxide HCl	up to 100 mg	IM, IV	J1990
Chloromycetin Sodium Succinate, *see* Chloramphenicol sodium succinate			
Chloroprocaine HCl	per 30 ml	VAR	J2400
Chlorpromazine HCl, oral	10 mg	ORAL	Q0171
	25 mg	ORAL	Q0172
Chloroquine HCl	up to 250 mg	IM	J0390
Chlorothiazide sodium	per 500 mg	IV	J1205
Chlorpromazine HCl	up to 50 mg	IM, IV	J3230
Chorex-5, *see* Chorionic gonadotropin			
Chorex-10, *see* Chorionic gonadotropin			
Chorignon, *see* Chorionic gonadotropin			
Chorionic gonadotropin	per 1,000 USP units	IM	J0725
Choron-10, *see* Chorionic gonadotropin			
Cidofovir	375 mg	IV	J0740
Cilastatin sodium, imipenem	per 250 mg	IV, IM	J0743
Cipro IV, *see* Ciprofloxacin			
Ciprofloxacin	200 mg	IV	J0706
Cisplatin, powder or solution	per 10 mg	IV	J9060
Cisplatin	50 mg	IV	J9062
Cladribine	per mg	IV	J9065
Claforan, *see* Cefotaxime sodium			
Clofarabine	1 mg		J9027
Clonidine HCl	1 mg	epidural	J0735
Cobex, *see* Vitamin B-12, cyanocobalamin			
Codeine phosphate	per 30 mg	IM, IV, SC	J0745
Codimal-A, *see* Brompheniramine maleate			
Cogentin, *see* Benztropine mesylate			
Colchicine	per 1 mg	IV	J0760
Colistimethate sodium	up to 150 mg	IM, IV	J0770
Coly-Mycin M, *see* Colistimethate sodium			
Compa-Z, *see* Prochlorperazine			
Compazine, *see* Prochlorperazine			
Cophene-B, *see* Brompheniramine maleate			
Copper contraceptive, intrauterine	—	OTH	J7300
Cordarone, *see* Amiodarone HCl			
Corgonject-5, *see* Chorionic gonadotropin			
Corticorelin ovine triflutate	per dose		J0795
Corticotropin	up to 40 units	IV, IM, SC	J0800
Cortrosyn, *see* Cosyntropin			
Cosmegen, *see* Dactinomycin			
Cosyntropin	per 0.25 mg	IM, IV	J0835
Cotranzine, *see* Prochlorperazine			

Cromolyn sodium, unit dose form	per 10 mg	INH	J7631
Crysticillin 300 A.S., *see* Penicillin G procaine			
Crysticillin 600 A.S., *see* Penicillin G procaine			
Cyclophosphamide	100 mg	IV	J9070
	200 mg	IV	J9080
	500 mg	IV	J9090
	1 g	IV	J9091
	2 g	IV	J9092
Cyclophosphamide, lyophilized	100 mg	IV	J9070
	200 mg	IV	J9080
	500 mg	IV	J9090
	1 g	IV	J9091
	2g	IV	J9092
Cyclophosphamide, oral	25 mg	ORAL	J8530
Cyclosporine, oral	25 mg	ORAL	J7515
	100 mg	ORAL	J7502
Cyclosporine, parenteral	250 mg	IV	J7516
Cytarabine	100 mg	SC, IV	J9100
	500 mg	SC, IV	J9110
Cytarabine liposome	10 mg		J9098
Cytomegalovirus immune globulin intravenous (human)	per vial	IV	J0850
Cytosar-U, *see* Cytarabine			
Cytovene, *see* Ganciclovir sodium			
Cytoxan, *see* Cyclophosphamide; cyclophosphamide, lyophilized; and cyclophosphamide, oral			

D

D-5-W, infusion	1000 cc	IV	J7070
Dacarbazine	100 mg	IV	J9130
	200 mg	IV	J9140
Daclizumab	25 mg	IV	J7513
Dactinomycin	0.5 mg	IV	J9120
Dalalone, *see* Dexamethasone sodium phosphate			
Dalalone L.A., *see* Dexamethasone acetate			
Dalteparin sodium	per 2500 IU	SC	J1645
Daptomycin	1 mg		J0878
Darbepoetin Alfa	1 mcg		J0881, J0882
Daunorubicin citrate, liposomal formulation	10 mg	IV	J9151
Daunorubicin HCl	10 mg	IV	J9150
DaunoXome, (*see* Daunorubicin citrate)			
DDAVP, *see* Desmopressin acetate			
Decadron Phosphate, *see* Dexamethasone sodium phosphate			
Decadron, *see* Dexamethasone sodium phosphate			
Decadron-LA, *see* Dexamethasone acetate			
Deca-Durabolin, *see* Nandrolone decanoate			
Decaject, *see* Dexamethasone sodium phosphate			
Decaject-L.A., *see* Dexamethasone acetate			
Decolone-50, *see* Nandrolone decanoate			
Decolone-100, *see* Nandrolone decanoate			
De-Comberol, *see* Testosterone cypionate and estradiol cypionate			

Deferoxamine mesylate	500 mg	IM, SC, IV	J0895
Dehist, *see* Brompheniramine maleate			
Deladumone, *see* Testosterone enanthate and estradiol valerate			
Deladumone OB, *see* Testosterone enanthate and estradiol valerate			
Delatest, *see* Testosterone enanthate			
Delatestadiol, *see* Testosterone enanthate and estradiol valerate			
Delatestryl, *see* Testosterone enanthate			
Delta-Cortef, *see* Prednisolone, oral			
Delestrogen, *see* Estradiol valerate			
Demadex, *see* Torsemide			
Demerol HCl, *see* Meperidine HCl			
Denileukin diftitox	300 mcg		J9160
DepAndro 100, *see* Testosterone cypionate			
DepAndro 200, *see* Testosterone cypionate			
DepAndrogyn, *see* Testosterone cypionate and estradiol cypionate			
DepGynogen, *see* Depo-estradiol cypionate			
DepMedalone 40, *see* Methylprednisolone acetate			
DepMedalone 80, *see* Methylprednisolone acetate			
Depo-estradiol cypionate	up to 5 mg	IM	J1000
Depogen, *see* Depo-estradiol cypionate			
Depoject, *see* Methylprednisolone acetate			
Depo-Medrol, *see* Methylprednisolone acetate			
Depopred-40, *see* Methylprednisolone acetate			
Depopred-80, *see* Methylprednisolone acetate			
Depo-Provera, *see* Medroxyprogesterone acetate			
Depotest, *see* Testosterone cypionate			
Depo-Testadiol, *see* Testosterone cypionate and estradiol cypionate			
Depotestogen, *see* Testosterone cypionate and estradiol cypionate			
Depo-Testosterone, *see* Testosterone cypionate			
Desferal Mesylate, *see* Deferoxamine mesylate			
Desmopressin acetate	1 mcg	IV, SC	J2597
Dexacen LA-8, *see* Dexamethasone acetate			
Dexacen-4, *see* Dexamethasone sodium phosphate			
Dexamethasone, concentrated form	per mg	INH	J7637
Dexamethasone, unit form	per mg	INH	J7638
Dexamethasone, oral	0.25mg		J8540
Dexamethasone acetate	1 mg	IM	J1094

Dexamethasone sodium phosphate	1 mg	IM, IV, OTH	J1100
Dexasone, *see* Dexamethasone sodium phosphate			
Dexasone L.A., *see* Dexamethasone acetate			
Dexferrum, *see* Iron dextran			
Dexone, *see* Dexamethasone sodium phosphate			
Dexone LA, *see* Dexamethasone acetate			
Dexrazoxane HCl	250 mg	IV	J1190
Dextran 40	500 ml	IV	J7100
Dextran 75	500 ml	IV	J7110
Dextrose 5%/normal saline solution	500 ml = 1 unit	IV	J7042
Dextrose/water (5%)	500 ml = 1 unit	IV	J7060
D.H.E. 45, *see* Dihydroergotamine			
Diamox, *see* Acetazolamide sodium			
Diazepam	up to 5 mg	IM, IV	J3360
Diazoxide	up to 300 mg	IV	J1730
Dibent, *see* Dicyclomine HCl			
Dicyclomine HCl	up to 20 mg	IM	J0500
Didronel, *see* Etidronate disodium			
Diethylstilbestrol diphosphate	250 mg	IV	J9165
Diflucan, see Fluconazole			
Digoxin	up to 0.5 mg	IM, IV	J1160
Digoxin immune Fab (ovine)	per vial		J1162
Dihydrex, *see* Diphenhydramine HCl			
Dihydroergotamine mesylate	per 1 mg	IM, IV	J1110
Dilantin, *see* Phenytoin sodium			
Dilaudid, *see* Hydromorphone HCl			
Dilocaine, *see* Lidocaine HCl			
Dilomine, *see* Dicyclomine HCl			
Dilor, *see* Dyphylline			
Dimenhydrinate	up to 50 mg	IM, IV	J1240
Dimercaprol	per 100 mg	IM	J0470
Dimethyl sulfoxide, *see* DMSO, Dimethyl sulfoxide			
Dinate, *see* Dimenhydrinate			
Dioval, *see* Estradiol valerate			
Dioval 40, *see* Estradiol valerate			
Dioval XX, *see* Estradiol valerate			
Diphenacen-50, *see* Diphenhydramine HCl			
Diphenhydramine HCl, injection	up to 50 mg	IV, IM	J1200
Diphenhydramine HCl, oral	50 mg	ORAL	Q0163
Dipyridamole	per 10 mg	IV	J1245
Disotate, *see* Endrate ethylenediamine-tetra-acetic acid			
Di-Spaz, *see* Dicyclomine HCl			
Ditate-DS, *see* Testosterone enanthate and estradiol valerate			
Diuril Sodium, *see* Chlorothiazide sodium			
D-Med 80, *see* Methylprednisolone acetate			
DMSO, Dimethyl sulfoxide	50%, 50 ml	OTH	J1212
Dobutamine HCl	per 250 mg	IV	J1250
Dobutrex, *see* Dobutamine HCl			
Docetaxel	20 mg	IV	J9170
Dolasetron mesylate, injection	10 mg	IV	J1260
Dolasetron mesylate, tablets	100 mg	ORAL	Q0180
Dolophine HCl, *see* Methadone HCl			
Dommanate, *see* Dimenhydrinate			
Dopamine HCl	40 mg		J1265
Dornase alpha, unit dose form	per mg	INH	J7639
Doxercalciferol	1 mcg	IV	J1270
Doxil, *see* Doxorubicin HCl, lipid			
Doxorubicin HCl	10 mg	IV	J9000
Doxorubicin HCl, all lipid	10 mg	IV	J9001
Dramamine, *see* Dimenhydrinate			
Dramanate, *see* Dimenhydrinate			
Dramilin, *see* Dimenhydrinate			
Dramocen, *see* Dimenhydrinate			
Dramoject, *see* Dimenhydrinate			
Dronabinol, oral	2.5 mg	ORAL	Q0167
Dronabinol, oral	5 mg	ORAL	Q0168
Droperidol	up to 5 mg	IM, IV	J1790
Drug administered through a metered dose inhaler		INH	J3535
Droperidol and fentanyl citrate	up to 2 ml ampule	IM, IV	J1810
DTIC-Dome, *see* Dacarbazine			
Dua-Gen L.A., *see* Testosterone enanthate and estradiol valerate cypionate			
Duoval P.A., *see* Testosterone enanthate and estradiol valerate			
Durabolin, *see* Nandrolone phenpropionate			
Duraclon, *see* Clonidine HCl			
Dura-Estrin, *see* Depo-estradiol cypionate			
Duracillin A.S., *see* Penicillin G procaine			
Duragen-10, *see* Estradiol valerate			
Duragen-20, *see* Estradiol valerate			
Duragen-40, *see* Estradiol valerate			
Duralone-40, *see* Methylprednisolone acetate			
Duralone-80, *see* Methylprednisolone acetate			
Duralutin, *see* Hydroxyprogesterone caproate			
Duramorph, *see* Morphine sulfate			
Duratest-100, *see* Testosterone cypionate			
Duratest-200, *see* Testosterone cypionate			
Duratestrin, *see* Testosterone cypionate and estradiol cypionate			
Durathate-200, *see* Testosterone enanthate			
Dymenate, *see* Dimenhydrinate			
Dyphylline	up to 500 mg	IM	J1180

E

Edetate calcium disodium	up to 1000 mg	IV, SC, IM	J0600
Edetate disodium	per 150 mg	IV	J3520
Elavil, *see* Amitriptyline HCl			
Ellence, *see* Epirubicin HCl			
Elliott's B solution	1 ml	OTH	J9175
Elspar, *see* Asparaginase			
Emete-Con, *see* Benzquinamide			
Eminase, *see* Anistreplase			
Enbrel, *see* Etanercept			
Endrate ethylenediamine-tetra-acetic acid, *see* Edetate disodium			
Enovil, *see* Amitriptyline HCl			
Enoxaparin sodium	10 mg	SC	J1650
Epinephrine, adrenalin	up to 1 ml ampule	SC, IM	J0170
Epirubicin hydrochloride	2 mg		J9178
Epoetin alfa	1000 units		Q4055
Epoprostenol	0.5 mg	IV	J1325
Eptifibatide, injection	5 mg	IM, IV	J1327
Ergonovine maleate	up to 0.2 mg	IM, IV	J1330
Ertapenem sodium	500 mg		J1335
Erythromycin lactobionate	500 mg	IV	J1364
Estra-D, *see* Depo-estradiol cypionate			
Estra-L 20, *see* Estradiol valerate			
Estra-L 40, *see* Estradiol valerate			
Estra-Testrin, *see* Testosterone enanthate and estradiol valerate			
Estradiol Cypionate, *see* Depo-estradiol cypionate			
Estradiol L.A., *see* Estradiol valerate			
Estradiol L.A. 20, *see* Estradiol valerate			
Estradiol L.A. 40, *see* Estradiol valerate			
Estradiol valerate	up to 10 mg	IM	J1380
	up to 20 mg	IM	J1390
	up to 40 mg	IM	J0970
Estro-Cyp, *see* Depo-estradiol cypionate			
Estrogen, conjugated	per 25 mg	IV, IM	J1410
Estroject L.A., *see* Depo-estradiol cypionate			
Estrone	per 1 mg	IM	J1435
Estrone 5, *see* Estrone			
Estrone Aqueous, *see* Estrone			
Estronol, *see* Estrone			
Estronol-L.A., *see* Depo-estradiol cypionate			
Etanercept, injection	25 mg	IM, IV	J1438
Ethanolamine	100 mg		J1430
Ethyol, *see* Amifostine			
Etidronate disodium	per 300 mg	IV	J1436
Etopophos, *see* Etoposide			
Etoposide	10 mg	IV	J9181
	100 mg	IV	J9182
Etoposide, oral	50 mg	ORAL	J8560
Everone, *see* Testosterone enanthate			

F

Factor VIIa (coagulation factor, recombinant)	1 mcg	IV	J7189
Factor VIII (anti-hemophilic factor, human)	per IU	IV	J7190
Factor VIII (anti-hemophilic factor, porcine)	per IU	IV	J7191
Factor VIII (anti-hemophilic factor, recombinant)	per IU	IV	J7192
Factor IX (anti-hemophilic factor, purified, non-recombinant)	per IU	IV	Q0160
Factor IX (anti-hemophilic factor, recombinant)	per IU	IV	Q0161
Factor IX, complex	per IU	IV	J7194
Factors, other hemophilia clotting	per IU	IV	J7196
Factrel, *see* Gonadorelin HCl			
Feiba VH Immuno, *see* Factors, other hemophilia clotting			
Fentanyl citrate	0.1 mg	IM, IV	J3010
Ferrlecit, *see* Sodium ferric-gluconate complex in sucrose injection			
Filgrastim (G-CSF)	300 mcg	SC, IV	J1440
	480 mcg	SC, IV	J1441
Flexoject, *see* Orphenadrine citrate			
Flexon, *see* Orphenadrine citrate			
Flolan, *see* Epoprostenol			
Floxuridine	500 mg	IV	J9200
Fluconazole	200 mg	IV	J1450
Fludara, *see* Fludarabine phosphate			
Fludarabine phosphate	50 mg	IV	J9185
Flunisolide inhalation solution, unit dose form	per mg	INH	J7641
Fluorouracil	500 mg	IV	J9190
Folex, *see* Methotrexate sodium			
Folex PFS, *see* Methotrexate sodium			
Follutein, *see* Chorionic gonadotropin			
Fomepizole	1.5 mg		J1451
Fomivirsen sodium	1.65 mg	Intraocular	J1452
Fondaparinux sodium	0.5 mg		J1652
Formoterol	12 mcg	INH	J7640
Fortaz, *see* Ceftazidime			
Foscarnet sodium	per 1,000 mg	IV	J1455
Foscavir, *see* Foscarnet sodium			
Fosphenytoin	50 mg		Q2009
FUDR, *see* Floxuridine			
Fulvestrant	25 mg		J9395
Fungizone Intravenous, *see* Amphotericin B			
Furomide M.D., *see* Furosemide			
Furosemide	up to 20 mg	IM, IV	J1940

G

Gallium nitrate	1 mg		J1457
Gamastan, *see* Gamma globulin and Immune globulin			
Gamma globulin	1 cc	IM	J1460
	2 cc	IM	J1470
	3 cc	IM	J1480
	4 cc	IM	J1490
	5 cc	IM	J1500
	6 cc	IM	J1510
	7 cc	IM	J1520
	8 cc	IM	J1530
	9 cc	IM	J1540
	10 cc	IM	J1550
	over 10 cc	IM	J1560
Gammar, *see* Gamma globulin and immune globulin			

Gammar-IV, *see* Immune globulin intravenous (human)			
Gamulin RH, *see* Rho(D) immune globulin			
Ganciclovir, implant	4.5 mg	OTH	J7310
Ganciclovir sodium	500 mg	IV	J1570
Garamycin, gentamicin	up to 80 mg	IM, IV	J1580
Gatifloxacin	10 mg	IV	J1590
Gefitinib	250 mg		J8565
Gemcitabine HCl	200 mg	IV	J9201
Gemtuzumab ozogamicin	5 mg	IV	J9300
Gentamicin Sulfate, *see* Garamycin, gentamicin			
Gentran, *see* Dextran 40			
Gentran 75, *see* Dextran 75			
Gesterol 50, *see* Progesterone			
Glatiramer acetate	20 mg		J1595
Glucagon HCl	per 1 mg	SC, IM, IV	J1610
Glukor, *see* Chorionic gonadotropin			
Glycopyrrolate, concentrated form	per 1 mg	INH	J7642
Glycopyrrolate, unit dose form	per 1 mg	INH	J7643
Gold sodium thiomalate	up to 50 mg	IM	J1600
Gonadorelin HCl	per 100 mcg	SC, IV	J1620
Gonic, *see* Chorionic gonadotropin			
Goserelin acetate implant	per 3.6 mg	SC	J9202
Granisetron HCl, injection	100 mcg	IV	J1626
Granisetron HCl, oral	1 mg	ORAL	Q0166
Gynogen L.A. "A10," *see* Estradiol valerate			
Gynogen L.A. "A20," *see* Estradiol valerate			
Gynogen L.A. "A40," *see* Estradiol valerate			

H

Haldol, *see* Haloperidol			
Haloperidol	up to 5 mg	IM, IV	J1630
Haloperidol decanoate	per 50 mg	IM	J1631
Hectorol, *see* Doxercalciferol			
Hemin	1 mg		J1640
Hemofil M, *see* Factor VIII			
Hemophilia clotting factors (e.g., anti-inhibitors)	per IU	IV	J7198
Hemophilia clotting factors, NOC	per IU	IV	J7199
Hepatitis B vaccine			Q3021-Q3023
Hep-Lock, *see* Heparin sodium (heparin lock flush)			
Heparin sodium	1,000 units	IV, SC	J1644
Heparin sodium (heparin lock flush)	10 units	IV	J1642
Herceptin, *see* Trastuzumab			
Hexadrol Phosphate, *see* Dexamethasone sodium phosphate			
Histaject, *see* Brompheniramine maleate			
Histerone 50, *see* Testosterone suspension			
Histerone 100, *see* Testosterone suspension			
Histrelin acetate	10 mg		J1675
Histrelin implant	50 mg		J9225
Hyalgan, *see* Sodium hyaluronate			
Hyaluronidase	up to 150 units	SC, IV	J3470

Hyaluronidase, ovine			J3471, J3472
Hyate:C, *see* Factor VIII (anti-hemophilic factor, porcine)			
Hybolin Improved, *see* Nandrolone phenpropionate			
Hybolin Decanoate, *see* Nandrolone decanoate			
Hycamtin, *see* Topotecan			
Hydralazine HCl	up to 20 mg	IV, IM	J0360
Hydrate, *see* Dimenhydrinate			
Hydrocortisone acetate	up to 25 mg	IV, IM, SC	J1700
Hydrocortisone sodium phosphate	up to 50 mg	IV, IM, SC	J1710
Hydrocortisone succinate sodium	up to 100 mg	IV, IM, SC	J1720
Hydrocortone Acetate, *see* Hydrocortisone acetate			
Hydrocortone Phosphate, *see* Hydrocortisone sodium phosphate			
Hydromorphone HCl	up to 4 mg	SC, IM, IV	J1170
Hydroxyzine HCl	up to 25 mg	IM	J3410
Hydroxyzine pamoate	25 mg	ORAL	Q0177
	50 mg	ORAL	Q0178
Hylan G-F 20	16 mg	OTH	J7320
Hyoscyamine sulfate	up to 0.25 mg	SC, IM, IV	J1980
Hyperstat IV, *see* Diazoxide			
Hyper-Tet, *see* Tetanus immune globulin, human			
HypRho-D, *see* Rho(D) immune globulin			
Hyrexin-50, *see* Diphenhydramine HCl			
Hyzine-50, *see* Hydroxyzine HCl			

I

Ibutilide fumarate	1 mg	IV	J1742
Idamycin, *see* Idarubicin HCl			
Idarubicin HCl	5 mg	IV	J9211
Ifex, *see* Ifosfamide			
Ifosfamide	per 1 g	IV	J9208
Ilotycin, *see* Erythromycin gluceptate			
Imferon, *see* Iron dextran			
Imiglucerase	per unit	IV	J1785
Imitrex, *see* Sumatriptan succinate			
Immune globulin	per 500 mg	IV	J1561
Immune globulin, intravenous, powder	500 mg	IV	J1566
Immune globulin, intravenous, liquid	500 mg	IV	J1567
Immunosuppressive drug, not otherwise classified			J7599
Imuran, *see* Azathioprine			
Inapsine, *see* Droperidol			
Inderal, *see* Propranolol HCl			
Infed, *see* Iron dextran			
Infergen, *see* Interferon alfa-1			
Infliximab, injection	10 mg	IM, IV	J1745
Innohep, *see* Tinzarparin			
Innovar, *see* Droperidol with fentanyl citrate			
Insulin	5 units	SC	J1815
Insulin lispro	50 units	SC	J1817

131

Intal, *see* Cromolyn sodium or Cromolyn sodium, compounded

Integrilin, injection, *see* Eptifibatide

Interferon alphacon-1, recombinant	1 mcg	SC	J9212
Interferon alfa-2a, recombinant	3 million units	SC, IM	J9213
Interferon alfa-2b, recombinant	1 million units	SC, IM	J9214
Interferon alfa-n3 (human leukocyte derived)	250,000 IU	IM	J9215
Interferon beta-1a	33 mcg	IM	J1825
	11 mcg	IM	Q3025
	11 mcg	SC	Q3026
Interferon beta-1b	0.25 mg	SC	J1830
Interferon gamma-1b	3 million units	SC	J9216

Intrauterine copper contraceptive, *see* Copper contraceptive, intrauterine

Ipratropium bromide, unit dose form	per mg	INH	J7644
Irinotecan	20 mg	IV	J9206
Iron dextran	50 mg		J1751, J1752
Iron sucrose	1 mg	IV	J1756
Irrigation solution for Tx of bladder calculi	per 50 ml	OTH	Q2004

Isocaine HCl, *see* Mepivacaine

Isoetharine HCl, concentrated form	per mg	INH	J7648
Isoetharine HCl, unit dose form	per mg	INH	J7649
Isoproterenol HCl, concentrated form	per mg	INH	J7658
Isoproterenol HCl, unit dose form	per mg	INH	J7659

Isuprel, *see* Isoproterenol HCl

Itraconazole	50 mg	IV	J1835

J

Jenamicin, *see* Garamycin, gentamicin

K

Kabikinase, *see* Streptokinase

Kaleinate, *see* Calcium gluconate

Kanamycin sulfate	up to 75 mg	IM, IV	J1850
Kanamycin sulfate	up to 500 mg	IM, IV	J1840

Kantrex, *see* Kanamycin sulfate

Keflin, *see* Cephalothin sodium

Kefurox, *see* Cufuroxime sodium

Kefzol, *see* Cefazolin sodium

Kenaject-40, *see* Triamcinolone acetonide

Kenalog-10, *see* Triamcinolone acetonide

Kenalog-40, *see* Triamcinolone acetonide

Kestrone 5, *see* Estrone

Ketorolac tromethamine	per 15 mg	IM, IV	J1885

Key-Pred 25, *see* Prednisolone acetate

Key-Pred 50, *see* Prednisolone acetate

Key-Pred-SP, *see* Prednisolone sodium phosphate

K-Flex, *see* Orphenadrine citrate

Klebcil, *see* Kanamycin sulfate

Konate-HP, *see* Factor VIII

Kogenate, *see* Factor VIII

Konakion, *see* Vitamin K, phytonadione, etc.

Konyne 80, *see* Factor IX, complex

Kutapressin	up to 2 ml	SC, IM	J1910

Kytril, *see* Granisetron HCl

L

L.A.E. 20, *see* Estradiol valerate

Laetrile, Amygdalin, vitamin B-17			J3570

Lanoxin, *see* Digoxin

Largon, *see* Propiomazine HCl

Laronidase	0.1 mg		J1931

Lasix, *see* Furosemide

L-Caine, *see* Lidocaine HCl

Lepirudin	50 mg		J1945
Leucovorin calcium	per 50 mg	IM, IV	J0640

Leukine, *see* Sargramostim (GM-CSF)

Leuprolide acetate (for depot suspension)	3.75 mg	IM	J1950
Leuprolide acetate	7.5 mg	IM	J9217
Leuprolide acetate	per 1 mg	IM	J9218
Leuprolide acetate implant	65 mg		J9219

Leustatin, *see* Cladribine

Levalbuterol, concentrated form	0.5 mg	INH	J7612
Levalbuterol, unit form	0.5 mg	INH	J7614

Levaquin I.U., *see* Levofloxacin

Levocarnitine	per 1 gm	IV	J1955

Levo-Dromoran, *see* Levorphanol tartrate

Levofloxacin	250 mg	IV	J1956
Levonorgestrel implant			J7306
Levonorgestrel releasing intrauterine contraceptive	52 mg	OTH	J7302
Levorphanol tartrate	up to 2 mg	SC, IV	J1960

Levsin, *see* Hyoscyamine sulfate

Levulan Kerastick, *see* Aminolevulinic acid HC1

Librium, *see* Chlordiazepoxide HCl

Lidocaine HCl	10 mg	IV	J2001

Lidoject-1, *see* Lidocaine HCl

Lidoject-2, *see* Lidocaine HCl

Lincocin, *see* Lincomycin HCl

Lincomycin HCl	up to 300 mg	IV	J2010
Linezolid	200 mg	IV	J2020

Liquaemin Sodium, *see* Heparin sodium

Lioresal, *see* Baclofen

LMD (10%), *see* Dextran 40

Lovenox, *see* Enoxaparin sodium

Lorazepam	2 mg	IM, IV	J2060

Lufyllin, *see* Dyphylline

Luminal Sodium, *see* Phenobarbital sodium

Lunelle, *see* Medroxyprogesterone acetate/estradiol cypionate

Lupron, *see* Leuprolide acetate			
Lymphocyte immune globulin anti-thymocyte globulin, equine	250 mg	IV	J7504
anti-thymocyte, globulin, rabbit	25 mg	IV	J7511
Lyophilized, *see* Cyclophosphamide, lyophilized			

M

Magnesium sulfate	500 mg		J3475
Mannitol	25% in 50 ml	IV	J2150
Marmine, *see* Dimenhydrinate			
Maxipime, *see* Cefepime hydrochloride			
Mechlorethamine HCl (nitrogen mustard), HN2	10 mg	IV	J9230
Medralone 40, *see* Methylprednisolone acetate			
Medralone 80, *see* Methylprednisolone acetate			
Medrol, *see* Methylprednisolone			
Medroxyprogesterone acetate	50 mg	IM	J1051
	150 mg	IM	J1055
Medroxyprogesterone acetate/estradiol cypionate	5 mg/25 mg	IV	J1056
Mefoxin, *see* Cefoxitin sodium			
Melphalan HCl	50 mg	IV	J9245
Melphalan, oral	2 mg	ORAL	J8600
Menoject LA, *see* Testosterone cypionate and estradiol cypionate			
Mepergan Injection, *see* Meperidine and promethazine HCl			
Meperidine HCl	per 100 mg	IM, IV, SC	J2175
Meperidine and promethazine HCl	up to 50 mg	IM, IV	J2180
Mepivacaine HCL	per 10 ml	VAR	J0670
Meropenem	100 mg		J2185
Mesna	200 mg	IV	J9209
Mesnex, *see* Mesna			
Metaprel, *see* Metaproterenol sulfate			
Metaproterenol sulfate, concentrated form	per 10 mg	INH	J7668
Metaproterenol sulfate, unit dose form	per 10 mg	INH	J7669
Metaraminol bitartrate	per 10 mg	IV, IM, SC	J0380
Metastron, *see* Strontium-89 chloride			
Metacholine chloride	1 mg		J7674
Methadone HCl	up to 10 mg	IM, SC	J1230
Methergine, *see* Methylergonovine maleate			
Methocarbamol	up to 10 ml	IV, IM	J2800
Methotrexate, oral	2.5 mg	ORAL	J8610
Methotrexate sodium	5 mg	IV, IM, IT, IA	J9250
	50 mg	IV, IM, IT, IA	J9260
Methotrexate LPF, *see* Methotrexate sodium			
Methylergonovine maleate	up to 0.2 mg	IM, IV	J2210
Methyldopate HCl	up to 250 mg	IV	J0210
Methylene blue	1 ml		A9535
Methylergonovine maleate	up to 0.2 mg		J2210
Methylprednisolone, oral	per 4 mg	ORAL	J7509
Methylprednisolone acetate	20 mg	IM	J1020
	40 mg	IM	J1030
	80 mg	IM	J1040

Methylprednisolone sodium succinate	up to 40 mg	IM, IV	J2920
	up to 125 mg	IM, IV	J2930
Metoclopramide HCl	up to 10 mg	IV	J2765
Miacalcin, *see* Calcitonin-salmon			
Midazolam HCl	per 1 mg	IM, IV	J2250
Milrinone lactate	5 mg	IV	J2260
Mirena, *see* Levonorgestrel releasing intrauterine contraceptive			
Mithracin, *see* Plicamycin			
Mitomycin	5 mg	IV	J9280
	20 mg	IV	J9290
	40 mg	IV	J9291
Mitoxantrone HCl	per 5 mg	IV	J9293
Monocid, *see* Cefonicid sodium			
Monoclate-P, *see* Factor VIII			
Monoclonal antibodies, parenteral	5 mg	IV	J7505
Mononine, *see* Factor IX, purified, non-recombinant			
Morphine sulfate	up to 10 mg	IM, IV, SC	J2270
	100 mg	IM, IV, SC	J2271
Morphine sulfate, preservative-free	per 10 mg	IM, IV, SC	J2275
Moxifloxacin	100 mg		J2280
M-Prednisol-40, *see* Methylprednisolone acetate			
M-Prednisol-80, *see* Methylprednisolone acetate			
Mucomyst, *see* Acetylcysteine or Acetylcysteine, compounded			
Mucosol, *see* Acetylcysteine			
Muromonab-CD3	5 mg	IV	J7505
Muse, *see* Alprostadil			
Mustargen, *see* Mechlorethamine HCl			
Mutamycin, *see* Mitomycin			
Mycophenolic acid	180 mg		J7518
Mycophenolate mofetil	250 mg	ORAL	J7517
Myleran, *see* Busulfan			
Mylotarg, *see* Gemtuzumab ozogamicin			
Myobloc, *see* Botulinum toxin type B			
Myochrysine, *see* Gold sodium thiomalate			
Myolin, *see* Orphenadrine citrate			

N

Nalbuphine HCl	per 10 mg	IM, IV, SC	J2300
Naloxone HCl	per 1 mg	IM, IV, SC	J2310
Nandrobolic L.A., *see* Nandrolone decanoate			
Nandrolone decanoate	up to 50 mg	IM	J2320
	up to 100 mg	IM	J2321
	up to 200 mg	IM	J2322
Narcan, *see* Naloxone HCl			
Naropin, *see* Ropivacaine HCl			
Nasahist B, *see* Brompheniramine maleate			
Nasal vaccine inhalation		INH	J3530
Natalizumab	1 mg		Q4079
Navane, *see* Thiothixene			
Navelbine, *see* Vinorelbine tartrate			
ND Stat, *see* Brompheniramine maleate			
Nebcin, *see* Tobramycin sulfate			
NebuPent, *see* Pentamidine isethionate			

Nembutal Sodium Solution, *see* Pentobarbital sodium			
Neocyten, *see* Orphenadrine citrate			
Neo-Durabolic, *see* Nandrolone decanoate			
Neoquess, *see* Dicyclomine HCl			
Neosar, *see* Cyclophosphamide			
Neostigmine methylsulfate	up to 0.5 mg	IM, IV, SC	J2710
Neo-Synephrine, *see* Phenylephrine HCl			
Nervocaine 1%, *see* Lidocaine HCl			
Nervocaine 2%, *see* Lidocaine HCl			
Nesacaine, *see* Chloroprocaine HCl			
Nesacaine-MPF, *see* Chloroprocaine HCl			
Nesiritide	0.1 mg		J2325
Neumega, *see* Oprelvekin			
Neupogen, *see* Filgrastim (G-CSF)			
Neutrexin, *see* Trimetrexate glucuronate			
Nipent, *see* Pentostatin			
Nordryl, *see* Diphenhydramine HCl			
Norflex, *see* Orphenadrine citrate			
Norzine, *see* Thiethylperazine maleate			
Not otherwise classified drugs			J3490
Not otherwise classified drugs	other than INH, administered thru DME		J7799
Not otherwise classified drugs	INH, administered thru DME		J7699
Not otherwise classified drugs, anti-neoplastic	—		J9999
Not otherwise classified drugs, chemotherapeutic		ORAL	J8999
Not otherwise classified drugs, immunosuppressive	—		J7599
Not otherwise classified drugs, nonchemotherapeutic		ORAL	J8499
Novantrone, *see* Mitoxantrone HCl			
Novo Seven, *see* Factor VIIa			
NPH, *see* Insulin			
Nubain, *see* Nalbuphine HCl			
Nulicaine, *see* Lidocaine HCl			
Numorphan, *see* Oxymorphone HCl			
Numorphan H.P., *see* Oxymorphone HCl			

O

Octreotide Acetate, injection	1 mg	IM	J2353
	25 mcg	IV, SQ	J2354
Oculinum, *see* Botulinum toxin type A			
O-Flex, *see* Orphenadrine citrate			
Omalizumab	5 mg		J2357
Omnipen-N, *see* Ampicillin			
Oncaspar, *see* Pegaspargase			
Oncovin, *see* Vincristine sulfate			

Ondansetron HCl, oral	8 mg	ORAL	Q0179
Oprelvekin	5 mg	SC	J2355
Oraminic II, *see* Brompheniramine maleate			
Ormazine, *see* Chlorpromazine HCl			
Orphenadrine citrate	up to 60 mg	IV, IM	J2360
Orphenate, *see* Orphenadrine citrate			
Or-Tyl, *see* Dicyclomine			
Oxacillin sodium	up to 250 mg	IM, IV	J2700
Oxaliplatin	0.5 mg		J9263
Oxymorphone HCl	up to 1 mg	IV, SC, IM	J2410
Oxytetracycline HCl	up to 50 mg	IM	J2460
Oxytocin	up to 10 units	IV, IM	J2590

P

Paclitaxel	30 mg	IV	J9265
Paclitaxel protein-bound particles	1 mg		J9264
Palifermin	50 mcg		J2425
Palonosetron HCl	25 mcg		J2469
Pamidronate disodium	per 30 mg	IV	J2430
Papaverine HCl	up to 60 mg	IV, IM	J2440
Paragard T 380 A, *see* Copper contraceptive, intrauterine			
Paraplatin, *see* Carboplatin			
Paricalcitol, injection	1 mcg	IV, IM	J2501
Pegademase bovine	25 IU		J2504
Pegaptinib	0.3 mg		J2503
Pegaspargase	per single dose vial	IM, IV	J9266
Pegfilgrastim	6 mg		J2505
Pemetrexed	10 mg		J9305
Penicillin G benzathine	up to 600,000 units	IM	J0560
	up to 1,200,000 units	IM	J0570
	up to 2,400,000 units	IM	J0580
Penicillin G benzathine and penicillin G procaine	up to 600,000 units	IM	J0530
	up to 1,200,000 units	IM	J0540
	up to 2,400,000 units	IM	J0550
Penicillin G potassium	up to 600,000 units	IM, IV	J2540
Penicillin G procaine, aqueous	up to 600,000 units	IM, IV	J2510
Pentamidine isethionate	per 300 mg	INH	J2545
Pentastarch, 10%	100 ml		J2513
Pentazocine HCl	up to 30 mg	IM, SC, IV	J3070
Pentobarbital sodium	per 50 mg	IM, IV, OTH	J2515
Pentostatin	per 10 mg	IV	J9268
Permapen, *see* Penicillin G benzathine			
Perphenazine, injection	up to 5 mg	IM, IV	J3310
Perphenazine, tablets	4 mg	ORAL	Q0175
	8 mg	ORAL	Q0176
Persantine IV, *see* Dipyridamole			
Pfizerpen, *see* Penicillin G potassium			
Pfizerpen A.S., *see* Penicillin G procaine			
Phenazine 25, *see* Promethazine HCl			
Phenazine 50, *see* Promethazine HCl			

Phenergan, *see* Promethazine HCl			
Phenobarbital sodium	up to 120 mg	IM, IV	J2560
Phentolamine mesylate	up to 5 mg	IM, IV	J2760
Phenylephrine HCl	up to 1 ml	SC, IM, IV	J2370
Phenytoin sodium	per 50 mg	IM, IV	J1165
Photofrin, *see* Porfimer sodium			
Phytonadione (Vitamin K)	per 1 mg	IM, SC, IV	J3430
Piperacillin/Tazobactam Sodium, injection	1.125 g	IV	J2543
Pitocin, *see* Oxytocin			
Plantinol AQ, *see* Cisplatin			
Plas + SD, *see* Plasma, pooled multiple donor			
Plasma, cryoprecipitate reduced	each unit		P9044
Plasma, pooled multiple donor, frozen, each unit		IV	P9023
Platinol, *see* Cisplatin			
Plicamycin	2,500 mcg	IV	J9270
Polocaine, *see* Mepivacaine			
Polycillin-N, *see* Ampicillin			
Porfimer Sodium	75 mg	IV	J9600
Potassium chloride	per 2 mEq	IV	J3480
Pralidoxime chloride	up to 1 g	IV, IM, SC	J2730
Predalone-50, *see* Prednisolone acetate			
Predcor-25, *see* Prednisolone acetate			
Predcor-50, *see* Prednisolone acetate			
Predicort-50, *see* Prednisolone acetate			
Prednisone	per 5 mg	ORAL	J7506
Prednisolone, oral	5 mg	ORAL	J7510
Prednisolone acetate	up to 1 ml	IM	J2650
Predoject-50, *see* Prednisolone acetate			
Pregnyl, *see* Chorionic gonadotropin			
Premarin Intravenous, *see* Estrogen, conjugated			
Prescription, chemotherapeutic, not otherwise specified		ORAL	J8999
Prescription, nonchemotherapeutic, not otherwise specified		ORAL	J8499
Primacor, *see* Milrinone lactate			
Primaxin I.M., *see* Cilastatin sodium, imipenem			
Primaxin I.V., *see* Cilastatin sodium, imipenem			
Priscoline HCl, *see* Tolazoline HCl			
Pro-Depo, *see* Hydroxyprogesterone Caproate			
Procainamide HCl	up to 1 g	IM, IV	J2690
Prochlorperazine	up to 10 mg	IM, IV	J0780
Prochlorperazine maleate, oral	5 mg	ORAL	Q0164
	10 mg	ORAL	Q0165
Profasi HP, *see* Chorionic gonadotropin			
Profilnine Heat-Treated, *see* Factor IX			
Progestaject, *see* Progesterone			
Progesterone	per 50 mg		J2675
Prograf, *see* Tacrolimus, oral or parenteral			
Prokine, *see* Sargramostim (GM-CSF)			
Prolastin, *see* Alpha 1-proteinase inhibitor (human)			
Proleukin, *see* Aldesleukin			
Prolixin Decanoate, *see* Fluphenazine decanoate			
Promazine HCl	up to 25 mg	IM	J2950
Promethazine HCl, injection	up to 50 mg	IM, IV	J2550
Promethazine HCl, oral	12.5 mg	ORAL	Q0169
	25 mg	ORAL	Q0170
Pronestyl, *see* Procainamide HCl			
Proplex T, *see* Factor IX			
Proplex SX-T, *see* Factor IX			
Propranolol HCl	up to 1 mg	IV	J1800
Prorex-25, *see* Promethazine HCl			
Prorex-50, *see* Promethazine HCl			
Prostaphlin, *see* Procainamide HCl			
Prostigmin, *see* Neostigmine methylsulfate			
Protamine sulfate	per 10 mg	IV	J2720
Protirelin	per 250 mcg	IV	J2725
Prothazine, *see* Promethazine HCl			
Protopam Chloride, *see* Pralidoxime chloride			
Proventil, *see* Albuterol sulfate, compounded			
Prozine-50, *see* Promazine HCl			
Pulmicort Respules, *see* Budesonide			
Pyridoxine HCl	100 mg		J3415

Q

Quelicin, *see* Succinylcholine chloride			
Quinupristin/dalfopristin	500 mg (150/350)	IV	J2770

R

Ranitidine HCl, injection	25 mg	IV, IM	J2780
Rapamune, *see* Sirolimus			
Rasburicase	0.5 mg		J2783
Recombinate, *see* Factor VIII			
Redisol, *see* Vitamin B-12 cyanocobalamin			
Regitine, *see* Phentolamine mesylate			
Reglan, *see* Metoclopramide HCl			
Regular, *see* Insulin			
Relefact TRH, *see* Protirelin			
Remicade, *see* Infliximab, injection			
Reo Pro, *see* Abciximab			
Rep-Pred 40, *see* Methylprednisolone acetate			
Rep-Pred 80, *see* Methylprednisolone acetate			
RespiGam, *see* Respiratory Syncytial Virus			
Respiratory Syncytial Virus Immune-globulin	50 mg	IV	J1565
Retavase, *see* Reteplase			
Reteplase	18.8 mg	IV	J2993
Retrovir, *see* Zidovudine			
Rheomacrodex, *see* Dextran 40			
Rhesonativ, *see* Rho(D) immune globulin, human			
Rheumatrex Dose Pack, *see* Methotrexate, oral			

Rho(D) immune globulin, human	1 dose package, 300 mcg	IM	J2790
	1 dose package, 50 mcg	IM	J2798
Rho(D)immune globulin (human), solvent detergent	100 IU	IV	J2792
RhoGAM, *see* Rho(D) immune globulin, human			
Ringer's lactate infusion	up to 1,000 cc	IV	J7120
Risperidone	0.5 mg		J2794
Rituxan, *see* Rituximab			
Rituximab	100 mg	IV	J9310
Robaxin, *see* Methocarbamol			
Rocephin, *see* Ceftriaxone sodium			
Roferon-A, *see* Interferon alfa-2A, recombinant			
Ropivacaine HCl	1 mg		J2795
Rubex, *see* Doxorubicin HCl			
Rubramin PC, *see* Vitamin B-12 cyanocobalamin			

S

Saline solution	5% dextrose, 500 ml	IV	J7042
	infusion, 250 cc	IV	J7050
	infusion, 1,000 cc	IV	J7030
Saline solution, sterile	500 ml = 1 unit	IV, OTH	J7040
	up to 5 cc	IV, OTH	J7051
Sandimmune, *see* Cyclosporine			
Sandoglobulin, *see* Immune globulin intravenous (human)			
Sandostatin Lar Depot, *see* Octreotide			
Sargramostim (GM-CSF)	50 mcg	IV	J2820
Secobarbital sodium	up to 250 mg	IM, IV	J2860
Seconal, *see* Secobarbital sodium			
Selestoject, *see* Betamethasone sodium phosphate			
Sermorelin acetate	0.5 mg		Q0515
Sincalide	5 mcg		J2805
Sinusol-B, *see* Brompheniramine maleate	per 2 ml	IV	J2912
Sirolimus	1 mg	ORAL	J7520
Sodium chloride, 0.9%	per 2 ml		J2912
Sodium ferricgluconate in sucrose	12.5 mg		J2916
Sodium hyaluronate	20–25 mg	OTH	J7317
Solganal, *see* Aurothioglucose			
Solu-Cortef, *see* Hydrocortisone sodium phosphate			J1710
Solu-Medrol, *see* Methylprednisolone sodium succinate			
Solurex, *see* Dexamethasone sodium phosphate			
Solurex LA, *see* Dexamethasone acetate			
Somatrem	1 mg		J2940
Somatropin	1 mg		J2941
Sparine, *see* Promazine			
Spasmoject, *see* Dicyclomine HCl			
Spectinomycin HCl	up to 2 g	IM	J3320
Sporanox, *see* Itraconazole			

Staphcillin, *see* Methicillin sodium			
Stilphostrol, *see* Diethylstilbestrol diphosphate			
Streptase, *see* Streptokinase			
Streptokinase	per 250,000 IU	IV	J2995
Streptomycin Sulfate, *see* Streptomycin			
Streptomycin	up to 1 g	IM	J3000
Streptozocin	1 gm	IV	J9320
Strontium-89 chloride	per 10 ml	IV	J3005
Sublimaze, *see* Fentanyl citrate			
Succinylcholine chloride	up to 20 mg	IV, IM	J0330
Sumatriptan succinate	6 mg	SC	J3030
Supartz *see* Sodium hyaluronate			
Surostrin, *see* Succinycholine chloride			
Sus-Phrine, *see* Adrenalin, epinephrine			
Synercid, *see* Quinupristin/dalfopristin			
Synkavite, *see* Vitamin K, phytonadione, etc.			
Syntocinon, *see* Oxytocin			
Synvisc, *see* Hylan G-F 20			
Sytobex, *see* Vitamin B-12 cyanocobalamin			

T

Tacrolimus, oral	per 1 mg	ORAL	J7507
Tacrolimus, parenteral	5 mg		J7515
Talwin, *see* Pentazocine HCl			
Taractan, *see* Chlorprothixene			
Taxol, *see* Paclitaxel			
Taxotere, *see* Docetaxel			
Tazidime, *see* Ceftazidime			
Technetium TC Sestamibi	per dose		A9500
TEEV, *see* Testosterone enanthate and estradiol valerate			
Temozolomide	5 mg	ORAL	J8700
Tenecteplase	50 mg		J3100
Teniposide	50 mg		Q2017
Tequin, *see* Gatifloxacin			
Terbutaline sulfate	up to 1 mg	SC, IV	J3105
Terbutaline sulfate, concentrated form	per 1 mg	INH	J7680
Terbutaline sulfate, unit dose form	per 1 mg	INH	J7681
Teriparatide	10 mcg		J3110
Terramycin IM, *see* Oxytetracycline HCl			
Testa-C, *see* Testosterone cypionate			
Testadiate, *see* Testosterone enanthate and estradiol valerate			
Testadiate-Depo, *see* Testosterone cypionate			
Testaject-LA, *see* Testosterone cypionate			
Testaqua, *see* Testosterone suspension			
Test-Estro Cypionates, *see* Testosterone cypionate and estradiol cypionate			
Test-Estro-C, *see* Testosterone cypionate and estradiol cypionate			
Testex, *see* Testosterone propionate			

Testoject-50, *see* Testosterone suspension

Testoject-LA, *see* Testosterone cypionate

Testone LA 200, *see* Testosterone enanthate

Testone LA 100, *see* Testosterone enanthate

Testosterone Aqueous, *see* Testosterone suspension

Drug	Amount	Route	Code
Testosterone enanthate and estradiol valerate	up to 1 cc	IM	J0900
Testosterone enanthate	up to 100 mg	IM	J3120
	up to 200 mg	IM	J3130
Testosterone cypionate	up to 100 mg	IM	J1070
	1 cc, 200 mg	IM	J1080
Testosterone cypionate and estradiol cypionate	up to 1 ml	IM	J1060
Testosterone propionate	up to 100 mg	IM	J3150
Testosterone suspension	up to 50 mg	IM	J3140

Testradiol 90/4, *see* Testosterone enanthate and estradiol valerate

Testrin PA, *see* Testosterone enanthate

Drug	Amount	Route	Code
Tetanus immune globulin, human	up to 250 units	IM	J1670
Tetracycline	up to 250 mg	IM, IV	J0120
Thallous Chloride TL 201	per MCI		A9505

Theelin Aqueous, *see* Estrone

Drug	Amount	Route	Code
Theophylline	per 40 mg	IV	J2810

TheraCys, *see* BCG live

Drug	Amount	Route	Code
Thiamine HCl	100 mg		J3411
Thiethylperazine maleate, injection	up to 10 mg	IM	J3280
Thiethylperazine maleate, oral	10 mg	ORAL	Q0174
Thiotepa	15 mg	IV	J9340

Thorazine, *see* Chlorpromazine HCl

Thymoglobulin, *see* Immune globulin, anti-thymocyte

Thypinone, *see* Protirelin

Thyrogen, *see* Thyrotropin Alfa

Drug	Amount	Route	Code
Thyrotropin Alpha, injection	0.9 mg	IM, SC	J3240

Tice BCG, *see* BCG live

Ticon, *see* Trimethobenzamide HCl

Tigan, *see* Trimethobenzamide HCl

Tiject-20, *see* Trimethobenzamide HCl

Drug	Amount	Route	Code
Tinzarparin	1000 IU	SC	J1655
Tirofiban hydrochloride, injection	12.5 mg	IM, IV	J3246

TNKase, *see*, Tenecteplase

Tobi, *see* Tobramycin, inhalation solution

Drug	Amount	Route	Code
Tobramycin, inhalation solution	300 mg	INH	J7682
Tobramycin sulfate	up to 80 mg	IM, IV	J3260

Tofranil, *see* Imipramine HCl

Drug	Amount	Route	Code
Tolazoline HCl	up to 25 mg	IV	J2670
Topotecan	4 mg	IV	J9350

Toradol, *see* Ketorolac tromethamine

Torecan, *see* Thiethylperazine maleate

Tornalate, *see* Bitolterol mesylate

Drug	Amount	Route	Code
Torsemide	10 mg/ml	IV	J3265

Totacillin-N, *see* Ampicillin

Drug	Amount	Route	Code
Trastuzumab	10 mg	IV	J9355
Treprostinil	1 mg		Q4077

Tri-Kort, *see* Triamcinolone acetonide

Triam-A, *see* Triamcinolone acetonide

Drug	Amount	Route	Code
Triamcinolone, concentrated form	per 1 mg	INH	J7683
Triamcinolone, unit dose	per 1 mg	INH	J7684
Triamcinolone acetonide	per 10 mg	IM	J3301
Triamcinolone diacetate	per 5 mg	IM	J3302
Triamcinolone hexacetonide	per 5 mg	VAR	J3303
Triflupromazine HCl	up to 20 mg	IM, IV	J3400

Trilafon, *see* Perphenazine

Trilog, *see* Triamcinolone acetonide

Trilone, *see* Triamcinolone diacetate

Drug	Amount	Route	Code
Trimethobenzamide HCl, injection	up to 200 mg	IM	J3250
Trimethobenzamide HCl, oral	250 mg	ORAL	Q0173
Trimetrexate glucuronate	per 25 mg	IV	J3305
Triptorelin Pamoate	3.75 mg		J3315

Trisenox, *see* Arsenic trioxide

Trobicin, *see* Spectinomycin HCl

Trovan, *see* Alatrofloxacin mesylate

Tysabri, *see* Natalizumab

U

Ultrazine-10, *see* Prochlorperazine

Unasyn, *see* Ampicillin sodium/sulbactam sodium

Drug	Amount	Route	Code
Unclassified drugs (*see also* Not elsewhere classified)			J3490
Unspecified oral antiemetic			Q0181
Urea	up to 40 gm	IV	J3350

Ureaphil, *see* Urea

Urecholine, *see* Bethanechol chloride

Drug	Amount	Route	Code
Urofollitropin	75 IU		J3355
Urokinase	5,000 IU vial	IV	J3364
	250,000 IU vial	IV	J3365

V

V-Gan 25, *see* Promethazine HCl

V-Gan 50, *see* Promethazine HCl

Valergen 10, *see* Estradiol valerate

Valergen 20, *see* Estradiol valerate

Valergen 40, *see* Estradiol valerate

Valertest No. 1, *see* Testosterone enanthate and estradiol valerate

Valertest No. 2, *see* Testosterone enanthate and estradiol valerate

Valium, *see* Diazepam

Drug	Amount	Route	Code
Valrubicin, intravesical	200 mg	OTH	J9357

Valstar, *see* Valrubicin

Vancocin, *see* Vancomycin HCl

Vancoled, *see* Vancomycin
HCl

Vancomycin HCl	up to 500 mg	IV, IM	J3370

Vasoxyl, *see* Methoxamine
HCl
Velban, *see* Vinblastine sulfate
Velsar, *see* Vinblastine sulfate
Venofer, *see* Iron sucrose
Ventolin, *see* Albuterol sulfate
VePesid, *see* Etoposide and Etoposide, oral
Versed, *see* Midazolam HCl

Verteporfin	15 mg	IV	J3396

Vesprin, *see* Trifluromazine
HCl
Viadur, *see* Leuprolide acetate implant

Vinblastine sulfate	1 mg	IV	J9360

Vincasar PFS, *see* Vincristine sulfate

Vincristine sulfate	1 mg	IV	J9370
	2 mg	IV	J9375
	5 mg	IV	J9380
Vinorelbine tartrate	per 10 mg	IV	J9390

Vistaject-25, *see* Hydroxyzine
HCl
Vistaril, *see* Hydroxyzine
HCl
Vistide, *see* Cidofovir
Visudyne, *see* Verteporfin

Vitamin K, phytonadione, menadione, menadiol sodium diphosphate	per 1 mg	IM, SC, IV	J3430
Vitamin B-12 cyanocobalamin	up to 1,000 mcg	IM, SC	J3420
Von Willebrand factor complex, human	per IU	IV	J7188
Voriconazole	10 mg		J3465

W

Wehamine, *see* Dimenhydrinate
Wehdryl, *see* Diphenhydramine HCl
Wellcovorin, *see* Leucovorin calcium
Win Rho SD, *see* Rho(D)immune globulin (human), solvent detergent
Wyamine Sulfate, *see* Mephentermine sulfate
Wycillin, *see* Penicillin G procaine
Wydase, *see* Hyaluronidase

X

Xeloda, *see* Capecitabine
Xopenex, *see* Albuterol
Xylocaine HCl, *see* Lidocaine HCl

Z

Zanosar, *see* Streptozocin
Zantac, *see* Ranitidine HCl
Zemplar, *see* Paricalcitol
Zenapax, *see* Daclizumab
Zetran, *see* Diazepam

Ziconotide	1 mcg	IV	J2278
Zidovudine	10 mg	IV	J3485

Zinacef, *see* Cefuroxime sodium

Ziprasidone Mesylate	10 mg		J3486

Zithromax, *see* Azithromycin dihydrate
Zithromax I.V., *see* Azithromycin, injection
Zofran, *see* Ondansetron HCl
Zoladex, *see* Goserelin acetate implant

Zoledronic Acid			J3487

Zolicef, *see* Cefazolin sodium
Zosyn, *see* Piperacillin
Zyvox, *see* Linezolid

A

Abarelix, J0128

Abciximab, J0130

Abdomen
dressing holder/binder, A4462
pad, low profile, L1270
supports, pendulous, L0920, L0930

Abduction control, each, L2624

Abduction rotation bar, foot, L3140–L3170

Absorption dressing, A6251–A6256

Access system, A4301

Accessories
ambulation devices, E0153–E0159
artificial kidney and machine (*see also* ESRD), E1510–E1699
beds, E0271–E0280, E0300–E0326
wheelchairs, E0950–E1030, E1050–E1298, E2300–E2399, K0001–K0109

Acetazolamide sodium, J1120

Acetylcysteine, inhalation solution, J7608

Acetylcysteine, injection, J0132

Acyclovir, J0133

Adalimumab, J0135

Adenosine, J0150, J0152

Adhesive, A4364
disc or foam pad, A5126
remover, A4365, A4455
support, breast prosthesis, A4280
tape, A4454, A6265

Administrative, Miscellaneous and Investigational, A9000–A9999

Adrenalin, J0170

Aerosol
compressor, E0571, E0572
compressor filter, K0178–K0179
mask, K0180

AFO, E1815, E1830, L1900–L1990, L4392, L4396

Agalsidase beta, J0180

Aggrastat, J3245

A-hydroCort, J1710

Air ambulance (*see also* Ambulance), A0030, A0040

Air bubble detector, dialysis, E1530

Air fluidized bed, E0194

Air pressure pad/mattress, E0176, E0186, E0197

Air travel and nonemergency transportation, A0140

Alarm, pressure, dialysis, E1540

Alatrofloxacin mesylate, J0200

Albumin, human, P9041, P9042

Albuterol, all formulations, inhalation solution, concentrated, J7611

Albuterol, all formulations, inhalation solution, unit dose, J7613

Albuterol, all formulations, inhalation solution, J7620

Alcohol, A4244

Alcohol wipes, A4245

Aldesleukin (IL2), J9015

Alefacept, J0215

Alemtuzumab, J9010

Alert device, A9280

Alginate dressing, A6196–A6199

Alglucerase, J0205

Alpha-1-proteinase inhibitor, human, J0256

Alprostadil
injection, J0270
urethral suppository, J0275

Alteplase recombinant, J2997

Alternating pressure mattress/pad, A4640, E0180, E0181, E0277

Ambulance, A0021–A0999
air, A0430, A0431, A0435, A0436
disposable supplies, A0382–A0398
oxygen, A0422

Ambulation device, E0100–E0159

Amikacin Sulfate, J0278

Aminolevulinic acid HCl, J7308

Aminophylline, J0280

Amiodarone HCl, J0282

Amitriptyline HCl, J1320

Ammonia N-13, A9526

Ammonia test paper, A4774

Amniotic membrane, V2790

Amobarbital, J0300

Amphotericin B, J0285

Amphotericin B Lipid Complex, J0287–J0289

Ampicillin sodium, J0290

Ampicillin sodium/sulbactam sodium, J0295

Amputee
adapter, wheelchair, E0959
prosthesis, L5000–L7510, L7520, L7900, L8400–L8465
stump sock, L8470–L8490
wheelchair, E1170–E1190, E1200, K0100

Amygdalin, J3570

Anesthesia
dialysis, A4735

Anistreplase, J0350

Ankle splint, recumbent, K0126–K0130

Ankle-foot orthosis (AFO), L1900–L1990, L2106–L2116, L4392, L4396

Anterior-posterior-lateral orthosis, L0520, L0550–L0565, L0700, L0710

Anterior-posterior-lateral-rotary orthosis, L0340–L0440

Anterior-posterior orthosis, L0320, L0330, L0530

Antiemetic, oral, Q0163–Q0181, J8498, J8597

Anti-hemophilic factor (Factor VIII), J7190–J7192

Anti-inhibitors, per I.U., J7198

Anti-neoplastic drug, NOC, J9999

Antithrombin III, J7197

Apnea monitor, E0608

Appliance
cleaner, A5131
pneumatic, E0655–E0673

Aprotinin, J0365

Aqueous
shunt, L8612
sterile, J7051

Arbutamine HCl, J0395

Arch support, L3040–L3100
intralesional, J3302

Arm, wheelchair, E0973

Arsenic trioxide, J9017

Artificial
cornea, L8609
kidney machines and accessories (*see also* Dialysis), E1510–E1699
larynx, L8500

Asparaginase, J9020

Assessment
audiologic, V5008–V5020
cardiac output, M0302
speech, V5362–V5364

Astramorph, J2275

Atropine, inhalation solution, concentrated, J7635

Atropine, inhalation solution, unit dose, J7636

Atropine sulfate, J0460

Audiologic assessment, V5008–V5020

Aurothioglucose, J2910

Azacitidine, J9025

Azathioprine, J7500, J7501

Azithromycin injection, J0456

B

Back supports, L0500–L0960
Baclofen, J0475, J0476
Bacterial sensitivity study, P7001
Bag
    drainage, A4357
    irrigation supply, A4398
    urinary, A5112, A4358
Bandage, A4441–A4456
Basiliximab, J0480
Bathtub
    chair, E0240
    stool or bench, E0245, E0247–E0248
    transfer rail, E0246
    wall rail, E0241, E0242
Battery, K0082–K0087, L7360, L7364–
    L7368
    charger, E1066, K0088, K0089, L7362,
      L7366
    replacement for blood glucose moni-
      tor, A4233–A4234
    replacement for cochlear impant de-
      vice, L8623–L8624
    replacement for TENS, A4630
    ventilator, A4611–A4613
    wheelchair, A4631
BCG live, intravesical, J9031
Beclomethasone inhalation solution, J7622
Bed
    air fluidized, E0194
    cradle, any type, E0280
    drainage bag, bottle, A4357, A5102
    hospital, E0250–E0270, E0298–E0301
    pan, E0275, E0276
    rail, E0305, E0310
    safety enclosure frame/canopy, E0316
Below knee suspension sleeve, L5674,
    L5675
Belt
    extremity, E0945
    ostomy, A4367
    pelvic, E0944
    safety, K0031
    wheelchair, E0978, E0979
Bench, bathtub (see also Bathtub),
    E0245
Benefix, see Factor IX, Q0161

Benesch boot, L3212–L3214
Benztropine, J0515
Betadine, A4246, A4247
Betameth, J0704
Betamethasone inhalation solution, J7624
Betamethasone acetate and betametha-
    sone sodium phosphate, J0702
Betamethasone sodium phosphate, J0704
Bethanechol chloride, J0520
Bevacizumab, J9035
Bicarbonate dialysate, A4705
Bifocal, glass or plastic, V2200–V2299
Bilirubin (phototherapy) light, E0202
Binder, A4465
Biofeedback device, E0746
Bioimpedance, electrical, cardiac output,
    M0302
Biperiden lactate, J0190
Bitolterol mesylate, inhalation solution,
    concentrated, J7628
Bitolterol mesylate, inhalation solution,
    unit dose, J7629
Bivalirudin, J0583
Bladder calculi irrigation solution,
    Q2004
Bladder capacity test, ultrasound, G0050
Bleomycin sulfate, J9040
Blood
    Congo red, P2029
    fresh frozen plasma, P9017
    glucose monitor, E0607, E2100, E2101
    glucose test, A4253
    granulocytes, pheresis, P9050
    leak detector, dialysis, E1560
    leukocyte poor, P9016
    mucoprotein, P2038
    platelets, P9019
    platelets, irradiated, P9032
    platelets, leukocytes reduced, P9031
    platelets, leukocytes reduced, irradi-
      ated, P9033
    platelets, pheresis, P9034
    platelets, pheresis, irradiated, P9036
    platelets, pheresis, leukocytes reduced,
      P9035
    platelets, pheresis, leukocytes reduced,
      irradiated, P9037

    pressure monitor, A4660, A4663, A4670
    pump, dialysis, E1620
    red blood cells, deglycerolized, P9039
    red blood cells, irradiated, P9038
    red blood cells, leukocytes reduced,
      P9016
    red blood cells, leukocytes reduced, ir-
      radiated, P9040
    red blood cells, washed, P9022
    strips, A4253
    supply, P9010–P9022
    testing supplies, A4770
    tubing, A4750, A4755
Blood collection devices accessory,
    A4257, E0620
Body jacket
    lumbar-sacral orthosis (spinal), L0500–
      L0565, L0600, L0610
    scoliosis, L1300, L1310
Body sock, L0984
Bond or cement, ostomy skin, A4364
Bone mineral density study, G0062,
    G0063
Boot
    pelvic, E0944
    surgical, ambulatory, L3260
Bortezomib, J9041
Botulinum toxin type A, J0585
Botulinum toxin type B, J0587
Brachytherapy radioelements, Q3001
Brachytherapy source, A9670
Breast prosthesis, L8000–L8035, L8600
Breast prosthesis, adhesive skin sup-
    port, A4280
Breast pump
    accessories, A4281-4286
    electric, any type, E0603
    heavy duty, hospital grade, E0604
    manual, any type, E0602
Breathing circuit, A4618
Brompheniramine maleate, J0945
Budesonide inhalation solution, J7626,
    J7627, J7633
Buprenorphine hydrochloride, J0592
Bus, nonemergency transportation,
    A0110
Butorphanol tartrate, J0595

C

Cabergoline, oral, J8515
Caffeine citrate, J0706
Calcitriol, J0636
Calcitonin-salmon, J0630
Calcium disodium edetate, J0600
Calcium gluconate, J0610
Calcium glycerophosphate and calcium lactate, J0620
Calcium lactate and calcium glycerophosphate, J0620
Calcium leucovorin, J0640
Calibrator solution, A4256
Cane, E0100, E0105
    accessory, A4636, A4637
Canister, disposable, used with suction pump, A7000
Canister, non-disposable, used with suction pump, A7001
Cannula, nasal, A4615
Capecitabine, oral, J8520, J8521
Carbon filter, A4680
Carboplatin, J9045
Cardia Event, recorder, implantable, E0616
Cardiokymography, Q0035
Cardiovascular services, M0300–M0302
Carmustine, J9050
Case management, T1016, T1017
Caspofungin acetate, J0637
Cast
    hand restoration, L6900–L6915
    materials, special, A4590
    plaster, L2102, L2122
    supplies, A4580, A4590, Q4001–Q4051
    synthetic, L2104, L2124
    thermoplastic, L2106, L2126
Caster, front, for power wheelchair, K0099
Caster, wheelchair, E0997, E0998
Catheter, A4300–A4365
    anchoring device, A5200, A4333, A4334
    cap, disposable (dialysis), A4860
    external collection device, A4327–A4330, A4347, K0410, K0411
    implanted, A7042, A7043
    indwelling, A4338–A4346
    indwelling, insertion of, G0002
    insertion tray, A4354
    intermittent with insertion supplies, A4353
    irrigation supplies, A4355, K0409
    male external, A4324, A4325, A4348
    oropharyngeal suction, A4628
    starter set, A4329
    trachea (suction), A4609–A4610, A4624
    transtracheal oxygen, A4608
Catheterization, specimen collection, P9612, P9615
Cefazolin sodium, J0690
Cefepime HC1, J0692
Cefotaxime sodium, J0698
Ceftazidime, J0713
Ceftizoxime sodium, J0715
Ceftriaxone sodium, J0696
Cefuroxime sodium, J0697
CellCept, K0412
Cellular therapy, M0075
Cement, ostomy, A4364
Centrifuge, A4650
Cephalin Flocculation, blood, P2028
Cephalothin sodium, J1890
Cephapirin sodium, J0710

Cervical
    halo, L0810–L0830
    head harness/halter, E0942
    orthosis, L0100–L0200
    pillow, E0943
    traction, E0855
Cervical cap contraceptive, A4261
Cervical-thoracic-lumbar-sacral orthosis (CTLSO), L0700, L0710
Cetuximab, J9055
Chair
    adjustable, dialysis, E1570
    commode with seat lift, E0169
    lift, E0627
    rollabout, E1031
    sitz bath, E0160–E0162
Chelation therapy, M0300
Chemical endarterectomy, M0300
Chemistry and toxicology tests, P2028–P3001
Chemotherapy
    administration, Q0083–Q0085 (hospital reporting only)
    drug, oral, not otherwise classified, J8999
    drugs (see also drug by name), J9000–J9999
Chest shell (cuirass), E0457
Chest Wall Oscillation System, E0483
    hose, replacement, A7026
    vest, replacement, A7025
Chest wrap, E0459
Chin cup, cervical, L0150
Chin strap (for positive airway pressure device), K0186
Chloramphenicol sodium succinate, J0720
Chlordiazepoxide HCl, J1990
Chloromycetin Sodium Succinate, J0720
Chloroprocaine HCl, J2400
Chloroquine HCl, J0390
Chlorothiazide sodium, J1205
Chlorpromazine HCl, J3230
Chorionic gonadotropin, J0725
Chromic phosphate P32 suspension, A9564
Chromium CR-51 sodium chromate, A9553
Cidofovir, J0740
Cilastatin sodium, imipenem, J0743
Ciprofloxacin, for intravenous infusion, J0744
Cisplatin, J9060, J9062
Cladribine, J9065
Clamp
    dialysis, A4910, A4918, A4920
    external urethral, A4356
Cleanser, wound, A6260
Cleansing agent, dialysis equipment, A4790
Clofarabine, J9027
Clonidine, J0735
Clotting time tube, A4771
Clubfoot wedge, L3380
Cochlear prosthetic implant, L8614
    accessories, L8615–L8617
    batteries, L8620–L8622
    replacement, L8619
Codeine phosphate, J0745
Colchicine, J0760
Colistimethate sodium, J0770
Collagen
    skin test, G0025
    urinary tract implant, L8603
    wound dressing, A6020–A6024
Collar, cervical
    multiple post, L0180–L0200
    nonadjust (foam), L0120

Collection device for nebulizer, K0177
Coly-Mycin M, J0770
Comfort items, A9190
Commode, E0160–E0175
    chair, E0170–E0171
    lift, E0625, E0172
    pail, E0167
    seat, wheelchair, E0968
Composite dressing, A6200–A6205
Compressed gas system, E0424–E0480, L3902
Compression bandage, A4460
Compression burn garment, A6501–A6512
Compression stockings, A6530–A6549
Compressor, E0565, E0570, E0571, E0572, E0650–E0652, E1375
    filter, aerosol, K0178–K0179
Concentrator, oxygen, E1377–E1385
Conductivity meter, bath, dialysis, E1550
Congo red, blood, P2029
Contact layer, A6206–A6208
Contact lens, V2500–V2599
Continent device, A5081, A5082
Continuous positive airway pressure (CPAP) device, E0601
    compressor, K0269
    intermittent assist, E0452
    nasal application accessories, K0184
Contraceptive
    cervical cap, A4261
    condoms, A4267, A4268
    diaphragm, A4266
    intrauterine, copper, J7300
    intrauterine, levonorgestrel releasing, J7302
    levonorgestrel, implants and supplies, A4260
    patch, J7304
    spermicide, A4269
    vaginal ring, J7303
Contracts, maintenance, ESRD, A4890
Contrast material
    injection during MRI, A4643
    low osmolar, A4644–A4646
Corneal tissue processing, V2785
Corrugated tubing, used with nebulizer, K0175, K0176
Corset, spinal orthosis, L0970–L0976
Corticorelin ovine triflutate, J0795
Corticotropin, J0800
Corvert, see Ibutilide fumarate
Cosyntropin, J0835
Cough stimulating device, E0482
Cover, wound
    alginate dressing, A6196–A6198
    collagen dressing, A6020
    foam dressing, A6209–A6214
    hydrocolloid dressing, K0234–K0239
    hydrogel dressing, A0242–A0248
    non-contact wound warming cover, and accessory, A6000, E0231, E0232
    specialty absorptive dressing, A6251–A6256
CPAP (continuous positive airway pressure) device, E0601
    chin strap, K0186
    compressor, K0269
    filter, K0188, K0189
    headgear, K0185
    humidifier, A7046, K0193, K0268
    intermittent assist, E0452, K0194
    nasal application accessories, K0183, K0184
    tubing, K0187

Cradle, bed, E0280
Crib, E0300
Cromolyn sodium, inhalation solution, unit dose, J7631
Crutches, E0110–E0118
  accessories, A4635–A4637, K0102
Cryoprecipitate, each unit, P9012
CTLSO, L1000–L1120, L0700, L0710
Cuirass, E0457
Culture sensitivity study, P7001
Cushion, wheelchair, E0962–E0965, E0977
Cyanocobalamin Cobalt CO57, A9559
Cycler dialysis machine, E1594
Cyclophosphamide, J9070–J9092
Cyclophosphamide, lyophilized, J9093–J9097
Cyclophosphamide, oral, J8530
Cyclosporine, J7502, J7515, J7516
Cylinder tank carrier, K0104
Cytarabine, J9110
Cytarabine liposome, J9098
Cytomegalovirus immune globulin (human), J0850

D

Dacarbazine, J9130, J9140
Daclizumab, J7513
Dactinomycin, J9120
Dalalone, J1100
Dalteparin sodium, J1645
Daptomycin, J0878
Darbepoetin Alfa, J0881–J0882
Daunorubicin citrate, J9151
Daunorubicin HCl, J9150
DaunoXome, see Daunorubicin citrate
Decubitus care equipment, E0176–E0199
Deferoxamine mesylate, J0895
Defibrillator, external, E0617, K0606
  battery, K0607
  electrode, K0609
  garment, K0608
Deionizer, water purification system, E1615
Delivery/set-up/dispensing, A9901
Denileukin diftitox, J9160
Depo-estradiol cypionate, J1000
Desmopressin acetate, J2597
Detector, blood leak, dialysis, E1560
Device, water collection (for nebulizer), K0177
Dexamethasone acetate, J1094
Dexamethasone, inhalation solution, concentrated, J7637
Dexamethasone, inhalation solution, unit dose, J7638

Dexamethasone, oral, J8540
Dexamethasone sodium phosphate, J1100
Dextran, J7100
Dextrose
  saline (normal), J7042
  water, J7060, J7070
Dextrostick, A4772
Diagnostic
  radiology services, R0070–R5999
Dialysate concentrate additives, A4765
Dialysate solution, A4700, A4705, A4728
Dialysate testing solution, A4760
Dialysis
  air bubble detector, E1530
  bath conductivity, meter, E1550
  chemicals/antiseptics solution, A4674
  continuous ambulatory peritoneal dialysis (CAPD) supply kit, A4900
  continuous cycling peritoneal dialysis (CCPD) supply kit, A4901
  disposable cycler set, A4671
  equipment, E1510–E1702
  extension line, A4672–A4673
  filter, A4680
  fluid barrier, E1575
  forceps, A4910
  kit, A4820, A4914
  measuring cylinder, A4921
  pressure alarm, E1540
  shunt, A4740
  supplies, A4650–A4927
  thermometer, A4910
  tourniquet, A4910
  unipuncture control system, E1580
  venous pressure clamp, A4918
Dialyzer, A4690
  holder, A4919
Diaper, T1500, T4521–T4540
Diaper, adult incontinence garment, A4520
Diazepam, J3360
Diazoxide, J1730
Dicyclomine HCl, J0500
Diethylstilbestrol diphosphate, J9165
Digoxin, J1160
Digoxin immune fab (ovine), J1162
Dihydroergotamine mesylate, J1110
Dimenhydrinate, J1240
Dimercaprol, J0470
Dimethyl sulfoxide (DMSO), J1212
Diphenhydramine HCl, J1200
Dipyridamole, J1245
Disarticulation
  lower extremities, prosthesis, L5000–L5999
  upper extremities, prosthesis, L6000–L6692
Disposable supplies, ambulance, A0382, A0384, A0392–A0398

Distilled water (for nebulizer), K0182
DMSO, J1212
Dobutamine HCl, J1250
Docetaxel, J9170
Dolasetron mesylate, J1260
Dome and mouthpiece (for nebulizer), A7016
Dopamine HCl, J1265
Dornase alpha, inhalation solution, unit dose form, J7639
Doxercalciferol, J1270
Doxil, J9001
Doxorubicin HCl, J9000, J9001
Drainage
  bag, A4347, A4357, A4358
  board, postural, E0606
  bottle, A5102
Dressing (see also Bandage), A6020–A6406
  alginate, A6196–A6199
  collagen, A6020–A6024
  composite, A6200–A6205
  contact layer, A6206–A6208
  foam, A6209–A6215
  gauze, A6216–A6230, A6402–A6406
  holder/binder, A4462
  hydrocolloid, A6234–A6241
  hydrogel, A6242–A6248
  specialty absorptive, A6251–A6256
  tape, A4454, A6265
  transparent film, A6257–A6259
  tubular, A6457
Droperidol, J1790
  and fentanyl citrate, J1810
Dropper, A4649
Drugs (see also Table of Drugs)
  administered through a metered dose inhaler, J3535
  chemotherapy, J8500–J9999
  dispensing fee for DME drugs, E0590
  disposable delivery system, 5 ml or less per hour, A4306
  disposable delivery system, 50 ml or greater per hour, A4305
  immunosuppressive, J7500–J7599
  infusion supplies, A4230–A4232, A4221, A4222
  inhalation solutions, J7608–J7699
  not otherwise classified, J3490, J7599, J7699, J7799, J8499, J8999, J9999
  prescription, oral, J8499, J8999
Dry pressure pad/mattress, E0179, E0184, E0199
Durable medical equipment (DME), E0100–E1830, K Codes
Duraclon, see Clonidine
Dyphylline, J1180

E

Ear mold, V5264
Echocardiography injectable contrast material, A9700
Edetate calcium disodium, J0600
Edetate disodium, J3520
Eggcrate dry pressure pad/mattress, E0179, E0184, E0199
Elastic
    bandage, A4460
    gauze, A6263, A6405
Elbow
    disarticulation, endoskeletal, L6450
    orthosis (EO), E1800, L3700–L3740, L3760
    protector, E0191
Electrical work, dialysis equipment, A4870
Electrocardiogram strips,
    monitoring, G0004–G0007
    physician interpretation, G0016
    tracing, G0015
    transmission, G0015, G0016
Electrodes, per pair A4556
Elevating leg rest, K0195
Elliott's b solution, J9175
EMG, E0746
Eminase, J0350
Endarterectomy, chemical, M0300
Endoscope sheath, A4270
Endoskeletal system, addition, L5858, L5856–L5857, L5925
Enoxaparin sodium, J1650
Enteral
    feeding supply kit (syringe) (pump) (gravity), B4034–B4036
    formulae, B4149–B4156
    nutrition infusion pump (with alarm) (without), B9000, B9002
Epinephrine, J0170
Epirubicin HCl, J9178
Epoetin alpha, J0885–J0886
Epoprostenol, J1325
Ergonovine maleate, J1330
Ertapenem sodium, J1335
Erythromycin lactobionate, J1364
ESRD (End Stage Renal Disease; see also Dialysis)
    machines and accessories, E1500–E1699
    plumbing, A4870
    supplies, A4651–A4929
Estrogen conjugated, J1410
Estrone (5, Aqueous), J1435
Ethanolamine oleate, J1430
Etidronate disodium, J1436
Etoposide, J9181, J9182
Etoposide, oral, J8560
Exercise equipment, A9300
External
    ambulatory infusion pump, E0781, E0784
    power, battery components, L7360–L7499
    power, elbow, L7160–L7191
    urinary supplies, A4356–A4359
Extremity belt/harness, E0945

Eye
    case, V2756
    lens (contact) (spectacle), V2100–V2615
    pad, A4610–A4612
    prosthetic, V2623, V2629
    service (miscellaneous), V2700–V2799

F

Faceplate, ostomy, A4361, K0428
Face tent, oxygen, A4619
Factor VIIA coagulation factor, recombinant, J7189
Factor VIII, anti-hemophilic factor, J7190–J7192
Factor IX, J7193, J7194, J7195
Family Planning Education, H1010
Fecal leukocyte examination, G0026
Fentanyl citrate, J3010
Fentanyl citrate and droperidol, J1810
Fern test, Q0114
Filgrastim (G-CSF), J1440, J1441
Filler, wound
    alginate dressing, A6199
    foam dressing, A6215
    hydrocolloid dressing, A6240, A6241
    hydrogel dressing, A6248
    not elsewhere classified, A6261, A6262
Film, transparent (for dressing), A6257–A6259
Filter
    aerosol compressor, A7014
    CPAP device, K0188, K0189
    dialysis carbon, A4680
    ostomy, A4368
    tracheostoma, A4481
    ultrasonic generator, A7014
Fistula cannulation set, A4730
Flowmeter, E0440, E0555, E0580
Floxuridine, J9200
Fluconazole, injection, J1450
Fludarabine phosphate, J9185
Fluid barrier, dialysis, E1575
Flunisolide inhalation solution, J7641
Fluorodeoxyglucose F-18 FDG, A9552
Fluorouracil, J9190
Foam dressing, A6209–A6215
Foam pad adhesive, A5126
Folding walker, E0135, E0143
Foley catheter, A4312–A4316, A4338–A4346
Fomepizole, J1451
Fomivirsen sodium intraocular, J1452
Fondaparinux sodium, J1652
Footdrop splint, L4398
Footplate, E0175, E0970, L3031
Footwear, orthopedic, L3201–L3265
Forceps, dialysis, A4910
Forearm crutches, E0110, E0111
Formoterol, J7640
Foscarnet sodium, J1455
Fosphenytoin, Q2009
Fracture
    bedpan, E0276
    frame, E0920, E0930, E0946–E0948
    orthosis, L2102–L2136, L3980–L3986
    orthotic additions, L2180–L2192, L3995
Fragmin, see Dalteparin sodium
Frames (spectacles), V2020, V2025

Fulvestrant, J9395
Furosemide, J1940

G

Gadolinium, A4647
Gait trainer, E8000–E8002
Gallium Ga 67, A9556
Gallium nitrate, J1457
Gamma globulin, J1460–J1561
Ganciclovir, implant, J7310
Ganciclovir sodium, J1570
Garamycin, J1580
Gas system
    compressed, E0424, E0425
    gaseous, E0430, E0431, E0441, E0443
    liquid, E0434–E0440, E0442, E0444
Gastrostomy/jejunostomy tubing, B4084
Gastrostomy tube, B4085
Gatifloxacin, J1590
Gauze (see also Bandage)
    elastic, A6263, A6405
    impregnated, A6222–A6230, A6231–A6233, A6266
    nonelastic, A6264, A6406
    nonimpregnated, A6216–A6221, A6402–A6404
Gefitinib, J8565
Gel
    conductive, A4558
    pressure pad, E0178, E0185, E0196
Gemcitabine HCl, J9201
Gemtuzumab ozogamicin, J9300
Generator
    implantable neurostimulator, E0751
    ultrasonic with nebulizer, E0574
Gentamicin (Sulfate), J1580
Glasses
    air conduction, V5070
    binaural, V5120–V5150
    bone conduction, V5080
    frames, V2020, V2025
    hearing aid, V5230
Glatiramer acetate, Q2010
Gloves, A4927
Glucagon HCl, J1610
Glucose monitor with integrated lancing/blood sample collection, E2101
Glucose monitor with integrated voice synthesizer, E2100
Glucose test strips, A4253, A4772
Gluteal pad, L2650
Glycopyrrolate, inhalation solution concentrated, J7642
Glycopyrrolate, inhalation solution, unit dose, J7643
Gold sodium thiomalate, J1600
Gomco drain bottle, A4912
Gonadorelin HCl, J1620
Goserelin acetate implant (see also Implant), J9202
Grab bar, trapeze, E0910, E0940
Grade-aid, wheelchair, E0974
Granisetron HCl, J1626
Gravity traction device, E0941
Gravlee jet washer, A4470

H

Hair analysis (excluding arsenic), P2031
Hallus-Valgus dynamic splint, L3100
Hallux prosthetic implant, L8642
Haloperidol, J1630
  decanoate, J1631
Halo procedures, L0810–L0860
Halter, cervical head, E0942
Hand finger orthosis, prefabricated, L3923
Hand restoration, L6900–L6915
  partial prosthesis, L6000–L6020
  orthosis (WHFO), E1805, E1825, L3800–L3805, L3900–L3954
  rims, wheelchair, E0967
Handgrip (cane, crutch, walker), A4636
Harness, E0942, E0944, E0945
Harvard pressure clamp, dialysis, A4920
Headgear (for positive airway pressure device), K0185
Hearing devices, V5000–V5299, L8614
Heat
  application, E0200–E0239
  infrared heating pad system, A4639, E0221
  lamp, E0200, E0205
  pad, E0210, E0215, E0237, E0238, E0249
Heater (nebulizer), E1372
Heel
  elevator, air, E0370
  protector, E0191
  shoe, L3430–L3485
  stabilizer, L3170
Helicopter, ambulance (see also Ambulance)
Helmet, cervical, L0100, L0110
Helmet, head, E0701
Hemin, J1640
Hemi-wheelchair, E1083–E1086
Hemipelvectomy prosthesis, L5280, L5340
Hemodialysis
  kit, A4820
  machine, E1590
Hemodialyzer, portable, E1635
Hemofil M, J7190
Hemoglobin, Q0116
Hemophilia clotting factor, J7190–J7198
Hemophilia clotting factor, NOC, J7199
Hemostats, A4850
Hemostix, A4773
Heparin infusion pump, dialysis, E1520
Heparin lock flush, J1642
Heparin sodium, A4800, J1644
Hepatitis B vaccine, Q3021–Q3023
Hep-Lock (U/P), J1642
Hexalite, A4590
High osmolar contrast material, Q9958–Q9964
Hip
  disarticulation prosthesis, L5250, L5270, L5330
  orthosis (HO), L1600–L1690
Hip-knee-ankle-foot orthosis (HKAFO), L2040–L2090
Histrelin acetate, J1675
Histrelin implant, J9225
HKAFO, L2040–L2090
Home Health Agency Services, T0221
Hot water bottle, E0220
Humidifier, A7046, E0550–E0563
Hyaluronate, sodium, J7317
Hyaluronidase, J3470
Hyaluronidase, ovine, J3471–J3472
Hydralazine HCl, J0360
Hydraulic patient lift, E0630

Hydrocollator, E0225, E0239
Hydrocolloid dressing, A6234–A6241
Hydrocortisone
  acetate, J1700
  sodium phosphate, J1710
  sodium succinate, J1720
Hydrogel dressing, A6242–A6248, A6231–A6233
Hydromorphone, J1170
Hydroxyzine HCl, J3410
Hylan G-F 20, J7320
Hyoscyamine Sulfate, J1980
Hyperbaric oxygen chamber, topical, A4575
Hypertonic saline solution, J7130

I

Ibutilide Fumarate, J1742
Ice
  cap, E0230
  collar, E0230
Idarubicin HCl, J9211
Ifosfamide, J9208
Imiglucerase, J1785
Immune globulin intravenous, J1566–J1567
Immunosuppressive drug, not otherwise classified, J7599
Implant
  access system, A4301
  aqueous shunt, L8612
  breast, L8600
  cochlear, L8614, L8619
  collagen, urinary tract, L8603
  contraceptive, A4260
  ganciclovir, J7310
  hallux, L8642
  indium III-in Pentetreotide, Q3008
  infusion pump, programmable, E0783, E0786
  joint, L8630, L8641, L8658
  lacrimal duct, A4262, A4263
  metacarpophalangeal joint, L8630
  metatarsal joint, L8641
  neurostimulator electrodes, E0752
  neurostimulator pulse generator, E0756, L8681–L8688
  neurostimulator radiofrequency receiver, E0757
  not otherwise specified, L8699
  ocular, L8610
  ossicular, L8613
  osteogenesis stimulator, E0749
  percutaneous access system, A4301
  replacement implantable intraspinal catheter, E0785
  synthetic, urinary, L8606
  urinary tract, L8603, L8606
  vascular graft, L8670
Impregnated gauze dressing, A6222–A6230, K0535–K0537
Incontinence
  appliances and supplies, A4310–A4355, A4356–A4360, A5071–A5075, A5102–A5114, K0280, K0281
  products, A4521–A4538
  treatment system, E0740
Indium In-111 carpromab pendetide, A9507
Indium In-111 ibritumomab tiuxetan, A9542
Indium In-111 oxyquinoline, A9547
Indium In-111 pentetate, A9548
Indium In-111 pentetreotide, A9565
Indium In-111 satumomab, A4642

Indwelling catheter insertion, G0002
Infliximab injection, J1745
Infusion
  pump, ambulatory, with administrative equipment, E0781
  pump, heparin, dialysis, E1520
  pump, implantable, E0782, E0783
  pump, implantable, refill kit, A4220
  pump, insulin, E0784
  pump, mechanical, reusable, E0779, E0780
  pump, uninterrupted infusion of Epiprostenol, K0455
  supplies, A4221, A4222, A4230–A4232
  therapy, other than chemotherapeutic drugs, Q0081
Inhalation solution (see also drug name), J7608–J7699
Injections (see also drug name), J0120–J7320
  contrast material, during MRI, A4643
  supplies for self-administered, A4211
Insertion, indwelling catheter, G0002
Insertion tray, A4310–A4316
Insulin, J1815, J1817
Insulin lispro, K0548
Interferon
  Alpha, J9212–J9215
  Beta-1a, J1825, Q3025–Q3026
  Beta-1b, J1830
  Gamma, J9216
Intermittent
  assist device with continuous positive airway pressure device, E0470–E0472
  peritoneal dialysis system, E1592
  positive pressure breathing (IPPB) machine, E0500
Interphalangeal joint, prosthetic implant, L8658, L8659
Interscapular thoracic prosthesis
  endoskeletal, L6570
  upper limb, L6350–L6370
Intraconazole, J1835
Intraocular lenses, V2630–V2632
Intrapulmonary percussive ventilation system, E0481
Intrauterine copper contraceptive, J7300
Iodine iobenguane sulfate I-131, A9508
Iodine I-123 sodium iodide, A9516, A9517
Iodine I-125 serum albumin, A9532
Iodine I-125 sodium iothalamate, A9554
Iodine I-131 iodinated serum albumin, A9524
Iodine I-131 sodium iodide capsule, A9528
Iodine I-131 sodium iodide solution, A9529–A9531
Iodine I-131 tositumomab, A9544–A9545
Iodine swabs/wipes, A4247
IPD
  supply kit, A4905
  system, E1592
IPPB machine, E0500
Ipratropium bromide, inhalation solution, unit dose, J7644
Irinotecan, J9206
Iron Dextran, J1751, J1752
Iron sucrose, J1756
Irrigation/evacuation system, bowel
  control unit, E0350
  disposable supplies for, E0352
Irrigation solution for bladder calculi, Q2004
Irrigation supplies, A4320–A4323, A4355, A4397–A4400
Isoetharine HCL, inhalation solution, concentrated, J7648

Isoetharine HCL, inhalation solution, unit dose, J7649
Isolates, B4150, B4152
Isoproterenol HCL, inhalation solution, concentrated, J7658
Isoproterenol HCL, inhalation solution, unit dose, J7659
IV pole, each, E0776, K0105

J

Jacket
    body (LSO) (spinal), L0500–L0565
    scoliosis, L1300, L1310
Jenamicin, J1580
Joint supportive device/garment, A4464

K

Kanamycin sulfate, J1840, J1850
Kartop patient lift, toilet or bathroom
    (*see also* Lift), E0625
Ketorolac thomethamine, J1885
Kidney
    ESRD supply, A4650–A4927
    system, E1510
    wearable artificial, E1632
Kits
    continuous ambulatory peritoneal dialysis (CAPD), A4900
    continuous cycling peritoneal dialysis (CCPD), A4901
    dialysis, A4910
    enteral feeding supply (syringe) (pump) (gravity), B4034–B4036
    fistula cannulation (set), A4730
    intermittent peritoneal dialysis (IPD) supply, A4905
    parenteral nutrition, B4220–B4224

surgical dressing (tray), A4550
tracheostomy, A4625
Knee
    disarticulation, prosthesis, L5150, L5160
    joint, miniature, L5826
    orthosis (KO), E1810, L1800–L1885
Knee-ankle-foot orthosis (KAFO), L2000–L2039, L2126–L2136
    addition, high strength, lightweight material, L2755
Kutapressin, J1910
Kyphosis pad, L1020, L1025

L

Laboratory tests
    chemistry, P2028–P2038
    microbiology, P7001
    miscellaneous, P9010–P9615, Q0111–Q0115
    toxicology, P3000–P3001, Q0091
Lacrimal duct implant
    permanent, A4263
    temporary, A4262
Lactated Ringer's infusion, J7120
Laetrile, J3570
Lancet, A4258, A4259
Laronidase, J1931
Larynx, artificial, L8500
Laser blood collection device and accessory, E0620, A4257
Lead investigation, T1029
Lead wires, per pair, A4557
Leg
    bag, A4358, A5105, A5112
    extensions for walker, E0158
    rest, elevating, K0195
    rest, wheelchair, E0990
    strap, replacement, A5113–A5114

Legg Perthes orthosis, L1700–L1755
Lens
    aniseikonic, V2118, V2318
    contact, V2500–V2599
    eye, V2100–V2615, V2700–V2799
    intraocular, V2630–V2632
    low vision, V2600–V2615
    progressive, V2781
Lepirudin, J1945
Leucovorin calcium, J0640
Leukocyte examination, fecal, G0026
Leukocyte poor blood, each unit, P9016
Leuprolide acetate, J1950, J9217, J9218, J9219
Levalbuterol, all formulations, inhalation solution, J7617
Levalbuterol, all formulations, inhalation solution, concentrated, J7612
Levalbuterol, all formulations, inhalation solution, unit dose, J7614
Levocarnitine, J1955
Levofloxacin, J1956
Levonorgestrel, (contraceptive), implants and supplies, J7306
Levorphanol tartrate, J1960
Lidocaine HCl, J2001
Lift
    patient (includes seat lift), E0621–E0635
    shoe, L3300–L3334
Lincomycin HCl, J2010
Linezolid, J2020
Liquid barrier, ostomy, A4363
Lodging, recipient, escort nonemergency transport, A0180, A0200
Lorazepam, J2060
Low osmolar contrast material, Q9945–Q9951
LSO, L0621–L0640
Lubricant, A4402, A4332
Lumbar flexion, L0540
Lumbar-sacral orthosis (LSO), L0621–L0640
Lymphocyte immune globulin, J7504, J7511

M

Magnesium sulphate, J3475
Maintenance contract, ESRD, A4890
Manipulation of spine, chiropractic, A2000
Mannitol, J2150
Mask
   aerosol, K0180
   oxygen, A4620, A4621
Mastectomy
   bra, L8000
   form, L8020
   prosthesis, L8030, L8600
   sleeve, L8010
Mattress
   air pressure, E0186
   alternating pressure, E0277
   dry pressure, E0184
   gel pressure, E0196
   hospital bed, E0271, E0272
   non-powered, pressure reducing, E0373
   overlay, E0371–E0372
   powered, pressure reducing, E0277
   water pressure, E0187
Measuring cylinder, dialysis, A4921
Mechlorethamine HCl, J9230
Medical and surgical supplies, A4206–A8999
Medroxyprogesterone acetate, J1051, J1055
Medroxyprogesterone acetate/estradiol cypionate, J1056
Melphalan HCl, J9245
Melphalan, oral, J8600
Meperidine, J2175
Meperidine and promethazine, J2180
Mepivacaine HCl, J0670
Meropenem, J2185
Mesna, J9209
Metabolically active tissue, Q0184
Metabolically active D/E tissue, Q0185
Metacarpophalangeal joint, prosthetic implant, L8630, L8631
Metaproterenol sulfate, inhalation solution, concentrated, J7668
Metaproterenol sulfate, inhalation solution, unit dose, J7669
Metaraminol bitartrate, J0380
Metatarsal joint, prosthetic implant, L8641
Meter, bath conductivity, dialysis, E1550
Methacholine chloride, J7674
Methadone HCl, J1230
Methocarbamol, J2800
Methotrexate, oral, J8610
Methotrexate sodium, J9250, J9260
Methyldopate HCl, J0210
Methylene blue, A9535
Methylergonovine maleate, J2210
Methylprednisolone
   acetate, J1020–J1040
   oral, J7509
   sodium succinate, J2920, J2930

Metoclopramide HCl, J2765
Microbiology test, P7001
Midazolam HCl, J2250
Mileage, ambulance, A0380, A0390
Mini-bus, nonemergency transportation, A0120
Milrinone lactate, J2260
Mitomycin, J9280–J9291
Mitoxantrone HCl, J9293
Modalities, with office visit, M0005–M0008
Moisture exchanger for use with invasive mechanical ventilation, A4483
Moisturizer, skin, A6250
Monitor
   apnea, E0608
   blood glucose, E0607, E0609
   blood pressure, A4670
   pacemaker, E0610, E0615
Monitoring and recording, EKG, G0004–G0007
Monoclonal antibodies, J7505
Mononine, Q0160
Morphine sulfate, J2270, J2271
   sterile, preservative-free, J2275
Mouthpiece (for respiratory equipment), A4617
   and dome (for nebulizer), K0181
Moxifloxacin, J2280
MRI contrast material, A4643
Mucoprotein, blood, P2038
Multiaxial ankle, L5986
Multidisciplinary services, H2000–H2001, T1023–T1028
Multiple post collar, cervical, L0180–L0200
Multi-Podus type AFO, L4396
Muromonab-CD3, J7505
Mycophenolate mofetil, J7517
Mycophenolic acid, J7518

N

Nalbuphine HCl, J2300
Naloxone HCl, J2310
Nandrolone
   decanoate, J2320–J2322
Narrowing device, wheelchair, E0969
Nasal application device, K0183
Nasal pillows/seals (for nasal application device), K0184
Nasal vaccine inhalation, J3530
Nasogastric tubing, B4081, B4082
Natalizumab, Q4079
Nebulizer, E0570–E0585
   aerosol compressor, E0571
   aerosol mask, A7015
   corrugated tubing, disposable, A7010
   corrugated tubing, non-disposable, A7011
   distilled water, K0182
   drug dispensing fee, E0590
   filter, disposable, A7013
   filter, non-disposable, A7014

   heater, E1372
   large volume, disposable, prefilled, A7008
   large volume, disposable, unfilled, A7007
   not used with oxygen, durable, glass, A7017
   pneumatic, administration set, A7003, A7005, A7006
   pneumatic, nonfiltered, A7004
   portable, E0570
   small volume, A7003–A7005
   ultrasonic, E0575
   ultrasonic, dome and mouthpiece, A7016
   ultrasonic, reservoir bottle, non-disposable, A7009
   water collection device, large volume nebulizer, A7012
Needle, A4215
   dialysis, A4655
   non-coring, A4212
   with syringe, A4206–A4209
Negative pressure wound therapy pump, E2402
   accessories, A6550
Neonatal transport, ambulance, base rate, A0225
Neostigmine methylsulfate, J2710
Nerve stimulator with batteries, E0765
Nesiritide injection, J2324
Neuromuscular stimulator, E0745
Neurostimulator
   electrodes, E0753
   programmer, E0754
   pulse generator, E0756, L8681–L8688
   receiver, E0757
   transmitter, E0758
Nitrogen N-13 ammonia, A9526
Nonchemotherapy drug, oral, NOS, J8499
Noncovered services, A9270
Nonelastic gauze, A6264, A6406
Nonemergency transportation, A0080–A0210
Nonimpregnated gauze dressing, A6216–A6221, A6402–A6404
Nonmetabolic active tissue, Q0183
Nonprescription drug, A9150
Not otherwise classified drug, J3490, J7599, J7699, J7799, J8499, J8999, J9999, Q0181
NPH, J1820
NTIOL category 1, Q1001
NTIOL category 2, Q1002
NTIOL category 3, Q1003
NTIOL category 4, Q1004
NTIOL category 5, Q1005
Nursing care, T1030–T1031
Nutrition
   enteral infusion pump, B9000, B9002
   parenteral infusion pump, B9004, B9006
   parenteral solution, B4164–B5200

O

P

Pacemaker monitor, E0610, E0615
Paclitaxel, J9265
Paclitaxel protein-bound particles, J9264
Pad
   gel pressure, E0178, E0185, E0196
   heat, E0210, E0215, E0217, E0238, E0249
   orthotic device interface, E1820
   sheepskin, E0188, E0189
   water circulating cold with pump, E0218
   water circulating heat with pump, E0217
   water circulating heat unit, E0249
   wheelchair, low pressure and positioning, E0192
Pail, for use with commode chair, E0167
Palate, prosthetic implant, L8618
Palifermin, J2425
Palonosetron HCl, J2469
Pamidronate disodium, J2430
Pan, for use with commode chair, E0167
Papanicolaou (Pap) screening smear, P3000, P3001, Q0091
Papaverine HCl, J2440
Paraffin, A4265
Paraffin bath unit, E0235
Paramagnetic contrast material, (Gadolinium), A4647
Paramedic intercept, rural, Q0186
Parenteral nutrition
   administration kit, B4224
   pump, B9004, B9006
   solution, B4164–B5200
   supply kit, B4220, B4222
Paricalcitol, J2501
Parking fee, nonemergency transport, A0170
Paste, conductive, A4558
Patella, prosthetic implant, L8640
Pathology and laboratory tests, miscellaneous, P9010–P9615
Patient support system, E0636
PEFR, peak expiratory flow rate meter, A4614
Pegademase bovine, J2504
Pegaptanib, J2503
Pegaspargase, J9266
Pegfilgrastim, J2505
Pelvic belt/harness/boot, E0944
Pemetrexed, J9305
Penicillin
   G benzathine/G benzathine and penicillin G procaine, J0530–J0580
   G potassium, J2540
   G procaine, aqueous, J2510
Pentamidine isethionate, J2545
Pentastarch, 10% solution, J2513
Pentazocine HCl, J3070
Pentobarbital sodium, J2515
Pentostatin, J9268
Percussor, E0480
Percutaneous access system, A4301
Perflexane lipid microspheres, Q9955
Perflutren lipid microspheres, Q9957
Peroneal strap, L0980
Peroxide, A4244
Perphenazine, J3310
Personal care services, T1019–T1021
Personal comfort item, A9190

Pessary, A4561, A4562
PET myocardial perfusion imaging, G0030–G0047
Phenobarbital sodium, J2560
Phentolamine mesylate, J2760
Phenylephrine HCl, J2370
Phenytoin sodium, J1165
Phisohex solution, A4246
Photofrin, see Porfimer sodium
Phototherapy light, E0202
Phytonadione, J3430
Pillow, cervical, E0943
Pinworm examination, Q0113
Plasma
   multiple donor, pooled, frozen, P9023
   protein fraction, P9018
   single donor, fresh frozen, P9017
Plastazote, L3002, L3252, L3253, L3265, L5654–L5658
Platelet
   concentrate, each unit, P9019
   rich plasma, each unit, P9020
Platform attachment
   forearm crutch, E0153
   walker, E0154
Plicamycin, J9270
Plumbing, for home ESRD equipment, A4870
Pneumatic
   appliance, E0655–E0673, L4350–L4380
   compressor, E0650–E0652
   splint, L4350–L4380
   tire, wheelchair, E0953
   ventricular assist device, Q0480–Q0505
Pneumatic nebulizer
   administration set, small volume, filtered, A7006
   administration set, small volume, non-filtered, A7003
   administration set, small volume, non-filtered, non-disposable, A7005
   small volume, disposable, A7004
Porfimer, J9600
Portable
   equipment transfer, R0070–R0076
   hemodialyzer system, E1635
   nebulizer, E1375
   x-ray equipment, Q0092
Positioning seat, T5001
Positive airway pressure device, accessories, A7030–A7039, E0561–E0562
Positive expiratory pressure device, E0484
Post-coital examination, Q0115
Post-voiding residual, ultrasound, G0050
Postural drainage board, E0606
Potassium chloride, J3480
Potassium hydroxide (KOH) preparation, Q0112
Pouch
   fecal collection, A4330
   ostomy, A4375–A4378, A5051–A5054, A5061–A5065
   urinary, A4379–A4383, A5071–A5075
Pralidoxime chloride, J2730
Prednisolone
   acetate, J2650
   oral, J7506, J7510

Prednisone, J7506
Preparation kits, dialysis, A4914
Preparatory prosthesis, L5510–L5595
   chemotherapy, J8999
   nonchemotherapy, J8499
Pressure
   alarm, dialysis, E1540
   pad, A4640, E0176–E0199
   ventilator, E0454
Procainamide HCl, J2690
Prochlorperazine, J0780
Prolotherapy, M0076
Promazine HCl, J2950
Promethazine HCl, J2550
Promethazine and meperidine, J2180
Propranolol HCl, J1800
Prosthesis
   artificial larynx battery/accessory, L8505
   breast, L8000–L8035, L8600
   eye, L8610, L8611, V2623–V2629
   fitting, L5400–L5460, L6380–L6388
   foot/ankle one piece system, L5979
   hand, L6000–L6020, L6025
   implants, L8600–L8690
   larynx, L8500
   lower extremity, L5700–L5999, L8640–L8642
   mandible, L8617
   maxilla, L8616
   maxillofacial, provided by a non-physician, L8040–L8048
   miscellaneous service, L8499
   ocular, V2623–V2629
   repair of, L7520, L8049
   socks (shrinker, sheath, stump sock), L8400–L8485
   taxes, orthotic/prosthetic/other, L9999
   tracheo-esophageal, L8507-L8509
   upper extremity, L6000–L6999
   vacuum erection system, L7900
   voice amplifier, E1904
Prosthetic additions
   lower extremity, L5610–L5999
   upper extremity, L6600–L7405
Protamine sulfate, J2720
Protectant, skin, A6250
Protector, heel or elbow, E0191
Protirelin, J2725
Pulse generator, E2120
Pump
   alternating pressure pad, E0182
   ambulatory infusion, E0781
   ambulatory insulin, E0784
   blood, dialysis, E1620
   breast, E0602-E0604
   enteral infusion, B9000, B9002
   external infusion, E0779
   heparin infusion, E1520
   implantable infusion, E0782, E0783
   implantable infusion, refill kit, A4220
   infusion, supplies, A4230, A4232, K0110–K0111
   negative pressure wound therapy, K0538
   parenteral infusion, B9004, B9006
   suction, portable, E0600
   suction, supplies, K0190–K0192
   water circulating pad, E0236
Purification system, A4880, E1610, E1615
Pyridoxine HCl, J3415

Q

Quad cane, E0105
Quinupristin/dalfopristin, J2770

R

Rack/stand, oxygen, E1355
Radial head, prosthetic implant, L8620
Radioelements for brachytherapy, Q3001
Radiofrequency transmitter, E0758, E0759
Radiology service, R0070–R0076
Radiopharmaceutical diagnostic imaging agent, A4641, A4642, A9500, A9507, A9512–A9532, Q3002–Q3004
Radiopharmaceutical, therapeutic, A9600, A9605
Rail
    bathtub, E0241, E0242, E0246
    bed, E0305, E0310
    toilet, E0243

Rasburicase, J2783
Reaching/grabbing device, A9281
Reciprocating peritoneal dialysis system, E1630
Red blood cells, P9021, P9022
Reduction pneumoplasty, G0061
Regular insulin, J1820
Regulator, oxygen, E1353
Repair
    contract, ESRD, A4890
    durable medical equipment, E1340
    maxillofacial prosthesis, L8049
    orthosis, L4000–L4130
    prosthetic, L7500, L7510, K0285
Replacement
    battery, A4254, A4630, A4631
    components, ESRD machine, E1640
    pad (alternating pressure), A4640
    tanks, dialysis, A4880
    tip for cane, crutches, walker, A4637
    underarm pad for crutches, A4635
Reservoir bottle (for ultrasonic nebulizer), K0174
RespiGam, *see* Respiratory syncytial virus immune globulin

Respiratory
    Heated humidifier used with PAP, K0531
    Invasive assist with backup, K0534
    Noninvasive assist with backup, K0533
    Noninvasive assist without backup, K0532
Respiratory syncytial virus immune globulin, J1565
Restraint, any type, E0710
Reteplase, J2993
Rho(D) immune globulin, human, J2788, J2790, J2792
Rib belt, thoracic, A4572, L0210, L0220
Ringer's lactate infusion, J7120
Ring, ostomy, A4404
Risperidone, J2794
Rituximab, J9310
Robin-Aids, L6000, L6010, L6020, L6855, L6860
Rocking bed, E0462
Rollabout chair, E1031
Ropivacaine Hcl, J2795
Rubidium Rb-82, A9555

S

Sacral nerve stimulation test lead, A4290
Sacroiliac orthosis, L0600–L0620
Safety belt/pelvic strap, each, K0031
Safety equipment, E0700
   vest, wheelchair, E0980
Saline
   hypertonic, J7130
   solution, J7030–J7050, A4216–A4218
Samarium SM 153 Lexidronamm, A9605
Sandimmune, K0418
Sargramostim (GM-CSF), J2820
Scale, dialysis, A4910
Scissors, dialysis, A4910
Scoliosis, L1000–L1499
   additions, L1010–L1120, L1210–L1290
Sealant
   skin, A6250
Seat
   attachment, walker, E0156
   insert, wheelchair, E0992
   lift (patient), E0621, E0627–E0629
   upholstery, wheelchair, E0975
Secobarbital sodium, J2860
Secretin, J2850
Semen analysis, G0027
Sensitivity study, P7001
Sermorelin acetate, Q0515
Serum clotting time tube, A4771
SEWHO, L3960–L3974
Sheepskin pad, E0188, E0189
Shoes
   arch support, L3040–L3100
   for diabetics, A5500–A5508
   insert, L3000–L3030
   lift, L3300–L3334
   miscellaneous additions, L3500–L3595
   orthopedic, L3201–L3265
   positioning device, L3140–L3170
   transfer, L3600–L3649
   wedge, L3340–L3485
Shoulder
   disarticulation, prosthetic, L6300–L6320, L6550
   orthosis (SO), L3650–L3675
   spinal, cervical, L0100–L0200
   spinal, DME, K0112–K0116
Shoulder-elbow-wrist-hand orthosis (SEWHO), L3960–L3969
Shunt accessory for dialysis, A4740
   aqueous, L8612
Sigmoidoscopy, cancer screening, G0104, G0106
Sincalide, J2805

Sirolimus, J7520
Sitz bath, E0160–E0162
Skin
   barrier, ostomy, A4362, A4363, A4369–A4374, A4385–A4386, A5120
   bond or cement, ostomy, A4364
   sealant, protectant, moisturizer, A6250
   test, collagen, G0025
Sling, A4565
   patient lift, E0621, E0630, E0635
Social worker, nonemergency transport, A0160
Sock
   body sock, L0984
   prosthetic sock, L8420–L8435, L8470, L8480, L8485
   stump sock, L8470–L8485
Sodium
   chloride injection, J2912
   ferric gluconate complex in sucrose, J2916
   hyaluronate, J7315, J7317
   phosphate P32, A9563
   succinate, J1720
Solution
   calibrator, A4256
   dialysate, A4700, A4705, A4760
   elliott's b, J9175
   enteral formulae, B4149–B4156
   irrigation, A4323
   parenteral nutrition, B4164–B5200
Somatrem, J2940
Somatropin, J2941
Sorbent cartridge, ESRD, E1636
Specialty absorptive dressing, A6251–A6256
Spectinomycin HCl, J3320
Speech assessment, V5362–V5364
Speech generating device, E2500–E2599
Spinal orthosis
   anterior-posterior, L0320, L0330, L0530
   anterior-posterior-lateral, L0520, L0550–L0565
   anterior-posterior-lateral-rotary, L0340–L0440
   cervical, L0100–L0200
   cervical-thoracic-lumbar-sacral (CTLSO), L0700, L0710
   DME, K0112–K0116
   halo, L0810–L0830
   lumbar flexion, L0540
   lumbar-sacral (LSO), L0500–L0565
   multiple post collar, L0180–L0200
   sacroiliac, L0600–L0620

   scoliosis, L1000–L1499
   torso supports, L0900–L0960
Splint, A4570, L3100, L4350–L4380
   ankle, L4390–L4398
   dynamic, E1800, E1805, E1810, E1815, E1825, E1830, E1840
   footdrop, L4398
Spoke protectors, each, K0065
Static progressive stretch, E1801, E1806, E1811, E1816, E1818, E1821
Sterile cefuroxime sodium, J0697
Sterile water, A4216–A4217
Stimulators
   neuromuscular, E0744, E0745
   osteogenesis, electrical, E0747–E0749
   ultrasound, E0760
   salivary reflex, E0755
Stomach tube, B4083
Streptokinase, J2995
Streptomycin, J3000
Streptozocin, J9320
Strip, blood glucose test, A4253, A4772
   urine reagent, A4250
Strontium-89 chloride, supply of, A9600
Stump sock, L8470–L8485
Stylet, A4212
Succinylcholine chloride, J0330
Suction pump
   canister, K0190–K0191
   gastric, home model, E2000
   portable, E0600
   respiratory, home model, E0600
   tubing, K0192
Sumatriptan succinate, J3030
Supply/accessory/service, A9900
Support
   arch, L3040–L3090
   cervical, L0100–L0200
   spinal, L0900–L0960
   stockings, L8100–L8239
   suspension sleeve, BK, L5674, L5675
Surgical
   boot, L3208–L3211
   brush, dialysis, A4910
   dressing, A6196–A6406, Q0183–Q0185
   stocking, A4490–A4510
   supplies, A4649
   tray, A4550
Swabs, betadine or iodine, A4247
Syringe, A4213
   dialysis, A4655
   with needle, A4206–A4209

T

Tables, bed, E0274, E0315
Tacrolimus, oral, J7507
Tacrolimus, parenteral, J7515
Tape, A4454, A6265, K0265
Taxi, nonemergency transportation, A0100
Technetium TC 99M Arcitumomab, A9549
Technetium TC 99M Bicisate, A9557, Q3003
Technetium TC 99M Depreotide, A9536, A9511
Technetium TC 99M Disofenin, A9510
Technetium TC 99M Exametazine, A9521
Technetium TC 99M Fanolesomab, A9566
Technetium TC 99M Glucepatate, A9550
Technetium TC 99M–Labeled–labeled red blood cells, A9560, Q3010
Technetium TC 99M Macroaggregated albumin, A9540
Technetium TC 99M Mebrofenin, A9537
Technetium TC 99M Mertiatide, A9562
Technetium TC 99M Oxidronate, A9561, Q3009
Technetium TC 99M Pentetate, A9539, A9567
Technetium TC 99M Pertechnetate, A9512
Technetium TC 99M Pyrophosphate, A9538
Technetium TC 99M Sestamibi, A9500
Technetium TC 99M Succimer, A9551
Technetium TC 99M Sulfur colloid, A9541
TEEV, J0900
Telehealth, Q3014
Telehealth transmission, T1014
Temozolomide, oral, J8700
Tenecteplase, J3100
Teniposide, Q2017
TENS, A4595, E0720–E0749
Tent, oxygen, E0455
Terbutaline sulfate, J3105
Terbutaline sulfate, inhalation solution, concentrated, J7680
Terbutaline sulfate, inhalation solution, unit dose, J7681
Teriparatide, J3110
Terminal devices, L6700–L6895
Testosterone
    aqueous, J3140
    cypionate and estradiol cypionate, J1060
    enanthate, J3120, J3130
    enanthate and estradiol valerate, J0900
    propionate, J3150
    suspension, J3140
Tetanus immune globulin, human, J1670
Tetracycline, J0120
Thallous chloride TL 201, A9505
Theophylline, J2810
Therapeutic lightbox, A4634, E0203
Therapy
    activity, Q0082
    occupational, H5300
    physical (evaluation/treatment), Q0086
Thermometer, A4931–A4932
Thermometer, dialysis, A4910

Thiamine HCl, J3411
Thiethylperazine maleate, J3280
Thiotepa, J9340
Thoracic-hip-knee-ankle (THKAO), L1500–L1520
Thoracic-lumbar-sacral orthosis (TLSO)
    scoliosis, L1200–L1290
    spinal, K0618–K0619, L0430–L0492
Thoracic orthosis, L0210
Thymol turbidity, blood, P2033
Thyrotropin, Alfa, J3240
Tinzarparin, sodium, J1655
Tip (cane, crutch, walker) replacement, A4637
Tire, wheelchair, E0996, E0999, E1000
Tirofiban, J3246
Tissue-based surgical dressings, Q0183–Q0185
Tissue of human origin, J7340, J7342, J7350
TLSO, L0430–L0492, L1200–L1290
Tobramycin, inhalation solution, unit dose, J7682
Tobramycin sulfate, J3260
Toilet accessories, E0167–E0179, E0243, E0244, E0625
Tolazoline HCl, J2670
Toll, nonemergency transport, A0170
Tool kit, dialysis, A4910
Topical hyperbaric oxygen chamber, A4575
Topotecan, J9350
Torsemide, J3265
Torso support, L0900–L0960
Tourniquet, dialysis, A4910
Tracheostoma heat moisture exchange system, A7501–A7509
Tracheostomy
    care kit, A4629
    filter, A4481
    speaking valve, L8501
    supplies, A4623, A4629, A7523–A7524
    tube, A7520–A7522
Tracheotomy mask or collar, A7525–A7526
Traction device, ambulatory, E0830
Traction equipment, E0840–E0948
Transcutaneous electrical nerve stimulator (TENS), E0720–E0749
Transducer protector, dialysis, E1575
Transfer board or device, E0972
Transfer (shoe orthosis), L3600–L3640
Transfer system with seat, E1035
Transparent film (for dressing), A6257–A6259
Transportation
    ambulance, A0021–A0999, Q3019–Q3020
    corneal tissue, V2785
    EKG (portable), R0076
    handicapped, A0130
    nonemergency, A0080–A0210, T2001–T2005
    service, including ambulance, A0021–A0999, T2006
    taxi, nonemergency, A0100
    toll, nonemergency, A0170
    volunteer, nonemergency, A0080, A0090
    x-ray (portable), R0070, R0075
Transtracheal oxygen catheter, A7018
Trapeze bar, E0910–E0912, E0940
Trapezium, prosthetic implant, L8625

Tray
    insertion, A4310–A4316
    irrigation, A4320
    surgical (see also kits), A4550
    wheelchair, E0950
Treprostinil, J3285
Triamcinolone, J3301–J3303
    acetonide, J3301
    diacetate, J3302
    hexacetonide, J3303
    inhalation solution, concentrated, J7683
    inhalation solution, unit dose, J7684
Trifluromazine HCl, J3400
Trifocal, glass or plastic, V2300–V2399
Trimethobenzamide HCl, J3250
Trimetrexate glucuronate, J3305
Triptorelin pamoate, J3315
Truss, L8300–L8330
Tube/Tubing
    anchoring device, A5200
    blood, A4750, A4755
    corrugated, for nebulizer, K0175, K0176
    CPAP device, K0187
    drainage extension, A4331
    gastrostomy, B4084, B4085, B4086
    irrigation, A4355
    laryngectomy, A4622
    nasogastric, B4081, B4082
    oxygen, A4616
    serum clotting time, A4771
    stomach, B4083
    suction pump, each, A7002
    tire, K0064, K0068, K0078, K0091, K0093, K0095, K0097
    tracheostomy, A4622
    urinary drainage, K0280

U

Ultrasonic nebulizer, E0575
Ultrasonic nebulizer reservoir bottle, K0174
Ultrasound bladder capacity test, G0050
Ultrasound bone mineral study, G0133
Ultraviolet cabinet, E0690
Ultraviolet light therapy system, A4633, E0691–E0694
Unclassified drug, J3490
Unipuncture control system, dialysis, E1580
Upper extremity addition, locking elbow, L6693
Upper extremity fracture orthosis, L3980–L3999
Upper limb prosthesis, L6000–L7499
Urea, J3350
Ureterostomy supplies, A4454–A4590
Urethral suppository, Alprostadil, J0275
Urinal, E0325, E0326
Urinary
    catheter, A4338-A4346, A4351-A4353, K0410, K0411
    collection and retention (supplies), A4310–A4359, K0407, K0408, K0410, K0411
    tract implant, collagen, L8603
    tract implant, synthetic, L8606
Urine
    sensitivity study, P7001
    tests, A4250
Urofollitropin, J3355
Urokinase, J3364, J3365
U-V lens, V2755

V

Vabra aspirator, A4480
Vaccination, administration
  hepatitis B, G0010
  influenza virus, G0008
  pneumococcal, G0009
Vancomycin HCl, J3370
Vaporizer, E0605
Vascular
  catheter (appliances and supplies),
    A4300–A4306
  graft material, synthetic, L8670
Vasoxyl, J3390
Venipuncture, routine specimen collection, G0001
Venous pressure clamp, dialysis, A4918
Ventilator
  battery, A4611–A4613
  moisture exchanger, disposable, A4483
  negative pressure, E0460
  volume, stationary or portable, E0450,
    E0461–E0464
Ventricular assist device, Q0480–Q0505
Verteporfin, J3396
Vest, safety, wheelchair, E0980
Vinblastine sulfate, J9360
Vincristine sulfate, J9370–J9380
Vinorelbine tartrate, J9390
Vision service, V2020–V2799
Vitamin B-12 cyanocobalamin, J3420
Vitamin K, J3430
Voice amplifier, L8510
Voice prosthesis, L8511–L8514
Von Willebrand Factor Complex, human, J7188
Voriconazole, J3465

W

Waiver, T2012–T2050
Walker, E0130–E0149
  accessories, A4636, A4637
  attachments, E0153–E0159

Walking splint, L4386
Water
  collection device (for nebulizer),
    K0177
  distilled (for nebulizer), A7018
  pressure pad/mattress, E0177, E0187,
    E0198
  purification system (ESRD), E1610,
    E1615
  softening system (ESRD), E1625
  sterile, A4712, A4714, A4319
  tanks (dialysis), A4880
Wedges, shoe, L3340–L3420
Wet mount, Q0111
Wheel attachment, rigid pickup walker,
  E0155
Wheelchair, E0950–E1298, K0001–
  K0108
  accessories, E0192, E0950–E1030,
    E1065–E1069, E2300–E2399
  amputee, E1170–E1200
  back, fully reclining, manual, E1226
  battery, A4631
  bearings, K0452
  component or accessory, not otherwise
    specified, K0108
  cushions, E2601–E2619
  motorized, E1210–E1213
  narrowing device, E0969
  power add-on, E0983–E0984
  shock absorber, E1015–E1018
  specially sized, E1220, E1230
  stump support system, K0551
  tire, E0996, E0999, E1000
  transfer board or device, E0972
  tray, K0107
  van, nonemergency, A0130
  youth, E1091
WHFO with inflatable air chamber,
  L3807
WHO, wrist extension, L3914
Whirlpool equipment, E1300–
  E1310

Wipes, A4245, A4247
Wound cleanser, A6260
Wound cover
  alginate dressing, A6196–A6198
  collagen dressing, A6020–A6024
  foam dressing, A6209–A6214
  hydrocolloid dressing, A6234–A6239
  hydrogel dressing, A6242–A6247
  non-contact wound warming cover,
    and accessory, E0231, E0232
  specialty absorptive dressing, A6251–
    A6256
Wound filler
  alginate dressing, A6199
  collagen based, A6010
  foam dressing, A6215
  hydrocolloid dressing, A6240, A6241
  hydrogel dressing, A6248
  not elsewhere classified, A6261, A6262
Wound pouch, A6154
Wrist
  disarticulation prosthesis, L6050, L6055
  hand/finger orthosis (WHFO), E1805,
    E1825, L3800–L3954

X

Xenon Xe 133, Q3004
X-ray equipment, portable, Q0092,
  R0070, R0075
Xylocaine HCl, J2000

Z

Zidovudine, J3485
Ziprasidone mesylate, J3486
Zoledronic acid, J3487

MEDICARE CARRIERS MANUAL (MCM), SELECT

CENTERS FOR MEDICARE AND MEDICAID SERVICES (CMS) INTERNET-ONLY MANUALS (IOM)

The CMS manuals underwent a major transformation as the paper-based manuals were phased out and the new internet-only manuals (IOM) were implemented. The internet-only manuals are the official copy of the manuals and will be maintained in the CMS central office.

Effective October 1, 2003, the CMS will no longer issue program memoranda (PMs) containing new policies and procedure as this information will be contained in the IOM.

The paper-based Coverage Issue Manual (CIM) is replaced by the internet-only National Coverage Determinations Manual (NCD). The NCD is organized by categories such as supplies and medical procedures. The manual contains Chapter 1, which outlines the CMS determinations regarding coverage, and Chapter 2, which contains the HCPCS codes that correlate to each of the CMS determinations. CPT categories are also used in Chapter 2 of the manual.

The paper-based Medicare Carriers Manual (MCM) was replaced by the internet-only manual, publications 100. The CMS Manual System includes the following functional areas:

Pub 100	Introduction
Pub 100-01	Medicare General Information, Eligibility, and Entitlement
Pub 100-02	Medicare Benefit Policy
Pub 100-03	Medicare National Coverage Determinations
Pub 100-04	Medicare Claims Processing
Pub 100-05	Medicare Secondary Payer
Pub 100-06	Medicare Financial Management
Pub 100-07	Medicare State Operations
Pub 100-08	Medicare Program Integrity
Pub 100-09	Medicare Contractor Beneficiary and Provider Communications
Pub 100-10	Medicare Quality Improvement Organization
Pub 100-11	Reserved
Pub 100-12	State Medicaid
Pub 100-13	Medicate State Children's Health Insurance Program
Pub 100-14	Medicare End Stage Renal Disease Network
Pub 100-15	Medicare State Buy-In
Pub 100-16	Medicare Managed Care
Pub 100-17	Medicare Business Partners Systems Security
Pub 100-18	Reserved
Pub 100-19	Demonstrations
Pub 100-20	One-Time Notification
Pub 100-21	Recurring Update Notification

The CMS web site contains the latest IOM at www.cms.gov/manuals/.

To assist in the transformation, the CMS has provided crosswalks indication the location of the paper-based material and the new location of the material in the internet-based manual. Following is a crosswalk for the CIM to NCD.

MEDICARE NATIONAL COVERAGE DETERMINATIONS (NCD) MANUAL

Crosswalk CIM to NCD Sections—The column on the far right (column 3) is in CIM sequence. Column 1 shows the NDC Manual section. Note that the sections in the NCD are in CPT category sequence and not in Medicare benefit category sequence.

NCD Section	Title	CIM Section
310.1	Routine Costs in Clinical Trails	CIM 30-1
10.8.1	Stem Cell Transplantation	CIM 35.30.1
100.7	Colonic Irrigation	CIM 35-1
20.29	Hyperbaric Oxygen Therapy	CIM 35-10
80.2	Photodynamic Therapy	CIM 35-100
250.4	Treatment of Actinic Keratosis	CIM 35-101
160.25	Multiple Electroconvulsive Therapy (MECT)	CIM 35-103
260.5	Intestinal and Multivisceral Transplantation	CIM 35-104
230.3	Sterilization	CIM 35-11
140.4	Plastic Surgery to Correct "Moon Face"	CIM 35-12
150.7	Prolotherapy; Joint Sclerotherapy, and Ligamentous Injections with Sclerosing Agents	CIM 35-13
70.1	Consultations With a Beneficiary's Family and Associates	CIM 35-14
240.7	Postural Drainage Procedures and Pulmonary Exercises	CIM 35-15
80.11	Vitrectomy	CIM 35-16
160.1	Induced Lesions of Nerve Tracts	CIM 35-17
30.4	Electrosleep Therapy	CIM 35-18
30.6	Intravenous Histamine Therapy	CIM 35-19
150.1	Manipulation	CIM 35-2
160.2	Treatment of Motor Function Disorders with Electric Nerve Stimulation	CIM 35-20
10.3	Inpatient Hospital Pain Rehabilitation Programs	CIM 35-21
10.4	Outpatient Hospital Pain Rehabilitation Programs	CIM 35-21.1
130.1	Inpatient Hospital Stays for the Treatment of Alcoholism	CIM 35-22
130.2	Outpatient Hospital Services for Treatment of Alcoholism	CIM 35-22
130.6	Treatment of Drug Abuse (Chemical Dependency)	CIM 35-22.2
130.5	Treatment of Alcoholism and Drug Abuse in a Freestanding Clinic	CIM 35-22.3
130.3	Chemical Aversion Therapy for Treatment of Alcoholism	CIM 35-23
130.4	Electrical Aversion Therapy for Treatment of Alcoholism	CIM 35-23.1
230.4	Diagnosis and Treatment of Impotence	CIM 35-24
20.10	Cardiac Rehabilitation Programs	CIM 35-25
40.5	Treatment of Obesity	CIM 35-26
30.1	Biofeedback Therapy	CIM 35-27
30.1.1	Biofeedback Therapy For The Treatment Of Urinary Incontinence	CIM 35-27.1
50.5	Oxygen Treatment of Inner Ear/Carbon Therapy	CIM 35-29
240.3	Heat Treatment, Including the Use of Diathermy and Ultra-Sound for Pulmonary Conditions	CIM 35-3
110.8	Blood Platelet Transfusions	CIM 35-30
270.4	Treatment Of Decubitus Ulcers	CIM 35-31
100.8	Intestinal By-Pass Surgery	CIM 35-33
230.2	Uroflowmetric Evaluations	CIM 35-33
20.23	Fabric Wrapping of Abdominal Aneurysms	CIM 35-34
20.28	Therapeutic Embolization	CIM 35-35
20.01	Vertebral Artery Surgery	CIM 35-37
20.2	Extracranial-Intracranial (EC-IC) Arterial Bypass Surgery	CIM 35-37
110.15	Ultrafiltration, Hemoperfusion and Hemofiltration	CIM 35-38
80.6	Intraocular Photography	CIM 35-39
50.8	Ultrasonic Surgery	CIM 35-4
100.1	Gastric Bypass Surgery for Obesity	CIM 35-40
150.5	Diathermy Treatment	CIM 35-41
130.7	Withdrawal Treatments for Narcotic Addictions	CIM 35-42

NCD Section	Title	CIM Section
10.1	Use Of Visual Tests Prior To And General Anesthesia During Cataract Surgery	CIM 35-44
20.25	Cardiac Catheterization Performed in Other Than a Hospital Setting	CIM 35-45
160.3	Assessing Patients Suitability for Electrical Nerve Stimulation	CIM 35-46
160.7.1	Assessing Patients Suitability for Electrical Nerve Stimulation Therapy	CIM 35-46
140.2	Breast Reconstruction Following Mastectomy	CIM 35-47
150.2	Osteogenic Stimulator	CIM 35-48
160.11	Osteogenic Stimulation	CIM 35-48
110.1	Hyperthermia for Treatment of Cancer	CIM 35-49
30.8	Cellular Therapy	CIM 35-5
50.7	Cochleostomy with Neurovascular Transplant for Meniere's Disease	CIM 35-50
130.8	Hemodialysis for Treatment of Schizophrenia	CIM 35-51
140.5	Laser Procedures	CIM 35-52
260.1	Adult Liver Transplantation	CIM 35-53
260.2	Pediatric Liver Transplantation	CIM 35-53.1
80.7	Refractive Keratoplasty	CIM 35-54
240.6	Transvenous (Catheter) Pulmonary Embolectomy	CIM 35-55
150.8	Fluidized Therapy Dry Heat for Certain Musculoskeletal Disorders	CIM 35-56
160.8	Electroencephalographic Monitoring During Surgical Procedures Involving the Cerebral Vasculature	CIM 35-57
160.9	Electroencephalographic (EEG) Monitoring During Open-Heart Surgery	CIM 35-57.1
20.3	Thoracic Duct Drainage (TDD) In Renal Transplants	CIM 35-58
100.2	Endoscopy	CIM 35-59
30.2	Thermogenic Therapy	CIM 35-6
110.14	Apheresis (Therapeutic Pheresis)	CIM 35-60
140.3	Transsexual Surgery	CIM 35-61
160.14	Invasive Intracranial Pressure Monitoring	CIM 35-62
50.6	Tinnitus Masking	CIM 35-63
20.21	Chelation Therapy for Treatment of Atherosclerosis	CIM 35-64
100.6	Gastric Freezing	CIM 35-65
250.1	Treatment of Psoriasis	CIM 35-66
170.2	Melodic Intonation Therapy	CIM 35-67
100.9	Implantation of Anti-Gastroesophageal Reflux Device	CIM 35-69
20.18	Carotid Body Resection/Carotid Body Denervation	CIM 35-7
40.3	Closed-Loop Blood Glucose Control Device (CBGCD)	CIM 35-70
110.16	Nonselective (Random) Transfusions and Living Related Donor Specific Transfusions (DST) in Kidney Transplantation	CIM 35-71
160.15	Electrotherapy for Treatment of Facial Nerve Palsy (Bell's Palsy)	CIM 35-72
100.10	Injection Sclerotherapy for Esophageal Variceal Bleeding	CIM 35-73
20.20	External Counterpulsation (ECP) for Severe Angina	CIM 35-74
20.11	Intraoperative Ventricular Mapping	CIM 35-75
150.4	Neuromuscular Electrical Stimulator (NMES) in the Treatment of Disuse Atrophy	CIM 35-77
160.12	Neuromuscular Electrical Stimulation (NMES) in the Treatment of Disuse Atrophy	CIM 35-77
20.12	Diagnostic Endocardial Electrical Stimulation (Pacing)	CIM 35-78

NCD Section	Title	CIM Section
10.6	Anesthesia in Cardiac Pacemaker Surgery	CIM 35-79
20.8.3	Anesthesia in Cardiac Pacemaker Surgery	CIM 35-79
30.3	Acupuncture	CIM 35-8
230.1	Treatment of Kidney Stones	CIM 35-81
260.3	Pancreas Transplants	CIM 35-82
100.3	24-Hour Ambulatory Esophegeal pH Monitoring	CIM 35-83
160.4	Steroetactic Cingulotomy as a Means of Psychosurgery	CIM 35-84
20.4	Implantation of Automatic Defibrillators	CIM 35-85
100.11	Gastric Balloon for Treatment of Obesity	CIM 35-86
260.9	Heart Transplants	CIM 35-87
110.4	Extracorporeal Photopheresis	CIM 35-88
170.3	Speech Pathology Services for the Treatment of Dysphagia	CIM 35-89
80.10	Phaco-Emulsification Procedure (Cataract Extraction)	CIM 35-9
20.5	Extracorporeal Immunoadsorption (ECI) Using Protein A Columns	CIM 35-90
100.13	Laproscopic Cholecystectomy	CIM 35-91
30.5	Transcendental Meditation	CIM 35-92
240.1	Lung Volume Reduction Surgery (Reduction Pneumoplasty)	CIM 35-93
20.6	Transmyocardial Revascularization (TMR)	CIM 35-94
20.26	Partial Ventriculectomy	CIM 35-95
230.9	Cryosurgery of Prostate	CIM 35-96
160.16	Vertebral Axial Decompression (VAX-D)	CIM 35-97
270.1	Electrostimulation in the Treatment of Wounds	CIM 35-98
140.1	Abortion	CIM 35-99
160.17	L-Dopa	CIM 45-1
30.7	Laetrile and Related Substances	CIM 45-10
10.5	Autogenous Epidural Blood Graft	CIM 45-11
270.5	Porcine Skin and Gradient Pressure Dressings	CIM 45-12
70.3	Physician's Office Within an Institution—Coverage of Services and Supplies Incident to a Physician's Services	CIM 45-15
110.2	Certain Drugs Distributed by the National Cancer Institute	CIM 45-16
160.20	Transfer Factor For Treatment of Multiple Sclerosis	CIM 45-17
110.5	Granulocyte Transfusions	CIM 45-18
10.2	Transcutaneous Electrical Nerve Stimulation (TENS) for Acute Post-Operative Pain	CIM 45-19
20.22	Ethylenediamine-Tetra-Acetic (EDTA) Chelation Therapy for Treatment of Atherosclerosis	CIM 45-20
110.6	Scalp Hypothermia During Chemotherapy to Prevent Hair Loss	CIM 45-21
260.7	Lymphocyte Immune Globulin, Anti-Thymocyte Globulin (Equine)	CIM 45-22
230.12	Dimethyl Sulfoxide (DMSO)	CIM 45-23
110.3	Anti-Inhibitor Coagulant Complex (AICC)	CIM 45-24
160.13	Supplies Used in the Delivery of Transcutaneous Electrical Nerve Stimulation (TENS) and Neuromuscular Electrical Stimulation (NMES)	CIM 45-25
270.3	Platelet-Derived Wound Healing Formula	CIM 45-26
110.7	Blood Transfusions	CIM 45-27
110.9	Antigens Prepared for Sublingual Administration	CIM 45-28
110.10	Intravenous Iron Therapy	CIM 45-29

NCD Section	Title	CIM Section
40.4	Insulin Syringe	CIM 45-3
80.3	Photosensitive Drugs	CIM 45-30
250.3	Intravenous Immune Globulin For The Treatment Of Autoimmune Mucutaneous Blistering Diseases	CIM 45-31
230.19	Levocarnitine for Use in the Treatment of Carnitine Deficiency in ESRD Patients	CIM 45-32
150.6	Vitamin B12 Injections to Strengthen Tendons; Ligaments; etc; of the Foot	CIM 45-4
80.1	Hydrophilic Contact Lens for Corneal Bandage	CIM 45-7
70.2.1	Services Provided for the Diagnosis and Treatment of Diabetic Sensory Neuropathy with Loss of Protective Sensation (aka Diabetic Peripheral Neuropathy)	CIM 50.8.1
20.8.1	Cardiac Pacemaker Evaluation Services	CIM 50-1
20.8.1.1	Transtelephonic Monitoring of Cardiac Pacemakers	CIM 50-1
230.6	Vabra Aspirator	CIM 50-10
220.1	Computerized Tomography	CIM 50-12
220.2	Magnetic Resonance Imaging	CIM 50-13
220.3	Magnetic Resonance Angiography	CIM 50-14
20.15	Electrocardiographic Services	CIM 50-15
250.2	Hemorheograph	CIM 50-16
190.4	Electron Microscope	CIM 50-18
70.4	Pronouncement of Death	CIM 50-19
110.13	Cytotoxic Food Tests	CIM 50-2
190.2	Diagnostic Pap Smears	CIM 50-20
230.11	Diagnostic Pap Smears	CIM 50-20
210.2	Screening Pap Smears and Pelvic Examinations for Early Detection of Cervical or Vaginal Cancer	CIM 50-20.1
220.4	Mammograms	CIM 50-21
110.12	Challenge Ingestion Food Testing	CIM 50-22
190.1	Histocompatibility Testing	CIM 50-23
190.6	Hair Analysis	CIM 50-24
100.4	Esophageal Manometry	CIM 50-25
260.6	Dental Examination Prior to Kidney Transplantation	CIM 50-26
220.7	Xenon Scan	CIM 50-27
70.5	Hospital and Skilled Nursing Facility Admission Diagnostic Procedures	CIM 50-28
190.3	Cytogenetic Studies	CIM 50-29
20.13	HIS Bundle Study	CIM 50-3
220.8	Nuclear Radiology Procedure	CIM 50-30
160.10	Evoked Response Tests	CIM 50-31
20.7	Percutaneous Transluminal Angioplasty (PTA)	CIM 50-32
300.1	Obsolete or Unreliable Diagnostic Tests	CIM 50-34
190.5	Sweat Test	CIM 50-35
220.6	Positron Emission Tomography (PET) Scans	CIM 50-36
20.17	Noninvasive Tests of Carotid Function	CIM 50-37
80.8	Endothelial Cell Photography	CIM 50-38
160.21	Telephone Transmission of EEGs	CIM 50-39
160.22	Ambulatory EEG Monitoring	CIM 50-39.1
230.5	Gravlee Jet Washer	CIM 50-4
160.5	Sterotaxic Depth Electrode Implantation	CIM 50-40
190.7	Human Tumor Stem Cell Drug Sensitivity Assays	CIM 50-41
20.19	Ambulatory Blood Pressure Monitoring	CIM 50-42
220.9	Digital Subtraction Angiography	CIM 50-43
150.3	Bone (Mineral) Density Studies	CIM 50-44
190.8	Lymphocyte Mitogen Response Assays	CIM 50-45
30.9	Transillumination Light Scanning or Diaphanography	CIM 50-46
20.27	Cardiointegram (CIG) as an Alternative to Stress Test or Thallium Stress Test	CIM 50-47
220.10	Portable Hand-Held X-Ray Instrument	CIM 50-48
80.9	Computer Enhanced Perimetry	CIM 50-49

NCD Section	Title	CIM Section
220.11	Thermography	CIM 50-5
20.24	Displacement Cardiography	CIM 50-50
100.5	Diagnostic Breath Analyses	CIM 50-51
190.9	Serologic Testing for Acquired Immunodeficiency Syndrome (AIDS)	CIM 50-52
110.11	Food Allergy Testing and Treatment	CIM 50-53
20.16	Cardiac Output Monitoring By Electrical Bioimpedance	CIM 50-54
210.1	Prostate Cancer Screening Tests	CIM 50-55
190.11	Home Prothrombin Time INR Monitoring for Anticoagulation Management	CIM 50-56
160.23	Current Perception Threshold/Sensory Nerve Conduction Threshold Test (sNCT)	CIM 50-57.1
220.12	Single Photon Emission Computed Tomograph (SPECT)	CIM 50-58
220.13	Percutaneous Image-Guided Breast Biopsy	CIM 50-59
20.14	Plethysmography	CIM 50-6
220.5	Ultrasound Diagnostic Procedures	CIM 50-7
70.2	Consultation Services Rendered By a Podiatrist in a Skilled Nursing Facility	CIM 50-8
100.12	Gastrophotography	CIM 50-9
230.7	Water Purification and Softening Systems Used in Conjunction with Home Dialysis	CIM 55-1
230.13	Peridex CAPD Filter Set	CIM 55-2
230.14	Ultrafiltration Monitor	CIM 55-3
40.2	Home Blood Glucose Monitors	CIM 60-11 and CIM 60-14
280.14	Infusion Pumps	CIM 60-14
280.5	Safety Roller	CIM 60-15
280.6	Pneumatic Compression Devices	CIM 60-16
240.4	Continuous Positive Airway Pressure (CPAP)	CIM 60-17
280.7	Hospital Beds	CIM 60-18
280.8	Air-Fluidized Bed	CIM 60-19
280.13	Transcutaneous Electrical Nerve Stimulators (TENS)	CIM 60-20
240.5	Intrapulmonary Percussive Ventilator (IPV)	CIM 60-21
160.18	Vagus Nerve Stimulation for Treatment of Seizures	CIM 60-22
50.1	Speech Generating Devices	CIM 60-23
230.8	Non-Implantable Pelvic Flood Electrical Stimulator	CIM 60-24
270.2	Noncontact Normothermic Wound Therapy (NNWT)	CIM 60-25
280.2	White Cane for Use by a Blind Person	CIM 60-3
240.2	Home Use of Oxygen	CIM 60-4
280.9	Power Operated Vehicles That May Be Used as Wheelchairs	CIM 60-5
280.3	Specially Sized Wheelchairs	CIM 60-6
20.8.2	Self-Contained Pacemaker Monitors	CIM 60-7
280.4	Seat Lift	CIM 60-8
280.1	Durable Medical Equipment Reference List	CIM 60-9
80.5	Scleral Shell	CIM 65.3
80.4	Hydrophilic Contact Lenses	CIM 65-1
180.2	Enteral and Parenteral Nutritional Therapy	CIM 65-10
230.16	Bladder Stimulators (Pacemakers)	CIM 65-11
160.19	Phrenic Nerve Stimulator	CIM 65-13
50.3	Cochlear Implantation	CIM 65-14
20.9	Artificial Hearts and Related Devices	CIM 65-16
50.4	Tracheostomy Speaking Valve	CIM 65-165
230.17	Urinary Drainage Bags	CIM 65-17
230.18	Sacral Nerve Stimulation for Urinary Incontinence	CIM 65-18
160.24	Deep Brain Stimulation for Essential Tremor and Parkinson's Disease	CIM 65-19

NCD Section	Title	CIM Section
230.15	Electrical Continence Aid	CIM 65-2
160.6	Carotid Sinus Nerve Stimulator	CIM 65-4
50.2	Electronic Speech Aids	CIM 65-5
20.8	Cardiac Pacemakers	CIM 65-6
80.12	Intraocular Lenses (IOLs)	CIM 65-7
160.7	Electrical Nerve Stimulators	CIM 65-8
230.10	Incontinence Control Devices	CIM 65-9
280.11	Corset Used as Hernia Support	CIM 70-1
280.12	Sykes Hernia Control	CIM 70-2
280.10	Prosthetic Shoe	CIM 70-3
170.1	Institutional and Home Care Patient Education Programs	CIM 80-1
40.1	Diabetes Outpatient Self-Management Training	CIM 80-2
180.1	Medical Nutrition Therapy	CIM 80-3
290.1	Home Health Visits to a Blind Diabetic	CIM 90-1
290.2	Home Health Nurses' Visits to Patients Requiring Heparin Injections	CIM 90-2

The crosswalk for the Medicare Carriers Manual (MCM) is too extensive to display in this text, but can be accessed at www.cms.hhs.gov/manuals/.

102, Chapter 15

20.1—Physician Expense for Surgery, Childbirth, and Treatment for Infertility

(Rev. 1, 10-01-03)

B3-2005.l

A. Surgery and Childbirth

Skilled medical management is covered throughout the events of pregnancy, beginning with diagnosis, continuing through delivery and ending after the necessary postnatal care. Similarly, in the event of termination of pregnancy, regardless of whether terminated spontaneously or for therapeutic reasons (i.e., where the life of the mother would be endangered if the fetus were brought to term), the need for skilled medical management and/or medical services is equally important as in those cases carried to full term. After the infant is delivered and is a separate individual, items and services furnished to the infant are not covered on the basis of the mother's eligibility.

Most surgeons and obstetricians bill patients an all-inclusive package charge intended to cover all services associated with the surgical procedure or delivery of the child. All expenses for surgical and obstetrical care, including preoperative/prenatal examinations and tests and post-operative/postnatal services, are considered incurred on the date of surgery or delivery, as appropriate. This policy applies whether the physician bills on a package charge basis, or itemizes the bill separately for these items.

Occasionally, a physician's bill may include charges for additional services not directly related to the surgical procedure or the delivery. Such charges are considered incurred on the date the additional services are furnished.

The above policy applies only where the charges are imposed by one physician or by a clinic on behalf of a group of physicians. Where more than one physician imposes charges for surgical or obstetrical services, all preoperative/prenatal and post-operative/postnatal services performed by the physician who performed the surgery or delivery are considered incurred on the date of the surgery or delivery. Expenses for services rendered by other physicians are considered incurred on the date they were performed.

B. Treatment for Infertility

Reasonable and necessary services associated with treatment for infertility are covered under Medicare. Infertility is a condition sufficiently at variance with the usual state of health to make it appropriate for a person who normally is expected to be fertile to seek medical consultation and treatment.

50—DRUGS AND BIOLOGICALS

(Rev. 1, 10-01-03)

B3-2049, A3-3112.4.B, HO-230.4.B

The Medicare program provides limited benefits for outpatient drugs. The program covers drugs that are furnished "incident to" a physician's service provided that the drugs are not usually self-administered by the patients who take them.

Generally, drugs and biologicals are covered only if all of the following requirements are met:

- They meet the definition of drugs or biologicals (see §50.1);
- They are of the type that are not usually self-administered. (see §50.2);
- They meet all the general requirements for coverage of items as incident to a physician's services (see §§50.1 and 50.3);
- They are reasonable and necessary for the diagnosis or treatment of the illness or injury for which they are administered according to accepted standards of medical practice (see §50.4);
- They are not excluded as noncovered immunizations (see §50.4.4.2); and
- They have not been determined by the FDA to be less than effective. (See §§50.4.4).

Medicare Part B does generally not cover drugs that can be self-administered, such as those in pill form, or are used for self-injection. However, the statute provides for the coverage of some self-administered drugs. Examples of self-administered drugs that are covered include blood-clotting factors, drugs used in immunosuppressive therapy, erythropoietin for dialysis patients, osteoporosis drugs for certain homebound patients, and certain oral cancer drugs. (See §110.3 for coverage of drugs, which are necessary to the effective use of Durable Medical Equipment (DME) or prosthetic devices.)

50.1—Definition of Drug or Biological

(Rev. 1, 10-01-03)

B3-2049.1

Drugs and biologicals must be determined to meet the statutory definition. Under the statute §1861(t)(1), payment may be made for a drug or biological only where it is included, or approved for inclusion, in the latest official edition of the United States Pharmacopoeia National Formulary (USP-NF), the United States Pharmacopoeia-Drug Information (USD-DI), or the American Dental Association (AOA) Guide to Dental Therapeutics, except for those drugs and biologicals unfavorably evaluated in the ADA Guide to Dental Therapeutics. The inclusion of an item in the USP DI does not necessarily mean that the item is a drug or biological. The USP DI is a database of drug information developed by the U.S. Pharmacopoeia but maintained by Micromedex, which contains medically accepted uses for generic and brand name drug products. Inclusion in such reference (or approval by a hospital committee) is a necessary condition for a product to be considered a drug or biological under the Medicare program, however, it is not enough. Rather, the product must also meet all other program requirements to be determined to be a drug or biological. Combination drugs are also included in the definition of drugs if the combination itself or all of the therapeutic ingredients of the combination are included, or approved for inclusion, in any of the above drug compendia.

Drugs and biologicals are considered approved for inclusion in a compendium if approved under the established procedure by the professional organization responsible for revision of the compendium.

50.2—Determining Self-Administration of Drug or Biological

(Rev. 1, 10-01-03)

AB-02-072, AB-02-139, B3-2049.2

The Medicare program provides limited benefits for outpatient prescription drugs. The program covers drugs that are furnished "incident to" a physician's service provided that the drugs are not usually self-administered by the patients who take them. Section 112 of the Benefits, Improvements & Protection Act of 2000 (BIPA) amended sections 1861(s)(2)(A) and 1861(s)(2)(B) of the Act to redefine this exclusion. The prior statutory language referred to those drugs "which cannot be self-administered." Implementation of the BIPA provision requires interpretation of the phrase "not usually self-administered by the patient".

A—Policy

Fiscal intermediaries and carriers are instructed to follow the instructions below when applying the exclusion for drugs that are usually self-administered by the patient. Each individual contractor must make its own individual determination on each drug. Contractors must continue to apply the policy that not only the drug is medically reasonable and necessary for any individual claim, but also that the route of administration is medically reasonable and necessary. That is, if a drug is available in both oral and injectable forms, the injectable form of the drug must be medically reasonable and necessary as compared to using the oral form.

For certain injectable drugs, it will be apparent due to the nature of the condition(s) for which they are administered or the usual course of treatment for those conditions, they are, or are not, usually self-administered. For example, an injectable drug used to treat migraine headaches is usually self-administered. On the other hand, an injectable drug, administered at the same time as chemotherapy, used to treat anemia secondary to chemotherapy is not usually self-administered.

B—Administered

The term "administered" refers only to the physical process by which the drug enters the patient's body. It does not refer to whether the process is supervised by a medical professional (for example, to observe proper technique or side-effects of the drug). Only injectable (including intravenous) drugs are eligible for inclusion under the "incident to" benefit. Other routes of administration including, but not limited to, oral drugs, suppositories, topical medications are all considered to be usually self-administered by the patient.

C—Usually

For the purposes of applying this exclusion, the term "usually" means more than 50 percent of the time for all Medicare beneficiaries who use the drug. Therefore, if a drug is self-administered by more than 50 percent of Medicare beneficiaries, the drug is excluded from coverage and the contractor may not make any Medicare payment for it. In arriving at a single determination as to whether a drug is usually self-administered, contractors should make a separate determination for each indication for a drug as to whether that drug is usually self-administered.

After determining whether a drug is usually self-administered for each indication, contractors should determine the relative contribution of each indication to total use of the drug (i.e., weighted average) in order to make an overall determination as to whether the drug is usually self-administered. For example, if a drug has three indications, is not self-administered for the first indication, but is self administered for the second and third indications, and the first indication makes up 40 percent of total usage, the second indication makes up 30 percent of total usage, and the third indication makes up 30 percent of total usage, then the drug would be considered usually self-administered.

Reliable statistical information on the extent of self-administration by the patient may not always be available. Consequently, CMS offers the following guidance for each contractor's consideration in making this determination in the absence of such data:

1. Absent evidence to the contrary, presume that drugs delivered intravenously are not usually self-administered by the patient.

2. Absent evidence to the contrary, presume that drugs delivered by intramuscular injection are not usually self-administered by the patient. (Avonex, for example, is delivered by intramuscular injection, not usually self-administered by the patient.) The contractor may consider the depth and nature of the particular

intramuscular injection in applying this presumption. In applying this presumption, contractors should examine the use of the particular drug and consider the following factors:

3. Absent evidence to the contrary, presume that drugs delivered by subcutaneous injection are self-administered by the patient. However, contractors should examine the use of the particular drug and consider the following factors:

A. **Acute Condition**—Is the condition for which the drug is used an acute condition? If so, it is less likely that a patient would self-administer the drug. If the condition were longer term, it would be more likely that the patient would self-administer the drug.

B. **Frequency of Administration**—How often is the injection given? For example, if the drug is administered once per month, it is less likely to be self-administered by the patient. However, if it is administered once or more per week, it is likely that the drug is self-administered by the patient.

In some instances, carriers may have provided payment for one or perhaps several doses of a drug that would otherwise not be paid for because the drug is usually self-administered. Carriers may have exercised this discretion for limited coverage, for example, during a brief time when the patient is being trained under the supervision of a physician in the proper technique for self-administration. Medicare will no longer pay for such doses. In addition, contractors may no longer pay for any drug when it is administered on an outpatient emergency basis, if the drug is excluded because it is usually self-administered by the patient.

D—Definition of Acute Condition

For the purposes of determining whether a drug is usually self-administered, an acute condition means a condition that begins over a short time period, is likely to be of short duration and/or the expected course of treatment is for a short, finite interval. A course of treatment consisting of scheduled injections lasting less than two weeks, regardless of frequency or route of administration, is considered acute. Evidence to support this may include Food and Drug administration (FDA) approval language, package inserts, drug compendia, and other information.

E—By the Patient

The term "by the patient" means Medicare beneficiaries as a collective whole. The carrier includes only the patients themselves and not other individuals (that is, spouses, friends, or other caregivers are not considered the patient). The determination is based on whether the drug is self-administered by the patient a majority of the time that the drug is used on an outpatient basis by Medicare beneficiaries for medically necessary indications. The carrier ignores all instances when the drug is administered on an inpatient basis.

The carrier makes this determination on a drug-by-drug basis, not on a beneficiary-by-beneficiary basis. In evaluating whether beneficiaries as a collective whole self-administer, individual beneficiaries who do not have the capacity to self-administer any drug due to a condition other than the condition for which they are taking the drug in question are not considered. For example, an individual afflicted with paraplegia or advanced dementia would not have the capacity to self-administer any injectable drug, so such individuals would not be included in the population upon which the determination for self-administration by the patient was based. Note that some individuals afflicted with a less severe stage of an otherwise debilitating condition would be included in the population upon which the determination for "self-administered by the patient" was based; for example, an early onset of dementia.

F—Evidentiary Criteria

Contractors are only required to consider the following types of evidence: peer reviewed medical literature, standards of medical practice, evidence-based practice guidelines, FDA approved label, and package inserts. Contractors may also consider other evidence submitted by interested individuals or groups subject to their judgment.

Contractors should also use these evidentiary criteria when reviewing requests for making a determination as to whether a drug is usually self-administered, and requests for reconsideration of a pending or published determination.

Please note that prior to the August 1, 2002, one of the principal factors used to determine whether a drug was subject to the self-administered exclusion was whether the FDA label contained instructions for self-administration. However, CMS notes that under the new standard, the fact that the FDA label includes instructions for self-administration is not, by itself, a determining factor that a drug is subject to this exclusion.

G—Provider Notice of Noncovered Drugs

Contractors must describe on their Web site the process they will use to determine whether a drug is usually self-administered and thus does not meet the "incident to" benefit category. Contractors must publish a list of the injectable drugs that are subject to the self-administered exclusion on their Web site, including the data and rationale that led to the determination. Contractors will report the workload associated with developing new coverage statements in CAFM 21208.

Contractors must provide notice 45 days prior to the date that these drugs will not be covered. During the 45-day time period, contractors will maintain existing medical review and payment procedures. After the 45-day notice, contractors may deny payment for the drugs subject to the notice.

Contractors must not develop local medical review policies (LMRPs) for this purpose because further elaboration to describe drugs that do not meet the 'incident to' and the 'not usually self-administered" provisions of the statute are unnecessary. Current LMRPs based solely on these provisions must be withdrawn. LMRPs that address the self-administered exclusion and other information may be reissued absent the self-administered drug exclusion material. Contractors will report this workload in CAFM 21206. However, contractors may continue to use and write LMRPs to describe reasonable and necessary uses of drugs that are not usually self-administered.

H—Conferences Between Contractors

Contractors' Medical Directors may meet and discuss whether a drug is usually self-administered without reaching a formal consensus. Each contractor uses its discretion as to whether or not it will participate in such discussions. Each contractor must make its own individual determinations, except that fiscal intermediaries may, at their discretion, follow the determinations of the local carrier with respect to the self-administered exclusion.

I—Beneficiary Appeals

If a beneficiary's claim for a particular drug is denied because the drug is subject to the "self-administered drug" exclusion, the beneficiary may appeal the denial. Because it is a "benefit category" denial and not a denial based on medical necessity, an Advance Beneficiary Notice (ABN) is not required. A "benefit category" denial (i.e., a denial based on the fact that there is no benefit category under which the drug may be covered) does not trigger the financial liability protection provisions of Limitation On Liability (under §1879 of the Act). Therefore, physicians or providers may charge the beneficiary for an excluded drug.

J—Provider and Physician Appeals

A physician accepting assignment may appeal a denial under the provisions found in Chapter 29 of the Medicare Claims Processing Manual.

K—Reasonable and Necessary

Carriers and fiscal intermediaries will make the determination of reasonable and necessary with respect to the medical appropriateness of a drug to treat the patient's condition. Contractors will continue to make the determination of whether the intravenous or injection form of a drug is appropriate as opposed to the oral form. Contractors will also continue to make the determination as to whether a physician's office visit was reasonable and necessary. However, contractors should not make a determination of whether it was reasonable and necessary for the patient to choose to have his or her drug administered in the physician's office or outpatient hospital setting. That is, while a physician's office visit may not be reasonable and necessary in a specific situation, in such a case an injection service would be payable.

L—Reporting Requirements

Each carrier and intermediary must report to CMS, every September 1 and March 1, its complete list of injectable drugs that the contractor has determined are excluded when furnished incident to a physician's service on the basis that the drug is usually self-administered. The CMS anticipates that contractors will review injectable drugs on a rolling basis and publish their list of excluded drugs as it is developed. For example, contractors should not wait to publish this list until every drug has been reviewed. Contractors must send their exclusion list to the following e-mail address: drugdata@cms.hhs.gov a template that CMS will provide separately, consisting of the following data elements in order:

1. Carrier Name
2. State
3. Carrier ID#
4. HCPCS
5. Descriptor
6. Effective Date of Exclusion
7. End Date of Exclusion
8. Comments

Any exclusion list not provided in the CMS mandated format will be returned for correction.

To view the presently mandated CMS format for this report, open the file located at:
http://cms.hhs.gov/manuals/pm_trans/AB02_139a.zip

50.3—Incident-to Requirements
(Rev. 1, 10-01-03)
B3-2049.3

In order to meet all the general requirements for coverage under the incident-to provision, an FDA approved drug or biological must:

- Be of a form that is not usually self-administered;
- Must be furnished by a physician; and
- Must be administered by the physician, or by auxiliary personnel employed by the physician and under the physician's personal supervision.

The charge, if any, for the drug or biological must be included in the physician's bill, and the cost of the drug or biological must represent an expense to the physician. Drugs and biologicals furnished by other health professionals may also meet these requirements. (See §§170, 180, 190 and 200 for specific instructions.)

Whole blood is a biological, which cannot be self-administered and is covered when furnished incident to a physician's services. Payment may also be made for blood fractions if all coverage requirements are satisfied and the blood deductible has been met.

50.4—Reasonableness and Necessity
(Rev. 1, 10-01-03)
B3-2049.4

50.4.1—Approved Use of Drug
(Rev. 1, 10-01-03)
B3-2049.4

Use of the drug or biological must be safe and effective and otherwise reasonable and necessary. (See the Medicare Benefit Policy Manual, Chapter 16, "General Exclusions from Coverage," §20.) Drugs or biologicals approved for marketing by the Food and Drug Administration (FDA) are considered safe and effective for purposes of this requirement when used for indications specified on the labeling. Therefore, the program may pay for the use of an FDA approved drug or biological, if:

- It was injected on or after the date of the FDA's approval;

- It is reasonable and necessary for the individual patient; and
- All other applicable coverage requirements are met.

The carrier, DMERC, or intermediary will deny coverage for drugs and biologicals which have not received final marketing approval by the FDA unless it receives instructions from CMS to the contrary. For specific guidelines on coverage of Group C cancer drugs, see the Medicare National Coverage Determinations Manual

If there is reason to question whether the FDA has approved a drug or biological for marketing, the carrier or intermediary must obtain satisfactory evidence of FDA's approval. Acceptable evidence includes:

- A copy of the FDA's letter to the drug's manufacturer approving the new drug application (NDA);
- A listing of the drug or biological in the FDA's "Approved Drug Products" or "FDA Drug and Device Product Approvals";
- A copy of the manufacturer's package insert, approved by the FDA as part of the labeling of the drug, containing its recommended uses and dosage, as well as possible adverse reactions and recommended precautions in using it; or
- Information from the FDA's Web site.

When necessary, the Regional Office (RO) may be able to help in obtaining information.

50.4.2—Unlabeled Use of Drug

(Rev. 1, 10-01-03)

B3-2049.3

An unlabeled use of a drug is a use that is not included as an indication on the drug's label as approved by the FDA. FDA approved drugs used for indications other than what is indicated on the official label may be covered under Medicare if the carrier determines the use to be medically accepted, taking into consideration the major drug compendia, authoritative medical literature and/or accepted standards of medical practice. In the case of drugs used in an anti-cancer chemotherapeutic regimen, unlabeled uses are covered for a medically accepted indication as defined in §50.5.

These decisions are made by the contractor on a case-by-case basis.

50.4.3—Examples of Not Reasonable and Necessary

(Rev. 1, 10-01-03)

B3-2049.4

Determinations as to whether medication is reasonable and necessary for an individual patient should be made on the same basis as all other such determinations (i.e., with the advice of medical consultants and with reference to accepted standards of medical practice and the medical circumstances of the individual case). The following guidelines identify three categories with specific examples of situations in which medications would not be reasonable and necessary according to accepted standards of medical practice:

1—Not for Particular Illness

Medications given for a purpose other than the treatment of a particular condition, illness, or injury are not covered (except for certain immunizations). Charges for medications, e.g., vitamins, given simply for the general good and welfare of the patient and not as accepted therapies for a particular illness are excluded from coverage.

2—Injection Method Not Indicated

Medication given by injection (parenterally) is not covered if standard medical practice indicates that the administration of the medication by mouth (orally) is effective and is an accepted or preferred method of administration. For example, the accepted standard of medical practice for the treatment of certain diseases is to initiate therapy with parenteral penicillin and to complete therapy with oral penicillin. Carriers exclude the entire charge for penicillin injections given after the initiation of therapy if oral penicillin is indicated unless there are special medical circumstances that justify additional injections.

3—Excessive Medications

Medications administered for treatment of a disease and which exceed the frequency or duration of injections indicated by accepted standards of medical practice are not covered. For example, the accepted standard of medical practice in the maintenance treatment of pernicious anemia is one vitamin B-12 injection per month. Carriers exclude the entire charge for injections given in excess of this frequency unless there are special medical circumstances that justify additional injections.

Carriers will supplement the guidelines as necessary with guidelines concerning appropriate use of specific injections in other situations. They will use the guidelines to screen out questionable cases for special review, further development, or denial when the injection billed for would not be reasonable and necessary. They will coordinate any type of drug treatment review with the Quality Improvement Organization (QIO).

If a medication is determined not to be reasonable and necessary for diagnosis or treatment of an illness or injury according to these guidelines, the carrier excludes the entire charge (i.e., for both the drug and its administration). Also, carriers exclude from payment any charges for other services (such as office visits) which were primarily for the purpose of administering a noncovered injection (i.e., an injection that is not reasonable and necessary for the diagnosis or treatment of an illness or injury).

50.4.4—Payment for Antigens and Immunizations

(Rev. 1, 10-01-03)

50.4.4.1—Antigens

(Rev. 1, 10-01-03)

B3-2049.4

Payment may be made for a reasonable supply of antigens that have been prepared for a particular patient if: (1) the antigens are prepared by a physician who is a doctor of medicine or osteopathy, and (2) the physician who prepared the antigens has examined the patient and has determined a plan of treatment and a dosage regimen.

Antigens must be administered in accordance with the plan of treatment and by a doctor of medicine or osteopathy or by a properly instructed person (who could be the patient) under the supervision of the doctor. The associations of allergists that CMS consulted advised that a reasonable supply of antigens is considered to be not more than a 12-month supply of antigens that has been prepared for a particular patient at any one time. The purpose of the reasonable supply limitation is to assure that the antigens retain their potency and effectiveness over the period in which they are to be administered to the patient. (See §§20.2 and 50.2.)

50.4.4.2—Immunizations

(Rev. 1, 10-01-03)

A3-3157.A, B3-2049.4, HO-230.4.C

Vaccinations or inoculations are excluded as immunizations unless they are directly related to the treatment of an injury or direct exposure to a disease or condition, such as anti-rabies treatment, tetanus antitoxin or booster vaccine, botulin antitoxin, antivenin sera, or immune globulin. In the absence of injury or direct exposure, preventive immunization (vaccination or inoculation) against such diseases as smallpox, polio, diphtheria, etc., is not covered. However, pneumococcal, hepatitis B, and influenza virus vaccines are exceptions to this rule. (See items A, B, and C below.) In cases where a vaccination or inoculation is excluded from coverage, related charges are also not covered.

A—Pneumococcal Pneumonia Vaccinations

A3-3157.A.1, HO-230.4.C.1

Effective for services furnished on or after May 1, 1981, the Medicare Part B program covers pneumococcal pneumonia vaccine and its administration when furnished in compliance with any applicable State law by any provider of services or any entity or individual with a supplier number. This includes revaccination of patients at highest risk of pneumococcal infection. Typically, these vaccines are administered once in a lifetime except for persons at highest risk. Effective July 1, 2000, Medicare does not require for coverage purposes that a doctor of medicine or osteopathy order the vaccine. Therefore, the beneficiary may receive the vaccine upon request without a physician's order and without physician supervision.

An initial vaccine may be administered only to persons at high risk (see below) of pneumococcal disease. Revaccination may be administered only to persons at highest risk of serious pneumococcal infection and those likely to have a rapid decline in pneumococcal antibody levels, provided that at least five years have [passed since the previous doe of pneumococcal vaccine.

Persons at high risk for whom an initial vaccine may be administered include all people age 65 and older; immunocompetent adults who are at increased risk of pneumococcal disease or its complications because of chronic illness (e.g., cardiovascular disease, pulmonary disease, diabetes mellitus, alcoholism, cirrhosis, or cerebrospinal fluid leaks); and individuals with compromised immune systems (e.g., splenic dysfunction or anatomic asplenia, Hodgkin's disease, lymphoma, multiple myeloma, chronic renal failure, HIV infection, nephrotic syndrome, sickle cell disease, or organ transplantation).

Persons at highest risk and those most likely to have rapid declines in antibody levels are those for whom revaccination may be appropriate. This group includes persons with functional or anatomic asplenia (e.g., sickle cell disease, splenectomy), HIV infection, leukemia, lymphoma, Hodgkin's disease, multiple myeloma, generalized malignancy, chronic renal failure, nephrotic syndrome, or other conditions associated with immunosuppression such as organ or bone marrow transplantation, and those receiving immunosuppressive chemotherapy. It is not appropriate for routine revaccination of people age 65 or older that are not at highest risk.

Those administering the vaccine should not require the patient to present an immunization record prior to administering the pneumococcal vaccine, nor should they feel compelled to review the patient's complete medical record if it is not available. Instead, provided that the patient is competent, it is acceptable to rely on the patient's verbal history to determine prior vaccination status. If the patient is uncertain about his or her vaccination history in the past five years, the vaccine should be given. However, if the patient is certain he/she was were vaccinated in the last five years, the vaccine should not be given. If the patient is certain that the vaccine was given more than five years ago, revaccination is covered only if the patient is at high risk.

B—Hepatitis B Vaccine

Effective for services furnished on or after September 1, 1984, P.L. 98-369 provides coverage under Part B for hepatitis B vaccine and its administration, furnished to a Medicare beneficiary who is at high or intermediate risk of contracting hepatitis B. This coverage is effective for services furnished on or after September 1, 1984. High-risk groups currently identified include (see exception below):

- ESRD patients;
- Hemophiliacs who receive Factor VIII or IX concentrates;
- Clients of institutions for the mentally retarded;
- Persons who live in the same household as an Hepatitis B Virus (HBV) carrier;
- Homosexual men; and
- Illicit injectable drug abusers.

Intermediate risk groups currently identified include:

- Staff in institutions for the mentally retarded; and
- Workers in health care professions who have frequent contact with blood or blood-derived body fluids during routine work.

EXCEPTION: Persons in both of the above-listed groups in paragraph B, would not be considered at high or inter-mediate risk of contracting hepatitis B, however, if there were laboratory evidence positive for antibodies to hepatitis B. (ESRD patients are routinely tested for hepatitis B antibodies as part of their continuing monitoring and therapy.)

For Medicare program purposes, the vaccine may be administered upon the order of a doctor of medicine or osteopathy, by a doctor of medicine or osteopathy, or by home health agencies, skilled nursing facilities, ESRD facilities, hospital outpatient departments, and persons recognized under the incident to physicians' services provision of law.

A charge separate from the ESRD composite rate will be recognized and paid for administration of the vaccine to ESRD patients.

C—Influenza Virus Vaccine

Effective for services furnished on or after May 1, 1993, the Medicare Part B program covers influenza virus vaccine and its administration when furnished in compliance with any applicable State law by any provider of services or any entity or individual with a supplier number. Typically, these vaccines are administered once a year in the fall or winter. Medicare does not require, for coverage purposes, that a doctor of medicine or osteopathy order the vaccine. Therefore, the beneficiary may receive the vaccine upon request without a physician's order and without physician supervision.

50.4.5—Unlabeled Use for Anti-Cancer Drugs

(Rev. 1, 10-01-03)

B3-2049.4.C

Effective January 1, 1994, unlabeled uses of FDA approved drugs and biologicals used in an anti-cancer chemotherapeutic regimen for a medically accepted indication are evaluated under the conditions described in this paragraph. A regimen is a combination of anti-cancer agents which has been clinically recognized for the treatment of a specific type of cancer. An example of a drug regimen is: Cyclophosphamide + vincristine + prednisone (CVP) for non-Hodgkin's lymphoma.

In addition to listing the combination of drugs for a type of cancer, there may be a different regimen or combinations which are used at different times in the history of the cancer (induction, prophylaxis of CNS involvement, post remission, and relapsed or refractory disease). A protocol may specify the combination of drugs, doses, and schedules for administration of the drugs. For purposes of this provision, a cancer treatment regimen includes drugs used to treat toxicities or side effects of the cancer treatment regimen when the drug is administered incident to a chemotherapy treatment.

Contractors must not deny coverage based solely on the absence of FDA approved labeling for the use, if the use is supported by one of the following and the use is **not** listed as "not indicated" in any of the three compendia. (See note at the end of this subsection.)

A—American Hospital Formulary Service Drug Information

Drug monographs are arranged in alphabetical order within therapeutic classifications. Within the text of the monograph, information concerning indications is provided; including both labeled and unlabeled uses. Unlabeled uses are identified with daggers. The text must be analyzed to make a determination whether a particular use is supported.

B—American Medical Association Drug Evaluations

Drug evaluations are organized into sections and Chapters that are based on therapeutic classifications. The evaluation of a drug provides information concerning indications, including both labeled and unlabeled uses. Unlabeled uses are not specifically identified as such. The text must be analyzed to make a determination whether a particular use is supported. In making these determinations, also refer to the "AMA Drug Evaluations Subscription," Volume III, section 17 (Oncolytic Drugs), Chapter 1 (Principles of Cancer Chemotherapy), tables 1 and 2.

Table 1, Specific Agents Used In Cancer Chemotherapy, lists the anti-neoplastic agents which are currently available for use in various cancers. The indications presented in this table for a particular anti-cancer drug include labeled and unlabeled uses (although they are not identified as such). Any indication appearing in this table is considered to be a medically accepted use.

Table 2, Clinical Responses To Chemotherapy, lists some of the currently preferred regimens for various cancers. The table headings include (1) type of cancer, (2) drugs or regimens currently preferred, (3) alternative or secondary drugs or regimens, and (4) other drugs or regimens with reported activity.

A regimen appearing under the preferred or alternative/secondary headings is considered to be a medically accepted use.

A regimen appearing under the heading "Other Drugs or Regimens With Reported Activity" is considered to be for a medically accepted use provided:

• The preferred and alternative/secondary drugs or regimens are contraindicated;
• A preferred and/or alternative/secondary drug or regimen was used but was not tolerated or was ineffective; or
• There was tumor progression or recurrence after an initial response.

C—United States Pharmacopoeia Drug Information (USPDI)

Monographs are arranged in alphabetic order by generic or family name. Indications for use appear as accepted, unaccepted, or insufficient data. An indication is considered to be a medically accepted use only if the indication is listed as accepted. Unlabeled uses are identified with brackets. A separate indications index lists all indications included in USPDI along with the medically accepted drugs used in treatment or diagnosis.

D—A Use Supported by Clinical Research That Appears in Peer Reviewed Medical Literature

This applies only when an unlabeled use does not appear in any of the compendia or is listed as insufficient data or investigational. If an unlabeled use of a drug meets these criteria, the carrier will contact the compendia to see if a report regarding this use is forthcoming. If a report is forthcoming, the carrier uses this information as a basis for making decisions. The compendium process for making decisions concerning unlabeled uses is very thorough and continuously updated. Peer reviewed medical literature includes scientific, medical, and pharmaceutical publications in which original manuscripts are published, only after having been critically reviewed for scientific accuracy, validity, and reliability by unbiased independent experts. This does not include in-house publications of pharmaceutical manufacturing companies or abstracts (including meeting abstracts).

In determining whether there is supportive clinical evidence for a particular use of a drug, carrier medical staff (in consultation with local medical specialty groups) will evaluate the quality of the evidence in published peer reviewed medical literature. When evaluating this literature, they will consider (among other things) the following:

• The prevalence and life history of the disease when evaluating the adequacy of the number of subjects and the response rate. While a 20 percent response rate may be adequate for highly prevalent disease states, a lower rate may be adequate for rare diseases or highly unresponsive conditions.
• The effect on the patient's well-being and other responses to therapy that indicate effectiveness, e.g., a significant increase in survival rate or life expectancy or an objective and significant decrease in the size of the tumor or a reduction in symptoms related to the tumor. Stabilization is not considered a response to therapy.
• The appropriateness of the study design. The carrier will consider:

1. Whether the experimental design in light of the drugs and conditions under investigation is appropriate to address the investigative question. (For example, in some clinical studies, it may be unnecessary or not feasible to use randomization, double blind trials, placebos, or crossover.);

2. That nonrandomized clinical trials with a significant number of subjects may be a basis for supportive clinical evidence for determining accepted uses of drugs; and

3. That case reports are generally considered uncontrolled and anecdotal information and do not provide adequate supportive clinical evidence for determining accepted uses of drugs.

The carrier will use peer reviewed medical literature appearing in the following publications:

• American Journal of Medicine;
• Annals of Internal Medicine;
• The Journal of the American Medical Association;
• Journal of Clinical Oncology;
• Blood;
• Journal of the National Cancer Institute;
• The New England Journal of Medicine;
• British Journal of Cancer;
• British Journal of Hematology;
• British Medical Journal;
• Cancer;
• Drugs;
• European Journal of Cancer (formerly the European Journal of Cancer and Clinical Oncology);
• Lancet; or
• Leukemia.

The carrier is not required to maintain copies of these publications. If a claim raises a question about the use of a drug for a purpose not included in the FDA approved labeling or the compendia, the carrier will ask the physician to submit copies of relevant supporting literature.

Unlabeled uses may also be considered medically accepted if determined by the carrier to be medically accepted generally as safe and effective for the particular use.

NOTE: If a use is identified as not indicated by CMS or the FDA, or if a use is specifically identified as not indicated in one or more of the three compendia mentioned or if the carrier determines, based on peer reviewed medical literature, that a particular use of a drug is not safe and effective, the off-label usage is not supported and, therefore, the drug is not covered.

50.4.6—Less Than Effective Drug
(Rev. 1, 10-01-03)

B3-2049.4.C.5

This is a drug that has been determined by the Food and Drug Administration (FDA) to lack substantial evidence of effectiveness for all labeled indications. Also, a drug that has been the subject of a Notice of an Opportunity for a Hearing (NOOH) published in the "Federal Register" before being withdrawn from the market, and for which the Secretary has not determined there is a compelling justification for its medical need, is considered less than effective. This includes any other drug product that is identical, similar, or related. Payment may not be made for a less than effective drug.

Because the FDA has not yet completed its identification of drug products that are still on the market, existing FDA efficacy decisions must be applied to all similar products once they are identified.

50.4.7—Denial of Medicare Payment for Compounded Drugs Produced in Violation of Federal Food, Drug, and Cosmetic Act
(Rev. 1, 10-01-03)

B3-2049.4.C.6

The Food and Drug Administration (FDA) has found that, from time to time, firms established as retail pharmacies engage in mass production of compounded drugs, beyond the normal scope of pharmaceutical practice, in violation of the Federal Food, Drug, and Cosmetic Act (FFDCA). By compounding drugs on a large scale, a company may be operating as a drug manufacturer within the meaning of the FFDCA, without complying with requirements of that law. Such companies may be manufacturing drugs which are subject to the new drug application (NDA) requirements of the FFDCA, but for which FDA has not approved an NDA or which are misbranded or adulterated. If the FDA has not approved the manufacturing and processing procedures used by these facilities, the FDA has no assurance that the drugs these companies are producing are safe and effective. The safety and effectiveness issues pertain to such factors as chemical stability, purity, strength, bioequivalency, and biovailability.

Section 1862(a)(1)(A) of the Act requires that drugs must be reasonable and necessary in order to by covered under Medicare. This means, in the case of drugs, the FDA must approve them for marketing. Section 50.4.1 instructs carriers and intermediaries to deny coverage for drugs that have not received final marketing approval by the FDA, unless instructed otherwise by CMS. The Medicare Benefit Policy Manual, Chapter 16, "General Exclusions from Coverage," §180, instructs carriers to deny coverage of services related to the use of noncovered drugs as well. Hence, if DME or a prosthetic device is used to administer a noncovered drug, coverage is denied for both the nonapproved drug and the DME or prosthetic device.

In those cases in which the FDA has determined that a company is producing compounded drugs in violation of the FFDCA, Medicare does not pay for the drugs because they do not meet the FDA approval requirements of the Medicare program. In addition, Medicare does not pay for the DME or prosthetic device used to administer such a drug if FDA determines that a required NDA has not been approved or that the drug is misbranded or adulterated.

The CMS will notify the carrier when the FDA has determined that compounded drugs are being produced in violation of the FFDCA. The carrier does not stop Medicare payment for such a drug unless it is notified that it is appropriate to do so through a subsequent instruction. In addition, if the carrier or Regional Offices (ROs) become aware that other companies are possibly operating in violation of the FFDCA, the carrier or RO notifies:

Centers for Medicare & Medicaid Services
Center for Medicare Management
7500 Security Blvd.
Baltimore, MD 21244-1850

50.5—Self-Administered Drugs and Biologicals

(Rev. 1, 10-01-03)

B3-2049.5

Medicare Part B does not cover drugs that are usually self-administered by the patient unless the statute provides for such coverage. The statute explicitly provides coverage, for blood clotting factors, drugs used in immunosuppressive therapy, erythropoietin for dialysis patients, certain oral anti-cancer drugs and anti-emetics used in certain situations.

50.5.1—Immunosuppressive Drugs

(Rev. 1, 10-01-03)

A3-3112.4.B.3, HO-230.4.B.3, AB-01-10

Until January 1, 1995, immunosuppressive drugs were covered under Part B for a period of one year following discharge from a hospital for a Medicare covered organ transplant. The CMS interpreted the 1-year period after the date of the transplant procedure to mean 365 days from the day on which an inpatient is discharged from the hospital. Beneficiaries are eligible to receive additional Part B coverage **within** 18 months after the discharge date for drugs furnished in 1995; **within** 24 months for drugs furnished in 1996; **within** 30 months for drugs furnished in 1997; and **within** 36 months for drugs furnished after 1997.

For immunosuppressive drugs furnished on or after December 21, 2000, this time limit for coverage is eliminated.

Covered drugs include those immunosuppressive drugs that have been specifically labeled as such and approved for marketing by the FDA. (This is an exception to the standing drug policy which

permits coverage of FDA approved drugs for **nonlabeled** uses, where such uses are found to be reasonable and necessary in an individual case.)

Covered drugs also include those prescription drugs, such as prednisone, that are used in conjunction with immunosuppressive drugs as part of a therapeutic regimen reflected in FDA approved labeling for immunosuppressive drugs. Therefore, antibiotics, hypertensives, and other drugs that are not directly related to rejection are not covered.

The FDA has identified and approved for marketing the following specifically labeled immunosuppressive drugs. They are:

Sandimmune (cyclosporine), Sandoz Pharmaceutical;
Imuran (azathioprine), Burroughs Wellcome;
Atgam (antithymocyte globulin), Upjohn;
Orthoclone OKT3 (Muromonab-CD3), Ortho Pharmaceutical;
Prograf (tacrolimus), Fujisawa USA, Inc;
Celicept (mycophenolate mefetil, Roche Laboratories;
Daclizumab (Zenapax);
Cyclophosphamide (Cytoxan);
Prednisone; and
Prednosolone.

The CMS expects contractors to keep informed of FDA additions to the list of the immunosuppressive drugs.

50.5.2—Erythropoietin (EPO)

(Rev. 1, 10-01-03)

A3-3112.4.B.4, HO-230.4.B.4

The statute provides that EPO is covered for the treatment of anemia for patients with chronic renal failure who are on dialysis. Coverage is available regardless of whether the drug is administered by the patient or the patient's caregiver. EPO is a biologically engineered protein which stimulates the bone marrow to make new red blood cells.

NOTE: Non-ESRD patients who are receiving EPO to treat anemia induced by other conditions such as chemotherapy or the drug zidovudine (commonly called AZT) must meet the coverage requirements in §50.

EPO is covered for the treatment of anemia for patients with chronic renal failure who are on dialysis when:

• It is administered in the renal dialysis facility; or
• It is self-administered in the home by any dialysis patient (or patient caregiver) who is determined competent to use the drug and meets the other conditions detailed below.

NOTE: Payment may not be made for EPO under the incident to provision when EPO is administered in the renal dialysis facility.

Also, in the office setting, reimbursement will be made for the administration charge only for non-ESRD patients receiving EPO.

50.5.2.1—Requirements for Medicare Coverage for EPO

(Rev. 1, 10-01-03)

B3-2049.5

Medicare covers EPO and items related to its administration for dialysis patients who use EPO in the home when the following conditions are met:

A—Patient Care Plan

A dialysis patient who uses EPO in the home must have a current care plan (a copy of which must be maintained by the designated backup facility for Method II patients) for monitoring home use of EPO that includes the following:

1. Review of diet and fluid intake for aberrations as indicated by hyperkalemia and elevated blood pressure secondary to volume overload;

2. Review of medications to ensure adequate provision of supplemental iron;

3. Ongoing evaluations of hematocrit and iron stores;

4. Reevaluation of the dialysis prescription taking into account the patient's increased appetite and red blood cell volume;

5. Method for physician and facility (including backup facility for Method II patients) follow-up on blood tests and a mechanism (such as a patient log) for keeping the physician informed of the results;

6. Training of the patient to identify the signs and symptoms of hypotension and hypertension; and

7. The decrease or discontinuance of EPO if hypertension is uncontrollable.

B—Patient Selection

The dialysis facility, or the physician responsible for all dialysis-related services furnished to the patient, must make a comprehensive assessment that includes the following:

1. **Preselection Monitoring**—The patient's hematocrit (or hemoglobin), serum iron, transferrin saturation, serum ferritin, and blood pressure must be measured.

2. **Conditions the Patient Must Meet**—The assessment must find that the patient meets the following conditions:

a. Is a dialysis patient;

b. Has a hematocrit (or comparable hemoglobin level) that is as follows:

• For a patient who is initiating EPO treatment, no higher than 30 percent unless there is medical documentation showing the need for EPO despite a hematocrit (or comparable hemoglobin level) higher than 30 percent. Patients with severe angina, severe pulmonary distress, or severe hypotension may require EPO to prevent adverse symptoms even if they have higher hematocrit or hemoglobin levels.

• For a patient who has been receiving EPO from the facility or the physician, between 30 and 36 percent.

c. Is under the care of:

• A physician who is responsible for all dialysis-related services and who prescribes the EPO and follows the drug labeling instructions when monitoring the EPO home therapy; and

• A renal dialysis facility that establishes the plan of care and monitors the progress of the home EPO therapy.

3. The assessment must find that the patient or a caregiver meets the following conditions:

• Is trained by the facility to inject EPO and is capable of carrying out the procedure;

• Is capable of reading and understanding the drug labeling; and

• Is trained in, and capable of observing, aseptic techniques.

4. **Care and Storage of Drug**—The assessment must find that EPO can be stored in the patient's residence under refrigeration and that the patient is aware of the potential hazard of a child's having access to the drug and syringes.

C—Responsibilities of Physician or Dialysis Facility

(Rev. 1, 10-01-03)

HO-230.4.B.4.c

The patient's physician or dialysis facility must:

• Develop a protocol that follows the drug label instructions;
• Make the protocol available to the patient to ensure safe and effective home use of EPO;
• Through the amounts prescribed, ensure that the drug on hand at any time does not exceed a 2-month supply;
• Maintain adequate records to allow quality assurance for review by the Network and State Survey Agencies. For Method II patients, current records must be provided to and maintained by the designated backup facility; and
• The dialysis facility must submit claims for EPO, if the facility provides it.

See the Medicare Claims Processing Manual, Chapter 11, "End Stage Renal Disease," for instructions for billing and processing claims for EPO under Method 1 and Method 2. Note that hematocrit readings are required on claims. It is expected that the ESRD facility or hospital outpatient department will maintain the following information in each patient's medical record to permit the review of the medical necessity of EPO.

1. Diagnostic coding;
2. Most recent creatinine prior to initiation of EPO therapy;
3. Date of most recent creatinine prior to initiation of EPO therapy;
4. Most recent hematocrit (HCT) prior to initiation of EPO therapy;
5. Date of most recent hematocrit (HCT) prior to initiation of EPO therapy;
6. Dosage in units/kg;
7. Weight in kgs; and
8. Number of units administered.

50.5.2.2—Medicare Coverage of Epoetin Alfa (Procrit) for Preoperative Use

(Rev. 1, 10-01-03)

PM-AB-99-59, Dated 8/1/99

This instruction pertains exclusively to the preoperative surgical indication of the drug Procrit, in which it is administered to specific patients prior to surgery to reduce risk of transfusion. It does not affect Medicare policies related to other Food and Drug Administration (FDA) approved uses of Procrit. **It is not a national coverage decision**.

Procrit as Preventive Service

The carrier may determine that Procrit is covered for individuals who:

1. Are undergoing hip or knee surgery
2. Have an anemia with a hemoglobin between 10 and 13 mg/dL;
3. Are not a candidate for autologous blood transfusion;
4. Are expected to lose more than 2 units of blood; and
5. Have had a workup so that their anemia appears to be that of chronic disease.

The preoperative use of Procrit may be afforded to these individuals when carriers, exercising their discretion, determine that this treatment is reasonable and necessary. In other cases, Procrit is considered a preventive service and therefore not covered.

50.5.3—Oral Anti-Cancer Drugs

(Rev. 1, 10-01-03)

A3-3112.4.B.5, HO-230.4.B.5

Effective January 1, 1994, Medicare Part B coverage is extended to include oral anti-cancer drugs that are prescribed as anti-cancer chemotherapeutic agents providing they have the same active ingredients and are used for the same indications as anti-cancer chemotherapeutic agents which would be covered if they were not self-administered and they were furnished incident to a physician's service as drugs and biologicals.

For an oral anti-cancer drug to be covered under Part B, it must:

• Be prescribed by a physician or other practitioner licensed under State law to prescribe such drugs as anti-cancer chemotherapeutic agents;
• Be a drug or biological that has been approved by the Food and Drug Administration (FDA);
• Have the same active ingredients as a non-self-administrable anti-cancer chemotherapeutic drug or biological that is covered when furnished incident to a physician's service. The oral anti-cancer drug and the non-self-administrable drug must have the same chemical/generic name as indicated by the FDA's "Approved Drug Products" (Orange Book), "Physician's Desk Reference" (PDR), or an authoritative drug compendium;
• Be used for the same indications, including unlabeled uses, as the non-self-administrable version of the drug; and
• Be reasonable and necessary for the individual patient.

50.5.4—Oral Anti-Nausea (Anti-Emetic) Drugs

(Rev. 1, 10-01-03)

PM AB-97-26

Effective January 1, 1998, Medicare also covers self-administered anti-emetics which are necessary for the administration and absorption of the anti-neoplastic chemotherapeutic agents when a high likelihood of vomiting exists. The anti-emetic drug is covered as a necessary means for administration of the antineoplastic chemotherapeutic agents. Oral drugs prescribed for use with the primary drug, which enhance the anti-neoplastic effect of the primary drug or permit the patient to tolerate the primary anti-neoplastic drug in higher doses for longer periods are not covered. Self-administered anti-emetics to reduce the side effects of nausea and vomiting brought on by the primary drug are not included beyond the administration necessary to achieve drug absorption.

Section 1861(s)(2) of the Act extends coverage to oral anti-emetic drugs that are used as full replacement for intravenous dosage forms of a cancer regimen under the following conditions:

- Coverage is provided only for oral drugs approved by the Food and Drug Administration (FDA) for use as anti-emetics;
- The oral anti-emetic must either be administered by the treating physician or in accordance with a written order from the physician as part of a cancer chemotherapy regimen;
- Oral anti-emetic drugs administered with a particular chemotherapy treatment must be initiated within two hours of the administration of the chemotherapeutic agent and may be continued for a period not to exceed 48 hours from that time;
- The oral anti-emetic drugs provided must be used as a full therapeutic replacement for the intravenous anti-emetic drugs that would have otherwise been administered at the time of the chemotherapy treatment.

Only drugs pursuant to a physician's order at the time of the chemotherapy treatment qualify for this benefit. The dispensed number of dosage units may not exceed a loading dose administered within two hours of the treatment, plus a supply of additional dosage units not to exceed 48 hours of therapy.

Oral drugs that are not approved by the FDA for use as anti-emetics and which are used by treating physicians adjunctively in a manner incidental to cancer chemotherapy are not covered by this benefit and are not reimbursable within the scope of this benefit.

It is recognized that a limited number of patients will fail on oral anti-emetic drugs. Intravenous anti-emetics may be covered (subject to the rules of medical necessity) when furnished to patients who fail on oral anti-emetic therapy.

More than one oral anti emetic drug may be prescribed and may be covered for concurrent use if needed to fully replace the intravenous drugs that otherwise would be given.

50.5.5—Hemophilia Clotting Factors

(Rev. 1, 10-01-03)

A3-3112.4.B.2, HO-230.4.B.2

Section 1861(s)(2)(I) of the Act provides Medicare coverage of blood clotting factors for hemophilia patients competent to use such factors to control bleeding without medical supervision, and items related to the administration of such factors. Hemophilia, a blood disorder characterized by prolonged coagulation time, is caused by deficiency of a factor in plasma necessary for blood to clot. For purposes of Medicare Part B coverage, hemophilia encompasses the following conditions:

- Factor VIII deficiency (classic hemophilia);
- Factor IX deficiency (also termed plasma thromboplastin component (PTC) or Christmas factor deficiency); and
- Von Willebrand's disease.

Claims for blood clotting factors for hemophilia patients with these diagnoses may be covered if the patient is competent to use such factors without medical supervision.

The amount of clotting factors determined to be necessary to have on hand and thus covered under this provision is based on the historical utilization pattern or profile developed by the contractor for each patient. It is expected that the treating source, e.g., a family physician or comprehensive hemophilia diagnostic and treatment center, have such information. From this data, the contractor is able to anticipate and make reasonable projections concerning the quantity of clotting factors the patient will need over a specific period of time. Unanticipated occurrences involving extraordinary events, such as automobile accidents or inpatient hospital stays, will change this base line data and should be appropriately considered. In addition, changes in a patient's medical needs over a period of time require adjustments in the profile.

80—REQUIREMENTS FOR DIAGNOSTIC X-RAY, DIAGNOSTIC LABORATORY, AND OTHER DIAGNOSTIC TESTS

(Rev. 1, 10-01-03)

B3-2070

This section describes the levels of physician supervision required for furnishing the technical component of diagnostic tests for a Medicare beneficiary who is not a hospital inpatient or outpatient. Section 410.32(b) of the Code of Federal Regulations (CFR) requires that diagnostic tests covered under §1861(s)(3) of the Act (the Act) and payable under the physician fee schedule, with certain exceptions listed in the regulation, have to be performed under the supervision of an individual meeting the definition of a physician (§1861(r) of the Act) to be considered reasonable and necessary and, therefore, covered under Medicare. The regulation defines these levels of physician supervision for diagnostic tests as follows:

General Supervision—means the procedure is furnished under the physician's overall direction and control, but the physician's presence is not required during the performance of the procedure. Under general supervision, the training of the nonphysician personnel who actually performs the diagnostic procedure and the maintenance of the necessary equipment and supplies are the continuing responsibility of the physician.

Direct Supervision—in the office setting means the physician must be present in the office suite and immediately available to furnish assistance and direction throughout the performance of the procedure. It does not mean that the physician must be present in the room when the procedure is performed.

Personal Supervision—means a physician must be in attendance in the room during the performance of the procedure.

One of the following numerical levels is assigned to each CPT or HCPCS code in the Medicare Physician Fee Schedule Database:

0   Procedure is not a diagnostic test or procedure is a diagnostic test which is not subject to the physician supervision policy.

1   Procedure must be performed under the general supervision of a physician.

2   Procedure must be performed under the direct supervision of a physician.

3   Procedure must be performed under the personal supervision of a physician.

4   Physician supervision policy does not apply when procedure is furnished by a qualified, independent psychologist or a clinical psychologist; otherwise must be performed under the general supervision of a physician.

5   Physician supervision policy does not apply when procedure is furnished by a qualified audiologist; otherwise must be performed under the general supervision of a physician.

6   Procedure must be performed by a physician or by a physical therapist (PT) who is certified by the American Board of Physical Therapy Specialties (ABPTS) as a qualified electrophysiologic clinical specialist and is permitted to provide the procedure under State law.

6a Supervision standards for level 66 apply; in addition, the

PT with ABPTS certification may supervise another PT but only the PT with ABPTS certification may bill.

7a Supervision standards for level 77 apply; in addition, the PT with ABPTS certification may supervise another PT but only the PT with ABPTS certification may bill.

9 Concept does not apply.

21 Procedure must be performed by a technician with certification under general supervision of a physician; otherwise must be performed under direct supervision of a physician.

22 Procedure may be performed by a technician with on-line real-time contact with physician.

66 Procedure must be performed by a physician or by a PT with ABPTS certification and certification in this specific procedure.

77 Procedure must be performed by a PT with ABPTS certification or by a PT without certification under direct supervision of a physician, or by a technician with certification under general supervision of a physician.

Nurse practitioners, clinical nurse specialists, and physician assistants are not defined as physicians under §1861(r) of the Act. Therefore, they may not function as supervisory physicians under the diagnostic tests benefit (§1861(s)(3) of the Act). However, when these practitioners personally perform diagnostic tests as provided under §1861(s)(2)(K) of the Act, §1861(s)(3) does not apply and they may perform diagnostic tests pursuant to State scope of practice laws and under the applicable State requirements for physician supervision or collaboration.

Because the diagnostic tests benefit set forth in §1861(s)(3) of the Act is separate and distinct from the incident to benefit set forth in §1861(s)(2) of the Act, diagnostic tests need not meet the incident to requirements. Diagnostic tests may be furnished under situations that meet the incident to requirements but this is not required. However, carriers must not scrutinize claims for diagnostic tests utilizing the incident to requirements.

80.1—Clinical Laboratory Services

(Rev. 1, 10-01-03)

B3-2070.1

Section 1833 and 1861 of the Act provides for payment of clinical laboratory services under Medicare Part B. Clinical laboratory services involve the biological, microbiological, serological, chemical, immunohematological, hematological, biophysical, cytological, pathological, or other examination of materials derived from the human body for the diagnosis, prevention, or treatment of a disease or assessment of a medical condition. Laboratory services must meet all applicable requirements of the Clinical Laboratory Improvement Amendments of 1988 (CLIA), as set forth at 42 CFR part 493. Section 1862(a)(1)(A) of the Act provides that Medicare payment may not be made for services that are not reasonable and necessary. Clinical laboratory services must be ordered and used promptly by the physician who is treating the beneficiary as described in 42CFR410.32(a), or by a qualified nonphysician practitioner, as described in 42CFR410.32(a)(3).

See the Medicare Claims Processing Manual Chapter 16 for related claims processing instructions.

80.1.1—Certification Changes

(Rev. 1, 10-01-03)

B3-2070.1.E

Each page of the lists of approved specialties also includes a column "Certification Changed" in which the following codes are used:

"C" indicates a change in the laboratory's approved certification since the preceding listing.

"A" discloses an accretion.

"TERM"—Laboratory not approved for payment after the indicated date which follows the code. The reason for termination also is given in the following codes:

1. Involuntary termination—no longer meets requirements
2. Voluntary withdrawal
3. Laboratory closed, merged with other interests, or organizational change
4. Ownership change with new ownership participating under different name
5. Ownership change with new owner not participating
6. Change in ownership—new provider number assigned
7. Involuntary termination—failure to abide by agreement
8. Former "emergency" hospital now fully participating

80.1.2—Carrier Contacts With Independent Clinical Laboratories

(Rev. 1, 10-01-03)

B3-2070.1.F

An important role of the carrier is as a communicant of necessary information to independent clinical laboratories. Experience has shown that the failure to inform laboratories of Medicare regulations and claims processing procedures may have an adverse effect on prosecution of laboratories suspected of fraudulent activities with respect to tests performed by, or billed on behalf of, independent laboratories. United States Attorneys often have to prosecute under a handicap or may simply refuse to prosecute cases where there is no evidence that a laboratory has been specifically informed of Medicare regulations and claims processing procedures.

Carriers must follow the Provider Education and Training (PET) guidelines to assure that laboratories are aware of Medicare regulations and the carrier's policy when any changes are made in coverage policy or claims processing procedures. The PET guidelines require carriers to use various methods of communication (such as print, Internet, face-to-face instruction). Newsletters/bulletins that contain program and billing information must be produced at least quarterly and posted on the carrier Web site where duplicate copies may be obtained.

Some items which should be communicated to laboratories and responsibilities that laboratories are required to perform are:

- The requirements to have the same fee schedule for Medicare and private patients;
- To specify whether the tests are manual or automated;
- To document fully the medical necessity for pickup of specimens from a skilled nursing facility or a beneficiary's home, and
- In cases when a laboratory service is referred from one independent laboratory to another independent laboratory, to identify the laboratory actually performing the test.

Additionally, when carrier professional relations representatives make personal contacts with particular laboratories, the representative should prepare and retain reports of contact indicating dates, persons present, and issues discussed. Finally, carriers should inform independent laboratories that the Medicare National Coverage Determinations Manual as well as other guidelines contained in the manual for determining medical necessity are on the Web site. Carriers should also publish local guidelines on its Web site; the carrier should not duplicate national instructions here. Timely paper or electronic communications concerning the Internet publications to independent laboratories new to the carrier's service area are essential.

80.1.3—Independent Laboratory Service to a Patient in the Patient's Home or an Institution

(Rev. 1, 10-01-03)

B3-2070.1.G

Where it is medically necessary for an independent laboratory to visit a patient to obtain a specimen, the service would be covered in the following circumstances:

1—Patient Confined to Home

If a patient is confined to the home or other place of residence used as his or her home (see §60.4.1 for the definition of a "homebound patient"), medical necessity would exist (e.g., where a laboratory technician draws a blood specimen). However, where the specimen is a type which would require only the services of a messenger and would not require the skills of a laboratory technician, e.g., urine or sputum, a specimen pickup service would not be considered medically necessary.

2—Place of Residence is an Institution

Medical necessity could also exist where the patient's place of residence is an institution, including a skilled nursing facility that does not perform venipunctures. This would apply even though the institution meets the basic definition of a skilled nursing facility and would not ordinarily be considered a beneficiary's home. (This policy is intended for independent laboratories only and does not expand the range of coverage of services to homebound patients under the incident to provision.) A trip by an independent laboratory technician to a facility (other than a hospital) for the purpose of performing a venipuncture is considered medically necessary only if:

a. The patient was confined to the facility; and

b. The facility did not have on duty personnel qualified to perform this service.

When facility personnel actually obtained and prepared the specimens for the independent laboratory to pick them up, the laboratory provides this pickup service as a service to the facility in the same manner as it does for physicians.

110—DURABLE MEDICAL EQUIPMENT—GENERAL

(Rev. 1, 10-01-03)

B3-2100, A3-3113, HO-235, HHA-220

Expenses incurred by a beneficiary for the rental or purchases of durable medical equipment (DME) are reimbursable if the following three requirements are met:

- The equipment meets the definition of DME (§110.1);
- The equipment is necessary and reasonable for the treatment of the patient's illness or injury or to improve the functioning of his or her malformed body member (§110.1); and
- The equipment is used in the patient's home.

The decision whether to rent or purchase an item of equipment generally resides with the beneficiary, but the decision on how to pay rests with CMS. For some DME, program payment policy calls for lump sum payments and in others for periodic payment. Where covered DME is furnished to a beneficiary by a supplier of services other than a provider of services, the DMERC makes the reimbursement. If a provider of services furnishes the equipment, the intermediary makes the reimbursement. The payment method is identified in the annual fee schedule update furnished by CMS.

The CMS issues quarterly updates to a fee schedule file that contains rates by HCPCS code and also identifies the classification of the HCPCS code within the following categories.

Category Code	Definition
IN	Inexpensive and Other Routinely Purchased Items
FS	Frequently Serviced Items
CR	Capped Rental Items
OX	Oxygen and Oxygen Equipment
OS	Ostomy, Tracheostomy & Urological Items
SD	Surgical Dressings
PO	Prosthetics & Orthotics
SU	Supplies
TE	Transcutaneous Electrical Nerve Stimulators

The DMERCs, carriers, and intermediaries, where appropriate, use the CMS files to determine payment rules. See the Medicare Claims Processing Manual, Chapter 20, "Durable Medical Equipment, Surgical Dressings and Casts, Orthotics and Artificial Limbs, and Prosthetic Devices," for a detailed description of payment rules for each classification.

Payment may also be made for repairs, maintenance, and delivery of equipment and for expendable and nonreusable items essential to the effective use of the equipment subject to the conditions in §110.2.

See the Medicare Benefit Policy Manual, Chapter 11, "End Stage Renal Disease," for hemodialysis equipment and supplies.

110.1—Definition of Durable Medical Equipment

(Rev. 1, 10-01-03)

B3-2100.1, A3-3113.1, HO-235.1, HHA-220.1, B3-2100.2, A3-3113.2, HO-235.2, HHA-220.2

Durable medical equipment is equipment which:

- Can withstand repeated use;
- Is primarily and customarily used to serve a medical purpose;
- Generally is not useful to a person in the absence of an illness or injury; and
- Is appropriate for use in the home.

All requirements of the definition must be met before an item can be considered to be durable medical equipment.

The following describes the underlying policies for determining whether an item meets the definition of DME and may be covered.

A—Durability

An item is considered durable if it can withstand repeated use, i.e., the type of item that could normally be rented. Medical supplies of an expendable nature, such as incontinent pads, lambs wool pads, catheters, ace bandages, elastic stockings, surgical facemasks, irrigating kits, sheets, and bags are not considered "durable" within the meaning of the definition. There are other items that, although durable in nature, may fall into other coverage categories such as supplies, braces, prosthetic devices, artificial arms, legs, and eyes.

B—Medical Equipment

Medical equipment is equipment primarily and customarily used for medical purposes and is not generally useful in the absence of illness or injury. In most instances, no development will be needed to determine whether a specific item of equipment is medical in nature. However, some cases will require development to determine whether the item constitutes medical equipment. This development would include the advice of local medical organizations (hospitals, medical schools, medical societies) and specialists in the field of physical medicine and rehabilitation. If the equipment is new on the market, it may be necessary, prior to seeking professional advice, to obtain information from the supplier or manufacturer explaining the design, purpose, effectiveness and method of using the equipment in the home as well as the results of any tests or clinical studies that have been conducted.

1. **Equipment Presumptively Medical**—Items such as hospital beds, wheelchairs, hemodialysis equipment, iron lungs, respirators, intermittent positive pressure breathing machines, medical regulators, oxygen tents, crutches, canes, trapeze bars, walkers, inhalators, nebulizers, commodes, suction machines, and traction equipment presumptively constitute medical equipment. (Although hemodialysis equipment is covered as a prosthetic device (§120), it also meets the definition of DME, and reimbursement for the rental or purchase of such equipment for use in the beneficiary's home will be made only under the provisions for payment applicable to DME. See the Medicare Benefit Policy Manual, Chapter 11, "End Stage Renal Disease," §30.1, for coverage of home use of hemodialysis.) NOTE: There is a wide variety in types of respirators and suction machines. The DMERC's medical staff should determine whether the apparatus specified in the claim is appropriate for home use.

2. **Equipment Presumptively Nonmedical**—Equipment which is primarily and customarily used for a nonmedical purpose may not be considered "medical" equipment for which payment can be made under the medical insurance program. This is true even though the item has some remote medically related use. For example, in the case of a cardiac patient, an air conditioner might

possibly be used to lower room temperature to reduce fluid loss in the patient and to restore an environment conducive to maintenance of the proper fluid balance. Nevertheless, because the primary and customary use of an air conditioner is a nonmedical one, the air conditioner cannot be deemed to be medical equipment for which payment can be made.

Other devices and equipment used for environmental control or to enhance the environmental setting in which the beneficiary is placed are not considered covered DME. These include, for example, room heaters, humidifiers, dehumidifiers, and electric air cleaners. Equipment which basically serves comfort or convenience functions or is primarily for the convenience of a person caring for the patient, such as elevators, stairway elevators, and posture chairs, do not constitute medical equipment. Similarly, physical fitness equipment (such as an exercycle), first-aid or precautionary-type equipment (such as preset portable oxygen units), self-help devices (such as safety grab bars), and training equipment (such as Braille training texts) are considered nonmedical in nature.

3. **Special Exception Items**—Specified items of equipment may be covered under certain conditions even though they do not meet the definition of DME because they are not primarily and customarily used to serve a medical purpose and/or are generally useful in the absence of illness or injury. These items would be covered when it is clearly established that they serve a therapeutic purpose in an individual case and would include:

a. Gel pads and pressure and water mattresses (which generally serve a preventive purpose) when prescribed for a patient who had bed sores or there is medical evidence indicating that they are highly susceptible to such ulceration; and

b. Heat lamps for a medical rather than a soothing or cosmetic purpose, e.g., where the need for heat therapy has been established.

In establishing medical necessity for the above items, the evidence must show that the item is included in the physician's course of treatment and a physician is supervising its use.

NOTE: The above items represent special exceptions and no extension of coverage to other items should be inferred

C—Necessary and Reasonable

Although an item may be classified as DME, it may not be covered in every instance. Coverage in a particular case is subject to the requirement that the equipment be necessary and reasonable for treatment of an illness or injury, or to improve the functioning of a malformed body member. These considerations will bar payment for equipment which cannot reasonably be expected to perform a therapeutic function in an individual case or will permit only partial therapeutic function in an individual case or will permit only partial payment when the type of equipment furnished substantially exceeds that required for the treatment of the illness or injury involved.

See the Medicare Claims Processing Manual, Chapter 1, "General Billing Requirements;" §60, regarding the rules for providing advance beneficiary notices (ABNs) that advise beneficiaries, before items or services actually are furnished, when Medicare is likely to deny payment for them. ABNs allow beneficiaries to make an informed consumer decision about receiving items or services for which they may have to pay out-of-pocket and to be more active participants in their own health care treatment decisions.

1. **Necessity for the Equipment**—Equipment is necessary when it can be expected to make a meaningful contribution to the treatment of the patient's illness or injury or to the improvement of his or her malformed body member. In most cases the physician's prescription for the equipment and other medical information available to the DMERC will be sufficient to establish that the equipment serves this purpose.

2. **Reasonableness of the Equipment**—Even though an item of DME may serve a useful medical purpose, the DMERC or intermediary must also consider to what extent, if any, it would be reasonable for the Medicare program to pay for the item pre-

scribed. The following considerations should enter into the determination of reasonableness:

1. Would the expense of the item to the program be clearly disproportionate to the therapeutic benefits which could ordinarily be derived from use of the equipment?

2. Is the item substantially more costly than a medically appropriate and realistically feasible alternative pattern of care?

3. Does the item serve essentially the same purpose as equipment already available to the beneficiary?

3. **Payment Consistent With What is Necessary and Reasonable**—Where a claim is filed for equipment containing features of an aesthetic nature or features of a medical nature which are not required by the patient's condition or where there exists a reasonably feasible and medically appropriate alternative pattern of care which is less costly than the equipment furnished, the amount payable is based on the rate for the equipment or alternative treatment which meets the patient's medical needs.

The acceptance of an assignment binds the supplier-assignee to accept the payment for the medically required equipment or service as the full charge and the supplier-assignee cannot charge the beneficiary the differential attributable to the equipment actually furnished.

4. **Establishing the Period of Medical Necessity**—Generally, the period of time an item of durable medical equipment will be considered to be medically necessary is based on the physician's estimate of the time that his or her patient will need the equipment. See the Medicare Program Integrity Manual, Chapters 5 and 6, for medical review guidelines.

D—Definition of a Beneficiary's Home

B3-2100.3, A3-3113.6, HO-235.6, HHA-220.3

For purposes of rental and purchase of DME a beneficiary's home may be his/her own dwelling, an apartment, a relative's home, a home for the aged, or some other type of institution. However, an institution may not be considered a beneficiary's home if it:

- Meets at least the basic requirement in the definition of a hospital, i.e., it is primarily engaged in providing by or under the supervision of physicians, to inpatients, diagnostic and therapeutic services for medical diagnosis, treatment, and care of injured, disabled, and sick persons, or rehabilitation services for the rehabilitation of injured, disabled, or sick persons; or
- Meets at least the basic requirement in the definition of a skilled nursing facility, i.e., it is primarily engaged in providing to inpatients skilled nursing care and related services for patients who require medical or nursing care, or rehabilitation services for the rehabilitation of injured, disabled, or sick persons.

Thus, if an individual is a patient in an institution or distinct part of an institution which provides the services described in the bullets above, the individual is not entitled to have separate Part B payment made for rental or purchase of DME. This is because such an institution may not be considered the individual's home. The same concept applies even if the patient resides in a bed or portion of the institution not certified for Medicare.

If the patient is at home for part of a month and, for part of the same month is in an institution that cannot qualify as his or her home, or is outside the U.S., monthly payments may be made for the entire month. Similarly, if DME is returned to the provider before the end of a payment month because the beneficiary died in that month or because the equipment became unnecessary in that month, payment may be made for the entire month.

110.2—Repairs, Maintenance, Replacement, and Delivery

(Rev. 1, 10-01-03)

B3-2100.4, A3-3113.3, HO-235.3, HHA-220.4

Under the circumstances specified below, payment may be made for repair, maintenance, and replacement of medically required DME which the beneficiary owns or is purchasing, including equipment which had been in use before the user enrolled in Part B of the program.

A—Repairs

B3-2100.4, A3-3113.3A, HO-235.3A

Repairs to equipment, which a beneficiary is purchasing or already owns are covered when necessary to make the equipment serviceable. A service charge may include the use of "loaner" equipment where this is required. If the expense for repairs exceeds the estimated expense of purchasing or renting another item of equipment for the remaining period of medical need, no payment can be made for the amount of the excess. (See subsection C where claims for repairs suggest malicious damage or culpable neglect.)

B—Maintenance

B3-2100.4, A3-3113.3.B, HO-235.3.B

Routine periodic servicing, such as testing, cleaning, regulating, and checking of the beneficiary's equipment, is not covered. The owner is expected to perform such routine maintenance rather than a retailer or some other person who charges the beneficiary. Normally, purchasers of DME are given operating manuals which describe the type of servicing an owner may perform to properly maintain the equipment. Thus, hiring a third party to do such work is for the convenience of the beneficiary and is not covered.

However, more extensive maintenance which, based on the manufacturers' recommendations, is to be performed by authorized technicians, is covered as repairs. This might include, for example, breaking down sealed components and performing tests which require specialized testing equipment not available to the beneficiary.

For capped rental items which have reached the 15-month rental cap, contractors pay claims for maintenance and servicing fees after 6 months have passed from the end of the final paid rental month or from the end of the period the item is no longer covered under the supplier's or manufacturer's warranty, whichever is later. See the Medicare Claims Processing Manual, Chapter 20, "Durable Medical Equipment, Prosthetics and Orthotics, and Supplies (DMEPOS)," for additional instruction and an example.

C—Replacement

B3-2100.4, A3-3113.3.C, HO-235.3.C

Replacement of equipment is covered in cases which the beneficiary owns or is purchasing is covered in cases of loss or irreparable damage or wear and when required because of a change in the patient's condition. Expenses for replacement required because of loss or irreparable damage may be reimbursed without a physician's order when in the judgment of the DMERC the equipment as originally ordered, considering the age of the order, still fills the patient's medical needs. However, claims involving replacement equipment necessitated because of wear or a change in the patient's condition must be supported by a current physician's order.

If a capped rental item of equipment has been in continuous use by the patient, on either a rental or purchase basis, for the equipment's useful lifetime or if the item is lost or irreparably damaged, the patient may elect to obtain a new piece of equipment. The contractor determines the reasonable useful lifetime for capped rental equipment but in no case can it be less than five years. Computation of the useful lifetime is based on when the equipment is delivered to the beneficiary, not the age of the equipment.

Payment may not be made for items covered under a manufacturer's or supplier's warranty. (See the Medicare Claims Processing Manual, Chapter 20, "Durable Medical Equipment, Prosthetics and Orthotics, and Supplies (DMEPOS)," and the Medicare Benefit Policy Manual, Chapter 16, "General Exclusions from Coverage," in regard to payment for equipment replaced under a warranty.) Cases suggesting malicious damage, culpable neglect, or wrongful disposition of equipment should be investigated and denied where the DMERC determines that it is unreasonable to make program payment under the circumstances. DMERCs refer such cases to the program integrity specialist in the RO.

D—Delivery

B3-2100.4, A3-3113.3.D, HO-235.3.D

Delivery and service charges are covered, but the related payment is included in the fee schedule for the related item. Separate payment is not made.

However, where special circumstances apply, e.g., beneficiary lives in remote area, or equipment could not be obtained from a local dealer special consideration can be applied at the discretion of the DMERC/intermediary.

110.3—Coverage of Supplies and Accessories

(Rev. 1, 10-01-03)

B3-2100.5, A3-3113.4, HO-235.4, HHA-220.5

Payment may be made for supplies, e.g., oxygen, that are necessary for the effective use of durable medical equipment. Such supplies include those drugs and biologicals which must be put directly into the equipment in order to achieve the therapeutic benefit of the durable medical equipment or to assure the proper functioning of the equipment, e.g., tumor chemotherapy agents used with an infusion pump or heparin used with a home dialysis system. However, the coverage of such drugs or biologicals does not preclude the need for a determination that the drug or biological itself is reasonable and necessary for treatment of the illness or injury or to improve the functioning of a malformed body member.

In the case of prescription drugs, other than oxygen, used in conjunction with durable medical equipment, prosthetic, orthotics, and supplies (DMEPOS) or prosthetic devices, the entity that dispenses the drug must furnish it directly to the patient for whom a prescription is written. The entity that dispenses the drugs must have a Medicare supplier number, must possess a current license to dispense prescription drugs in the State in which the drug is dispensed, and must bill and receive payment in its own name. A supplier that is not the entity that dispenses the drugs cannot purchase the drugs used in conjunction with DME for resale to the beneficiary. Reimbursement may be made for replacement of essential accessories such as hoses, tubes, mouthpieces, etc., for necessary DME, only if the beneficiary owns or is purchasing the equipment.

110.4—Miscellaneous Issues Included in the Coverage of Equipment

(Rev. 1, 10-01-03)

B3-2100.6, A3-3113.5, HO-235.5, HHA-220.6

Payment can be made for the purchase of DME even though rental payments may have been made for prior months. This could occur where, because of a change in his/her condition, the beneficiary feels that it would be to his/her advantage to purchase the equipment rather than to continue to rent it.

A beneficiary may sell or otherwise dispose of equipment for which they have no further use, for example, because of recovery from the illness or injury that gave rise to the need for the equipment. (There is no authority for the program to repossess the equipment.) If after such disposal there is again medical need for similar equipment, payment can be made for the rental or purchase of that equipment.

However, where an arrangement is motivated solely by a desire to create artificial expenses to be met by the program and to realize a profit thereby, such expenses would not be covered under the program. The resolution of questions involving the disposition and subsequent acquisition of durable medical equipment must be made on a case-by-case basis.

Cases where it appears that there has been an attempt to create an artificial expense and realize a profit thereby should be developed and when appropriate denied. After adjudication the DMERC would refer such cases to the program integrity specialist in the RO.

When payments stop because the beneficiary's condition has changed and the equipment is no longer medically necessary, the beneficiary is responsible for the remaining noncovered charges. Similarly, when payments stop because the beneficiary dies, the beneficiary's estate is responsible for the remaining noncovered charges.

Contractors do not get involved in issues relating to ownership or title of property.

110.5—Incurred Expense Dates for Durable Medical Equipment

(Rev. 1, 10-01-03)

A3-3113.7.B, HO-235.7.B, B3-3011

The date of service on the claim must be the date that the beneficiary or authorized representative received the DMEPOS item. If the date of delivery is not specified on the bill, the contractor should assume, in the absence of evidence to the contrary, that the date of purchase was the date of delivery.

For mail order DMEPOS items, the date of service on the claim must be the shipping date.

The date of service on the claim must be the date that the DMEPOS item(s) was received by the nursing facility if the supplier delivered it or the shipping date if the supplier utilized a delivery/shipping service.

An exception to the preceding statements concerning the date of service on the claim occurs when items are provided in anticipation of discharge from a hospital or nursing facility. If a DMEPOS item is delivered to a patient in a hospital up to two days prior to discharge to home and it is for the benefit of the patient for purposes of fitting or training of the patient on its use, the supplier should bill the date of service on the claim as the date of discharge to home and should use POS=12.

See the Medicare Program Integrity Manual, Chapter 5, "Items and Services Having Special DMERC Review Considerations," for additional information pertaining to the date of service on the claim. Also see the Medicare Claims Processing Manual, Chapter 20, "Durable Medical Equipment, Surgical dressings and Casts, Orthotics and Artificial Limbs, and Prosthetic Devices," for additional DME billing and claims processing information.

110.6—Determining Months for Which Periodic Payments May Be Made for Equipment Used in an Institution

(Rev. 1, 10-01-03)

A3-3113.7.D, HO-235.7.C

If a patient uses equipment subject to the monthly payment rule in an institution, which does not qualify as his or her home, the used months during which the beneficiary was institutionalized are not covered.

110.7—No Payment for Purchased Equipment Delivered Outside the United States or Before Beneficiary's Coverage Began

(Rev. 1, 10-01-03)

A3-3113.7.C

In the case of equipment subject to the lump sum payment rules, the beneficiary must have been in the United States and must have had Medicare coverage at the time the item was delivered. Therefore, where an item of durable medical equipment paid for as a lump sum was delivered to an individual outside the United States or before his or her coverage period began, the entire expense of the item would be excluded from coverage. Payment cannot be made in such cases even though the individual later uses the item inside the United States or after his or her coverage begins.

If the individual is outside the U.S. for more than 30 days and then returns to the U.S., the DMERC determines medical necessity as in an initial case before resuming payments.

120—PROSTHETIC DEVICES

(Rev. 1, 10-01-03)

B3-2130, A3-3110.4, HO-228.4, A3-3111, HO-229

A—General

Prosthetic devices (other than dental) which replace all or part of an internal body organ (including contiguous tissue), or replace all or part of the function of a permanently inoperative or malfunctioning internal body organ are covered when furnished on a physician's order. This does not require a determination that there is no possibility that the patient's condition may improve sometime in the future. If the medical record, including the judgment of the attending physician, indicates the condition is of long and indefinite duration, the test of permanence is considered met. (Such a device may also be covered under §60.1 as a supply when furnished incident to a physician's service.)

Examples of prosthetic devices include artificial limbs, parenteral and enteral (PEN) nutrition, cardiac pacemakers, prosthetic lenses (see subsection B), breast prostheses (including a surgical brassiere) for postmastectomy patients, maxillofacial devices, and devices which replace all or part of the ear or nose. A urinary collection and retention system with or without a tube is a prosthetic device replacing bladder function in case of permanent urinary incontinence. The Foley catheter is also considered a prosthetic device when ordered for a patient with permanent urinary incontinence. However, chucks, diapers, rubber sheets, etc., are supplies that are not covered under this provision. Although hemodialysis equipment is a prosthetic device, payment for the rental or purchase of such equipment in the home is made only for use under the provisions for payment applicable to durable medical equipment.

An exception is that if payment cannot be made on an inpatient's behalf under Part A, hemodialysis equipment, supplies, and services required by such patient could be covered under Part B as a prosthetic device, which replaces the function of a kidney. See the Medicare Benefit Policy Manual, Chapter 11, "End Stage Renal Disease," for payment for hemodialysis equipment used in the home. See the Medicare Benefit Policy Manual, Chapter 1, "Inpatient Hospital Services," §10, for additional instructions on hospitalization for renal dialysis.

NOTE: Medicare does not cover a prosthetic device dispensed to a patient prior to the time at which the patient undergoes the procedure that makes necessary the use of the device. For example, the carrier does not make a separate Part B payment for an intraocular lens (IOL) or pacemaker that a physician, during an office visit prior to the actual surgery, dispenses to the patient for his or her use. Dispensing a prosthetic device in this manner raises health and safety issues. Moreover, the need for the device cannot be clearly established until the procedure that makes its use possible is successfully performed. Therefore, dispensing a prosthetic device in this manner is not considered reasonable and necessary for the treatment of the patient's condition.

Colostomy (and other ostomy) bags and necessary accouterments required for attachment are covered as prosthetic devices. This coverage also includes irrigation and flushing equipment and other items and supplies directly related to ostomy care, whether the attachment of a bag is required.

Accessories and/or supplies which are used directly with an enteral or parenteral device to achieve the therapeutic benefit of the prosthesis or to assure the proper functioning of the device may also be covered under the prosthetic device benefit subject to the additional guidelines in the Medicare National Coverage Determinations Manual.

Covered items include catheters, filters, extension tubing, infusion bottles, pumps (either food or infusion), intravenous (I.V.) pole, needles, syringes, dressings, tape, Heparin Sodium (parenteral only), volumetric monitors (parenteral only), and parenteral and enteral nutrient solutions. Baby food and other regular grocery products that can be blenderized and used with the enteral system are not covered. Note that some of these items, e.g., a food pump and an I.V. pole, qualify as DME. Although coverage of the enteral and parenteral nutritional therapy systems is provided on the basis of the prosthetic device benefit, the payment rules relating to lump sum or monthly payment for DME apply to such items.

The coverage of prosthetic devices includes replacement of and repairs to such devices as explained in subsection D.

Finally, the Benefits Improvement and Protection Act of 2000 amended §1834(h)(1) of the Act by adding a provision (1834 (h)(1)(G)(i)) that requires Medicare payment to be made for the replacement of prosthetic devices which are artificial limbs, or for the replacement of any part of such devices, without regard to continuous use or useful lifetime restrictions if an ordering physician determines that the replacement device, or replacement part of such a device, is necessary.

Payment may be made for the replacement of a prosthetic device that is an artificial limb, or replacement part of a device if the ordering physician determines that the replacement device or part is necessary because of any of the following:

1. A change in the physiological condition of the patient;

2. An irreparable change in the condition of the device, or in a part of the device; or

3. The condition of the device, or the part of the device, requires repairs and the cost of such repairs would be more than 60 percent of the cost of a replacement device, or, as the case may be, of the part being replaced.

This provision is effective for items replaced on or after April 1, 2001. It supersedes any rule that that provided a 5-year or other replacement rule with regard to prosthetic devices.

B—Prosthetic Lenses

The term "internal body organ" includes the lens of an eye. Prostheses replacing the lens of an eye include post-surgical lenses customarily used during convalescence from eye surgery in which the lens of the eye was removed. In addition, permanent lenses are also covered when required by an individual lacking the organic lens of the eye because of surgical removal or congenital absence. Prosthetic lenses obtained on or after the beneficiary's date of entitlement to supplementary medical insurance benefits may be covered even though the surgical removal of the crystalline lens occurred before entitlement.

1. **Prosthetic Cataract Lenses**—One of the following prosthetic lenses or combinations of prosthetic lenses furnished by a physician (see §30.4 for coverage of prosthetic lenses prescribed by a doctor of optometry) may be covered when determined to be reasonable and necessary to restore essentially the vision provided by the crystalline lens of the eye:
   • Prosthetic bifocal lenses in frames;
   • Prosthetic lenses in frames for far vision, and prosthetic lenses in frames for near vision; or
   • When a prosthetic contact lens(es) for far vision is prescribed (including cases of binocular and monocular aphakia), make payment for the contact lens(es) and prosthetic lenses in frames for near vision to be worn at the same time as the contact lens(es), and prosthetic lenses in frames to be worn when the contacts have been removed.

Lenses which have ultraviolet absorbing or reflecting properties may be covered, in lieu of payment for regular (untinted) lenses, if it has been determined that such lenses are medically reasonable and necessary for the individual patient.

Medicare does not cover cataract sunglasses obtained in addition to the regular (untinted) prosthetic lenses since the sunglasses duplicate the restoration of vision function performed by the regular prosthetic lenses.

2. **Payment for Intraocular Lenses (IOLs) Furnished in Ambulatory Surgical Centers (ASCs)**—Effective for services furnished on or after March 12, 1990, payment for intraocular lenses (IOLs) inserted during or subsequent to cataract surgery in a Medicare

certified ASC is included with the payment for facility services that are furnished in connection with the covered surgery.

Refer to the Medicare Claims Processing Manual, Chapter 14, "Ambulatory Surgical Centers," for more information.

3. **Limitation on Coverage of Conventional Lenses**—One pair of conventional eyeglasses or conventional contact lenses furnished after each cataract surgery with insertion of an IOL is covered.

C—Dentures

Dentures are excluded from coverage. However, when a denture or a portion of the denture is an integral part (built-in) of a covered prosthesis (e.g., an obturator to fill an opening in the palate), it is covered as part of that prosthesis.

D—Supplies, Repairs, Adjustments, and Replacement

Supplies are covered that are necessary for the effective use of a prosthetic device (e.g., the batteries needed to operate an artificial larynx). Adjustment of prosthetic devices required by wear or by a change in the patient's condition is covered when ordered by a physician. General provisions relating to the repair and replacement of durable medical equipment in §110.2 for the repair and replacement of prosthetic devices are applicable. (See the Medicare Benefit Policy Manual, Chapter 16, "General Exclusions from Coverage," §40.4, for payment for devices replaced under a warranty.) Replacement of conventional eyeglasses or contact lenses furnished in accordance with §120.B.3 is not covered.

Necessary supplies, adjustments, repairs, and replacements are covered even when the device had been in use before the user enrolled in Part B of the program, so long as the device continues to be medically required.

160—CLINICAL PSYCHOLOGIST SERVICES

(Rev. 1, 10-01-03)

B3-2150

A—Clinical Psychologist (CP) Defined

To qualify as a clinical psychologist (CP), a practitioner must meet the following requirements:

• Hold a doctoral degree in psychology;
• Be licensed or certified, on the basis of the doctoral degree in psychology, by the State in which he or she practices, at the independent practice level of psychology to furnish diagnostic, assessment, preventive, and therapeutic services directly to individuals.

B—Qualified Clinical Psychologist Services Defined

Effective July 1, 1990, the diagnostic and therapeutic services of CPs and services and supplies furnished incident to such services are covered as the services furnished by a physician or as incident to physician's services are covered. However, the CP must be legally authorized to perform the services under applicable licensure laws of the State in which they are furnished.

C—Types of Clinical Psychologist Services That May Be Covered

The CPs may provide the following services:

• Diagnostic and therapeutic services that the CP is legally authorized to perform in accordance with State law and/or regulation. Carriers pay all qualified CPs based on the physician fee schedule for the diagnostic and therapeutic services. (Psychological tests by practitioners who do not meet the requirements for a CP may be covered under the provisions for diagnostic tests as described in §80.2.
• Services and supplies furnished incident to a CP's services are covered if the requirements that apply to services incident to a physician's services, as described in §60 are met. These services must be:
   • Mental health services that are commonly furnished in CPs' offices;
   • An integral, although incidental, part of professional services performed by the CP;

- Performed under the direct personal supervision of the CP; i.e., the CP must be physically present and immediately available; and
- Furnished without charge or included in the CP's bill.

Any person involved in performing the service must be an employee of the CP (or an employee of the legal entity that employs the supervising CP) under the common law control test of the Act, as set forth in 20 CFR 404.1007 and §RS 2101.020 of the Retirement and Survivors Insurance part of the Social Security Program Operations Manual System.

Carriers are required to familiarize themselves with appropriate State laws and/or regulations governing a CP's scope of practice.

D—Noncovered Services

The services of CPs are not covered if the service is otherwise excluded from Medicare coverage even though a clinical psychologist is authorized by State law to perform them. For example, §1862(a)(1)(A) of the Act excludes from coverage services that are not "reasonable and necessary for the diagnosis or treatment of an illness or injury or to improve the functioning of a malformed body member." Therefore, even though the services are authorized by State law, the services of a CP that are determined to be not reasonable and necessary are not covered. Additionally, any therapeutic services that are billed by CPs under CPT psychotherapy codes that include medical evaluation and management services are not covered.

E—Requirement for Consultation

When applying for a Medicare provider number, a CP must submit to the carrier a signed Medicare provider/supplier enrollment form that indicates an agreement to the effect that, contingent upon the patient's consent, the CP will attempt to consult with the patient's attending or primary care physician in accordance with accepted professional ethical norms, taking into consideration patient confidentiality.

If the patient assents to the consultation, the CP must attempt to consult with the patient's physician within a reasonable time after receiving the consent. If the CP's attempts to consult directly with the physician are not successful, the CP must notify the physician within a reasonable time that he or she is furnishing services to the patient. Additionally, the CP must document, in the patient's medical record, the date the patient consented or declined consent to consultations, the date of consultation, or, if attempts to consult did not succeed, that date and manner of notification to the physician.

The only exception to the consultation requirement for CPs is in cases where the patient's primary care or attending physician refers the patient to the CP. Also, neither a CP nor a primary care nor attending physician may bill Medicare or the patient for this required consultation.

F—Outpatient Mental Health Services Limitation

All covered therapeutic services furnished by qualified CPs are subject to the outpatient mental health services limitation in Pub 100-1, Medicare General Information, Eligibility, and Entitlement Manual, Chapter 3, "Deductibles, Coinsurance Amounts, and Payment Limitations," §30, (i.e., only 62 1/2 percent of expenses for these services are considered incurred expenses for Medicare purposes). The limitation does not apply to diagnostic services.

G—Assignment Requirement

Assignment is required.

170—CLINICAL SOCIAL WORKER (CSW) SERVICES

(Rev. 1, 10-01-03)

B3-2152

See the Medicare Claims Processing Manual Chapter 12, Physician/Nonphysician Practitioners, §150, "Clinical Social Worker Services," for payment requirements.

A—Clinical Social Worker Defined

Section 1861(hh) of the Act defines a "clinical social worker" as an individual who:

- Possesses a master's or doctor's degree in social work;
- Has performed at least two years of supervised clinical social work; and
- Is licensed or certified as a clinical social worker by the State in which the services are performed; or
- In the case of an individual in a State that does not provide for licensure or certification, has completed at least 2 years or 3,000 hours of post master's degree supervised clinical social work practice under the supervision of a master's level social worker in an appropriate setting such as a hospital, SNF, or clinic.

B—Clinical Social Worker Services Defined

Section 1861(hh)(2) of the Act defines "clinical social worker services" as those services that the CSW is legally authorized to perform under State law (or the State regulatory mechanism provided by State law) of the State in which such services are performed for the diagnosis and treatment of mental illnesses. Services furnished to an inpatient of a hospital or an inpatient of a SNF that the SNF is required to provide as a requirement for participation are not included. The services that are covered are those that are otherwise covered if furnished by a physician or as incident to a physician's professional service.

C—Covered Services

Coverage is limited to the services a CSW is legally authorized to perform in accordance with State law (or State regulatory mechanism established by State law). The services of a CSW may be covered under Part B if they are:

- The type of services that are otherwise covered if furnished by a physician, or as incident to a physician's service. (See §30 for a description of physicians' services and §70 of Pub 100-1, the Medicare General Information, Eligibility, and Entitlement Manual, Chapter 5, for the definition of a physician.);
- Performed by a person who meets the definition of a CSW (See subsection A.); and
- Not otherwise excluded from coverage.

Carriers should become familiar with the State law or regulatory mechanism governing a CSW's scope of practice in their service area.

D—Noncovered Services

Services of a CSW are not covered when furnished to inpatients of a hospital or to inpatients of a SNF if the services furnished in the SNF are those that the SNF is required to furnish as a condition of participation in Medicare. In addition, CSW services are not covered if they are otherwise excluded from Medicare coverage even though a CSW is authorized by State law to perform them. For example, the Medicare law excludes from coverage services that are not "reasonable and necessary for the diagnosis or treatment of an illness or injury or to improve the functioning of a malformed body member."

E—Outpatient Mental Health Services Limitation

All covered therapeutic services furnished by qualified CSWs are subject to the outpatient psychiatric services limitation in Pub 100-1, Medicare General Information, Eligibility, and Entitlement Manual, Chapter 3, "Deductibles, Coinsurance Amounts, and Payment Limitations," §30, (i.e., only 62 1/2 percent of expenses for these services are considered incurred expenses for Medicare purposes). The limitation does not apply to diagnostic services.

F—Assignment Requirement

Assignment is required.

230—PRACTICE OF PHYSICAL THERAPY, OCCUPATIONAL THERAPY, AND SPEECH-LANGUAGE PATHOLOGY

(Rev. 36, Issued: 06-24-05, Effective: 06-06-05, Implementation: 06-06-05)

230.1—Practice of Physical Therapy

(Rev. 36, Issued: 06-24-05, Effective: 06-06-05, Implementation: 06-06-05)

A—General

Physical therapy services are those services provided within the scope of practice of physical therapists and necessary for the diagnosis and treatment of impairments, functional limitations, disabilities or changes in physical function and health status. (See Pub. 100-03, the Medicare National Coverage Determinations Manual, for specific conditions or services.)

B—Qualified Physical Therapist Defined

Reference: 42CFR484.4

A qualified physical therapist for program coverage purposes is a person who is licensed as a physical therapist by the state in which he or she is practicing and meets one of the following requirements:

- Has graduated from a physical therapy curriculum approved by (1) the American Physical Therapy Association, or by (2) the Committee on Allied Health Education and Accreditation of the American Medical Association, or (3) Council on Medical Education of the American Medical Association, and the American Physical Therapy Association; or
- Prior to January 1, 1966, (1) was admitted to membership by the American Physical Therapy Association, or (2) was admitted to registration by the American Registry of Physical Therapists, or (3) has graduated from a physical therapy curriculum in a 4-year college or university approved by a state department of education; or
- Has 2 years of appropriate experience as a physical therapist and has achieved a satisfactory grade on a proficiency examination conducted, approved or sponsored by the Public Health Service, except that such determinations of proficiency do not apply with respect to persons initially licensed by a state or seeking qualification as a physical therapist after December 31, 1977; or
- Was licensed or registered prior to January 1, 1966, and prior to January 1, 1970, had 15 years of full-time experience in the treatment of illness or injury through the practice of physical therapy in which services were rendered under the order and direction of attending and referring doctors of medicine or osteopathy; or
- If trained outside the United States, (1) was graduated since 1928 from a physical therapy curriculum approved in the country in which the curriculum was located and in which there is a member organization of the World Confederation for Physical Therapy, (2) meets the requirements for membership in a member organization of the World Confederation for Physical Therapy.

C—Services of Physical Therapy Support Personnel

Reference: 42CFR 484.4

A physical therapist assistant (PTA) is a person who is licensed as a physical therapist assistant, if applicable, by the State in which practicing, and

- Has graduated from a 2-year college-level program approved by the American Physical Therapy Association; or
- Has 2 years of appropriate experience as a physical therapist assistant, and has achieved a satisfactory grade on a proficiency examination conducted, approved, or sponsored by the U.S. Public Health Service, except that these determinations of proficiency do not apply with respect to persons initially licensed by a State or seeking initial qualification as a PTA after December 31, 1977.

The services of PTAs used when providing covered therapy benefits are included as part of the covered service. These services are billed by the supervising physical therapist. PTAs may not provide evaluation services, make clinical judgments or decisions or take responsibility for the service. They act at the direction and under the supervision of the treating physical therapist and in accordance with state laws.

A physical therapist must supervise PTAs. The level and frequency of supervision differs by setting (and by state or local law). General supervision is required for PTAs in all settings except private practice (which requires direct supervision) unless state practice requirements are more stringent, in which case state or local requirements must be followed. See specific settings for details. For example, in clinics, rehabilitation agencies, and public

health agencies, 42CFR485.713 indicates that when a PTA provides services, either on or off the organization's premises, those services are supervised by a qualified physical therapist who makes an onsite supervisory visit at least once every 30 days or more frequently if required by state or local laws or regulation.

The services of a PTA shall not be billed as services incident to a physician/NPP's service, because they do not meet the qualifications of a therapist.

The cost of supplies (e.g., theraband, hand putty, electrodes) used in furnishing covered therapy care is included in the payment for the HCPCS codes billed by the physical therapist, and are, therefore, not separately billable. Separate coverage and billing provisions apply to items that meet the definition of brace in §130.

Services provided by aides, even if under the supervision of a therapist, are not therapy services in the outpatient setting and are not covered by Medicare. Although an aide may help the therapist by providing unskilled services, those services that are unskilled are not covered by Medicare and shall be denied as not reasonable and necessary if they are billed as therapy services.

D—Application of Medicare Guidelines to PT Services

This subsection will be used in the future to illustrate the application of the above guidelines to some of the physical therapy modalities and procedures utilized in the treatment of patients.

230.2—Practice of Occupational Therapy

(Rev. 36, Issued: 06-24-05, Effective: 06-06-05, Implementation: 06-06-05)

A—General

Occupational therapy services are those services provided within the scope of practice of occupational therapists and necessary for the diagnosis and treatment of impairments, functional disabilities or changes in physical function and health status. (See Pub. 100-03, the Medicare National Coverage Determinations Manual, for specific conditions or services.)

Occupational therapy is medically prescribed treatment concerned with improving or restoring functions which have been impaired by illness or injury or, where function has been permanently lost or reduced by illness or injury, to improve the individual's ability to perform those tasks required for independent functioning. Such therapy may involve:

The evaluation, and reevaluation as required, of a patient's level of function by administering diagnostic and prognostic tests;

The selection and teaching of task-oriented therapeutic activities designed to restore physical function; e.g., use of woodworking activities on an inclined table to restore shoulder, elbow, and wrist range of motion lost as a result of burns;

The planning, implementing, and supervising of individualized therapeutic activity programs as part of an overall "active treatment" program for a patient with a diagnosed psychiatric illness; e.g., the use of sewing activities which require following a pattern to reduce confusion and restore reality orientation in a schizophrenic patient;

The planning and implementing of therapeutic tasks and activities to restore sensory-integrative function; e.g., providing motor and tactile activities to increase sensory input and improve response for a stroke patient with functional loss resulting in a distorted body image;

The teaching of compensatory technique to improve the level of independence in the activities of daily living, for example:

- Teaching a patient who has lost the use of an arm how to pare potatoes and chop vegetables with one hand;
- Teaching an upper extremity amputee how to functionally utilize a prosthesis;
- Teaching a stroke patient new techniques to enable the patient to perform feeding, dressing, and other activities as independently as possible; or
- Teaching a patient with a hip fracture/hip replacement techniques of standing tolerance and balance to enable the patient to perform such functional activities as dressing and homemaking tasks.

The designing, fabricating, and fitting of orthotics and self-help devices; e.g., making a hand splint for a patient with rheumatoid arthritis to maintain the hand in a functional position or constructing a device which would enable an individual to hold a utensil and feed independently; or

Vocational and prevocational assessment and training, subject to the limitations specified in item B below.

Only a qualified occupational therapist has the knowledge, training, and experience required to evaluate and, as necessary, reevaluate a patient's level of function, determine whether an occupational therapy program could reasonably be expected to improve, restore, or compensate for lost function and, where appropriate, recommend to the physician/NPP a plan of treatment.

B—Qualified Occupational Therapist Defined

Reference: 42CFR484.4

A qualified occupational therapist for program coverage purposes is an individual who meets one of the following requirements:

- Is a graduate of an occupational therapy curriculum accredited jointly by the Committee on Allied Health Education of the American Medical Association and the American Occupational Therapy Association;
- Is eligible for the National Registration Examination of the American Occupational Therapy Association; or
- Has 2 years of appropriate experience as an occupational therapist, and has achieved a satisfactory grade on a proficiency examination conducted, approved, or sponsored by the U.S. Public Health Service, except that such determinations of proficiency do not apply with respect to persons initially licensed by a State or seeking initial qualification as an occupational therapist after December 31, 1977.

C—Services of Occupational Therapy Support Personnel

Reference: 42CFR 484.4

An occupational therapy assistant (OTA) is a person who:

- Meets the requirements for certification as an occupational therapy assistant established by the American Occupational Therapy Association; or
- Has 2 years of appropriate experience as an occupational therapy assistant and has achieved a satisfactory grade on a proficiency examination conducted, approved, or sponsored by the U.S. Public Health Service, except that such determinations of proficiency do not apply with respect to persons initially licensed by a State or seeking initial qualification as an occupational therapy assistant after December 31, 1977.

The services of OTAs used when providing covered therapy benefits are included as part of the covered service. These services are billed by the supervising occupational therapist. OTAs may not provide evaluation services, make clinical judgments or decisions or take responsibility for the service. They act at the direction and under the supervision of the treating occupational therapist and in accordance with state laws.

An occupational therapist must supervise OTAs. The level and frequency of supervision differs by setting (and by state or local law). General supervision is required for OTAs in all settings except private practice (which requires direct supervision) unless state practice requirements are more stringent, in which case state or local requirements must be followed. See specific settings for details. For example, in clinics, rehabilitation agencies, and public health agencies, 42CFR485.713 indicates that when an OTA provides services, either on or off the organization's premises, those services are supervised by a qualified occupational therapist who makes an onsite supervisory visit at least once every 30 days or more frequently if required by state or local laws or regulation.

The services of an OTA shall not be billed as services incident to a physician/NPP's service, because they do not meet the qualifications of a therapist.

The cost of supplies (e.g., looms, ceramic tiles, or leather) used in furnishing covered therapy care is included in the payment for the HCPCS codes billed by the occupational therapist and are, therefore, not separately billable. Separate coverage and billing provisions apply to items that meet the definition of brace in §130 of this manual.

Services provided by aides, even if under the supervision of a therapist, are not therapy services in the outpatient setting and are not covered by Medicare. Although an aide may help the therapist by providing unskilled services, those services that are unskilled are not covered by Medicare and shall be denied as not reasonable and necessary if they are billed as therapy services.

D—Application of Medicare Guidelines to Occupational Therapy Services

Occupational therapy may be required for a patient with a specific diagnosed psychiatric illness. If such services are required, they are covered assuming the coverage criteria are met. However, where an individual's motivational needs are not related to a specific diagnosed psychiatric illness, the meeting of such needs does not usually require an individualized therapeutic program. Such needs can be met through general activity programs or the efforts of other professional personnel involved in the care of the patient. Patient motivation is an appropriate and inherent function of all health disciplines, which is interwoven with other functions performed by such personnel for the patient. Accordingly, since the special skills of an occupational therapist are not required, an occupational therapy program for individuals who do not have a specific diagnosed psychiatric illness is not to be considered reasonable and necessary for the treatment of an illness or injury. Services furnished under such a program are not covered.

Occupational therapy may include vocational and prevocational assessment and training. When services provided by an occupational therapist are related solely to specific employment opportunities, work skills, or work settings, they are not reasonable or necessary for the diagnosis or treatment of an illness or injury and are not covered. However, carriers and intermediaries exercise care in applying this exclusion, because the assessment of level of function and the teaching of compensatory techniques to improve the level of function, especially in activities of daily living, are services which occupational therapists provide for both vocational and nonvocational purposes. For example, an assessment of sitting and standing tolerance might be nonvocational for a mother of young children or a retired individual living alone, but could also be a vocational test for a sales clerk. Training an amputee in the use of prosthesis for telephoning is necessary for everyday activities as well as for employment purposes. Major changes in life style may be mandatory for an individual with a substantial disability. The techniques of adjustment cannot be considered exclusively vocational or nonvocational.

230.3—Practice of Speech-Language Pathology

(Rev. 36, Issued: 06-24-05, Effective: 06-06-05, Implementation: 06-06-05)

A—General

Speech-language pathology services are those services provided within the scope of practice of speech-language pathologists and necessary for the diagnosis and treatment of speech and language disorders, which result in communication disabilities and for the diagnosis and treatment of swallowing disorders (dysphagia), regardless of the presence of a communication disability. (See Pub. 100-03, chapter 1, §170.3)

B—Qualified Speech-Language Pathologist Defined

A qualified speech-language pathologist for program coverage purposes meets one of the following requirements:

- The education and experience requirements for a Certificate of Clinical Competence in (speech-language pathology or audiology) granted by the American Speech-Language Hearing Association; or
- Meets the educational requirements for certification and is in the process of accumulating the supervised experience required for certification.

Speech-language pathologists may not enroll and submit claims directly to Medicare. The services of speech-language pathologists may be billed by providers such as rehabilitation agencies, HHAs, CORFs, hospices, outpatient departments of hospitals, and suppliers such as physicians, NPPs, physical and occupational therapists in private practice.

C—Services of Speech-Language Pathology Support Personnel

Services of speech-language pathology assistants are not recognized for Medicare coverage. Services provided by speech-language pathology assistants, even if they are licensed to provide services in their states, will be considered unskilled services and denied as not reasonable and necessary if they are billed as therapy services.

Services provided by aides, even if under the supervision of a therapist, are not therapy services and are not covered by Medicare. Although an aide may help the therapist by providing unskilled services, those services are not covered by Medicare and shall be denied as not reasonable and necessary if they are billed as therapy services.

D—Application of Medicare Guidelines to Speech-Language Pathology Services

1—Evaluation Services

Speech-language pathology evaluation services are covered if they are reasonable and necessary and not excluded as routine screening by §1862(a)(7) of the Act. The speech-language pathologist employs a variety of formal and informal speech, language, and dysphagia assessment tests to ascertain the type, causal factor(s), and severity of the speech and language or swallowing disorders. Reevaluation of patients for whom speech, language and swallowing were previously contraindicated is covered only if the patient exhibits a change in medical condition. However, monthly reevaluations; e.g., a Western Aphasia Battery, for a patient undergoing a rehabilitative speech-language pathology program, are considered a part of the treatment session and shall not be covered as a separate evaluation for billing purposes. Although hearing screening by the speech-language pathologist may be part of an evaluation, it is not billable as a separate service.

2—Therapeutic Services

The following are examples of common medical disorders and resulting communication deficits, which may necessitate active rehabilitative therapy. This list is not all-inclusive:

- Cerebrovascular disease such as cerebral vascular accidents presenting with dysphagia, aphasia/dysphasia, apraxia, and dysarthria;
- Neurological disease such as Parkinsonism or Multiple Sclerosis with dysarthria, dysphagia, inadequate respiratory volume/control, or voice disorder; or
- Laryngeal carcinoma requiring laryngectomy resulting in aphonia.

3—Aural Rehabilitation

Aural rehabilitation may be covered and medically necessary when it has been determined by a speech-language pathologist in collaboration with an audiologist that the beneficiary's current amplification options (hearing aid, other amplification device or cochlear implant) will not sufficiently meet the patient's functional communication needs.

Assessment for the need for aural rehabilitation may be done by a speech language pathologist and includes evaluation of comprehension and production of language in oral, signed or written modalities, speech and voice production, listening skills, speech reading, communications strategies, and the impact of the hearing loss on the patient/client and family.

Aural rehabilitation consists of treatment that focuses on comprehension, and production of language in oral, signed or written modalities; speech and voice production, auditory training, speech reading, multimodal (e.g., visual, auditory-visual, and tactile) training, communication strategies, education and counseling. In determining the necessity for treatment, the beneficiary's performance in both clinical and natural environment should be considered.

4—Dysphagia

Dysphagia, or difficulty in swallowing, can cause food to enter the airway, resulting in coughing, choking, pulmonary problems, aspiration or inadequate nutrition and hydration with resultant weight loss, failure to thrive, pneumonia and death. It is most often due to complex neurological and/or structural impairments including head and neck trauma, cerebrovascular accident, neuromuscular degenerative diseases, head and neck cancer, dementias, and encephalopathies. For these reasons, it is important that only qualified professionals with specific training and experience in this disorder provide evaluation and treatment.

The speech-language pathologist performs clinical and instrumental assessments and analyzes and integrates the diagnostic information to determine candidacy for intervention as well as appropriate compensations and rehabilitative therapy techniques. The equipment that is used in the examination may be fixed, mobile or portable. Professional guidelines recommend that the service be provided in a team setting with a physician/NPP who provides supervision of the radiological examination and interpretation of medical conditions revealed in it.

Swallowing assessment and rehabilitation are highly specialized services. The professional rendering care must have education, experience and demonstrated competencies. Competencies include but are not limited to: identifying abnormal upper aerodigestive tract structure and function; conducting an oral, pharyngeal, laryngeal and respiratory function examination as it relates to the functional assessment of swallowing; recommending methods of oral intake and risk precautions; and developing a treatment plan employing appropriate compensations and therapy techniques.

230.4—Services Furnished by a Physical or Occupational Therapist in Private Practice

(Rev. 36, Issued: 06-24-05, Effective: 06-06-05, Implementation: 06-06-05)

A—General

In order to qualify to bill Medicare directly as a therapist, each individual must be enrolled as a private practitioner and employed in one of the following practice types: an unincorporated solo practice, unincorporated partnership, unincorporated group practice, physician/NPP group or groups that are not professional corporations, if allowed by state and local law. Physician/NPP group practices may employ physical therapists in private practice (PTPP) and/or occupational therapists in private practice (OTPP) if state and local law permits this employee relationship.

For purposes of this provision, a physician/NPP group practice is defined as one or more physicians/NPPs enrolled with Medicare who may bill as one entity. For further details on issues concerning enrollment, see the provider enrollment Web site at www.cms.hhs.gov/providers/enrollment.

Private practice also includes therapists who are practicing therapy as employees of another supplier, of a professional corporation or other incorporated therapy practice. Private practice does not include individuals when they are working as employees of an institutional provider.

Services should be furnished in the therapist's or group's office or in the patient's home. The office is defined as the location(s) where the practice is operated, in the state(s) where the therapist (and practice, if applicable) is legally authorized to furnish services, during the hours that the therapist engages in the practice at that location. If services are furnished in a private practice office space, that space shall be owned, leased, or rented by the practice and used for the exclusive purpose of operating the practice. For example, a therapist in private practice may furnish aquatic therapy in a community center pool. As required in other settings (such as rehabilitation agencies and CORFs), the practice would have to rent or lease the pool for those hours, and the use of the pool during that time would have to be restricted to the therapist's patients, in order to recognize the pool as part of the therapist's own practice office during those hours. Therapists in private practice must be approved as meeting certain requirements, but do not execute a formal provider agreement with the Secretary.

If therapists who have their own Medicare Personal Identification number (PIN) or National Provider Identifier (NPI) are employed by therapist groups, physician/NPP groups, or groups that are not professional organizations, the requirement that therapy space be owned, leased, or rented may be satisfied by the group that employs the therapist. Each physical or occupational therapist employed by a group should enroll as a PT or OT in private practice.

When therapists with a Medicare PIN/NPI provide services in the physician's/NPP's office in which they are employed, and bill using their PIN/NPI for each therapy service, then the direct supervision requirement for PTAs and OTAs apply.

When the PT or OT who has a Medicare PIN/ NPI is employed in a physician's/NPP's office the services are ordinarily billed as services of the PT or OT, with the PT or OT identified on the claim as the supplier of services. However, services of the PT or OT who has a Medicare PIN/NPI may also be billed by the physician/NPP as services incident to the physician's/NPP's service. (See §230.5 for rules related to PTA and OTA services incident to a physician.) In that case, the physician/NPP is the supplier of service, the Unique Provider Identification Number (UPIN) or NPI of the physician/NPP (ordering or supervising, as indicated) is reported on the claim with the service and all the rules for incident to services (§230.5) must be followed.

B—Private Practice Defined

Reference: **Federal Register** November, 1998, pages 58863-58869; 42CFR 410.38(b)

The carrier considers a therapist to be in private practice if the therapist maintains office space at his or her own expense and furnishes services only in that space or the patient's home. Or, a therapist is employed by another supplier and furnishes services in facilities provided at the expense of that supplier.

The therapist need not be in full-time private practice but must be engaged in private practice on a regular basis; i.e., the therapist is recognized as a private practitioner and for that purpose has access to the necessary equipment to provide an adequate program of therapy.

The physical or occupational therapy services must be provided either by or under the direct supervision of the therapist in private practice. Each physical or occupational therapist in a practice should be enrolled as a Medicare provider. If a physical or occupational therapist is not enrolled, the services of that therapist must be directly supervised by an enrolled physical or occupational therapist. Direct supervision requires that the supervising private practice therapist be present in the office suite at the time the service is performed. These direct supervision requirements apply only in the private practice setting and only for physical therapists and occupational therapists and their assistants. In other outpatient settings, supervision rules differ. The services of support personnel must be included in the therapist's bill. The supporting personnel, including other therapists, must be W-2 or 1099 employees of the therapist in private practice or other qualified employer.

Coverage of outpatient physical therapy and occupational therapy under Part B includes the services of a qualified therapist in private practice when furnished in the therapist's office or the beneficiary's home. For this purpose, "home" includes an institution that is used as a home, but not a hospital, CAH or SNF, (**Federal Register** Nov. 2, 1998, pg 58869). Place of Service (POS) includes:

- 03/School, only if residential,
- 04/Homeless Shelter,
- 12/Home, other than a facility that is a private residence,
- 14/Group Home,
- 33/Custodial Care Facility.

C—Assignment

Reference: Nov. 2, 1998 **Federal Register**, pg. 58863
See also Pub. 100-04 chapter 1, 30.2.

When physicians, NPPs, PTPPs or OTPPs obtain provider numbers, they have the option of accepting assignment (participating) or not accepting assignment (nonparticipating). In contrast, providers, such as outpatient hospitals, SNFs, rehabilitation agencies, and CORFs, do not have the option. For these providers, assignment is mandatory.

If physicians/NPPs, PTPPs or OTPPs accept assignment (are participating), they must accept the Medicare Physician Fee Schedule amount as payment. Medicare pays 80% and the patient is responsible for 20%. In contrast, if they do not accept assignment, Medicare will only pay 95% of the fee schedule amount. However, when these services are not furnished on an assignment-related basis, the limiting charge applies. (See §1848(g)(2)(c) of the Act.)

NOTE: Services furnished by a therapist in the therapist's office under arrangements with hospitals in rural communities and public health agencies (or services provided in the beneficiary's home under arrangements with a provider of outpatient physical or occupational therapy services) are not covered under this provision. See section 230.6.

230.5—Physical Therapy, Occupational Therapy and Speech-Language Pathology Services Provided Incident to the Services of Physicians and (Rev. 36, Issued: 06-24-05, Effective: 06-06-05, Implementation: 06-06-05)

References: §1861(s)(2)(A) of the Act
42 CFR 410.10(b)
42 CFR 410.26
Pub. 100-02, ch. 15, § 60.

The Benefit. Therapy services have their own benefit under §1861 of the Social Security Act and shall be covered when provided according to the standards and conditions of the benefit described in Medicare manuals. The statute 1862(a)(20) requires that payment be made for a therapy service billed by a physician/NPP only if the service meets the standards and conditions--other than licensing--that would apply to a therapist. (For example, see coverage requirements in Pub. 100-08, chapter 13, §13.5.1(C), Pub. 100-04, chapter 5, and also the requirements of this manual, §220 and §230.

Incident to a Therapist. There is no coverage for services provided incident to the services of a therapist. Although PTAs and OTAs work under the supervision of a therapist and their services may be billed by the therapist, their services are covered under the benefit for therapy services and not by the benefit for services incident to a physician/NPP. The services furnished by PTAs and OTAs are not incident to the therapist's service.

Qualifications of Auxiliary Personnel. Therapy services appropriately billed incident to a physician's/NPP's service shall be subject to the same requirements as therapy services that would be furnished by a physical therapist, occupational therapist or speech-language pathologist in any other outpatient setting with one exception. When therapy services are performed incident to a physician's/NPP's service, the qualified personnel who perform the service do not need to have a license to practice therapy, unless it is required by state law. The qualified personnel must meet all the other requirements except licensure. Qualifications for therapists are found in 42CFR484.4 and in section 230.1, 230.2, and 230.3 of this manual. In effect, these rules require that the person who furnishes the service to the patient must, at least, be a graduate of a program of training for one of the therapy services as described above. Regardless of any state licensing that allows other health professionals to provide therapy services, Medicare is authorized to pay only for services provided by those trained specifically in physical therapy, occupational therapy or speech-language pathology. That means that the services of athletic trainers, massage therapists, recreation therapists, kinesiotherapists, low vision specialists or any other profession may not be billed as therapy services.

The services of PTAs and OTAs also may not be billed incident to a physician's/NPP's service. However, if a PT and PTA (or an OT and OTA) are both employed in a physician's office, the services of the PTA, when directly supervised by the PT or the services of the OTA, when directly supervised by the OT may be billed by the physician group as PT or OT services using the PIN/NPI of the enrolled PT (or OT). (See Section 230.4 for private practice rules on billing services performed in a physician's office.) If the PT or OT is not enrolled, Medicare shall not pay for the services of a PTA or OTA billed incident to the physician's service, because they do not meet the qualification standards in 42CFR484.4.

Therapy services provided and billed incident to the services of a physician/NPP also must meet all incident-to requirements in this manual in chapter 15, §60. Where the policies have different requirements, the more stringent requirement shall be met.

For example, when therapy services are billed as incident to a physician/NPP services, the requirement for direct supervision by the physician/NPP and other incident to requirements must be met, even though the service is provided by a licensed therapist who may perform the services unsupervised in other settings.

The mandatory assignment provision does not apply to therapy services furnished by a physician/NPP or "incident to" a physician's/NPP's service. However, when these services are not furnished on an assignment-related basis; the limiting charge applies.

For emphasis, following are some of the standards that apply to therapy services billed incident-to the services of a physician/NPP in the physician's/NPP's office or the beneficiary's residence.

  A. Therapy services provided to the beneficiary must be covered and payable outpatient rehabilitation services as described, for example, in this section as well as Pub. 100-08, chapter 13, §13.5.1.

  B. Therapy services must be provided by, or under the direct supervision of a physician (a doctor of medicine or osteopathy) or NPP who is legally authorized to practice therapy services by the state in which he or she performs such function or action. Direct supervision requirements are the same as in 42CFR410.32(b)(3). The supervisor must be present in the office suite and immediately available to furnish assistance and direction throughout the performance of the procedure. It does not mean that the physician/NPP must be present in the same room in the office where the service is performed.

  C. The services must be of a level of complexity that require that they be performed by a therapist or under the direct supervision of the therapist, physician/NPP who is licensed to perform them. Services that do not require the performance or supervision of the therapist, physician/NPP, are not considered reasonable or necessary therapy services even if they are performed or supervised by a physician/NPP or other qualified professional.

  D. Services must be furnished under a plan of treatment as in §220.1.2 of this chapter. The services provided must relate directly to the physician/NPP service to which it is incident.

230.6—Therapy Services Furnished Under Arrangements With Providers and Clinics

(Rev. 36, Issued: 06-24-05, Effective: 06-06-05, Implementation: 06-06-05)

References: See also Pub. 100-01, chapter 5, §10.3.

A—General

For rules regarding services provided under arrangement, see Pub. 100-01, chapter 5, §10.3.

A provider may have others furnish outpatient therapy (physical therapy, occupational therapy, or speech-language pathology) services through arrangements under which receipt of payment by the provider for the services discharges the liability of the beneficiary or any other person to pay for the service.

However, it is not intended that the provider merely serve as a billing mechanism for the other party. For such services to be covered the provider must assume professional responsibility for the services.

The provider's professional supervision over the services requires application of many of the same controls that are applied to services furnished by salaried employees. The provider must:

- Accept the patient for treatment in accordance with its admission policies;
- Maintain a complete and timely clinical record on the patient which includes diagnosis, medical history, orders, and progress notes relating to all services received;
- Maintain liaison with the attending physician/NPP with regard to the progress of the patient and to assure that the required plan of treatment is periodically reviewed by the physician/NPP;
- Secure from the physician/NPP the required certifications and recertifications; and
- Ensure that the medical necessity of such service is reviewed on a sample basis by the agency's staff or an outside review group.

In addition, when a provider provides outpatient services under an arrangement with others, such services must be furnished in accordance with the terms of a written contract, which provides for retention by the provider of responsibility for and control and supervision of such services. The terms of the contract should include at least the following:

- Provide that the therapy services are to be furnished in accordance with the plan of care established according to Medicare policies for therapy plans of care in Section 220.1.2 of this chapter;
- Specify the geographical areas in which the services are to be furnished;
- Provide that contracted personnel and services meet the same requirements as those which would be applicable if the personnel and services were furnished directly by the provider;
- Provide that the therapist will participate in conferences required to coordinate the care of an individual patient;
- Provide for the preparation of treatment records, with progress notes and observations, and for the prompt incorporation of such into the clinical records of the clinic;
- Specify the financial arrangements. The contracting organization or individual may not bill the patient or the health insurance program; and
- Specify the period of time the contract is to be in effect and the manner of termination or renewal.

B—Special Rules for Hospitals

- A hospital may bill Medicare for outpatient therapy (physical therapy, occupational therapy, or speech-language pathology) services that it furnishes to its outpatients either directly or under arrangements in the hospital's outpatient department. If a hospital furnishes medically necessary therapy services in its outpatient department to individuals who are registered as its outpatients, those services must be billed directly by the hospital using bill type 13X or 85X for critical access hospitals. Note that services provided to residents of a Medicare-certified SNF may not be billed by the hospital as services to its outpatients.
- When a hospital sends its therapists to the home of an individual who is registered as an outpatient of the hospital but who is unable, for medical reasons, to come to the hospital to receive medically necessary therapy services, the services must meet the requirements applicable to outpatient hospital therapy services, as set forth in the regulations and applicable Medicare manuals. The hospital may bill for those services directly using bill type 13X or 85X for critical access hospitals.
- If a hospital sends its therapists to provide therapy services to individuals who are registered as its outpatients and who are residing in the non-certified part of a SNF, or in another residential setting (e.g., a group home, assisted living facility or domiciliary care home), the hospital may bill for the services as hospital outpatient services if the services meet the requirements applicable to outpatient hospital therapy services, as set forth in the regulations and applicable Medicare manuals.
- A hospital may make an arrangement with another entity such as an Outpatient Rehab Facility (Rehabilitation Agency) or a private practice, to provide therapy services to individuals who are registered as outpatients of the hospital. These services must meet the requirements applicable to services furnished under arrangements and the requirements applicable to the outpatient hospital therapy services as set forth in the regulations and

applicable Medicare manuals. The hospital uses bill type 13X or 85X for critical access hospitals to bill for the services that another entity furnishes under arrangement to its outpatients.

- Where the provider is a public health agency or a hospital in a rural community, it may enter into arrangements to have outpatient physical therapy services furnished in the private office of a qualified physical therapist if the agency or hospital does not have the capacity to provide on its premises all of the modalities of treatment, tests, and measurements that are included in an adequate outpatient physical therapy program and the services and modalities which the public health agency or hospital cannot provide on its premises are not available on an outpatient basis in another accessible certified facility.
- In certain settings and under certain circumstances, hospitals may not bill Medicare for therapy services as services of the hospital:
  - If a hospital sends its therapists to provide therapy services to patients of another hospital, including a patient at an inpatient rehabilitation facility or a long term care facility, the services must be furnished under arrangements made with the hospital sending the therapists by the hospital having the patients and billed as hospital services by the facility whose patients are treated. These services would be subject to existing hospital bundling rules and would be paid under the payment method applicable to the hospital at which the individuals are patients.
  - A hospital may not send its therapists to provide therapy services to individuals who are receiving services from an HHA under a home health plan of care and bill for the therapy services as hospital outpatient services. For patients under a home health plan of care, payment for therapy services (unless provided by physicians/NPPs) is included or bundled into Medicare's episodic payment to the HHA, and those services must be billed by the HHA under the HHA consolidated billing rules. For patients receiving HHA services under an HHA plan of care, therapy services must be furnished directly or under arrangements made by the HHA, and only the HHA may bill for those services.
  - If a hospital sends its therapists to provide services under arrangements made by a SNF to residents of the Medicare-certified part of a SNF, SNF consolidated billing rules apply. For arrangements specific to SNF Part A, see Pub. 100-04, chapter 6, §10.4. This means that therapy services furnished to SNF residents in the Medicare-certified part of a SNF cannot be billed by any entity other than the SNF. Therefore, a hospital may not bill Medicare for PT/OT/SLP services furnished to residents of a Medicare-certified part of a SNF by its therapists as services of the hospital.

NOTE: If the SNF resident is in a covered Part A stay, the therapy services would be included in the SNF's global PPS per diem payment for the covered Part A stay itself. If the resident is in a noncovered stay (Part A benefits exhausted, no prior qualifying hospital stay, etc.), but remains in the Medicare-certified part of a SNF, the SNF would submit the Part B therapy bill to its fiscal intermediary.

SNF Setting	Applicable Rules	
Medicare Part A or B	Consolidated Billing Rules Apply?	Hospital May Bill For Outpatient Services?
Part A (Medicare Covered/PPS) Resident in Medicare-certified part of a SNF	Yes	No
Medicare Part B Resident in Medicare-certified part of a SNF	Yes	No
Medicare Part B Not a Resident in Medicare-certified part of a SNF	No	Yes

- A hospital may not send therapy staff to provide therapy services in non-residential health care settings and bill for the services as if they were provided at the hospital, even if the hospital owns the other facility or entity. Examples of such non-residential settings include CORFs, rehabilitation agencies, ORFs and offices of physicians/NPPs or other practitioners, such as physical therapists. For example, services furnished to patients of a CORF must be billed as CORF services and not as outpatient hospital services. Even if a CORF contracts with a hospital to furnish services to CORF patients, the hospital may not bill Medicare for the services as hospital outpatient services. However, the CORF could have the hospital furnish services to its patients under arrangements, in which case the CORF would bill for the services.

Psychiatric hospitals are treated the same as other hospitals for the purpose of therapy billing.

290—FOOT CARE

(Rev. 1, 10-01-03)

A3-3158, B3-2323, HO-260.9, B3-4120.1

A—Treatment of Subluxation of Foot

Subluxations of the foot are defined as partial dislocations or displacements of joint surfaces, tendons ligaments, or muscles of the foot. Surgical or nonsurgical treatments undertaken for the sole purpose of correcting a subluxated structure in the foot as an isolated entity are not covered.

However, medical or surgical treatment of subluxation of the ankle joint (talo-crural joint) is covered. In addition, reasonable and necessary medical or surgical services, diagnosis, or treatment for medical conditions that have resulted from or are associated with partial displacement of structures is covered. For example, if a patient has osteoarthritis that has resulted in a partial displacement of joints in the foot, and the primary treatment is for the osteoarthritis, coverage is provided

B—Exclusions from Coverage

The following foot care services are generally excluded from coverage under both Part A and Part B. (See §290.F and §290.G for instructions on applying foot care exclusions.)

1. **Treatment of Flat Foot**—The term "flat foot" is defined as a condition in which one or more arches of the foot have flattened out. Services or devices directed toward the care or correction of such conditions, including the prescription of supportive devices, are not covered.

2. **Routine Foot Care**—Except as provided above, routine foot care is excluded from coverage. Services that normally are considered routine and not covered by Medicare include the following:

   - The cutting or removal of corns and calluses;
   - The trimming, cutting, clipping, or debriding of nails; and
   - Other hygienic and preventive maintenance care, such as cleaning and soaking the feet, the use of skin creams to maintain skin tone of either ambulatory or bedfast patients, and any other service performed in the absence of localized illness, injury, or symptoms involving the foot.

3. **Supportive Devices for Feet**—Orthopedic shoes and other supportive devices for the feet generally are not covered. However, this exclusion does not apply to such a shoe if it is an integral part of a leg brace, and its expense is included as part of the cost of the brace. Also, this exclusion does not apply to therapeutic shoes furnished to diabetics.

C—Exceptions to Routine Foot Care Exclusion

1. **Necessary and Integral Part of Otherwise Covered Services**—In certain circumstances, services ordinarily considered to be routine may be covered if they are performed as a necessary and integral part of otherwise covered services, such as diagnosis and treatment of ulcers, wounds, or infections.

2. **Treatment of Warts on Foot**—The treatment of warts (including plantar warts) on the foot is covered to the same extent as services provided for the treatment of warts located elsewhere on the body.

3. **Presence of Systemic Condition**—The presence of a systemic condition such as metabolic, neurologic, or peripheral vascular disease may require scrupulous foot care by a professional that in the absence of such condition(s) would be considered routine (and, therefore, excluded from coverage). Accordingly, foot care that would otherwise be considered routine may be covered when systemic condition(s) result in severe circulatory embarrassment or areas of diminished sensation in the individual's legs or feet. (See subsection A.)

In these instances, certain foot care procedures that otherwise are considered routine (e.g., cutting or removing corns and calluses, or trimming, cutting, clipping, or debriding nails) may pose a hazard when performed by a nonprofessional person on patients with such systemic conditions. (See §290.G for procedural instructions.)

4. **Mycotic Nails**—In the absence of a systemic condition, treatment of mycotic nails may be covered.

The treatment of mycotic nails for an ambulatory patient is covered only when the physician attending the patient's mycotic condition documents that (1) there is clinical evidence of mycosis of the toenail, and (2) the patient has marked limitation of ambulation, pain, or secondary infection resulting from the thickening and dystrophy of the infected toenail plate.

The treatment of mycotic nails for a nonambulatory patient is covered only when the physician attending the patient's mycotic condition documents that (1) there is clinical evidence of mycosis of the toenail, and (2) the patient suffers from pain or secondary infection resulting from the thickening and dystrophy of the infected toenail plate.

For the purpose of these requirements, documentation means any written information that is required by the carrier in order for services to be covered. Thus, the information submitted with claims must be substantiated by information found in the patient's medical record. Any information, including that contained in a form letter, used for documentation purposes is subject to carrier verification in order to ensure that the information adequately justifies coverage of the treatment of mycotic nails.

D—Systemic Conditions That Might Justify Coverage

Although not intended as a comprehensive list, the following metabolic, neurologic, and peripheral vascular diseases (with synonyms in parentheses) most commonly represent the underlying conditions that might justify coverage for routine foot care.

- Diabetes mellitus*
- Arteriosclerosis obliterans (A.S.O., arteriosclerosis of the extremities, occlusive peripheral arteriosclerosis)
- Buerger's disease (thromboangiitis obliterans)
- Chronic thrombophlebitis*
- Peripheral neuropathies involving the feet—
  - Associated with malnutrition and vitamin deficiency*
    - Malnutrition (general, pellagra)
    - Alcoholism
    - Malabsorption (celiac disease, tropical sprue)
    - Pernicious anemia
  - Associated with carcinoma*
  - Associated with diabetes mellitus*
  - Associated with drugs and toxins*
  - Associated with multiple sclerosis*
  - Associated with uremia (chronic renal disease)*
  - Associated with traumatic injury
  - Associated with leprosy or neurosyphilis
  - Associated with hereditary disorders
    - Hereditary sensory radicular neuropathy
    - Angiokeratoma corporis diffusum (Fabry's)
    - Amyloid neuropathy

When the patient's condition is one of those designated by an asterisk (*), routine procedures are covered only if the patient is under the active care of a doctor of medicine or osteopathy who documents the condition.

E—Supportive Devices for Feet

Orthopedic shoes and other supportive devices for the feet generally are not covered. However, this exclusion does not apply to

such a shoe if it is an integral part of a leg brace, and its expense is included as part of the cost of the brace. Also, this exclusion does not apply to therapeutic shoes furnished to diabetics.

F—Presumption of Coverage

In evaluating whether the routine services can be reimbursed, a presumption of coverage may be made where the evidence available discloses certain physical and/or clinical findings consistent with the diagnosis and indicative of severe peripheral involvement. For purposes of applying this presumption the following findings are pertinent:

Class A Findings

- Nontraumatic amputation of foot or integral skeletal portion thereof.

Class B Findings

- Absent posterior tibial pulse;
- Advanced trophic changes as: hair growth (decrease or absence) nail changes (thickening) pigmentary changes (discoloration) skin texture (thin, shiny) skin color (rubor or redness) (Three required); and
- Absent dorsalis pedis pulse.

Class C Findings

- Claudication;
- Temperature changes (e.g., cold feet);
- Edema;
- Paresthesias (abnormal spontaneous sensations in the feet); and
- Burning.

The presumption of coverage may be applied when the physician rendering the routine foot care has identified:

1. A Class A finding;
2. Two of the Class B findings; or
3. One Class B and two Class C findings.

Cases evidencing findings falling short of these alternatives may involve podiatric treatment that may constitute covered care and should be reviewed by the intermediary's medical staff and developed as necessary.

For purposes of applying the coverage presumption where the routine services have been rendered by a podiatrist, the contractor may deem the active care requirement met if the claim or other evidence available discloses that the patient has seen an M.D. or D.O. for treatment and/or evaluation of the complicating disease process during the 6-month period prior to the rendition of the routine-type services. The intermediary may also accept the podiatrist's statement that the diagnosing and treating M.D. or D.O. also concurs with the podiatrist's findings as to the severity of the peripheral involvement indicated.

Services ordinarily considered routine might also be covered if they are performed as a necessary and integral part of otherwise covered services, such as diagnosis and treatment of diabetic ulcers, wounds, and infections.

G—Application of Foot Care Exclusions to Physician's Services

The exclusion of foot care is determined by the nature of the service. Thus, payment for an excluded service should be denied whether performed by a podiatrist, osteopath, or a doctor of medicine, and without regard to the difficulty or complexity of the procedure.

When an itemized bill shows both covered services and noncovered services not integrally related to the covered service, the portion of charges attributable to the noncovered services should be denied. (For example, if an itemized bill shows surgery for an ingrown toenail and also removal of calluses not necessary for the performance of toe surgery, any additional charge attributable to removal of the calluses should be denied.)

In reviewing claims involving foot care, the carrier should be alert to the following exceptional situations:

1. Payment may be made for incidental noncovered services performed as a necessary and integral part of, and secondary to, a covered procedure. For example, if trimming of toenails is re-

quired for application of a cast to a fractured foot, the carrier need not allocate and deny a portion of the charge for the trimming of the nails. However, a separately itemized charge for such excluded service should be disallowed. When the primary procedure is covered the administration of anesthesia necessary for the performance of such procedure is also covered.

2. Payment may be made for **initial** diagnostic services performed in connection with a specific symptom or complaint if it seems likely that its treatment would be covered even though the resulting diagnosis may be one requiring only noncovered care.

The name of the M.D. or D.O. who diagnosed the complicating condition must be submitted with the claim. In those cases, where active care is required, the approximate date the beneficiary was last seen by such physician must also be indicated.

NOTE: Section 939 of P.L. 96-499 removed "warts" from the routine foot care exclusion effective July 1, 1981.

Relatively few claims for routine-type care are anticipated considering the severity of conditions contemplated as the basis for this exception. Claims for this type of foot care should not be paid in the absence of convincing evidence that nonprofessional performance of the service would have been hazardous for the beneficiary because of an underlying systemic disease. The mere statement of a diagnosis such as those mentioned in §D above does not of itself indicate the severity of the condition. Where development is indicated to verify diagnosis and/or severity the carrier should follow existing claims processing practices which may include review of carrier's history and medical consultation as well as physician contacts.

The rules in §290.F concerning presumption of coverage also apply.

Codes and policies for routine foot care and supportive devices for the feet are not exclusively for the use of podiatrists. These codes must be used to report foot care services regardless of the specialty of the physician who furnishes the services. Carriers must instruct physicians to use the most appropriate code available when billing for routine foot care.

101, Chapter 3

20.5—Blood Deductibles (Part A and Part B)

(Rev. 1, 09-11-02)

Program payment may not be made for the first 3 pints of whole blood or equivalent units of packed red cells received under Part A and Part B combined in a calendar year. However, blood processing (e.g., administration, storage) is not subject to the deductible.

The blood deductibles are in addition to any other applicable deductible and coinsurance amounts for which the patient is responsible.

The deductible applies only to the first 3 pints of blood furnished in a calendar year, even if more than one provider furnished blood.

20.5.1—Part A Blood Deductible

(Rev. 1, 09-11-02)

Blood must be furnished on a Medicare covered day in a hospital or SNF to be counted under Part A. Blood furnished to an inpatient after benefits exhausted or before entitlement is not counted toward the combined deductible. Blood furnished during a lifetime extension election period is counted toward the combined A/B 3 pint total.

20.5.2—Part B Blood Deductible

(Rev. 1, 09-11-02)

Blood is furnished on an outpatient basis or is subject to the Part B blood deductible and is counted toward the combined limit. It should be noted that payment for blood may be made to the hospital under Part B only for blood furnished in an outpatient setting. Blood is not covered for inpatient Part B services.

20.5.3—Items Subject to Blood Deductibles

(Rev. 18, Issued: 03-04-05, Effective: 07-01-05, Implementation: 07-05-05)

The blood deductibles apply only to whole blood and packed red cells. The term whole blood means human blood from which none of the liquid or cellular components have been removed. Where packed red cells are furnished, a unit of packed red cells is considered equivalent to a pint of whole blood. Other components of blood such as platelets, fibrinogen, plasma, gamma globulin, and serum albumin are not subject to the blood deductible. However, these components of blood are covered as biologicals.

Refer to Pub. 100-04, Medicare Claims Processing Manual, Chapter 4, §231 regarding billing for blood and blood products under the Hospital Outpatient Prospective Payment System (OPPS).

20.5.4—Obligations of the Beneficiary to Pay for or Replace Deductible Blood

(Rev. 1, 09-11-02)

A provider may charge the beneficiary or a third party its customary charge for whole blood or units of packed red cells which are subject to either the Part A or Part B blood deductible, unless the individual, another person, or a blood bank replaces the blood or arranges to have it replaced.

20.5.4.1—Replacement of Blood

(Rev. 1, 09-11-02)

For replacement purposes, a pint of whole blood is considered equivalent to a unit of packed red cells. A deductible pint of whole blood or unit of packed red cells is considered replaced when a medically acceptable pint or unit is given or offered to the provider or, at the provider's request, to its blood supplier. Accordingly, where an individual or a blood bank offers blood as a replacement for a deductible pint or unit furnished a Medicare beneficiary, the provider may not charge the beneficiary for the blood, whether or not the provider or its blood supplier accepts the replacement offer. Thus a provider may not charge a beneficiary merely because it is the policy of the provider or its blood supplier not to accept blood from a particular source which has offered to replace blood on behalf of the beneficiary. However, a provider would not be barred from charging a beneficiary for deductible blood, if there is a reasonable basis for believing that replacement blood offered by or on behalf of the beneficiary would endanger the health of a recipient or that the prospective donor's health would be endangered by making a blood donation. Once a provider accepts a pint of replacement blood from a beneficiary or another individual acting on his/her behalf, the blood is deemed to have been replaced, and, the beneficiary may not be charged for the blood, even though the replacement blood is later found to be unfit and has to be discarded.

When a provider accepts blood donated in advance, in anticipation of need by a specific beneficiary, whether the beneficiary's own blood, that is, an autologous donation, or blood furnished by another individual or blood assurance group, such donations are considered replacement for pints or units subsequently furnished the beneficiary.

30—OUTPATIENT MENTAL HEALTH TREATMENT LIMITATION

(Rev. 1, 09-11-02)

Regardless of the actual expenses a beneficiary incurs for treatment of mental, psychoneurotic, and personality disorders while the beneficiary is not an inpatient of a hospital at the time such expenses are incurred, the amount of those expenses that may be recognized for Part B deductible and payment purposes is limited to 62.5 percent of the Medicare allowed amount for these services. The limitation is called the outpatient mental health treatment limitation. Since Part B deductible also applies the program pays for about half of the allowed amount recognized for mental health therapy services.

Expenses for diagnostic services (e.g., psychiatric testing and evaluation to diagnose the patient's illness) are not subject to this limitation. This limitation applies only to therapeutic services and to services performed to evaluate the progress of a course of treatment for a diagnosed condition.

30.3.5—Effect of Assignment Upon Purchase of Cataract Glasses From Participating Physician or Supplier on Claims Submitted to Carriers

(Rev. 1, 10-01-03)

B3-3045.4

A pair of cataract glasses is comprised of two distinct products: a professional product (the prescribed lenses) and a retail commercial product (the frames). The frames serve not only as a holder of lenses but also as an article of personal apparel. As such, they are usually selected on the basis of personal taste and style. Although Medicare will pay only for standard frames, most patients want deluxe frames. Participating physicians and suppliers cannot profitably furnish such deluxe frames unless they can make an extra (noncovered) charge for the frames even though they accept assignment.

Therefore, a participating physician or supplier (whether an ophthalmologist, optometrist, or optician) who accepts assignment on cataract glasses with deluxe frames may charge the Medicare patient the difference between his/her usual charge to private pay patients for glasses with standard frames and his/her usual charge to such patients for glasses with deluxe frames, in addition to the applicable deductible and coinsurance on glasses with standard frames, if all of the following requirements are met:

A. The participating physician or supplier has standard frames available, offers them for sale to the patient, and issues and ABN to the patient that explains the price and other differences between standard and deluxe frames. Refer to Chapter 30.

B. The participating physician or supplier obtains from the patient (or his/her representative) and keeps on file the following signed and dated statement:

Name of Patient   Medicare Claim Number

Having been informed that an extra charge is being made by the physician or supplier for deluxe frames, that this extra charge is not covered by Medicare, and that standard frames are available for purchase from the physician or supplier at no extra charge, I have chosen to purchase deluxe frames.

Signature   Date

C. The participating physician or supplier itemizes on his/her claim his/her actual charge for the lenses, his/her actual charge for the standard frames, and his/her actual extra charge for the deluxe frames (charge differential).

Once the assigned claim for deluxe frames has been processed, the carrier will follow the ABN instructions as described in §60.

30.3.6—Mandatory Assignment Requirement for Physician Office Laboratories on Claims Submitted to Carriers

(Rev. 1, 10-01-03)

B3-3045.5

A—General

No payment may be made for clinical diagnostic laboratory tests furnished by a physician or medical group unless the physician or medical group accepts assignment or claims payment under the indirect payment procedure. Carrier direct payment to a physician or group after the death of the beneficiary is considered assigned payment. Assignment may be accepted for the entire claim. See subsections B and C if a physician wishes to accept assignment only for laboratory services.

B—Submission of Non-EMC Claims

A nonparticipating physician or medical group who furnishes clinical diagnostic laboratory tests and other services to a benefici-

ary and accepts assignment only for the laboratory tests may either submit a separate (assigned) claim for them or a single claim that includes both the assigned tests and the other unassigned services. In the latter event, the claim must be annotated as unassigned in block 26 of the Form CMS-1500 and a special request for payment for the assigned tests written in block 25, as follows:

"I accept assignment for the clinical laboratory tests."

C—Submission of EMC Claims

A nonparticipating EMC physician or medical group who furnishes clinical diagnostic laboratory tests and other services and accepts assignment only for the laboratory tests may either submit a separate (assigned) data set for the tests or a single data set that includes both the assigned tests and the unassigned other services. In the latter event, the data set must include the unassigned indicator. The physician or group must have filed a blanket statement agreeing to accept assignment on all clinical diagnostic laboratory tests, not withstanding the inclusion of the unassigned indicator on electronic data sets.

D—Processing Claims

Carriers process as assigned all claims for clinical diagnostic laboratory tests as described above, including those submitted by a participating or non-participating physician or group either marked as unassigned or with no assignment option specified. Where, however, evidence clearly shows that the beneficiary or provider refuses to assign the claim, carriers should deny it. They split a claim containing assigned laboratory tests and other unassigned services.

E—Public Information

Carriers must inform all physicians and medical groups of this policy annually.

104, Chapter 1

30.2.10—Payment Under Reciprocal Billing Arrangements—Claims Submitted to Carriers

(Rev. 1, 10-01-03)

B3-3060.6

The patient's regular physician may submit the claim, and (if assignment is accepted) receive the Part B payment, for covered visit services (including emergency visits and related services) which the regular physician arranges to be provided by a substitute physician on an occasional reciprocal basis, if:

- The regular physician is unavailable to provide the visit services;
- The Medicare patient has arranged or seeks to receive the visit services from the regular physician;
- The substitute physician does not provide the visit services to Medicare patients over a continuous period of longer than 60 days; and
- The regular physician identifies the services as substitute physician services meeting the requirements of this section by entering in item 24d of Form CMS-1500 HCPCS code Q5 modifier (service furnished by a substitute physician under a reciprocal billing arrangement) after the procedure code. When Form CMS-1500 is next revised, provision will be made to identify the substitute physician by entering the unique physician identification number (UPIN) on the form and cross-referring the entry to the appropriate service line item(s) by number(s). Until further notice, the regular physician must keep on file a record of each service provided by the substitute physician, associated with the substitute physician's UPIN, and make this record available to the carrier upon request.

If the only substitution services a physician performs in connection with an operation are post-operative services furnished during the period covered by the global fee, these services need not be identified on the claim as substitution services.

A physician may have reciprocal arrangements with more than one physician. The arrangements need not be in writing.

The term "covered visit service" includes not only those services ordinarily characterized as a covered physician visit, but also any other covered items and services furnished by the substitute physician or by others as incident to the physician's services.

"Incident to" services furnished by staff of a substitute physician or regular physician are covered if furnished under the supervision of each.

A "continuous period of covered visit services" begins with the first day on which the substitute physician provides covered visit services to Medicare Part B patients of the regular physician, and ends with the last day the substitute physician provides services to these patients before the regular physician returns to work. This period continues without interruption on days on which no covered visit services are provided to patients on behalf of the regular physician or are furnished by some other substitute physician on behalf of the regular physician. A new period of covered visit services can begin after the regular physician has returned to work.

EXAMPLE

The regular physician goes on vacation on June 30, and returns to work on September 4. A substitute physician provides services to Medicare Part B patients of the regular physician on July 2, and at various times thereafter, including August 30 and September 2. The continuous period of covered visit services begins on July2 and runs through September 2, a period of 63 days. Since the September 2 services are furnished after the expiration of 60 days of the period, the regular physician is not entitled to bill and receive direct payment for them. The substitute physician must bill for these services in his/her own name. The regular physician may, however, bill and receive payment for the services that the substitute physician provides on his/her behalf in the period July 2 through August 30.

The requirements for the submission of claims under reciprocal billing arrangements are the same for assigned and unassigned claims.

A—Physician Medical Group Claims Under Reciprocal Billing Arrangements

The requirements of this section generally do not apply to the substitution arrangements among physicians in the same medical group where claims are submitted in the name of the group. On claims submitted by the group, the group physician who actually performed the service must be identified in the manner described in §30.2.13 with one exception. When a group member provides services on behalf of another group member who is the designated attending physician for a hospice patient, the Q5 modifier may be used by the designated attending physician to bill for services related to a hospice patient's terminal illness that were performed by another group member.

For a medical group to submit assigned and unassigned claims for the covered visit services of a substitute physician who is not a member of the group and for an independent physician to submit assigned and unassigned claims for the substitution services of a physician who is a member of a medical group, the following requirements must be met:

- The regular physician is unavailable to provide the visit services;
- The Medicare patient has arranged or seeks to receive the visit services from the regular physician; and
- The substitute physician does not provide the visit services to Medicare patients over a continuous period of longer than 60 days.

Substitute billing services are billed for each entity as follows:

- The medical group must enter in item 24d of Form CMS-1500 the HCPCS code modifier Q5 after the procedure code.
- The independent physician must enter in item 24 of Form CMS-1500 HCPCS code modifier Q5 after the procedure code.
- The designated attending physician for a hospice patient (receiving services related to a terminal illness) bills the Q5 modifier in item 24 of Form CMS-1500 when another group member covers for the attending physician.

- A record of each service provided by the substitute physician must be kept on file and associated with the substitute physician's UPIN. This record must be made available to the carrier upon request.
- In addition, the medical group physician for whom the substitution services are furnished must be identified by his/her provider identification number (PIN) in block 24k of the appropriate line item.

Physicians who are members of a group but who bill in their own names are treated as independent physicians for purposes of applying the requirements of this section.

Carriers should inform physicians of the compliance requirements when billing for services of a substitute physician. The physician notification should state that, in entering the Q5 modifier, the regular physician (or the medical group, where applicable) is certifying that the services are covered visit services furnished by the substitute physician identified in a record of the regular physician which is available for inspection, and are services for which the regular physician (or group) is entitled to submit the claim. Carriers should include in the notice that penalty for false certifications may be civil or criminal penalties for fraud. The physician's right to receive payment or to submit claims or accept any assignments may be revoked. The revocation procedures are set forth in §40.

If a line item includes the code Q5 certification, carriers assume that the claim meets the requirements of this section in the absence of evidence to the contrary. Carriers need not track the 60-day period or validate the billing arrangement on a prepayment basis, absent postpayment findings that indicate that the certifications by a particular physician may not be valid.

When carriers make Part B payment under this section, they determine the payment amount as though the regular physician provided the services. The identification of the substitute physician is primarily for purposes of providing an audit trail to verify that the services were furnished, not for purposes of the payment or the limiting charge. Also, notices of noncoverage are to be given in the name of the regular physician.

30.2.11—Physician Payment Under Locum Tenens Arrangements—Claims Submitted to Carriers—(Rev. 1, 10-01-03)

B3-3060.7

A—Background

It is a longstanding and widespread practice for physicians to retain substitute physicians to take over their professional practices when the regular physicians are absent for reasons such as illness, pregnancy, vacation, or continuing medical education, and for the regular physician to bill and receive payment for the substitute physician's services as though he/she performed them. The substitute physician generally has no practice of his/her own and moves from area to area as needed. The regular physician generally pays the substitute physician a fixed amount per diem, with the substitute physician having the status of an independent contractor rather than of an employee. These substitute physicians are generally called "locum tenens" physicians.

Section 125(b) of the Social Security Act Amendments of 1994 makes this procedure available on a permanent basis. Thus, beginning January 1, 1995, a regular physician may bill for the services of a locum tenens physicians. A regular physician is the physician that is normally scheduled to see a patient. Thus, a regular physician may include physician specialists (such as a cardiologist, oncologist, urologist, etc.).

B—Payment Procedure

A patient's regular physician may submit the claim, and (if assignment is accepted) receive the Part B payment, for covered visit services (including emergency visits and related services) of a locum tenens physician who is not an employee of the regular physician and whose services for patients of the regular physician are not restricted to the regular physician's offices, if:

- The regular physician is unavailable to provide the visit services;

- The Medicare beneficiary has arranged or seeks to receive the visit services from the regular physician;
- The regular physician pays the locum tenens for his/her services on a per diem or similar fee-for-time basis;
- The substitute physician does not provide the visit services to Medicare patients over a continuous period of longer than 60 days; and
- The regular physician identifies the services as substitute physician services meeting the requirements of this section by entering HCPCS code modifier Q6 (service furnished by a locum tenens physician) after the procedure code. When Form CMS-1500 is next revised, provision will be made to identify the substitute physician by entering his/her unique physician identification number (UPIN) to the carrier upon request.

If the only substitution services a physician performs in connection with an operation are post-operative services furnished during the period covered by the global fee, these services need not be identified on the claim as substitution services.

The requirements for the submission of claims under reciprocal billing arrangements are the same for assigned and unassigned claims.

C—Medical Group Claims Under Locum Tenens Arrangements

For a medical group to submit assigned and unassigned claims for the services a locum tenens physician provides for patients of the regular physician who is a member of the group, the requirements of subsection B must be met. For purposes of these requirements, per diem or similar fee-for-time compensation which the group pays the locum tenens physician is considered paid by the regular physician. Also, a physician who has left the group and for whom the group has engaged a locum tenens physician as a temporary replacement may bill for the temporary physician for up to 60 days. The group must enter in item 24d of Form CMS-1500 the HCPCS modifier Q6 after the procedure code. Until further notice, the group must keep on file a record of each service provided by the substitute physician, associated with the substitute physician's UPIN, and make this record available to the carrier upon request. In addition, the medical group physician for whom the substitution services are furnished must be identified by his/her provider identification number (PIN) on block 24k of the appropriate line item.

Physicians who are members of a group but who bill in their own names are generally treated as independent physicians for purposes of applying the requirements of subsection A for payment for locum tenens physician services. Compensation paid by the group to the locum tenens physician is considered paid by the regular physician for purposes of those requirements. The term "regular physician" includes a physician who has left the group and for whom the group has hired the locum tenens physician as a replacement.

104, Chapter 12

90.4.3—Claims Coding Requirements

(Rev. 280, Issued 08-13-04, Effective/Implementation: October 1, 2004 for the analysis and design phases for the MCS Maintainer and Contractors

January 1, 2005 for the coding, testing, and implementation phases for the MCS Maintainer and Contractors

January 1, 2005 for all phases for the VIPS Maintainers and Contractors)

B3-3350.3

For services with dates of service prior to January 1, 2005, physicians must indicate that their services were provided in an incentive-eligible rural or urban HPSA by using one of the following modifiers:

QB—physician providing a service in a rural HPSA; or
QU—physician providing a service in an urban HPSA.

For services with dates of service on or after January 1, 2005, the bonus will automatically be paid without the submission of a modifier for the following:

- When services are provided in a zip code area that fully falls within a full county HPSA.
- When services are provided in a zip code area that partially falls within a full county HPSA and has been determined to be dominant for the county by the USPS; and
- When services are provided within a zip code that fully falls within a partial county HPSA.

The submission of the QB or QU modifier will be required for the following:

- When services are provided in zip code areas that do not fully fall within a designated full county HPSA bonus area.
- When services are provided in a zip code area that partially falls within a full county HPSA but is not considered to be in that county based on the dominance decision made by the USPS.
- When services are provided in a zip code area that partially falls within a partial county HPSA.
- When services are provided in a zip code area that was not included in the automated file based on the date of the data run used to create the file.

In order to be considered for the bonus payment, the name, address, and zip code of where the service was rendered must be included on all electronic and paper claims submissions.

90.4.4—Payment

(Rev. 1, 10-01-03)

B3-3350.4

The incentive payment is 10 percent of the amount actually paid, **not** the approved amount. Carriers pay the incentive payment for services identified on either assigned or unassigned claims.

They do not include the incentive payment with each claim payment. Carriers should:

- Establish a quarterly schedule for issuing incentive payments. These payments are taxable and must be reported to the IRS.
- Prepare a list to accompany each payment. Include a line item for each assigned claim represented in the incentive check and a "summary" item showing the number of unassigned claims represented. The sum of the line items and the "summary" item should equal the amount of the check.

90.4.5—Services Eligible for HPSA and Physician Scarcity Bonus Payments

(Rev. 524, Issued: 04-15-05; Implementation and Effective Dates: 05-16-05)

B3-3350.5

A—Information in the Professional Component/Technical Component (PC/TC) Indicator Field of the Medicare Physician Fee Schedule Database

Carriers use the information in the Professional Component/Technical Component (PC/TC) indicator field of the Medicare Physician Fee Schedule Database to identify professional services eligible for HPSA and physician scarcity bonus payments. The following are the rules to apply in determining whether to pay the bonus on services furnished within a geographic HPSA or physician scarcity bonus area.

PC/TC Indicator	Bonus Payment Policy
0	Pay bonus
1	Globally billed. Only the professional component of this service qualifies for the bonus payment. The bonus cannot be paid on the technical component of globally billed services.

ACTION: Carriers return the service as unprocessable and notify the physician that the professional component must be re-billed if it is performed within a qualifying bonus area. If the technical component is the only component of the service that was performed in the bonus area, there wouldn't be a qualifying service.

PC/TC Indicator	Bonus Payment Policy
1	Professional Component (modifier 26). Carriers pay the bonus.
1	Technical Component (modifier TC). Carriers do not pay the bonus.
2	Professional Component only. Carriers pay the bonus.
3	Technical Component only. Carriers do not pay the bonus.
4	Global test only. Only the professional component of this service qualifies for the bonus payment.

ACTION: Carriers return the service as unprocessable. They instruct the provider to re-bill the service as separate professional and technical component procedure codes.

5	Incident to codes. Carriers do not pay the bonus.
6	Laboratory physician interpretation codes. Carriers pay the bonus.
7	Physical therapy service. Carriers do not pay the bonus.
8	Physician interpretation codes. Carriers pay the bonus.
9	Concept of PC/TC does not apply. Carriers do not pay the bonus.

NOTE: Codes that have a status of "X" on the Medicare Physician Fee Schedule Database (MFSDB) have been assigned PC/TC indicator 9 and are not considered physician services for MFSDB payment purposes. Therefore, neither the HPSA bonus payment nor the physician scarcity area will be paid for these codes.

B—Anesthesia Codes (CPT Codes 00100 Through 01999*) That Do Not Appear on the MFSDB

Anesthesia codes (CPT codes 00100 through 01999*) do not appear on the MFSDB. However, when a medically necessary anesthesia service is furnished within a HPSA or physician scarcity area by a physician, a HPSA bonus and/or physician scarcity bonus is payable.

To claim a bonus payment for anesthesia, physicians bill codes 00100 through 01999 with modifiers QY, QK, AD, AA, or GC to signify that the anesthesia service was performed by a physician along with the QB or QU modifier when required per section 90.4.3.

C—Mental Health Services

Physicians' professional mental health services rendered by the provider specialty of 26—psychiatry, are eligible for a HPSA bonus when rendered in a mental health HPSA. The service must have a PC/TC designation per the chart above. Should a zip code fall within both a primary care and mental health HPSA, only one bonus must be paid on the service.

104, Chapter 13

60—POSITRON EMISSION TOMOGRAPHY (PET) SCANS—GENERAL INFORMATION

(Rev. 527, Issued: 04-15-05, Effective: 01-28-05, Implementation: 04-18-05)

Positron emission tomography (PET) is a noninvasive imaging procedure that assesses perfusion and the level of metabolic activity in various organ systems of the human body. A positron camera (tomograph) is used to produce cross-sectional tomographic images which are obtained by detecting radioactivity from a radioactive tracer substance (radiopharmaceutical) that emits a radioactive tracer substance (radiopharmaceutical FDG) such as 2—[F-18] flouro-D-glucose FDG, that is administered intravenously to the patient.

The Medicare National Coverage Determinations (NCD) Manual, Chapter 1, §220.6, contains additional coverage instructions to indicate the conditions under which a PET scan is performed.

A—Definitions

For all uses of PET, excluding Rubidium 82 for perfusion of the heart, myocardial viability and refractory seizures, the following definitions apply:

- **Diagnosis::** PET is covered only in clinical situations in which the PET results may assist in avoiding an invasive diagnostic procedure, or in which the PET results may assist in determining the optimal anatomical location to perform an invasive diagnostic procedure. In general, for most solid tumors, a tissue diagnosis is made prior to the performance of PET scanning. PET scans following a tissue diagnosis are generally performed for the purpose of staging, rather than diagnosis. Therefore, the use of PET in the diagnosis of lymphoma, esophageal and colorectal cancers, as well as in melanoma, should be rare. PET is not covered for other diagnostic uses, and is not covered for screening (testing of patients without specific signs and symptoms of disease).
- **Staging and/or Restaging:** PET is covered in clinical situations in which (1) (a) the stage of the cancer remains in doubt after completion of a standard diagnostic workup, including conventional imaging (computed tomography, magnetic resonance imaging, or ultrasound) or, (b) the use of PET would also be considered reasonable and necessary if it could potentially replace one or more conventional imaging studies when it is expected that conventional study information is insufficient for the clinical management of the patient and, (2) clinical management of the patient would differ depending on the stage of the cancer identified.
- **Restaging:** PET will be covered for restaging: (1) after the completion of treatment for the purpose of detecting residual disease, (2) for detecting suspected recurrence, or metastasis, (3) to determine the extent of a known recurrence, or (4) if it could potentially replace one or more conventional imaging studies when it is expected that conventional study information is to determine the extent of a known recurrence, or if study information is insufficient for the clinical management of the patient. Restaging applies to testing after a course of treatment is completed and is covered subject to the conditions above.
- **Monitoring:** Use of PET to monitor tumor response during the planned course of therapy (i.e., when a change in therapy is anticipated).

B—Limitations

For staging and restaging: PET is covered in either/or both of the following circumstances:

- The stage of the cancer remains in doubt after completion of a standard diagnostic workup, including conventional imaging (computed tomography, magnetic resonance imaging, or ultrasound); and/or
- The clinical management of the patient would differ depending on the stage of the cancer identified. PET will be covered for restaging after the completion of treatment for the purpose of detecting residual disease, for detecting suspected recurrence, or to determine the extent of a known recurrence. Use of PET would also be considered reasonable and necessary if it could potentially replace one or more conventional imaging studies when it is expected that conventional study information is insufficient for the clinical management of the patient.

PET is not covered for other diagnostic uses, and is not covered for screening (testing of patients without specific symptoms). Use of PET to monitor tumor response during the planned course of therapy (i.e. when no change in therapy is being contemplated) is not covered.

60.1—Billing Instructions

(Rev. 527, Issued: 04-15-05, Effective: 01-28-05, Implementation: 04-18-05)

A—Billing and Payment Instructions or Responsibilities for Carriers

Claims for PET scan services must be billed on Form-CMS 1500 or the electronic equivalent with the appropriate HCPCS or CPT

---

code and diagnosis codes to the local carrier. Effective for claims received on or after July 1, 2001, PET modifiers were discontinued and are no longer a claims processing requirement for PET scan claims. Therefore, July 1, 2001, and after the MSN messages regarding the use of PET modifiers can be discontinued. The type of service (TOS) for the new PET scan procedure codes is TOS 4, Diagnostic Radiology. Payment is based on the Medicare Physician Fee Schedule.

B—Billing and Payment Instructions or Responsibilities for FIs

Claims for PET scan procedures must be billed to the FI on Form CMS-1450 (UB-92) or the electronic equivalent with the appropriate diagnosis and HCPCS "G" code or CPT code to indicate the conditions under which a PET scan was done. These codes represent the technical component costs associated with these procedures when furnished to hospital and SNF outpatients. They are paid as follows:

- under OPPS for hospitals subject to OPPS
- under current payment methodologies for hospitals not subject to OPPS
- on a reasonable cost basis for critical access hospitals.
- on a reasonable cost basis for skilled nursing facilities.

Institutional providers bill these codes under Revenue Code 0404 (PET Scan).

C—Frequency

In the absence of national frequency limitations, for all indications covered on and after July 1, 2001, contractors can, if necessary, develop frequency limitations on any or all covered PET scan services.

D—Post-Payment Review for PET Scans

As with any claim, but particularly in view of the limitations on this coverage, Medicare may decide to conduct post-payment reviews to determine that the use of PET scans is consistent with coverage instructions. Pet scanning facilities must keep patient record information on file for each Medicare patient for whom a PET scan claim is made. These medical records can be used in any post-payment reviews and must include the information necessary to substantiate the need for the PET scan. These records must include standard information (e.g., age, sex, and height) along with sufficient patient histories to allow determination that the steps required in the coverage instructions were followed. Such information must include, but is not limited to, the date, place and results of previous diagnostic tests (e.g., cytopathology and surgical pathology reports, CT), as well as the results and reports of the PET scan(s) performed at the center. If available, such records should include the prognosis derived from the PET scan, together with information regarding the physician or institution to which the patient proceeded following the scan for treatment or evaluation. The ordering physician is responsible for forwarding appropriate clinical data to the PET scan facility.

Effective for claims received on or after July 1, 2001, CMS no longer requires paper documentation to be submitted up front with PET scan claims. *Contractors shall be aware and advise providers of the specific documentation requirements for PET scans for dementia and neurodegenerative diseases. This information is outlined in section 60.12.* Documentation requirements such as physician referral and medical necessity determination are to be maintained by the provider as part of the beneficiary's medical record. This information must be made available to the carrier or FI upon request of additional documentation to determine appropriate payment of an individual claim.

60.2—Use of Gamma Cameras and Full Ring and Partial Ring PET Scanners for PET Scans

(Rev. 527, Issued: 04-15-05, Effective: 01-28-05, Implementation: 04-18-05)

See the Medicare National Coverage Determinations NCD Manual, Section 220.6, concerning 2-[F-18] Fluoro-D-Glucose (FDG) PET scanners and details about coverage.

On July 1, 2001, HCPCS codes G0210—G0230 were added to allow billing for all currently covered indications for FDG PET.

Although the codes do not indicate the type of PET scanner, these codes were used until January 1, 2002, by providers to bill for services in a manner consistent with the coverage policy.

Effective January 1, 2002, HCPCS codes G0210—G0230 were updated with new descriptors to properly reflect the type of PET scanner used. In addition, four new HCPCS codes became effective for dates of service on and after January 1, 2002, (G0231, G0232, G0233, G0234) for covered conditions that may be billed if a gamma camera is used for the PET scan. For services performed from January 1, 2002, through January 27, 2005, providers should bill using the revised HCPCS codes G0210—G0234. Beginning January 28, 2005 providers should bill using the appropriate CPT code.

60.2.1—Coverage for Myocardial Viability

(Rev. 1, 10-01-03)

AB-02-065

FDG PET is covered for the determination of myocardial viability following an inconclusive single photon computed tomography test (SPECT) from July 1, 2001, through September 30, 2002. Only full ring scanners are covered as the scanning medium for this service from July 1, 2001, through December 31, 2001. However, as of January 1, 2002, full and partial ring scanners are covered for myocardial viability following an inconclusive SPECT.

Beginning October 1, 2002, Medicare will cover FDG PET for the determination of myocardial viability as a primary or initial diagnostic study prior to revascularization, and will continue to cover FDG PET when used as a follow-up to an inconclusive SPECT. However, if a patient received a FDG PET study with inconclusive results, a follow-up SPECT is not covered. FDA full and partial ring PET scanners are covered.

In the event that a patient receives a SPECT with inconclusive results, a PET scan may be performed and covered by Medicare. However, a SPECT is not covered following a FDG PET with inconclusive results. See the Medicare National Coverage Determinations Manual for specific frequency limitations for Myocardial Viability following an inconclusive SPECT.

In the absence of national frequency limitations, contractors can, if necessary develop reasonable frequency limitations for myocardial viability.

Documentation that these conditions are met should be maintained by the referring physician as part of the beneficiary's medical record.

60.3—PET Scan Qualifying Conditions and HCPCS Code Chart

(Rev. 527, Issued: 04-15-05, Effective: 01-28-05, Implementation: 04-18-05)

Below is a summary of all covered PET Scan conditions, with effective dates.

NOTE: The G codes below except those a # can be used to bill for PET Scan services through January 27, 2005. Effective for dates of service on or after January 28, 2005, providers must bill for PET Scan services using the appropriate CPT codes. See section 60.3.1. The G codes with a # can continue to be used for billing after January 28, 2005 and these remain non-covered by Medicare. (**NOTE:** PET Scanners must be FDA-approved.)

Conditions	Coverage Effective Date	HCPCS/CPT Code
*Myocardial perfusion imaging (following previous PET G0030-G0047) single study, rest or stress (exercise and/or pharmacologic)	3/14/95	G0030
*Myocardial perfusion imaging (following previous PET G0030-G0047) multiple studies, rest or stress (exercise and/or pharmacologic)	3/14/95	G0031

Conditions	Coverage Effective Date	HCPCS/CPT Code
*Myocardial perfusion imaging (following rest SPECT, 78464); single study, rest or stress (exercise and/or pharmacologic)	3/14/95	G0032
*Myocardial perfusion imaging (following rest SPECT 78464); multiple studies, rest or stress (exercise and/or pharmacologic)	3/14/95	G0033
*Myocardial perfusion (following stress SPECT 78465); single study, rest or stress (exercise and/or pharmacologic)	3/14/95	G0034
*Myocardial Perfusion Imaging (following stress SPECT 78465); multiple studies, rest or stress (exercise and/or pharmacologic)	3/14/95	G0035
*Myocardial Perfusion Imaging (following coronary angiography 93510-93529); single study, rest or stress (exercise and/or pharmacologic)	3/14/95	G0036
*Myocardial Perfusion Imaging, (following coronary angiography), 93510-93529); multiple studies, rest or stress (exercise and/or pharmacologic)	3/14/95	G0037
*Myocardial Perfusion Imaging (following stress planar myocardial perfusion, 78460); single study, rest or stress (exercise and/or pharmacologic)	3/14/95	G0038
*Myocardial Perfusion Imaging (following stress planar myocardial perfusion, 78460); multiple studies, rest or stress (exercise and/or pharmacologic)	3/14/95	G0039
*Myocardial Perfusion Imaging (following stress echocardiogram 93350); single study, rest or stress (exercise and/or pharmacologic)	3/14/95	G0040
*Myocardial Perfusion Imaging (following stress echocardiogram, 93350); multiple studies, rest or stress (exercise and/or pharmacologic)	3/14/95	G0041
*Myocardial Perfusion Imaging (following stress nuclear ventriculogram 78481 or 78483); single study, rest or stress (exercise and/or pharmacologic)	3/14/95	G0042
*Myocardial Perfusion Imaging (following stress nuclear ventriculogram 78481 or 78483); multiple studies, rest or stress (exercise and/or pharmacologic)	3/14/95	G0043
*Myocardial Perfusion Imaging (following stress ECG, 93000); single study, rest or stress (exercise and/or pharmacologic)	3/14/95	G0044
*Myocardial perfusion (following stress ECG, 93000), multiple studies; rest or stress (exercise and/or pharmacologic)	3/14/95	G0045
*Myocardial perfusion (following stress ECG, 93015), single study; rest or stress (exercise and/or pharmacologic)	3/14/95	G0046
*Myocardial perfusion (following stress ECG, 93015); multiple studies, rest or stress (exercise and/or pharmacologic)	3/14/95	G0047
PET imaging regional or whole body; single pulmonary nodule	1/1/98	G0125

Conditions	Coverage Effective Date	HCPCS/CPT Code
Lung cancer, non-small cell (PET imaging whole body) Diagnosis, Initial Staging, Restaging	7/1/01	G0210 G0211 G0212
Colorectal cancer (PET imaging whole body) Diagnosis, Initial Staging, Restaging	7/1/01	G0213 G0214 G0215
Melanoma (PET imaging whole body) Diagnosis, Initial Staging, Restaging	7/1/01	G0216 G0217 G0218
Melanoma for non-covered indications	7/1/01	G0219
Lymphoma (PET imaging whole body) Diagnosis, Initial Staging, Restaging	7/1/01	G0220 G0221 G0222
Head and neck cancer; excluding thyroid and CNS cancers (PET imaging whole body or regional) Diagnosis, Initial Staging, Restaging	7/1/01	G0223 G0224 G0225
Esophageal cancer (PET imaging whole body) Diagnosis, Initial Staging, Restaging	7/1/01	G0226 G0227 G0228
Metabolic brain imaging for pre-surgical evaluation of refractory seizures	7/1/01	G0229
Metabolic assessment for myocardial viability following inconclusive SPECT study	7/1/01	G0230
Recurrence of colorectal or colorectal metastatic cancer (PET whole body, gamma cameras only)	1/1/02	G0231
Staging and characterization of lymphoma (PET whole body, gamma cameras only)	1/1/02	G0232
Recurrence of melanoma or melanoma metastatic cancer (PET whole body, gamma cameras only)	1/1/02	G0233
Regional or whole body, for solitary pulmonary nodule following CT, or for initial staging of non-small cell lung cancer (gamma cameras only)	1/1/02	G0234
Non-Covered Service	10/1/02	G0252
PET imaging, any site not otherwise specified	1/28/05	G0235
Initial diagnosis of breast cancer and/or surgical planning for breast cancer (e.g., initial staging of axillary lymph nodes), not covered (full- and partial-ring PET scanners only)		
Breast cancer, staging/restaging of local regional recurrence or distant metastases, i.e., staging/restaging after or prior to course of treatment (full- and partial-ring PET scanners only)	10/1/02	G0253
Breast cancer, evaluation of responses to treatment, performed during course of treatment (full- and partial-ring PET scanners only)	10/1/02	G0254
Myocardial imaging, positron emission tomography (PET), metabolic evaluation)	10/1/02	78459
Restaging or previously treated thyroid cancer of follicular cell origin following negative I-131 whole body scan (full- and partial-ring PET scanner only)	10/1/03	G0296
Tracer Rubidium**82 (Supply of Radiopharmaceutical Diagnostic Imaging Agent) (This is only billed through Outpatient Perspective Payment System, OPPS.) (Carriers must use HCPCS Code A4641).	10/1/03	Q3000

Conditions	Coverage Effective Date	HCPCS/CPT Code
Supply of Radiopharmaceutical Diagnostic Imaging Agent, Ammonia N-13	01/1/04	A9526
PET imaging, brain imaging for the differential diagnosis of Alzheimer's disease with aberrant features vs. fronto-temporal dementia	09/15/04	Appropriate CPT Code from section 60.3.1
PET Cervical Cancer Staging as adjunct to conventional imaging, other staging, diagnosis, restaging, monitoring	1/28/05	Appropriate CPT Code from section 60.3.1

*NOTE: Carriers must report A4641 for the tracer Rubidium 82 when used with PET scan codes G0030 through G0047.

**NOTE: Not FDG PET

***NOTE: For dates of service October 1, 2003, through December 31, 2003, use temporary code Q4078 for billing this radiopharmaceutical.

60.3.1—Appropriate CPT Codes Effective for PET Scans for Services Performed on or After January 28, 2005

(Rev. 527, Issued: 04-15-05, Effective: 01-28-05, Implementation: 04-18-05)

CPT Code	Description
78459	Myocardial imaging, positron emission tomography (PET), metabolic evaluation
78491	Myocardial imaging, positron emission tomography (PET), perfusion, single study at rest or stress
78492	Myocardial imaging, positron emission tomography (PET), perfusion, multiple studies at rest and/or stress

CPT Code	Description
78608	Brain imaging, positron emission tomography (PET); metabolic evaluation
78609	Brain imaging, positron emission tomography (PET); perfusion evaluation
78811	Tumor imaging, positron emission tomography (PET); limited area (eg, chest, head/neck)
78812	Tumor imaging, positron emission tomography (PET); skull base to mid thigh
78813	Tumor imaging, positron emission tomography (PET); whole body
78814	Tumor imaging, positron emission tomography (PET) with concurrently acquired computed tomography (CT) for attenuation correction and anatomical localization; limited area (e.g., chest, head/neck)
78815	Tumor imaging, positron emission tomography (PET) with concurrently acquired computed tomography (CT) for attenuation correction and anatomical localization; skull base to mid thigh
78816	Tumor imaging, positron emission tomography (PET) with concurrently acquired computed tomography (CT) for attenuation correction and anatomical localization; whole body

60.4—PET Scans for Imaging of the Perfu of the Heart Using Rubidium 82 (Rb 82)

(Rev. 223, Issued: 07-02-04) (Effective/Implementation: Not Applicable)

For dates of service on or after March 14, 1995, Medicare covers one PET scan for imaging of the perfusion of the heart using Rubidium 82 (Rb 82), provided that the following conditions are met:

- The PET is done at a PET imaging center with a PET scanner that has been approved by the FDA;
- The PET scan is a rest alone or rest with pharmacologic stress PET scan, used for noninvasive imaging of the perfusion of the heart for the diagnosis and management of patients with known or suspected coronary artery disease, using Rb 82; and
- Either the PET scan is used in place of, but not in addition to, a single photon emission computed tomography (SPECT) or the PET scan is used following a SPECT that was found inconclusive.

60.5—Expanded Coverage of PET Scan for Solitary Pulmonary Nodules (SPNs)

(Rev. 223, Issued: 07-02-04) (Effective/Implementation: Not Applicable)

For dates of service on or after January 1, 1998, Medicare expanded PET scan coverage to include characterization of solitary pulmonary nodules (SPNs).

60.6—Expanded Coverage of PET Scans Effective for Services on or after July 1, 1999

(Rev. 223, Issued: 07-02-04) (Effective/Implementation: Not Applicable)

Effective *for services performed on or after* July 1, 1999, Medicare expanded coverage of PET scans to include the evaluation of recurrent colorectal cancer in patients with rising levels of carinoembryonic antigen (CEA), for the staging of lymphoma (both Hodgkins and non-Hodgkins) when the PET scan substitutes for a gallium scan or lymphangiogram, and for the staging of recurrent melanoma prior to surgery, provided certain conditions are met. All three indications are covered only when using the radiopharmaceutical FDG-(2-[flourine-18]-fluoro-2-deoxy-D-glucose), and are further predicated on the legal availability of FDG for use in such scans.

60.7—Expanded Coverage of PET Scans Effective for Services on or After July 1, 2001

(Rev. 223, Issued: 07-02-04) (Effective/Implementation: Not Applicable)

See the Medicare National Coverage Determinations Manual, Section 220.6, for specific coverage criteria for PET Scans. Coverage is expanded for PET scans to include the following effective July 1, 2001:

- Scans performed with dedicated full-ring scanners will be covered. Gamma camera systems with at least a 1 inch thick crystal are eligible for coverage in addition to those already approved by CMS (FDA approved);
- The provider must maintain on file the doctor's referral and documentation that the procedure involved:
  - Only FDA approved drugs and devices and,
  - Did not involve investigational drugs, or procedures using investigational drugs, as determined by the FDA;
- The ordering physician is responsible for certifying the medical necessity of the study according to the conditions. The physician must have documentation in the beneficiary's medical record to support the referral supplied to the PET scan provider.

The following is a brief summary of the expanded coverage as of July 1, 2001:

- PET is covered for diagnosis, initial staging and restaging of non-small cell lung cancer (NSCLC).
- Usage of PET for colorectal cancer has been expanded to include diagnosis, staging, and restaging.
- Usage of PET for the initial staging, and restaging of both Hodgkin's and non-Hodgkin's disease.
- Usage of PET for the diagnosis, initial staging, and restaging of melanoma. **(PET Scans are NOT covered for the evaluation of regional nodes.)**
- Medicare covers PET for the diagnosis, initial staging, and restaging of esophageal cancer.
- Usage of PET for Head and Neck Cancers. **(PET scans for head and neck cancer is NOT covered for central nervous system or thyroid cancers.)**

- Usage of PET following an inconclusive single photon emission computed tomography (SPECT) only for myocardial viability. In the event that a patient has received a SPECT and the physician finds the results to be inconclusive, only then may a PET scan be ordered utilizing the proper documentation.
- Usage of PET for pre-surgical evaluation for patients with refractory seizures.

NOTE: Effective January 1, 2002, the definitions of HCPCS Codes G0210 through G0230 have been updated to properly reflect the type of PET scanner used.

60.8—Expanded Coverage of PET Scans for Breast Cancer Effective for Dates of Service on or After October 1, 2002

(Rev. 527, Issued: 04-15-05, Effective: 01-28-05, Implementation: 04-18-05)

Effective for dates of service on or after October 1, 2002, Medicare will cover FDG PET as an adjunct to other imaging modalities for staging and restaging for locoregional, recurrence or metastasis of *breast cancer.* Monitoring treatment of a locally advanced breast cancer tumor and metastatic breast cancer when a change in therapy is contemplated is also covered as an adjunct to other imaging modalities. The baseline PET study for monitoring should be done under the code for staging or restaging.

Medicare continues to have a national non-coverage determination for initial diagnosis of breast cancer and initial staging of axillary lymph nodes. Medicare coverage now includes PET as an adjunct to standard imaging modalities for staging patients with distant metastasis or restaging patients with locoregional recurrence or metastasis *of breast cancer*; as an adjunct to standard imaging modalities for monitoring for women with locally advanced and metastatic breast cancer when a change in therapy is contemplated.

CPT Codes for PET Scans Performed on or After October 1, 2002 for Breast Cancer

Contractors shall advise providers to use the appropriate CPT code from section 60.3.1 for covered breast cancer indications for services performed on or after January 28, 2005.

G0252 through G0254 are applicable codes for billing breast cancer PET scans performed on or after October 1, 2002.

NOTE: The NCD Manual contains a description of coverage. FDG Positron Emission Tomography is a minimally invasive diagnostic procedure using positron camera [tomograph] to measure the decay of radioisotopes such as FDG. The CMS determined that the benefit category for the requested indications fell under §1861(s)(3) of the Act diagnostic service.).

60.9—Coverage of PET Scans for Myocardial Viability

(Rev. 223, Issued: 07-02-04) (Effective/Implementation: Not Applicable)

FDG PET is covered for the determination of myocardial viability following an inconclusive single photon computed tomography test (SPECT) from July 1, 2001, through September 30, 2002. Only full ring scanners are covered as the scanning medium for this service from July 1, 2001, through December 31, 2001. However, as of January 1, 2002, full and partial ring scanners are covered for myocardial viability following an inconclusive SPECT.

Beginning October 1, 2002, Medicare will cover FDG PET for the determination of myocardial viability as a primary or initial diagnostic study prior to revascularization, and will continue to cover FDG PET when used as a follow-up to an inconclusive SPECT. However, if a patient received a FDG PET study with inconclusive results, a follow-up SPECT is not covered. FDA full and partial ring PET scanners are covered. In the event that a patient receives a SPECT with inconclusive results, a PET scan may be performed and covered by Medicare. However, a SPECT is not covered following a FDG PET with inconclusive results. See the Medicare National Coverage Determinations Manual, Section 220.6 for specific frequency limitations for Myocardial Viability following an inconclusive SPECT.

Documentation that these conditions are met should be maintained by the referring provider as part of the beneficiary's medical record.

HCPCS Code for PET Scan for Myocardial Viability

78459—Myocardial imaging, positron emission tomography (PET), metabolic evaluation

60.10—Coverage of PET Scans for PET Scan for Thyroid Cancer

(Rev. 527, Issued: 04-15-05, Effective: 01-28-05, Implementation: 04-18-05)

For services furnished on or after October 1, 2003, Medicare covers the use of FDG PET for thyroid cancer only for restaging of recurrent or residual thyroid cancers of follicular cell origin that have previously been treated by thyroidectomy and radioiodine ablation and have a serum thyroglobulin > 10ng/ml and negative I-131 whole body scan. Contractors shall advise providers to use the appropriate CPT code from section 60.3.1 for thyroid cancer for services performed on or after January 28, 2005.

HCPCS Code for Thyroid Cancer

G0296—PET imaging, full and partial ring PET scanner only, for restaging of reviously treated thyroid cancer of follicular cell origin following negative I-131 whole body scan.

60.11—Coverage of PET Scans for Perfusion of the Heart Using Ammonia N-13

Rev. 223, Issued: 07-02-04) (Effective/Implementation: Not Applicable)

Effective for service performed on or after October 1, 2003, PET scans performed at rest or with pharmacological stress used for noninvasive imaging of the perfusion of the heart for the diagnosis and management of patients with known or suspected coronary artery disease using the FDA-approved radiopharmaceutical ammonia N-13 are covered, provided the following requirements are met.

60.12—Coverage for PET Scans for Dementia and Neurodegenerative Diseases

(Rev. 527, Issued: 04-15-05, Effective: 01-28-05, Implementation: 04-18-05)

Effective for dates of service on or after September 15, 2004, Medicare will cover FDG PET scans for a differential diagnosis of fronto-temporal dementia (FTD) and Alzheimer's disease OR; its use in a CMS-approved practical clinical trial focused on the utility of FDG-PET in the diagnosis or treatment of dementing neurodegenerative diseases. Refer to Pub. 100-03 (National Coverage Determinations (NCD) Manual), section 220.6.13, for complete coverage conditions and clinical trial requirements.

A—Carrier and FI Billing Requirements for Pet Scan Claims for FDG-PET for the Differential Diagnosis of Fronto-temporal Dementia and Alzheimer's Disease:

CPT Code for PET Scans for Dementia and Neurodegenerative Diseases

Contractors shall advise providers to use the appropriate CPT code from section 60.3.1 for dementia and neurodegenerative diseases for services performed on or after January 28, 2005.

Diagnosis Codes for PET Scans for Dementia and Neurodegenerative Diseases

The contractor shall ensure one of the following appropriate diagnosis codes is present on claims for PET Scans for AD:

290.0, 290.10–290.13, 290.20–290.21, 290.3, 331.0, 331.11, 331.19, 331.2, 331.9, 780.93

Medicare contractors shall use an appropriate Medicare Summary Notice (MSN) message such as 16.48, "Medicare does not pay for this item or service for this condition" to deny claims when submitted with an appropriate CPT code from section 60.3.1 and with a diagnosis code other than the range of codes listed above.

Also, contractors shall use an appropriate Remittance Advice (RA) such as 11, "The diagnosis is inconsistent with the procedure."

Medicare contractors shall instruct providers to issue an Advanced Beneficiary Notice to beneficiaries advising them of potential financial liability prior to delivering the service if one of the appropriate diagnosis codes will not be present on the claim.

Provider Documentation Required with the PET Scan Claim

Medicare contractors shall inform providers to ensure the conditions mentioned in the NCD Manual, section 220.6.13, have been met. The information must also be maintained in the beneficiary's medical record:

- Date of onset of symptoms;
- Diagnosis of clinical syndrome (normal aging, mild cognitive impairment or MCI: mild, moderate, or severe dementia);
- Mini mental status exam (MMSE) or similar test score;
- Presumptive cause (possible, probably, uncertain AD);
- Any neuropsychological testing performed;
- Results of any structural imaging (MRI, CT) performed;
- Relevant laboratory tests (B12, thyroid hormone); and,
- Number and name of prescribed medications.

B—Carrier and FI Billing Requirements for FDG-PET Scans Claims for CMS-approved Neurodegenerative Disease Practical Clinical Trial

Carriers and FIs

Contractors should not receive claims for this service until the clinical trial centers have been identified. Once these centers are identified, CMS will list the centers on the CMS Web site.

Carriers Only

Carriers shall pay claims PET Scan G0336 for beneficiaries participating in a CMS-approved clinical trial submitted with the **QV** modifier. Refer to Pub. 100-03, NCD Manual, section 220.6, for complete policy and clinical trial requirements.

FIs Only

In order to pay claims for PET scans on behalf of beneficiaries participating in a CMS-approved clinical trial, FIs require providers to submit claims with ICD-9 code V70.7 in the second diagnosis position on the Form CMS-1450 (UB-92), or the electronic equivalent, with the appropriate principal diagnosis code and an appropriate CPT code from section 60.3.1. Refer to Publication 100-03, NCD Manual, section 220.6.13, for complete coverage policy and clinical trial requirements.

60.13—Billing Requirements for PET Scans for Specific Indications of Cervical Cancer for Services Performed on or After January 28, 2005

(Rev. 527, Issued: 04-15-05, Effective: 01-28-05, Implementation: 04-18-05)

Contractors shall accept claims for these services with the appropriate CPT code listed in section 60.3.1. Refer to Pub. 100-03, Section 220.6.14 for complete coverage guidelines for this new PET oncology indications. Implementation date for these CPT codes will be April 18, 2005.

60.14—Billing Requirements for PET Scans for Non-Covered Indications

(Rev. 527, Issued: 04-15-05, Effective: 01-28-05, Implementation: 04-18-05)

For services performed on or after January 28, 2005, contractors shall accept claims with the following HCPCS code for non-covered PET indications:

G0235: PET imaging, any site not otherwise specified

Short Descriptor: PET not otherwise specified

Type of Service: 4

NOTE: This code is for a non-covered service.

104, Chapter 18

50—PROSTATE CANCER SCREENING TESTS AND PROCEDURES

(Rev. 1, 10-01-03)

B3-4182, A3-3616

Sections 1861(s)(2)(P) and 1861(oo) of the Act (as added by §4103 of the Balanced Budget Act of 1997), provide for Medicare Part B coverage of certain prostate cancer screening tests subject to certain coverage, frequency, and payment limitations. Effective for services furnished on or after January 1, 2000, Medicare Part B covers prostate cancer screening tests/procedures for the early detection of prostate cancer. Coverage of prostate cancer screening tests includes the following procedures furnished to an individual for the early detection of prostate cancer:

- Screening digital rectal examination, and
- Screening prostate specific antigen (PSA) blood test.

Each test may be paid at a frequency of once every 12 months for men who have attained age 50 (i.e., starting at least one day after they have attained age 50), if at least 11 months have passed following the month in which the last Medicare-covered screening digital rectal examination was performed (for digital rectal exams) or PSA test was performed (for PSA tests).

50.1—Definitions

(Rev. 1, 10-01-03)

A3-3616.A.1 and 2

A—Screening Digital Rectal Examination

Screening digital rectal examination means a clinical examination of an individual's prostate for nodules or other abnormalities of the prostate. This screening must be performed by a doctor of medicine or osteopathy (as defined in §186l(r)(1) of the Act), or by a physician assistant, nurse practitioner, clinical nurse specialist, or by a certified nurse mid-wife (as defined in §1861(aa) and §1861(gg) of the Act), who is authorized under State law to perform the examination, fully knowledgeable about the beneficiary, and would be responsible for explaining the results of the examination to the beneficiary.

B—Screening Prostate Specific Antigen (PSA) Tests

Screening prostate specific antigen (PSA) is a test that measures the level of prostate specific antigen in an individual's blood. This screening must be ordered by the beneficiary's physician or by the beneficiary's physician assistant, nurse practitioner, clinical nurse specialist, or certified nurse midwife (the term "physician" is defined in §1861(r)(1) of the Act to mean a doctor of medicine or osteopathy and the terms "physician assistant, nurse practitioner, clinical nurse specialist, or certified nurse midwife" are defined in §1861(aa) and §1861(gg) of the Act) who is fully knowledgeable about the beneficiary, and who would be responsible for explaining the results of the test to the beneficiary.

50.2—Deductible and Coinsurance

(Rev. 1, 10-01-03)

B3-4182.3

The screening PSA test is a lab test to which neither deductible nor coinsurance apply.

Both deductible (if unmet) and coinsurance are applicable to screening rectal examinations.

50.3—Payment Method—FIs and Carriers

(Rev. 1, 10-01-03)

B3-4182.3, A3-3616.C

Screening PSA tests (G0103) are paid under the clinical diagnostic lab fee schedule.

---

*CPT only © 2004. *Current Procedural Terminology, 2005, Professional Edition*, American Medical Association. All Rights Reserved.

Screening rectal examinations (G0102) are paid under the MPFS except for the following bill types identified (FI only). Bill types not identified are paid under the MPFS.

12X = Outpatient Prospective Payment System
13X = Outpatient Prospective Payment System
14X = Outpatient Prospective Payment System
71X = Included in All Inclusive Rate
73X = Included in All Inclusive Rate
85X = Cost (Payment should be consistent with amounts paid for code 84153 or code 86316.)

RHCs and FQHCs should include the charges on the claims for future inclusion in encounter rate calculations.

50.3.1—Correct Coding Requirements for Carrier Claims

(Rev. 1, 10-01-03)

B3-4182.6

Billing and payment for a Digital Rectal Exam (DRE) (G0102) is bundled into the payment for a covered E/M service (CPT codes 99201–99456 and 99499)* when the two services are furnished to a patient on the same day. If the DRE is the only service or is provided as part of an otherwise noncovered service, HCPCS code G0102 would be payable separately if all other coverage requirements are met.

50.4—HCPCS, Revenue, and Type of Service Codes

(Rev. 1, 10-01-03)

The appropriate bill types for billing the FI on Form CMS-1450 or its electronic equivalent are 12X, 13X, 14X, 22X, 23X, 71X, 73X, 75X, and 85X.

HCPCS code G0102—for prostate cancer screening digital rectal examination.

- Carrier TOS is 1
- FI revenue code is 0770

HCPCS code G0103—for prostate cancer screening PSA tests

- Carrier TOS is 5
- FI revenue code is 030X

50.5—Diagnosis Coding

(Rev. 1, 10-01-03)

B3-4182.7

Prostate cancer screening digital rectal examinations and screening Prostate Specific Antigen (PSA) blood tests must be billed using screening ("V") code V76.44 (Special Screening for Malignant Neoplasms, Prostate).

50.6—Calculating Frequency

(Rev. 1, 10-01-03)

A3-3616.D and E, B3-4182.4, B3-4182.5

Calculating Frequency—To determine the 11-month period, the count starts beginning with the month after the month in which a previous test/procedure was performed.

EXAMPLE: The beneficiary received a screening prostate specific antigen test in January 2002. Start counts beginning February 2002. The beneficiary is eligible to receive another screening prostate specific antigen test in January 2003 (the month after 11 months have passed).

Common Working File (CWF) Edits

Beginning October 1, 2000, the following CWF edits were implemented for dates of service January 1, 2000, and later, for prostate cancer screening tests and procedures for the following:

- Age;
- Frequency;
- Sex; and
- Valid HCPCS code.

50.7—MSN Messages

(Rev. 1, 10-01-03)

B3-4182.8.B, A3-3616.F

If a claim for screening prostate specific antigen test or a screening digital rectal examination is being denied because of the age of the beneficiary, FIs use MSN message 18.13:

This service is not covered for patients under 50 years of age.

The Spanish version of this MSN message should read:

Este servicio no está cubierto hasta después de que el beneficiario cumpla 50 años.

Carriers use MSN Message 18.19:

This service is not covered until after the patient's 50th birthday.

The Spanish version of this MSN message should read:

Este servicio no está cubierto hasta después de que el beneficiario cumpla 50 años.

If the claim for screening prostate specific antigen test or screening digital rectal examination is being denied because the time period between the same test or procedure has not passed, FIs and carriers use MSN message 18.14:

Service is being denied because it has not been 12 months since your last test/procedure) of this kind.

The Spanish version of this MSN message should read:

Este servicio está siendo denegado ya que no han transcurrido (12, 24, 48) meses desde el último (examen/procedimiento) de esta clase.

50.8—Remittance Advice Notices

(Rev. 1, 10-01-03)

B3-4182.8, A3-3616.G

If the claim for a screening prostate antigen test or screening digital rectal examination is being denied because the patient is less than 50 years of age, ANSI X12N 835.

- Claim adjustment reason code 6 "the procedure/revenue code is inconsistent with the patient's age," at the line level; and
- Remark code M140 "Service is not covered until after the patient's 50th birthday, i.e., no coverage prior to the day after the 50th birthday."

If the claim for a screening prostate specific antigen test or screening digital rectal examination is being denied because the time period between the test/procedure has not passed, contractors use ANSI X12N 835 claim adjustment reason code 119 "Benefit maximum for this time period has been reached" at the line level.

If the claim for a screening prostate antigen test or screening digital rectal examination is being denied due to the absence of diagnosis code V76.44 on the claim, use ANSI X12N 835 claim adjustment reason code 47, "This (these) diagnosis(es) is (are) not covered, missing, or invalid."

50.18—Preventive Care

(Rev. 214, 06-25-04)

AB-02-010

18.1—Routine examinations and related services not covered.

18.2—This immunization and/or preventive care is not covered.

18.3—Screening mammography is not covered for women *under* 35 years of age.

18.4—This service is being denied because it has not been 12 months since your last examination of this kind. (NOTE: Insert appropriate number of months.)

18.6—A screening mammography is covered only once for women age 35—39.

18.7—Screening pap smears are covered only once every 24 months unless high risk factors are present.

18.12—Screening mammograms are covered annually for women 40 years of age and older.

18.13—This service is not covered for beneficiaries under 50 years of age.

18.14—Service is being denied because it has not been (12, 24, 48) months since your last (test/procedure) of this kind.

18.15—Medicare only covers this procedure for beneficiaries considered to be at high risk for colorectal cancer.

18.16—This service is being denied because payment has already been made for a similar procedure within a set time frame.

18.17—Medicare pays for a screening Pap smear and a screening pelvic examination once every 2 years unless high risk factors are present.

18.18—Medicare does not pay for this service separately since payment of it is included in our allowance for other services you received on the same day.

18.19—This service is not covered until after the beneficiary's 50th birthday

18.20—Medicare does not pay for both film and digital screening mammography performed on the same day.

18.21—Medicare does not pay for both film and digital diagnostic mammography performed on the same day.

51—CRYOSURGERY OF THE PROSTATE GLAND

(Rev. 260, Issued 07-30-04, Effective: 01-01-05/Implementation: 01-03-05)

Cryosurgery of the prostate gland, also known as cryosurgical ablation of the prostate (CAP), destroys prostate tissue by applying extremely cold temperatures in order to reduce the size of the prostate gland.

51.1—Coverage Requirements

(Rev. 260, Issued 07-30-04, Effective: 01-01-05/Implementation: 01-03-05)

Medicare covers cryosurgery of the prostate gland effective for claims with dates of service on or after July 1, 1999. The coverage is for:

1. Primary treatment of patients with clinically localized prostate cancer, Stages T1–T3 (diagnosis code is 185—malignant neoplasm of prostate).

2. Salvage therapy (effective for claims with dates of service on or after July 1, 2001 for patients:

    a. Having recurrent, localized prostate cancer;

    b. Failing a trial of radiation therapy as their primary treatment; and

    c. Meeting one of these conditions: State T2B or below; Gleason score less than 9 or; PSA less than 8 ng/ml.

51.2—Billing Requirements

(Rev. 260, Issued 07-30-04, Effective: 01-01-05/Implementation: 01-03-05)

Claims for cryosurgery for the prostate gland are to be submitted on Form CMS–1450 or electronic equivalent. This procedure can be rendered in an inpatient or outpatient hospital setting (types of bill (TOB) 11x 13x, 83x, and 85x).

The FI will look for the following when processing claims with cryosurgery services:

Diagnosis Code 185 (must be on all cryosurgical claims);

• For outpatient claims HCPCS 55873 and revenue code 0361, Cryosurgery ablation of localized prostate cancer, stages T1–T3 (includes ultrasonic guidance for interstital cryosurgery probe placement, postoperative irrigations and aspiration of sloughing tissue included) must be on all outpatient claims; and

For inpatient claims procedure code 60.62 (perineal prostatectomy—the definition includes cryoablation of prostate, cryostatec-

tomy of prostate, and radical cryosurgical ablation of prostate) must be on the claim.

51.3—Payment Requirements

(Rev. 260, Issued 07-30-04, Effective: 01-01-05/Implementation: 01-03-05)

This service may be paid as a primary treatment for patients with clinically localized prostate cancer, Stages T1–T3. The ultrasonic guidance associated with this procedure will not be paid for separately, but is bundled into the payment for the surgical procedure. When one provider has furnished the cryosurgical ablation and another the ultrasonic guidance, the provider of the ultrasonic guidance must seek compensation from the provider of the cryosurgical ablation.

Effective July 1, 2001, cryosurgery performed as salvage therapy, will be paid only according to the coverage requirements described above.

Type of facility and setting determines the basis of payment:

• For services performed on an inpatient or outpatient basis in a CAH, TOBs 11x and 85x: the FI will pay 101 percent of reasonable cost minus any applicable deductible and coinsurance.

• For services performed on an inpatient basis in short term acute care hospitals, (including those in Guam, America Samoa, Virgin Islands, Saipan, and Indian Health Services Hospitals) TOB 11x: the FI will pay the DRG payment minus any applicable deductible and coinsurance.

• For services performed on an outpatient basis in hospitals subject to the Outpatient PPS, TOB 13x: the FI will pay the assigned APC minus any applicable deductible and coinsurance.

• For outpatient services in hospitals that are exempt from OPPS (such as in American Samoa, Virgin Islands, Guam, and Saipan) TOBs 13x or 83x: the FI will pay reasonable cost subject to the ASC payment limitation for TOB 83x, minus any applicable deductible and coinsurance.

• For outpatient services in Indian Health Service hospitals TOBs 13x and 83x: the FI will pay reasonable cost subject to the ASC payment limitation for TOB 83x. minus any applicable deductible and coinsurance.

• For inpatient or outpatient services in hospitals in Maryland, make payment according to the State Cost Containment system.

For services performed on an inpatient basis: the hospitals exempt from inpatient acute care PPS shall be paid on reasonable cost basis, minus any applicable deductible and coinsurance.

104, Chapter 8

70—PAYMENT FOR HOME DIALYSIS

(Rev. 1, 10-01-03)

A3-3644, PRM-1-2706.1.E, PRM-1-2706.2, A3-3169, RO-2 3440.2, B3-4270.1

Home dialysis is dialysis performed by an appropriately trained dialysis patient at home. Hemodialysis, CCPD, IPD and CAPD may be performed at home. For all dialysis services furnished by an ESRD facility, the facility must accept assignment, and only the facility may be paid by the Medicare program. Method II suppliers can receive payment for patients selecting Method II. The Method II supplier must accept assignment. Method II suppliers receive payment for supplies and equipment only.

For purposes of home dialysis, a skilled nursing facility (SNF) may qualify as a beneficiary's home. The services are excluded from SNF consolidated billing for its inpatients. The home dialysis services are billed either by the ESRD facility or the supplier depending on the Method selection made by the beneficiary.

70.1—Method Selection for Home Dialysis Payment

(Rev. 1, 10-01-03)

B3-4271, PRM-1-2740.2

Medicare beneficiaries dialyzing at home can choose between two methods for Medicare program payment for care (exclusive of physician services), Method I or Method II as described below in §70.2.

When an ESRD beneficiary begins a course of home dialysis, he or she fills out the Form CMS-382, "ESRD Beneficiary Selection," to choose whether he or she wants to use Method I or Method II to obtain home dialysis equipment and supplies. Refer to http://www.cms.hhs.gov/forms/cms382.pdf for a copy of the ESRD Method Selection Form CMS-382, and the related instructions.

The beneficiary and or provider must:

- Furnish the information requested in items 1-6;
- Check only one block in items 7-9; and
- Enter the effective date at the bottom of item 7

The beneficiary must sign and date in items 11 and 12.

The facility sends the completed form to the FI. When the FI receives the correctly completed Form CMS-382, it must enter the beneficiary's choice into the common working file (CWF) within 30 days of receipt. The format is in Chapter 27. For method II selections, the FI must follow-up every 30 days until the method selection has been correctly entered.

If a claim is received by the Intermediary on behalf of a beneficiary for whom an initial election is not recorded on CWF, CWF informs the FI to return the claim to the provider. The provider must submit a copy of the completed Form CMS-382 prior to resubmitting the claim.

If a claim is received by the Intermediary on behalf of a beneficiary for whom Method I has been selected, CWF informs the FI to deny the claim.

DMERCs deny Method II claims where there is no method selection on file at CWF.

70.1.1—Change in Method

(Rev. 1, 10-01-03)

PRM-1-2740.2.D

Changes in method selection are effective January 1 of the year following the year in which the beneficiary requested the change. However, the FI may grant an exception in certain situations. The following is a sample list (i.e., not all-inclusive) of possible situations:

- Failure of a kidney transplant occurred within the past 6 months;
- Patient becomes confined to a nursing home or hospice;
- Home patient becomes an in-facility patient for any reason and then elects to go on home dialysis again after at least 6 full months in the center;
- Patient changes the place of residence to a location where the new facility does not recognize present method of payment and another facility is not available; or
- Patient is in a life threatening situation.

70.2—Prevention of Double Billing Under Method I and II

(Rev. 1, 10-01-03)

PRM-1-2740.3

Under Method I payment is made to the ESRD facility by the FI. Under Method II, payment is made to the facility for support services by the FI, but payment for home dialysis equipment and supplies is made to the supplier by the DMERC. The beneficiary's method and effective date are recorded on CWF.

The FI or contractor must pay claims in accordance with the documentation on the CWF record.

70.3—Overpayments

(Rev. 1, 10-01-03)

PRM-1-2740.4

Any overpayments that occur are subject to recovery following the usual Medicare program rules and procedures.

80—HOME DIALYSIS METHOD I BILLING TO THE INTERMEDIARY

(Rev. 1, 10-01-03)

A3-3644.A, PRM-1-2710, PRM-1-2710.4, A3-3169, RDF-318, RO2-3440, B3-4270, B3-4271

If the Medicare home dialysis patient chooses Method I, the dialysis facility with which the Medicare home patient is associated assumes responsibility for providing all home dialysis equipment and supplies, and home support services. For these services, the facility receives the same Medicare dialysis payment rate as it would receive for an in-facility patient under the composite rate system. The beneficiary is responsible for paying any unmet Part B deductible and the 20-percent coinsurance. After the beneficiary's Part B deductible is met, the FI pays 80 percent of the specific facility's composite rate for each in-facility outpatient maintenance dialysis treatment.

Under Method I items and services included in the composite rate must be furnished by the facility, either directly or under arrangement. The cost of an item or service is included under the composite rate unless specifically excluded. Therefore, the determination as to whether an item or service is covered under the composite rate payment does not depend on the frequency that dialysis patients require the item or service, or the number of patients who require it. If the facility fails to provide (either directly or under arrangement) any part of the items and services covered under the rate, the facility cannot be paid any amount for the items and services that it does furnish.

New items or services developed after the rate applicable for that particular year was computed are included in the composite rate payments. As such, ESRD facilities assume the responsibility for providing a dialysis service and must decide whether a particular item or service is medically appropriate and cost effective. Since the composite rate is adjusted, as necessary, based on the most recent cost data available to CMS, the costs of new items and services are taken into account in setting future rates. Similarly, any savings attributable to advancements in the treatment of ESRD accrue to the facility because no adjustment to any individual facility's rate is made.

80.1—Items and Services Included in the Composite Rate for Home Dialysis

(Rev. 1, 10-01-03)

A3-3169.1, PRM-1-2712

The following items are paid for and must be furnished under the composite rate. The facility may furnish them directly under arrangements, to all of its home dialysis patients. If the facility fails to furnish (either directly or under arrangements) any part of the items and services covered under the rate, then the facility cannot be paid any amount for the part of the items and services that the facility does furnish.

- Medically necessary dialysis equipment and dialysis support equipment;
- Home dialysis support services including the delivery, installation, maintenance, repair, and testing of home dialysis equipment, and home support equipment;
- Purchase and delivery of all necessary dialysis supplies;
- Routine ESRD related laboratory tests; and
- All dialysis services furnished by the facility's staff.

The following items and services are included in the composite rate and may not be billed separately when furnished by a dialysis facility:

- Staff time used to administer blood;
- Declotting of shunts and any supplies used to declot shunts by facility staff in the dialysis unit;
- Oxygen and the administration of oxygen furnished in the dialysis unit;
- Staff time used to administer separately billable parenteral items;
- Bicarbonate dialysate;
- Cardiac monitoring;

- Catheter changes (Ideal Loop);
- Suture removal;
- Dressing changes;
- Crash cart usage for cardiac arrest; or
- Staff time used to collect specimens for all laboratory tests.

Sometimes outpatient dialysis related services (e.g., declotting of shunts, suture removal, injecting separately billable ESRD related drugs) are furnished in a department of the hospital other than the dialysis unit (e.g., the emergency room). These services may be paid in addition to the composite rate only if the services could not be furnished in a dialysis facility or the dialysis unit of the hospital, due to the absence of specialized equipment or staff, which can be found only in the other department. In the case of emergency services furnished in the hospital emergency room (ER), the services are paid separately subject to the additional requirement that there is a sudden onset of a medical condition manifesting itself by acute symptoms of sufficient severity (including severe pain) such that the absence of immediate medical attention in the ER could reasonably be expected to result in either:

- Placing the patient's health in serious jeopardy;
- Causing serious impairment to bodily functions; or
- Causing serious dysfunction of any bodily organ or part.

These situations are rare and, in the absence of documentation to the contrary, these conditions are deemed to be not met.

80.2—General Intermediary Bill Processing Procedures for Method I Home Dialysis Services

(Rev. 1, 10-01-03)

A3-3644, CWF documentation

General instructions for completing the UB-92 or ANSI X12N formats are in Chapter 25. Instructions in §§50 and 50.3, above, apply to provider reporting of ESRD home dialysis services under Method I.

All home dialysis patients must have chosen either Method I or Method II.

The FI uses the method of election information provided in the "Method" field of CWF trailer 14 "ESRD Method Trailer" attached to the query response when an ESRD claim is submitted for approval.

If the beneficiary has elected Method I, the FI pays the facility the composite rate plus any additional billable services.

If the beneficiary has elected Method II, the facility is not paid the composite rate or for home dialysis supplies and equipment. Payment is made only for support, backup, and emergency dialysis services.

80.2.1—Required Billing Information for Method I Claims

(Rev. 1, 10-01-03)

A3-3644.2

Method I claims require the same information as listed in §50.3 above with the following changes.

FLs 24, 25, 26, 27, 28, 29 and 30. Condition Codes—Hospital-based and independent renal facilities complete these items. Note that one of the codes 71-76 is applicable for every bill. Special Program Indicator codes A0-A9 are not required.

Condition Code Structure (only codes effecting Medicare payment/processing are shown).

74—Home—Providers enter this code to indicate the billing is for a patient who received dialysis services at home, but code 75 below did not apply.

80.3—Calculating Payment for Intermittent Peritoneal Dialysis (IPD) for Method I Claims Submitted to the Intermediary

(Rev. 1, 10-01-03)

PRM-1-2709, PRM-1-2709.1.A, 2709.2, A3-3112.6

The value of a typical week of dialysis services generally serves as the maximum weekly payment; e.g., where, for nonmedical reasons, more frequent dialysis sessions of shorter duration are furnished.

While maintenance IPD is usually accomplished in sessions of 10-12 hours duration, three times per week, it is sometimes accomplished in fewer sessions of longer duration. The payment screens applicable to maintenance IPD, as well as the facility's actual payment for maintenance IPD, depends on the length of the dialysis session and the number of sessions furnished per week. If additional dialysis beyond the usual weekly maintenance dialysis is required because of special circumstances, the facility's claim for these extra services must be accompanied by a medical justification. Under these circumstances, additional payment may be made. In all cases, the Part B deductible and coinsurance apply.

A—Maintenance IPD Sessions of Less Than 20 Hours Duration

The payment screen applicable to a facility for maintenance IPD sessions of less than 20 hours duration is the same as the payment screen applicable to that facility for hemodialysis. (See §50.6.2, above.) However, in addition to the per dialysis payment screen, there is also a weekly maintenance IPD screen equal to three times the per treatment hemodialysis screen. For example, if the applicable hemodialysis payment screen for a facility is $150, then its maintenance IPD payment is $150 per dialysis session and $450 per week. Therefore, if the facility furnished two 12-hour IPD sessions to a patient in a week, its payment is based on a $300 payment screen for that week. If the facility furnished three or more 12-hour IPD sessions to a patient in a week, payment is based on a $450 weekly payment screen for that week.

B—Maintenance IPD Sessions of More Than 20 But Less Than 30 Hours Duration

Where maintenance IPD is accomplished in sessions of 20 hours or more duration but less than 30 hours, payment is made in accordance with the same weekly payment screen as described in subsection A. However, the individual dialysis session screen is equal to one and one half times the individual dialysis session screen derived in subsection A. Therefore, if the facility in the above example furnishes one 20-hour IPD session to a patient in a week, its payment is based on a $225 screen. Payment for two 20-hour maintenance IPD sessions to a patient in a week is based on a $450 screen for that week.

C—Maintenance IPD Sessions of 30 Hours or More Duration

Medical consultants indicate that patients undergoing IPD should be dialyzed more often than once per week. However, sometimes geographical considerations or other exigencies require a compromise to be made between optimum medical practice and patient convenience. In recognition of these special cases, IPD sessions of 30 hours or more duration are paid in accordance with the weekly payment screen described in subsection A. Therefore, if the facility in the above example furnished one 30-hour IPD session to a patient, it is paid in accordance with a $450 screen for that week.

Intermittent Peritoneal Dialysis (IPD) is furnished in a dialysis facility or at home. IPD in a facility is very impractical because of the great amount of time required; therefore, there are very few patients who receive IPD in the facility.

80.3.1—IPD at Home for Method I Claims Submitted to the Intermediary

(Rev. 1, 10-01-03)

PRM-1-2709.1.B

IPD in the home is accomplished according to any one of several schedules. The total weekly dialysis time varies from 50 to 80 hours. For example, home IPD may be furnished everyday for 10 hours per day, every other day for 15 hours per dialysis day, every night for 8 hours per night, etc. Regardless of the particular regimen used, under the composite rate home IPD is paid based on a weekly equivalence of three composite rates per week

With its FI's approval, a facility may be paid an equivalent daily rate equal to 3/7 of its usual composite rate.

80.4—Calculating Payment for Continuous Ambulatory Peritoneal Dialysis (CAPD) and Continuous Cycling Peritoneal Dialysis (CCPD) Under the Composite rate

(Rev. 1, 10-01-03)

PRM-1-2709.2, A3-3644.1

CAPD and CCPD are furnished on a continuous basis, not in discrete sessions and, therefore, are paid on a weekly or daily basis, not on a per treatment basis. Billing instructions require providers to report the number of days in the units field. A facility's daily payment rate is 1/7 of three times the composite rate for a single hemodialysis treatment.

The equivalent weekly or daily IPD or CAPD/CCPD payment does not depend upon the number of exchanges of dialysate fluid per day (typically 3-5) or the actual number of days per week that the patient undergoes dialysis. The weekly (or daily) rate is based on the equivalency of one week of IPD or CAPD/CCPD to one week of hemodialysis, regardless of the actual number of dialysis days or exchanges in that week.

All home dialysis support services, equipment and supplies necessary for home IPD or CAPD/CCPD are included in the composite rate payment. No support services, equipment or supplies may be paid in addition to the composite rate.

90—METHOD II BILLING

(Rev. 1, 10-01-03)

A3-3644.A, RO-2-3440.C, B3-4270, B3-4271, B3-4270.1, B3-4270.2, B3-34271, PRM-1-2740, A3-3644.3

Physicians and independent laboratories, must submit claims (Form CMS-1500 or electronic equivalent) to their local carrier for services furnished to end stage renal disease (ESRD) beneficiaries. Suppliers of Method II dialysis equipment and supplies will submit their claims (Form CMS-1500 or electronic equivalent) to the appropriate Durable Medical Equipment Regional Carriers (DMERCs). All ESRD facilities must submit their claims to their appropriate FI.

The amount of Medicare payment under Method II for home dialysis equipment and supplies may NOT exceed $1974.45 for continuous cycling peritoneal dialysis (CCPD) and $1490.85 for all other methods of dialysis.

All laboratory tests furnished to home dialysis patients who have selected payment Method II (see §70.1 above), are billed to and paid by the carrier at the fee schedule, if the tests are performed by an independent laboratory for an independent dialysis facility patient.

If the beneficiary elects to deal directly with a supplier and make arrangements for securing the necessary supplies and equipment to dialyze at home, and chooses Method II, he/she deals directly with a supplier of home dialysis equipment and supplies (this supplier is not a dialysis facility). A supplier other than a facility bills the DMERC. There can be only one supplier per beneficiary, and the supplier must accept assignment. The beneficiary is responsible for any unmet Part B deductible and the 20 percent coinsurance.

Only a supplier that is not a dialysis facility may submit a claim to a DMERC for home dialysis supplies and equipment. Suppliers will submit these claims on Form CMS-1500, or electronic equivalent. Under Method II, beneficiaries may not submit any claims and cannot receive payment for any benefits for home dialysis equipment and supplies.

The supplier must have a written agreement with a Medicare approved dialysis facility that will provide all necessary support, backup, and emergency dialysis services. The dialysis facility will not receive a regular per treatment payment for a patient who chooses Method II.

However, if the facility provides any support services, backup, and emergency dialysis services to a beneficiary who selects this option, the facility is reimbursed for the items or services it furnishes. Hospital-based facilities are paid the reasonable cost of support services, subject to the lesser of cost or charges provisions of §1833(a)(2)(A) of the Act. Independent facilities are paid on a reasonable charge basis for any home dialysis support services they furnish.

A—Description of Support Services

Support services specifically applicable to home patients include but are not limited to:

- Surveillance of the patient's home adaptation, including provisions for visits to the home in accordance with a written plan prepared and periodically reviewed by a team that includes the patient's physician and other professionals familiar with the patient's condition;
- Furnishing dialysis-related emergency services;
- Consultation for the patient with a qualified social worker and a qualified dietician;
- Maintaining a record-keeping system which assures continuity of care;
- Maintaining and submitting all required documentation to the ESRD network;
- Assuring that the water supply is of the appropriate quality;
- Assuring that the appropriate supplies are ordered on an ongoing basis;
- Arranging for the provision of all ESRD laboratory tests;
- Testing and appropriate treatment of water used in dialysis;
- Monitoring the functioning of dialysis equipment;
- All other necessary dialysis services as required under the ESRD conditions for coverage;
- Watching the patient perform CAPD and assuring that it is done correctly, and reviewing with the patient any aspects of the technique he/she may have forgotten, or informing the patient of modification in apparatus or technique;
- Documenting whether the patient has or has not had peritonitis that requires physician intervention or hospitalization, (unless there is evidence of peritonitis, a culture for peritonitis is not necessary);
- Inspection of the catheter site; and
- Since home dialysis support services include maintaining a medical record for each home dialysis patient, the Method II supplier must report to the support service dialysis facility within 30 days all items and services that it furnished to the patient so that the facility can record this information in the patient's medical record.

The services must be furnished in accordance with the written plan required for home dialysis patients. See the Medicare Benefit Policy Manual, Chapter 15, for coverage of telehealth services, and this manual, Chapter 12 for billing telehealth.

Each of the support services may be paid routinely at a frequency of once per month. Any support services furnished in excess of this frequency must be documented for being reasonable and necessary. For example, the patient may contract peritonitis and require an unscheduled connecting tube change.

B—Reasonableness Determinations

Support services (which include the laboratory services included under the composite rate for in-facility patients) are paid on a reasonable charge basis to independent facilities and a reasonable cost basis to hospital-based facilities, subject to the Method II payment cap (refer to §140). A reasonable cost/charge determination must be made for each individual support service furnished to home patients. With respect to the connecting tube change, facilities may bill Medicare for the personnel services required to change the connecting tube, but must look to the Method II supplier for payment for the connecting tube itself.

The payment cap is not a payment rate that is paid automatically each month. Accordingly, in no case may the FI routinely pay any monthly amount for support services without a claim that shows the services actually furnished.

104, Chapter 8

60.4.2—Epoetin Alfa (EPO) Supplier Billing Requirements (Method II) on the Form CMS-1500 and Electronic Equivalent

(Rev 118, 03-05-04)

A. Claims with dates of service prior to January 1, 2004:

For claims with dates of service prior to January 1, 2004, the correct EPO code to use is the one that indicates the patient's most recent hematocrit (HCT) (rounded to the nearest whole percent) or hemoglobin (Hgb) (rounded to the nearest g/dl) prior to the date of service of the EPO. For example, if the patient's most recent hematocrit was 20.5 percent, bill Q9921; if it was 28.4 percent, bill Q9928.

To convert actual hemoglobin to corresponding hematocrit for Q code reporting, multiply the Hgb value by 3 and round to the nearest whole number. For example, if Hgb = 8.4, report as Q9925 (8.4 × 3 = 25.2, rounded down to 25).

One unit of service of EPO is reported for each 1000 units dispensed. For example if 20,000 units are dispensed, bill 20 units. If the dose dispensed is not an even multiple of

1,000, rounded down for 1–499 units (e.g. 20,400 units dispensed = 20 units billed), round up for 500–999 units (e.g. 20,500 units dispensed = 21 units billed).

Q9920 Injection of EPO, per 1,000 units, at patient HCT of 20 or less
Q9921 Injection of EPO, per 1,000 units, at patient HCT of 21
Q9922 Injection of EPO, per 1,000 units, at patient HCT of 22
Q9923 Injection of EPO, per 1,000 units, at patient HCT of 23
Q9924 Injection of EPO, per 1,000 units, at patient HCT of 24
Q9925 Injection of EPO, per 1,000 units, at patient HCT of 25
Q9926 Injection of EPO, per 1,000 units, at patient HCT of 26
Q9927 Injection of EPO, per 1,000 units, at patient HCT of 27
Q9928 Injection of EPO, per 1,000 units, at patient HCT of 28
Q9929 Injection of EPO, per 1,000 units, at patient HCT of 29
Q9930 Injection of EPO, per 1,000 units, at patient HCT of 30
Q9931 Injection of EPO, per 1,000 units, at patient HCT of 31
Q9932 Injection of EPO, per 1,000 units, at patient HCT of 32
Q9933 Injection of EPO, per 1,000 units, at patient HCT of 33
Q9934 Injection of EPO, per 1,000 units, at patient HCT of 34
Q9935 Injection of EPO, per 1,000 units, at patient HCT of 35
Q9936 Injection of EPO, per 1,000 units, at patient HCT of 36
Q9937 Injection of EPO, per 1,000 units, at patient HCT of 37
Q9938 Injection of EPO, per 1,000 units, at patient HCT of 38
Q9939 Injection of EPO, per 1,000 units, at patient HCT of 39
Q9940 Injection of EPO, per 1,000 units, at patient HCT of 40 or above.

B. Claims with Dates of Service January 1, 2004 and after

The above codes were replaced effective January 1, 2004 by Q4055. This Q code is for the injection of EPO furnished to ESRD Beneficiaries on Dialysis. The new code does not include the hematocrit. See §60.7.

Q4055—Injection, Epoetin alfa, 1,000 units (for ESRD on Dialysis).

The DMERC shall return to provider (RTP) assigned claims for EPO, Q4055, that do not contain a HCT value. For unassigned claims, the DMERC shall deny claims for EPO, Q4055 that do not contain a HCT value.

DMERCs must use the following messages when payment for the injection (Q4055) does not meet the coverage criteria and is denied:

MSN Message 6.5—English: Medicare cannot pay for this injection because one or more requirements for coverage were not met

MSN Message 6.5—Spanish: Medicare no puede pagar por esta inyeccion porque uno o mas requisitos para la cubierta no fueron cumplidos. (MSN Message 6.5 in Spanish).

Adjustment Reason Code B:5 Payment adjusted because coverage/program guidelines were not met or were exceeded.

The DMERCs shall use the following messages when returning as unprocessable assigned claims without a HCT value:

ANSI Reason Code 16—Claim/service lacks information, which is needed for adjudication.

Additional information is supplied using remittance advice remarks codes whenever appropriate.

Remark Code M58—Missing/incomplete/invalid claim information. Resubmit claim after corrections.

Deductibles and coinsurance apply.

60.4.2.1—Other Information Required on the Form CMS-1500

(Rev 118, 03-05-04)

The following information is required for EPO. Incomplete assigned claims are returned to providers for completion. Incomplete unassigned claims are rejected. The rejection will be due to a lack of a HCT value. Note that when a claim is submitted on paper Form CMS-1500, these items are submitted on a separate document. It is not necessary to enter them into the claims processing system. This information is used in utilization review.

A. Diagnoses—The diagnoses must be submitted according to ICD-9-CM and correlated to the procedure. This information is in Item 21, of the Form CMS-1500.

B. Hematocrit (HCT)/Hemoglobin (Hgb)—There are special HCPCS codes for reporting the injection of EPO for claims with dates of service prior to January 1, 2004. These allow the simultaneous reporting of the patient's latest HCT or Hgb reading before administration of EPO.

The physician and/or staff are instructed to enter a separate line item for injections of EPO at different HCT/Hgb levels. The Q code for each line items is entered in Item 24D.

1. Code Q9920—Injection of EPO, per 1,000 units, at patient HCT of 20 or less/Hgb of 6.8 or less.

2. Codes Q9921 through Q9939—Injection of EPO, per 1,000 units, at patient HCT of 21 to 39/Hgb of 6.9 to 13.1. For HCT levels of 21 or more, up to a HCT of 39/Hgb of 6.9 to 13.1, a Q code that includes the actual HCT levels is used. To convert actual Hgb to corresponding HCT values for Q code reporting, multiply the Hgb value by 3 and round to the nearest whole number. Use the whole number to determine the appropriate Q code.

EXAMPLES: If the patient's HCT is 25/Hgb is 8.2-8.4, Q9925 must be entered on the claim. If the patient's HCT is 39/Hgb is 12.9-13.1, Q9939 is entered.

3. Code Q9940—Injection of EPO, per 1,000 units at patient HCT of 40 or above.

A single line item may include multiple doses of EPO administered while the patient's HCT level remained the same.

Codes Q9920-Q9940 will no longer be recognized by the system if submitted after March 31, 2004. If claims for dates of service prior to January 1, 2004 are submitted after March 31, 2004, then code Q4055 must be used.

C. Units Administered—The standard unit of EPO is 1,000. The number of 1,000 units administered per line item is included on the claim. The physician's office enters 1 in the units field for each multiple of 1,000 units. For example, if 12,000 units are administered, 12 is entered. This information is shown in Item 24G (Days/Units) on Form CMS-1500.

In some cases, the dosage for a single line item does not total an even multiple of 1,000. If this occurs, the physician's office rounds down supplemental dosages of 0 to 499 units to the prior 1,000 units. Supplemental dosages of 500 to 999 are rounded up to the next 1,000 units.

EXAMPLES

A patient's HCT reading on August 6 was 22/Hgb was 7.3. The patient received 5,000 units of EPO on August 7, August 9, and August 11, for a total of 15,000 units. The first line of Item 24 of Form CMS-1500 shows:

Dates of Service	Procedure Code	Days or Units
8/7–8/11	Q9922	15

On September 13, the patient's HCT reading increased to 27/Hgb increased to 9. The patient received 5,100 units of EPO on September 13, September 15, and September 17, for a total of 15,300 units. Since less than 15,500 units were given, the figure is rounded down to 15,000. This line on the claim form shows:

Dates of Service	Procedure Code	Days or Units
9/13–9/17	Q9927	15

On October 16, the HCT level increased to 33/Hgb increased to 11. The patient received doses of 4,850 units on October 16, October 18, and October 20 for a total of 14,550 units. Since more than 14,500 units were administered, the figure is rounded up to 15,000. Form CMS-1500 shows:

Dates of Service	Procedure Code	Days or Units
10/16–10/20	Q9933	15

NOTE: Creatinine and weight identified below are required on EPO claims as applicable.

D. Date of the Patient's most recent HCT or Hgb.

E. Most recent HCT or Hgb level—(prior to initiation of EPO therapy).

F. Date of most recent HCT or Hgb level—(prior to initiation of EPO therapy).

G. Patient's most recent serum creatinine—(within the last month, prior to initiation of EPO therapy).

H. Date of most recent serum creatinine—(prior to initiation of EPO therapy).

I. Patient's weight in kilograms

J. Patient's starting dose per kilogram—(The usual starting dose is 50-100 units per kilogram.)

60.4.2.2—Completion of Subsequent Form CMS-1500 Claims for EPO

(Rev 118, 03-05-04)

Subsequent claims are completed as initial claims in §60.4.2, except the following fields:

A. Diagnoses.

B. Hematocrit or Hemoglobin—For dates of service prior to January 1, 2004, this is indicated by the appropriate Q code. For dates of service January 1, 2004, and after, suppliers must indicate the beneficiary's hematocrit on the claim. (See 60.4.2.) Claims include an EJ modifier to the Q code. This allows the contractor to identify subsequent claims, which do not require as much information as initial claims and prevent unnecessary development.

C. Number of Units Administered—Subsequent claims may be submitted electronically.

60.4.3—Payment Amount for Epoetin Alfa (EPO)

(Rev. 373, Issued: 11-19-04, Effective: 01-01-05, Implementation: 01-03-05)

For Method I patients, the FI pays the facility $10 per 1,000 units of EPO administered, rounded to the nearest 100 units (i.e., $1.00 per 100 units). *Effective January 1, 2005, the cost of supplies to administer EPO may be billed to the FI. HCPCS A4657 and Revenue Code 270 should be used to capture the charges for syringes used in the administration of EPO.* Where EPO is furnished by a supplier that is not a facility, the DMERC pays at the same rate.

Prior to January 1, 1994, the Method I payment was $11 per 1,000 units. The statutory payment allowance for EPO is the only allowance for the drug and its administration. *Effective January 1, 2005, the cost of supplies to administer EPO may be billed to the FI.*

HCPCS A4657 and Revenue Code 270 should be used to capture the charges for syringes used in the administration of EPO.

Payment for medical supplies for the administration of EPO, whether in the home or in a facility, is included in the Medicare payment rate for EPO.

Physician payment is calculated through the drug payment methodology described in Chapter 17 of the Claims Processing Manual.

The composite rate add-on amount (the current $10 per 1,000 unit rate and the past $11 per 1,000 unit rate) is updated nationally by CMS. *Effective January 1, 2005, EPO will be paid based on the ASP Pricing File.* This add-on does not vary geographically and is the same for hospital-based and independent dialysis facilities.

EXAMPLE: The billing period is 2/1/94–2/28/94.

The facility provides the following:

Date	Units	Date	Units
2/1	3000	2/15	2500
2/4	3000	2/18	2500
2/6	3000	2/20	2560
2/8	3000	2/22	2500
2/11	2500	2/25	2000
2/13	2500	2/27	2000

Total 31,060 units

For value code 68, the facility enters 31,060. The 31,100 are used to determine the rate payable. This is 31,060 rounded to the nearest 100 units. The amount payable is 31.1 x $10 =$311.00. In their systems, FIs have the option of setting up payment of $1.00 per 100 units. *Effective January 1, 2005, EPO will be paid based on the ASP Pricing File.*

EXAMPLE: 311 × $1.00 = $311.00

If an ESRD beneficiary requires 10,000 units or more of EPO per administration, special documentation must accompany the claim. It must consist of a narrative report that addresses the following:

- Iron deficiency. Most patients need supplemental iron therapy while being treated, even if they do not start out iron deficient;
- Concomitant conditions such as infection, inflammation, or malignancy. These conditions must be addressed to assure that EPO has maximum effect;
- Unrecognized blood loss. Patients with kidney disease and anemia may easily have chronic blood loss (usually gastrointestinal) as a major cause of anemia. In those circumstances, EPO is limited in effectiveness;
- Concomitant hemolysis, bone morrow dysplasia, or refractory anemia for a reason other than renal disease, e.g., aluminum toxicity;
- Folic acid or vitamin B12 deficiencies;
- Circumstances in which the bone morrow is replaced with other tissue, e.g., malignancy or osteitis fibrosa cystica; and
- Patient's weight, the current dose required, a historical record of the amount that has been given, and the hematocrit response to date.

60.4.3.1—Payment for Epoetin Alfa (EPO) in Other Settings

(Rev 118, 03-05-04)

A3-3644

In the hospital inpatient setting, payment is included in the DRG.

In a skilled nursing facility (SNF), payment for EPO covered under the Part B EPO benefit is not included in the prospective payment rate for the resident's Medicare-covered SNF stay.

In a hospice, payment is included in the hospice per diem rate.

For a service furnished by a physician or incident to a physician's service, payment is made to the physician by the carrier in accordance with the rules for "incident to" services. When EPO is administered in the renal facility, the service is not an "incident to" service and not under the "incident to" provision.

60.4.3.2—Epoetin Alfa (EPO) Provided in the Hospital Outpatient Departments

(Rev. 373, Issued: 11-19-04, Effective: 01-01-05, Implementation: 01-03-05)

For patients with chronic renal failure who are not yet on a regular course of dialysis, EPO administered in a hospital outpatient department is paid under the Outpatient Prospective Payment System (OPPS).

Hospitals use type of bill 13X and report charges under revenue code 0636 with HCPCS code Q0136 and without value codes 48, 49, 68 or condition codes 70 through 76.

When ESRD patients come to the hospital for a medical emergency their dialysis related anemia may also require treatment. For patients with ESRD who are on a regular course of dialysis, EPO administered in a hospital outpatient department is paid using the statutory rate for EPO given to an ESRD beneficiary. *Effective January 1, 2005, EPO will be paid based on the ASP Pricing File.*

Hospitals use type of bill 13X and report charges under the respective revenue code 0634 for EPO less than 10,000 units and revenue code 0635 for EPO over 10,000 units with HCPCS code Q4055. The total number of units as a multiple of 1000 units is placed in the unit field. Value code 49 will contain the hematocrit value for the hospital outpatient visit.

60.4.4—Epoetin Alfa (EPO) Furnished to Home Patients

(Rev. 447, Issued: 01-21-05, Effective: 07-01-05, Implementation: 07-05-05)

B3-4270.1

Medicare covers EPO for dialysis patients who use EPO in the home, when requirements for a patient care plan and patient selection as described in the Medicare Benefit Policy Manual, Chapter 11, are met.

When EPO is prescribed for a home patient, it may be either administered in a facility, e.g., the one shown on the Form CMS-382 (ESRD Beneficiary Method Selection Form) or furnished by a facility or Method II supplier for self-administration to a home patient determined to be competent to administer this drug. For EPO furnished for self-administration to Method I and Method II home patients determined to be competent, the renal facility bills its FI and the Method II supplier bills its DMERC. No additional payment is made for training a prospective self-administering patient or retraining an existing home patient to self-administer EPO.

Method II patients who self-administer may obtain EPO only from either their Method II supplier, or a Medicare certified ESRD facility.

In this case, the DMERC makes payment at the same rate that applies to facilities. Program payment may not be made for EPO furnished by a physician to a patient for self-administration.

DMERCs pay for EPO for Method II ESRD beneficiaries only. DMERCs shall deny claims for EPO where the beneficiary is not a Method II home dialysis patient.

When denying line items for patients that are not Method II, use the following message on the remittance advice:

ANSI message 7011: Claim not covered by this payer contractor. You must send the claim to the correct payer contractor.

When denying line items for patients that are not Method II, use the following message on the Medicare Summary Notice (MSN):

English: 8.59—Durable Medical Equipment Regional Carriers pay for Epoetin Alfa and Darbepoetin Alfa only for Method II End Stage Renal Disease home dialysis patients.

Spanish: 8.59—Las Empresas Regionales de Equipo Médico Duradero pagan por los medicamentos Epoetina Alfa y Darbepoetina Alfa sólo a pacientes del Método II de diálisis con enfermedad renal en etapa final que están confinados al hogar.

60.4.4.1—Self Administered EPO Supply

(Rev. 1, 10-01-03)

B3-4270.1

Initially, facilities may bill for up to a 2-month supply of EPO for Method I beneficiaries who meet the criteria for selection for self-administration. After the initial two months' supply, the facility will bill for one month's supply at a time. Condition code 70 is used to indicate payment requested for a supply of EPO furnished a beneficiary. Usually, revenue code 0635 would apply since the supply would be over 10,000 units. Facilities leave FL 46, Units of Service, blank since they are not administering the drug. For value code 68, they enter the total amount of the supply.

60.5—Intradialytic Parenteral/Enteral Nutrition (IDPN)

(Rev. 1, 10-01-03)

PRM-1-2711.6

  A. General

Parenteral/enteral nutrition (PEN) administered during dialysis may be covered under Medicare, but it is not part of the Medicare ESRD benefit. Therefore, an ESRD facility or PEN supplier may bill Medicare separately from the composite rate for PEN solution if the patient meets all of the requirements for PEN coverage. (See Medicare Benefit Policy Manual for PEN coverage requirements.) If the ESRD facility bills, it does so as a PEN supplier and bills the appropriate DMERC.

  B. Staff Time

ESRD facility staff time used to administer PEN solution is not covered by Medicare, and, therefore, not included in the composite rate. (PEN is considered a self-administered therapy and generally administered in the patient's home.) Since it is not covered under Medicare, it is not part of the composite rate nor may a facility bill Medicare separately for it.

The costs of the staff time used for this purpose are allocated to a nonreimbursable cost center on the facility's Medicare ESRD facility cost report. If the facility cannot determine the cost of this service, any revenue the facility receives commensurate with the value of this service is used as an offset against the facility's cost.

Any payment the facility receives from the PEN supplier (e.g., for administration or record-keeping relating to the provision of parenteral nutritional therapy) is questionable under the Medicare program's anti-kickback provision.

60.6—Hepatitis B Vaccine Furnished to ESRD Patients

(Rev. 1, 10-01-03)

PRM-1-2711.4

The Medicare program covers hepatitis B vaccine and its administration when furnished to eligible beneficiaries in accordance with coverage rules. Payment may be made for both the vaccine and its administration (including staff time and supplies such as syringes). For coverage rules and HCPCS codes for billing, see Chapter 18. For payment rules see Chapter 17.

60.7—Darbepoetin Alfa (Aranesp) for ESRD Patients.

(Rev. 373, Issued: 11-19-04, Effective: 01-01-05, Implementation: 01-03-05)

Coverage rules Aranesp are explained in the Medicare Benefit Policy Manual, Chapter 11. For an explanation Method I ad Method II reimbursement for patients dialyzing at home see §40.1.

Intermediaries pay for Aranesp to ESRD facilities as a separately billable drug to the composite rate. No additional payment is made to administer Aranesp, whether in a facility or a home. *Effective January 1, 2005, the cost of supplies to administer Aranesp may be billed to the FI. HCPCS A4657 and Revenue Code 270 should be used to capture the charges for syringes used in the administration of Aranesp.*

If the beneficiary obtains Aranesp from a supplier for self-administration, the supplier bills the DMERC, and the DMERC pays in accordance with MMA Drug Payment Limits Pricing File.

Program payment may not be made to a physician for self-administration of Aranesp. When Aranesp is furnished by a physician as "incident to services," the carrier processes the claim.

For ESRD patients on maintenance dialysis treated in a physician's office, code Q4054, "injection, darbepoetin alfa, 1 mcg (for ESRD patients)," should continue to be used with the hematocrit included on the claim. (For ANSI 837 transactions, the hematocrit (HCT) value is reported in 2400 MEA03 with a qualifier of R2 in 2400 MEA02.) Claims without this information will be denied due to lack of documentation. Physicians who provide Aranesp for ESRD patients on maintenance dialysis must bill using code Q4054.

Darbepoetin Alfa Payment Methodology

Type of provider	Separately Billable	DMERC Payment	No Payment
In-facility freestanding and hospital based ESRD facility	X		
Self-administer Home Method I	X		
Self administer Home Method II		X	
Incident to physician in facility or for self-administration*			X

* Medicare pays for a drug if self-administered by a dialysis patient. When Aranesp is administered in a dialysis facility, the service is not an "incident to" service, and not under the "incident to" provision.

The Dialysis Outcomes Quality Initiative recommends a threshold hematocrit value range of 33 to 36 percent. National policy requires FIs and carriers to identify practitioners with an atypical number of patients with hematocrit levels above a 90-day rolling average of 37.5 percent for routine medical; review activities, such as provider education or pre-payment reviews. That is, medical documentation is not required for a single value over 36 percent. However, FIs and carriers must make a determination upon post payment review if the treating physician argues it is medically necessary to have a target hematocrit that is greater than 36 percent (which would then exceed the rolling average of 37.5 percent). These hematocrit requirements apply only to Aranesp furnished as an ESRD benefit under §1881(b) of the Social Security Act (the Act). Aranesp furnished incident to a physician's service is not included in this policy. Carriers have discretion for local policy for Aranesp furnished as "incident to service."

60.7.1—Darbepoetin Alfa (Aranesp) Facility Billing Requirements Using UB-92/Form CMS-1450

(Rev. 373, Issued: 11-19-04, Effective: 01-01-05, Implementation: 01-03-05)

CPCS code Q4054 is placed in FL 44. Revenue code 0636 is used to report for ESRD patients on maintenance dialysis.

The hematocrit reading taken prior to the last administration of Aranesp during the billing period must also be reported on the UB-92/Form CMS-1450 with value code 49.

The hematocrit reading is required. The FI must retain the hematocrit (HCT) reading in a format accessible to the claims process for use to average readings for a 90-day period on future claims.

The payment allowance for Aranesp is the only allowance for the drug and its administration when used for ESRD patients. *Effective January 1, 2005, the cost of supplies to administer Aranesp may be billed to the FI. HCPCS A4657 and Revenue Code 270 should be used to capture the charges for syringes used in the administration of Aranesp.* The maximum number of administrations of Aranesp for a billing cycle is 5 times in 30/ 31days.

60.7.2—Darbepoetin Alfa (Aranesp) Supplier Billing Requirements (Method II) on the Form CMS-1500 and Electronic Equivalent

(Rev 118, 03-05-04)

ESRD patients on dialysis can use Aranesp for the treatment of anemia effective January 1, 2004, the Q code for the injection of Aranesp for ESRD beneficiaries on dialysis, is Q4054.

Q4054—Injection, Darbepoetin alfa, 1 mcg (for ESRD on Dialysis).

Method II suppliers must use Item 19 on the CMS 1500 to place the most current HCT value (Q4054). Identify HCT as "HCT = the true value HCT". For 837P claims, the Method II supplier must supply the most current HCT value, when billing for darbepoetin alfa Q4054, in the 2400 MEA03 with a qualifier of R2 in 2400 MEA02.

DMERCs must apply coverage rules to Aranesp in the same manner that they apply them to EPO. DMERCs shall accept claims for Aranesp, Q4054, from suppliers that bill for Aranesp furnished to home patients for self-administration who have elected home dialysis and Method II payment.

DMERCs must accept HCPCS code Q4054 for Aranesp on the CMS-1500 or its electronic equivalent 837 P format. The DMERC shall return to provider (RTP) assigned claims for Aranesp, Q4054, that do not contain a HCT value. For unassigned claims, the DMERC shall deny claims for Aranesp, Q4054, that do not contain a HCT value.

Method II suppliers must place number of mcg's of Aranesp Q4054 administered in Item Field 24G Units on the CMS-1500 form, or 2400 SV104 of the 837P format. Method II suppliers must use Item 19 on the CMS 1500 to place the most current HCT value (Q4054). Identify HCT as "HCT = the true value HCT". For 837P claims, the Method II supplier must supply the most current HCT value, when billing for Aranesp Q4054, in the 2400 MEA03 with a qualifier of R2 in 2400 MEA02.

DMERCs must use the following messages when payment for the Aranesp injection (Q4054) does not meet the coverage criteria and is denied:

MSN Message 6.5—English: Medicare cannot pay for this injection because one or more requirements for coverage were not met

MSN Message 6.5—Spanish: Medicare no puede pagar por esta inyeccion porque uno o mas requisitos para la cubierta no fueron cumplidos. (MSN Message 6.5 in Spanish).

Adjustment Reason Code B:5 Payment adjusted because coverage/program guidelines were not met or were exceeded.

The DMERCs shall use the following messages when returning as unprocessable assigned claims without a HCT value:

ANSI Reason Code 16—Claim/service lacks information, which is needed for adjudication.

Additional information is supplied using remittance advice remarks codes whenever appropriate.

Remark Code M58—Missing/incomplete/invalid claim information. Resubmit claim after corrections.

Deductibles and coinsurance apply. DMERCs must pay for Aranesp (Q4054) based on the payment amount in the MMA Drug Payment Limits Pricing File. The contractor can obtain the rates from the CMS website, www.cms.hhs.gov/providers/drugs/default.asp.

60.7.2.1—Other Information Required on the Form CMS-1500 for Darbepoetin Alfa (Aranesp)

(Rev 118, 03-05-04)

The following information is required for Aranesp. Incomplete assigned claims are returned to providers for completion. Incomplete unassigned claims are rejected. The rejection will be due to a lack of a HCT value. Note that when a claim is submitted on paper Form CMS-1500, these items are submitted on a separate document. It is not necessary to enter them into the claims processing system. This information is used in utilization review.

A. Diagnoses—The diagnoses must be submitted according to ICD-9-CM and correlated to the procedure. This information is in Item 21, of the Form CMS-1500.

B. Date of the Patient's most recent HCT.

C. Most recent HCT (prior to initiation of Aranesp therapy).

D. Date of most recent HCT (prior to initiation of Aranesp therapy).

F. Patient's most recent serum creatinine—(within the last month, prior to initiation of Aranesp therapy).

G. Date of most recent serum creatinine—(prior to initiation of Aranesp therapy).

H. Patient's weight in kilograms

I. Patient's starting dose per kilogram

60.7.2.2—Completion of Subsequent Form CMS-1500 Claims for Darbepoetin Alfa (Aranesp)

(Rev 118, 03-05-04)

Subsequent claims are completed as initial claims in §60.7.2, except the following fields:

A. Diagnoses.

B. Hematocrit—For dates of service prior to January 1, 2004, this is indicated by the appropriate Q code. For dates of service January 1, 2004 and after, suppliers must indicate the beneficiary's hematocrit on the claim. (See 60.7.2). Claims include an EJ modifier to the Q code. This allows the contractor to identify subsequent claims, which do not require as much information as initial claims and prevent unnecessary development.

C. Number of Units Administered—Subsequent claims may be submitted electronically.

60.7.3—Payment Amount for Darbepoetin Alfa (Aranesp)

(Rev. 373, Issued: 11-19-04, Effective: 01-01-05, Implementation: 01-03-05)

For Method I patients, the FI pays the facility per one mcg of Aranesp administered, in accordance with the MMA Drug Payment Limits Pricing File rounded up to the next highest whole mcg. *Effective January 1, 2005, Aranesp will be paid based on the ASP Pricing File. Effective January 1, 2005, the cost of supplies to administer Aranesp may be billed to the FI. HCPCS A4657 and Revenue Code 270 should be used to capture the charges for syringes used in the administration of Aranesp.*

Physician payment is calculated through the drug payment methodology described in Chapter 17, of the Claims Processing Manual.

The coinsurance and deductible are based on the Medicare allowance payable, not on the provider's charges. The provider may not charge the beneficiary more than 20 percent of the Medicare Aranesp allowance. This rule applies to independent and hospital based renal facilities.

60.7.3.1—Payment for Darbepoetin Alfa (Aranesp) in Other Settings

(Rev 118, 03-05-04)

In the hospital inpatient setting, payment for Aranesp is included in the DRG.

In a skilled nursing facility (SNF), payment for Aranesp covered under the Part B EPO benefit is not included in the prospective payment rate for the resident's Medicare-covered SNF stay.

In a hospice, payment is included in the hospice per diem rate.

For a service furnished by a physician or incident to a physician's service, payment is made to the physician by the carrier in accordance with the rules for "incident to" services. When Aranesp is administered in the renal facility, the service is not an "incident to" service and not under the "incident to" provision.

60.7.3.2—Payment for Darbepoetin Alfa (Aranesp) in the Hospital Outpatient Department

(Rev. 373, Issued: 11-19-04, Effective: 01-01-05, Implementation: 01-03-05)

For patients with chronic renal failure who are not yet on a regular course of dialysis, Aranesp administered in a hospital outpatient department is paid under the OPPS.

Hospitals use bill type 13X and report charges under revenue code 0636, with HCPCS code Q0137 and without value codes 48, 49, 68 or condition codes 70-76.

When ESRD patients come to the hospital for a medical emergency their dialysis related anemia may also require treatment. For patients with ESRD who are on a regular course of dialysis, Aranesp administered in a hospital outpatient department is paid the MMA Drug Pricing File rate. *Effective January 1, 2005, Aranesp will be paid based on the ASP Pricing File.*

Hospitals use bill type 13X and report charges under revenue code 0636, with HCPCS code Q4054. The total number of units as a multiple of 1mcg is placed in the unit field. Value code 49 will contain the hematocrit value for the hospital outpatient visit.

In this case, the DMERC makes payment at the same rate that applies to facilities. Program payment may not be made for Aranesp furnished by a physician to a patient for self-administration.

60.7.4—Darbepoetin Alfa (Aranesp) Furnished to Home Patients

(Rev. 447, Issued: 01-21-05, Effective: 07-01-05, Implementation: 07-05-05)

B3-4270.1

Medicare covers Aranesp for dialysis patients who use Aranesp in the home, when requirements for a patient care plan and patient selection as described in the Medicare Benefit Policy Manual, Chapter 11, are met.

When Aranesp is prescribed for a home patient, it may be either administered in a facility, e.g., the one shown on the Form CMS-382 (ESRD Beneficiary Method Selection Form) or furnished by a facility or Method II supplier for self-administration to a home patient determined to be competent to administer this drug. For Aranesp furnished for self-administration to Method I and Method II home patients determined to be competent, the renal facility bills its FI and the Method II supplier bills its DMERC. No additional payment is made for training a prospective self-administering patient or retraining an existing home patient to self-administer Aranesp.

Method II home patients who self-administer may obtain Aranesp only from either their Method II supplier or a Medicare-certified ESRD facility.

In this case, the DMERC makes payment at the same rate that applies to facilities. Program payment may not be made for Aranesp furnished by a physician to a patient for self-administration.

DMERCs pay for Aranesp for Method II ESRD beneficiaries only. DMERCs shall deny claims for Aranesp where the beneficiary is not a Method II home dialysis patient.

When denying line items for patients that are not Method II, use the following message on the remittance advice:

ANSI message 7011: Claim not covered by this payer contractor. You must send the claim to the correct payer contractor.

When denying line items for patients that are not Method II, use the following message on the Medicare Summary Notice (MSN):

English: 8.59—Durable Medical Equipment Regional Carriers pay for Epoetin Alfa and Darbepoetin Alfa only for Method II End Stage Renal Disease home dialysis patients.

Spanish: 8.59—Las Empresas Regionales de Equipo Médico Duradero pagan por los medicamentos Epoetina Alfa y Darbepoetina Alfa sólo a pacientes del Método II de diálisis con enfermedad renal en etapa final que están confinados al hogar.

60.8—Shared Systems Changes for Medicare Part B Drugs for ESRD Independent Dialysis Facilities

(Rev. 257, Issued 07-30-04, Effective: 01-01-05, Implementation: 01-03-05)

Section 303 of the Medicare Prescription Drug, Improvement, and Modernization Act of 2003 (MMA) provides that the payment limits for ESRD-related drugs billed by differing types of facilities vary depending on the site of service. For calendar year 2005, the payment limits for Medicare Part B drugs will be updated on a quarterly basis. Therefore, Medicare Shared Systems (FISS) must be able to accommodate at least two payment limits for HCPCS drug codes per quarter effective for dates of service on or after January 1, 2005.

Fiscal intermediaries (FIs) shall use the 95 percent of the Average Wholesale Price (AWP) payment amount provided solely to pay independent dialysis facilities with type of bill (TOB) 72X for separately billable drugs furnished to ESRD beneficiaries. Specifically, the ESRD drug payment limit shall be used to determine payment for TOB 72X, but only for independent dialysis facilities with provider number in the range 2500-2899 (non-hospital renal facilities) and 2900-2999 (independent special purpose renal dialysis facilities).

104, Chapter 20

100.2.2—Evidence of Medical Necessity for Parenteral and Enteral Nutrition (PEN) Therapy

(Rev. 1, 10-01-03)

B3-3324, B3-4450

PEN coverage is determined by information provided by the treating physician and the PEN supplier. A completed certification of medical necessity (CMN) must accompany and support initial claims for PEN to establish whether coverage criteria are met and to ensure that the PEN therapy provided is consistent with the attending or ordering physician's prescription. Contractors ensure that the CMN contains pertinent information from the treating physician. Uniform specific medical data facilitate the review and promote consistency in coverage determinations and timelier claims processing.

The medical and prescription information on a PEN CMN can be most appropriately completed by the treating physician or from information in the patient's records by an employee of the physician for the physician's review and signature. Although PEN suppliers sometimes may assist in providing the PEN services, they cannot complete the CMN since they do not have the same access to patient information needed to properly enter medical or prescription information. Contractors use appropriate professional relations issuances, training sessions, and meetings to ensure that all persons and PEN suppliers are aware of this limitation of their role.

When properly completed, the PEN CMN includes the elements of a prescription as well as other data needed to determine whether Medicare coverage is possible. This practice will facilitate prompt delivery of PEN services and timely submittal of the related claim.

100.2.2.1—Scheduling and Documenting Certifications and Recertifications of Medical Necessity for PEN

(Rev. 1, 10-01-03)

A certification for PEN therapy must accompany the initial claim submitted. The initial certification is valid for six months. Contractors establish the schedule on a case-by-case basis for recertifying the need for PEN therapy. A change in prescription for a beneficiary past the initial certification period does not restart the certification process.

A period of medical necessity ends when PEN services are not medically required for 2 consecutive months. The entire certification process, if required, begins after 2 consecutive months have elapsed.

A revised certification or a change in prescription may impact on the payment levels of PEN services. A revised certification is appropriate when there is a change:

- In the treating physician's orders in the category of nutrients and/or calories prescribed;
- By more than one liter in the daily volume of parenteral solutions;
- From home-mix to pre-mix or pre-mix to home-mix parenteral solutions;
- From enteral to parenteral or parenteral to enteral therapy; or
- In the method of infusion (e.g., from gravity-fed to pump-fed).

100.2.2.2—Completion of the Elements of PEN CMN

(Rev. 1, 10-01-03)

The patient's name, address, and HICN and the nature of the certification (i.e., initial, renewed, or revised) must be entered on all certifications by the supplier, physician, or physician's designated employees. The supplier identifying information is required on all PEN certifications.

All medical and prescription information must be completed from the patient's records by the attending/ordering physician, or an employee of the physician authorized to act on the physician's behalf, and reviewed and signed by the physician.

1. Place of Service—The CMN must identify the site where the patient is receiving PEN services. A patient may receive services at home, in a nursing home setting (e.g., skilled nursing facility), or another site that must be indicated by the supplier/physician.

2. Patient's General Condition—The attending physician must complete information about the patient's age, height, and weight. The general condition of the patient also includes an estimated duration of therapy (i.e., in months, years, or for life), the ambulatory status, and whether the patient is conscious. The physician should also indicate food allergies/sensitivities, other medical treatments, therapies, and/or medical conditions that may affect the patient's nutritional needs.

3. Patient's Clinical Assessment—The attending physician must indicate all the diagnoses related to the PEN therapy and describe the patient's functional impairment of the digestive tract that precludes the enteral patient from swallowing and the parenteral patient from absorbing nutrients. The physician must certify that PEN therapy meets the requirement that a patient is not able to maintain weight and strength due to pathology or nonfunction of the ingestion system and that the enteral therapy serves as the source of nutrition for the patient who has a functioning digestive tract, but whose disability prevents ingestion of sufficient nutrients to the alimentary tract for metabolism. Nutritional supplements for patients capable of ingesting normally, even if required to maintain weight and strength, cannot be covered under the prosthetic device benefit. The physician must have a basis for certifying or recertifying the need for PEN services. The physician is expected to see the patient within 30 days prior to certifying or recertifying PEN services. However, if the physician did not see the patient, he/she must explain why and describe what other monitoring methods were used to evaluate the patient's PEN needs.

4. Patient's Nutritional Prescription—Subsequent to an examination of the patient and/or a review of the patient's medical information, the attending physician must complete the patient's nutritional requirements (prescription) to certify the PEN therapy provided.

For the parenteral patient, the CMN must contain the following information:

- The infusion frequency per week,
- The route of administration,
- A reason for the use of pre-mixed parenteral formulas,
- An explanation for the use of special formulas such as hepatic, renal, or stress formulas, and
- The amino acid/dextrose formula components of the parenteral solution mix.

Amino acids serve as a source of protein. Adult parenteral nutrition patients generally need 1 to 1.5 grams of protein per day for each kilogram (2.2 pounds) of body weight. Dextrose concentrations less than 10 percent must be explained by the physician. The physician must document the reason for using more than 12 units (@ 500ml per unit) of lipids per month.

Parenteral nutrition may be either "self-mixed" (i.e., the patient is taught to prepare the nutrient solution aseptically) or "pre-mixed" (i.e., the nutrient solution is prepared by trained professionals employed or contracted by the PEN supplier). The attending physician must provide information to justify the reason for "pre-mixed" parenteral nutrient solutions.

Renal dialysis patients sometimes undergo parenteral therapy to replace fluids and nutrients lost during dialysis. Patients are usually infused less than daily and parenteral feeding is often supplemental and, therefore, not covered as a PEN benefit. The renal dialysis patient must meet all the requirements for PEN coverage.

The attending physician must document that the patient, despite the need for renal dialysis, suffers from a permanently impaired functional impairment that precludes swallowing or absorption of nutrients.

For the enteral patient, the attending physician must include the following information on the CMN:

- The name of the nutrient product or nutrient category,
- The number of calories per day (100 calories = 1 unit),
- The frequency per day,
- The method of administration (i.e., syringe, gravity, or pump),
- The route of administration (i.e., nasogastric tube, gastrostomy tube, jejunostomy tube, percutaneous enteral gastrostomy tube, or naso-intestinal tube), and
- The reason for the use of a pump.

Categories of enteral nutrition are based on the composition and source of ingredients in each enteral nutrient product. Category IB of enteral nutrients contains products that are natural intact protein/protein isolates commonly known as blenderized nutrients. Additional documentation is required to justify the necessity of Category IB nutrients. The attending physician must provide sufficient information to indicate that the patient:

- Has an intolerance to nutritionally equivalent (semi-synthetic) products;
- Had a severe allergic reaction to a nutritionally equivalent (semi-synthetic) product; or
- Was changed to a blenderized nutrient to alleviate adverse symptoms expected to be of permanent duration with continued use of semi-synthetic products.

Enteral nutrient categories III through VI require additional medical justification for coverage. These categories represent formulas for special needs or use.

- Category III (code B4153): hydrolyzed protein/amino acids. These products contain a high nitrogen availability as a result of chemical treatment to reduce high molecular protein compounds into smaller molecules and amino acids that are easier to digest.
- Category IV (code B4154): defined formulas for special metabolic needs and conditions such as abnormal glucose tolerance, renal disease, liver disease, HIV, respiratory insufficiency, and malnutrition.
- Category V (code B4155): modular components (proteins, carbohydrates, fats).
- Category VI (code B4156): standardized nutrients. These products contain low residue ingredients.

If the patient exhibits a problem with any particular formula in Nutrient Category I (HCPCS B4150) or II (HCPCS B4152), the physician must document the unfavorable events that resulted in prescribing a higher category formula.

Generally, daily enteral intake of 750 to 2,000 calories is considered sufficient to maintain body weight. Patients with medical complications may require an intake outside the range. The attending physician must document the reason for prescribing less than 750 calories per day or more than 2000 calories per day.

Enteral nutrition may be administered by syringe, gravity, or pump. The attending physician must specify the reason that necessitates the use of an enteral feeding pump. Some enteral patients may experience complications associated with syringe or gravity method of administration. Contractors provide coverage for enteral pumps if the medical necessity is documented by the attending physician on the CMN. Examples of circumstances that indicate the need for a pump include, but are not limited to:

- Aspiration or Dumping Syndrome;
- Severe diarrhea remedied by regulated feeding;
- Insulin-dependent diabetics who require a flow rate of less than 100cc's per hour for proper regulation of nutrients;
- Patients with congestive heart failure who require a pump to prevent circulatory overload; or
- Patients with a jejunostomy tube for feeding.

The DMERC reviews the claims to ensure that the equipment for which payment is claimed is consistent with that prescribed (e.g., expect a claim for an I.V. pole, if a pump is used).

5. Attending Physician's Signature and Identification—A handwritten, original signature and date must be on each certification. The form must be dated to show reasonable association to the dates of active PEN therapy. The full name, address, telephone number (including area code), and Unique Physician Identification Number (UPIN) allows the contractor to determine if the prescriber is authorized to order Medicare services and facilitate claims development.

6. PEN Supplier's Identification—The PEN supplier's name, address, telephone number, and PEN identification number must be on each certification. This information allows the contractor to determine if the supplier is authorized to provide PEN supplies and facilitate claims development.

100.2.2.3—DMERC Review of Initial PEN Certifications

(Rev. 1, 10-01-03)

B3-4450

In reviewing the claim and the supporting data on the CMN, the DMERC compares certain items, especially pertinent dates of treatment. For example, the start date of PEN coverage cannot precede the date of physician certification. The estimated duration of therapy must be contained on the CMN. This information is used to verify that the test of permanence is met. Once coverage is established, the estimated length of need at the start of PEN services will determine the recertification schedule.

The information shown on the certification must support the need for PEN supplies as billed. A diagnosis must show a functional impairment that precludes the enteral patient from swallowing and the parenteral patient from absorbing nutrients.

Initial assigned claims with the following conditions are denied without development:

- Inappropriate or missing diagnosis or functional impairment;
- Estimated duration of therapy is less than 90 consecutive days;
- Duration of therapy is not listed;
- Supplies have not been provided;
- Supplies were provided prior to onset date of therapy; and
- Stamped physician's signature.

Unassigned claims are developed for missing or incomplete information.

A—Revised Certifications/Change in Prescription

A revised certification is required when:

- There is a change in the attending physician's orders in the category of nutrients and/or calories prescribed;
- There is a change by more than one liter in the daily volume of parenteral solutions;
- There is a change from home-mix to pre-mix or pre-mix to home-mix parenteral solutions;
- There is a change from enteral to parenteral or parenteral to enteral therapy; or
- There is a change in the method of infusion (e.g., from gravity-fed to pump-fed).

PEN payments are not adjusted unless a revised or renewed certification documents the necessity for the change. Payment levels for the most current certification or recertification may not be changed unless a prescription change is documented by a new recertification.

The DMERC may adjust the recertification schedule as needed.

104, Chapter 12

160.1—Payment

(Rev. 1, 10-01-03)

Diagnostic testing services are not subject to the outpatient mental health limitation. Refer to §210, below, for a discussion of the outpatient mental health limitation.

The diagnostic testing services performed by a psychologist (who is not a clinical psychologist) practicing independently of an institution, agency, or physician's office are covered as other diagnostic tests if a physician orders such testing. Medicare covers this type of testing as an outpatient service if furnished by any psychologist who is licensed or certified to practice psychology in the State or jurisdiction where he or she is furnishing services or, if the jurisdiction does not issue licenses, if provided by any practicing psychologist. (It is CMS' understanding that all States, the District of Columbia, and Puerto Rico license psychologists, but that some trust territories do not. Examples of psychologists, other than clinical psychologists, whose services are covered under this provision include, but are not limited to, educational psychologists and counseling psychologists.)

To determine whether the diagnostic psychological testing services of a particular independent psychologist are covered under Part B in States which have statutory licensure or certification, carriers must secure from the appropriate State agency a current listing of psychologists holding the required credentials. In States or territories which lack statutory licensing and certification, carriers must check individual qualifications as claims are submitted. Possible reference sources are the national directory of membership of the American Psychological Association, which provides data about the educational background of individuals and indicates which members are board-certified, and records and directories of the State or territorial psychological association. If qualification is dependent on a doctoral degree from a currently accredited program, carriers must verify the date of accreditation of the school involved, since such accreditation is not retroactive. If the reference sources listed above do not provide enough information (e.g., the psychologist is not a member of the association), carriers must contact the psychologist personally for the required information. Carriers may wish to maintain a continuing list of psychologists whose qualifications have been verified.

Medicare excludes expenses for diagnostic testing from the payment limitation on treatment for mental/psychoneurotic/personality disorders.

Carriers must identify the independent psychologist's choice whether or not to accept assignment when performing psychological tests.

Carriers must accept an independent psychologist claim only if the psychologist reports the name/UPIN of the physician who ordered a test.

Carriers pay nonparticipating independent psychologists at 95 percent of the physician fee schedule allowed amount. Carriers pay participating independent psychologists at 100 percent of the physician fee schedule allowed amount.

Independent psychologists are identified on the provider file by specialty code 62 and provider type 35.

170—CLINICAL PSYCHOLOGIST SERVICES

(Rev. 1, 10-01-03)

B3-2150

See Medicare Benefit Policy Manual, Chapter 15, for general coverage requirements.

Direct payment may be made under Part B for professional services. However, services furnished incident to the professional services of CPs to hospital patients remain bundled. Therefore, payment must continue to be made to the hospital (by the FI) for such "incident to" services.

170.1—Payment

(Rev. 1, 10-01-03)

B3-2150, B3-17001.1

All covered therapeutic services furnished by qualified CPs are subject to the outpatient mental health services limitation (i.e., only 62 1/2 percent of expenses for these services are considered incurred expenses for Medicare purposes). The limitation does not apply to diagnostic services. Refer to §210 below for a discussion of the outpatient mental health limitation.

Payment for the services of CPs is made on the basis of a fee schedule or the actual charge, whichever is less, and only on the basis of assignment.

CPs are identified by specialty code 68 and provider type 27. Modifier "AH" is required on CP services.

104, Chapter 16

10.2—General Explanation of Payment

(Rev. 1, 10-01-03)

B3-5114, HO-437, A3-3628, B3-5114.1, AB-03-076

Outpatient laboratory services can be paid in different ways:

• Physician Fee Schedule;
• Reasonable costs (Critical Access Hospitals (CAH) only);

NOTE: When the CAH bills a 14X bill type as a reference laboratory, the CAH is paid under the laboratory fee schedule.

• Laboratory Fee Schedule;
• Outpatient Prospective Payment System, (OPPS) except for most hospitals in the state of Maryland that are subject to waiver; or
• Reasonable Charge

Annually, CMS distributes a list of codes and indicates the payment method. Carriers and FIs pay as directed by this list. Neither deductible nor coinsurance applies to HCPCS codes paid under the laboratory fee schedule; further, deductible and coinsurance do not apply to HCPCS laboratory codes paid via reasonable cost to CAHs. The majority of outpatient laboratory services are paid under the laboratory fee schedule or the OPPS.

Carriers and FIs are responsible for applying the correct fee schedule for payment of clinical laboratory tests. FIs must determine which hospitals meet the criteria for payment at the 62 percent fee schedule. Only sole community hospitals with qualified hospital laboratories are eligible for payment under the 62 percent fee schedule. Generally, payment for diagnostic laboratory tests that are not subject to the clinical laboratory fee schedule is made in accordance with the reasonable charge or physician fee schedule methodologies (or reasonable costs for CAHs).

For Clinical Diagnostic Laboratory services denied due to frequency edits contractors must use standard health care adjustment reason code 151—"Payment adjusted because the payer deems the information submitted does not support this many services."

20—CALCULATION OF PAYMENT RATES—CLINICAL LABORATORY TEST FEE SCHEDULES

(Rev. 1, 10-01-03)

HO-437, A3-3628, PM AB-98-7, B3-5114.1

Under Part B, for services rendered on or after July 1, 1984, clinical laboratory tests performed in a physician's office, by an independent laboratory, or by a hospital laboratory for its outpatients are reimbursed on the basis of fee schedules. Current exceptions to this rule are CAH laboratory services as described in §10, and services provided by hospitals in the State of Maryland.

Medicare pays the lesser of:

• Actual charges;
• The fee schedule amount for the State or a local geographic area; or
• A national limitation amount (NLA) for the HCPCS code as provided by §1834(h) of the Act.

Annually, CMS furnishes to carriers and FIs the proper amount to pay for each HCPCS code for each local geographic area. This includes a calculation of whether a national limitation amount or the local fee schedule amount is to be used.

This information is available to the public on the CMS Web site in public use files.

20.1—Initial Development of Laboratory Fee Schedules

(Rev. 1, 10-01-03)

HO-437, A3-3628, B3-5114.1.C

Initially, each carrier established the fee schedules on a carrier-wide basis (not to exceed a statewide basis). If a carrier's area includes more than one State, the carrier established a separate fee schedule for each State. The carrier determined the fee schedule amount based on prevailing charges for laboratory billings by physicians and independent laboratories billing the carrier. Carriers set the fees at 60 percent of prevailing charges. FIs used the same fee schedules to pay outpatient hospital laboratory services. They set the fee at 62 percent of carrier prevailing charges. Subsequently, except for sole community hospitals, which continue to be paid at the 62 percent rate, FIs changed payments to hospital laboratories to the "60 percent fee schedule."

In 1994, CMS took over the annual update and distribution of clinical laboratory fee schedules. The CMS updates the fee schedule amounts annually to reflect changes in the Consumer Price Index (CPI) for all Urban Consumers (U.S. city average), or as otherwise specified by legislation.

Effective for hospital outpatient tests furnished by a hospital on or after April 1, 1988, to receive the 62 percent fee the hospital must be a sole community hospital. Otherwise, the fee is the "60 percent fee schedule." If a hospital is uncertain whether it meets the qualifications of a sole community hospital it can seek assistance from the FI or the RO.

For tests to hospital nonpatients, the fee is 60 percent of the carrier prevailing charge. If a hospital laboratory acts as an independent laboratory, i.e., performs tests for persons who are non-hospital patients; or if the hospital laboratory is not a qualified hospital laboratory, the services are reimbursed using the 60 percent fee schedule or the adjusted fee schedule, as appropriate.

See §10.1 for the definition of a hospital outpatient.

20.2—Annual Fee Schedule Updates

(Rev. 1, 10-01-03)

The CMS adjusts he fee schedule amounts annually to reflect changes in the Consumer Price Index (CPI) for all Urban Consumers (U.S. city average), or as otherwise specified by legislation. The CMS also determines, publishes for contractor use, and places on its web site, coding and pricing changes. A CMS issued temporary instruction informs contractors when and where the updates are published.

30—SPECIAL PAYMENT CONSIDERATIONS

(Rev. 1, 10-01-03)

30.1—Mandatory Assignment for Laboratory Tests

(Rev. 1, 10-01-03)

B3-5114.1

Unless a laboratory, physician, or medical group accepts assignment, the carrier makes no Part B payment for laboratory tests paid on the laboratory fee schedule. Laboratories, physicians, or medical groups that have entered into a participation agreement must accept assignment. Sanctions of double the violation charges, civil money penalties (up to $2,000 per violation), and/or exclusion from the program for a period of up to five years may be imposed on physicians and laboratories, with the exception of rural health clinic laboratories, that knowingly, willfully, and repeatedly bill patients on an unassigned basis. However, sole community physicians and physicians who are the sole source of an essential specialty in a community are not excluded from the program. Whenever a carrier is notified of a sanction action for this reason, the carrier does not pay for any laboratory services unless the services were furnished within 15 days after the date on the exclusion or suspension notice to the practitioner, and:

- It is the first claim filed for services rendered to that beneficiary after the date on the notice of suspension or exclusion; or

- It is filed with respect to services furnished within 15 days of the date on the first notice of denial of claims to the beneficiary. (Fifteen days are allowed for the notice to reach the beneficiary.)

Carriers refer questions on payment procedures to the Sanctions Coordinator in the RO.

Carriers process laboratory claims inadvertently submitted as unassigned as if they were assigned. (See §50.)

For purposes of this section, the term assignment includes assignment in the strict sense of the term as well as the procedure under which payment is made, after the death of the beneficiary, to the person or entity that furnished the service, on the basis of that person's or entity's agreement to accept the Medicare payment as the full charge or fee for the service.

104, Chapter 16

30.2—Deductible and Coinsurance Application for Laboratory Tests

(Rev. 1, 10-01-03)

B3-2462, B3-5114.1, A3-3215, HHA-160

Neither the annual cash deductible nor the 20 percent coinsurance apply to:

- Clinical laboratory tests performed by a physician, laboratory, or other entity paid on an assigned basis;
- Specimen collection fees; or
- Travel allowance related to laboratory tests (e.g., collecting specimen).

Codes on the physician fee schedule are generally subject to the Part B deductible and coinsurance, although exceptions may be noted for a given code in the MPFS or through formal Medicare instructions such as temporary instructions and requirements for specific services noted in this manual.

Any laboratory code paid at reasonable charge is subject to the Part B deductible and coinsurance, unless otherwise specified in the description of coverage and payment rules.

Neither deductible nor coinsurance is applied to payment for codes on the laboratory fee schedule that are made to CAHs.

30.3—Method of Payment for Clinical Laboratory Tests—Place of Service Variation

(Rev. 1, 10-01-03)

HO-437, A3-3628, B3-5114.1, PM A-01-31

The following apply in determining the amount of Part B payment for clinical laboratory tests, including those furnished under method II for ESRD beneficiaries:

Independent laboratory or a physician or medical group—Payment to an independent laboratory or a physician or medical group is the lesser of the actual charge, the fee schedule amount or the national limitation amount. Part B deductible and coinsurance do not apply.

Reference laboratory—For tests performed by a reference laboratory, the payment is the lesser of the actual charge by the billing laboratory, the fee schedule amount, or the national limitation amount. (See §50.5 for carrier jurisdiction details.) Part B deductible and coinsurance do not apply.

Outpatient or a nonpatient of the hospital—Payment to a hospital for tests furnished for an outpatient or a nonpatient of the hospital is the lesser of the actual charge, the 60 percent fee schedule amount, or the 60 percent NLA. Part B deductible and coinsurance do not apply.

Inpatient without Part A—Payment to a hospital for tests performed for an inpatient without Part A coverage is made on a reasonable cost basis and is subject to Part B deductible and coinsurance. Payment to a SNF inpatient without Part A coverage is made under the laboratory fee schedule.

Inpatient or SNF patient with Part A—Payment to a hospital for laboratory tests furnished to an inpatient whose stay is covered under Part A, is included in the PPS rate for PPS facilities or is made on a reasonable cost basis for non-PPS hospitals. Payment for lab services for beneficiaries in a Part A stay in a SNF, other than a swing bed in a CAH are included in the SNF PPS rate. For such services provided in a swing bed CAH, payment is made on a reasonable cost basis.

Sole community hospital—Payment to a sole community hospital for tests furnished for an outpatient of that hospital, is the least of the actual charge, the 62 percent fee schedule amount, or the 62 percent NLA. The Part B deductible and coinsurance do not apply.

Waived Hospitals—Payment to a hospital which has been granted a waiver of Medicare payment principles for outpatient services is subject to Part B deductible and coinsurance unless otherwise waived as part of an approved waiver. Specifically, laboratory fee schedules do not apply to laboratory tests furnished by hospitals in States or areas that have been granted demonstration waivers of Medicare reimbursement principles for outpatient services. The State of Maryland has been granted such demonstration waivers. This also may apply to hospitals in States granted approval for alternative payment methods for paying for hospital outpatient services under §1886(c) of the Act.

Critical Access Hospital—For a CAH being reimbursed under the "Standard Method" of reimbursement (See Chapter 4), payment for clinical laboratory services furnished as an outpatient service is made on a reasonable cost basis. Critical Access Hospitals choosing the "Standard Method" are paid under the fee schedule for services when they function as a reference laboratory (bill type 14X).

CAHs choosing the "Optional Method" of reimbursement (see Chapter 4) are reimbursed at reasonable cost for non-professional clinical laboratory services and at 115 percent of the fee schedule for professional clinical laboratory services.

Beneficiaries are not liable for any coinsurance, deductible, co-payment, or other cost sharing amount with respect to CAH clinical laboratory services.

Dialysis facility—Payment to a hospital-based or independent dialysis facility for laboratory tests included under the ESRD composite rate payment and performed for a patient of that facility, is included in the facility's composite rate payment for these tests and is subject to the Part B deductible and coinsurance. Laboratory tests that are not included under the ESRD composite rate payment; and are performed by an independent laboratory or a provider-based laboratory for dialysis patients of independent dialysis facilities or provider based facilities; are paid in addition to the composite rate payment and are subject to the fee schedule limits. This also applies to all laboratory tests furnished to home dialysis patients who have selected Payment Method II. These limits are 60 percent for all tests unless performed by a qualified hospital laboratory in a sole community hospital; in which case the 62 percent rate applies. The laboratory performing the tests must bill.

Rural health clinic—Payment to a rural health clinic (RHC) for laboratory tests performed for a patient of that clinic is not included in the all-inclusive rate and may be billed separately by the laboratory (including a laboratory that is part of a hospital that hosts a hospital based RHC). Payment for the laboratory service is not subject to Part B deductible and coinsurance. (See §40.4 for details on RHC billing.)

Enrolled in Managed Care—Payment to a participating health maintenance organization (HMO) or health care prepayment plan (HCPP) for laboratory tests provided to a Medicare beneficiary who is an enrolled member is included in the monthly capitation amount.

Nonenrolled Managed Care—Payment to a participating HMO or HCPP for laboratory tests performed for a patient who is not a member is the lesser of the actual charge, or the fee schedule, or the NLA. The Part B deductible and coinsurance do not apply.

Hospice—Payment to a hospice for laboratory tests performed by the hospice is included in the hospice rate.

30.4—Payment for Review of Laboratory Test Results by Physician

(Rev. 1, 10-01-03)

B3-5114.2

Reviewing results of laboratory tests, phoning results to patients, filing such results, etc., are Medicare covered services. Payment is included in the physician fee schedule payment for the evaluation and management (E and M) services to the patient. Visit services entail a wide range of components and activities that may vary somewhat from patient to patient. The CPT lists different levels of E and M services for both new and established patients and describes services that are included as E and M services. Such activities include obtaining, reviewing, and analyzing appropriate diagnostic tests.

40—BILLING FOR CLINICAL LABORATORY TESTS

(Rev. 1, 10-01-03)

40.1—Laboratories Billing for Referred Tests

(Rev. 85, 02-06-04)

B3-5114.1.E,

Section 1833(h)(5)(A) of the Act provides that a referring laboratory may bill for clinical laboratory diagnostic tests on the clinical laboratory fee schedule for Medicare beneficiaries performed by a reference laboratory only if the referring laboratory meets certain conditions. Payment may be made to the referring laboratory but only if one of the following conditions is met:

- the referring laboratory is located in, or is part of, a rural hospital;
- the referring laboratory is wholly owned by the entity performing such test, the referring laboratory wholly owns the entity performing such test, or both the referring laboratory and the entity performing such test are wholly-owned by a third entity; or
- the referring laboratory does not refer more than 30 percent of the clinical laboratory tests for which it receives requests for testing during the year (not counting referrals made under the wholly-owned condition described above).

In the case of a clinical laboratory test provided under an arrangement (as defined in §1861(w)(1)) made by a hospital, CAH or SNF, payment is made to the hospital or SNF.

Examples of 30 Percent Exception:

1. A laboratory receives requests for 200 tests, performs 139 tests, and refers 61 tests to a non-related laboratory. All tests referred to a non-related laboratory are counted. Thus, 30.5 percent (61/200) of the tests are considered tests referred to a non-related laboratory and, since this exceeds the 30 percent standard, the referring laboratory may not bill for any Medicare beneficiary laboratory tests referred to a non-related laboratory.

2. A laboratory receives requests for 200 tests, performs 139 tests and refers 15 to a related laboratory and 46 to a non-related laboratory. Only 23 percent of the tests were referred to non-related laboratories. Since this is less than 30 percent, the referring laboratory may bill for all tests.

If it is later found that a referring laboratory does not, in fact, meet an exception criterion, the carrier should recoup payment for the referred tests improperly billed. The RO shall take whatever action is necessary to correct the problem.

NOTE: This provision of §6111(b) of OBRA of 1989 has no effect on hospitals that are paid under §1833(h)(5)(A)(iii).

NOTE: Laboratory services provided to a SNF inpatient under Part A are billed by the SNF, not the laboratory, due to consolidated billing for SNFs.

Only one laboratory may bill for a referred laboratory service. It is the responsibility of the referring laboratory to ensure that the reference laboratory does not bill Medicare for the referred service when the referring laboratory does so (or intends to do so). In the event the reference laboratory bills or intends to bill Medicare, the referring laboratory may not do so.

40.1.1—Claims Information and Claims Forms and Formats

(Rev. 85, 02-06-04)

Claims for referred laboratory services may be made only by suppliers having specialty code 69, i.e., independent clinical laboratories. Claims for referred laboratory services made by other entities will be returned as unprocessable.

Independent laboratories shall use modifier 90 to identify all referred laboratory services. A claim for a referred laboratory service that does not contain the modifier 90 is returned as unprocessable if the claim can otherwise be identified as being for a referred service.

The name, address, and CLIA number of both the referring laboratory and the reference laboratory shall be reported on the claim.

40.1.1.1—Paper Claim Submission To Carriers

(Rev. 85, 02-06-04)

An independent clinical laboratory that elects to file a paper claim form shall file Form CMS-1500 for a referred laboratory service (as it would any laboratory service). The line item services must be submitted with a modifier 90.

An independent clinical laboratory that submits claims in paper format) may not combine non-referred (i.e., self-performed) and referred services on the same CMS 1500 claim form. When the referring laboratory bills for both non-referred and referred tests, it shall submit two separate claims, one claim for non-referred tests, the other for referred tests. If billing for services that have been referred to more than one laboratory, the referring laboratory shall submit a separate claim for each laboratory to which services were referred. (unless one or more of the reference laboratories are separately billing Medicare). A paper claim that contains both non-referred and referred tests is returned as unprocessable. When the referring laboratory is the billing laboratory, the reference laboratory's name and address shall be reported in item 32 on the CMS-1500 claim form to show where the service (test) was actually performed Also, the CLIA number of the reference laboratory shall be reported in item 23 on the CMS-1500 claim form. A paper claim that does not have the name and address of the reference laboratory in item 32 or the CLIA number of the reference laboratory in item 23 is returned as unprocessable.

EXAMPLE: A physician has ordered the ABC Laboratory to perform carcinoembryonic antigen (CEA) and hemoglobin testing for a patient. Since the ABC Laboratory is approved to perform tests only within the hematology LC level (which includes the hemoglobin test), it refers the CEA testing (which is a routine chemistry LC) to the XYZ laboratory.

Result: The ABC laboratory submits a claim for the hemoglobin test and reports its CLIA number in item 23 on the CMS-1500 form. Since the ABC laboratory referred the CEA test to the XYZ laboratory to perform, the ABC laboratory (billing laboratory) submits a second claim for the CEA testing, reporting XYZ's CLIA number in item 23 on the CMS-1500 form. The XYZ laboratory's name, and address is also reported in item 32 on Form CMS-1500 to show where the service (test) was actually rendered.

40.1.1.2—Electronic Claim Submission to Carriers

(Rev. 85, 02-06-04)

Electronic Claim Submission

American National Standards Institue (ANSI) X12N 837 (HIPAA version) format electronic claims:

CLIA number:

An ANSI claim for laboratory testing will require the presence of the performing (and billing) laboratory's CLIA number; if tests are referred to another laboratory, the CLIA number of the laboratory where the testing is rendered must also be on the claim. An ANSI electronic claim for laboratory testing must be submitted using the following format:

ANSI Electronic claim: the billing laboratory performs all laboratory testing.

The independent laboratory submits a single claim for CLIA-covered laboratory tests and reports the billing laboratory's number in:

X12N 837 (HIPAA version) loop 2300, REF02. REF01 = X4

ANSI Electronic claim: billing laboratory performs some laboratory testing; some testing is referred to another laboratory.

The ANSI electronic claim will not be split; CLIA numbers from both the billing and reference laboratories must be submitted on the same claim. The presence of the '90' modifier at the line item service identifies the referral tests. Referral laboratory claims are only permitted for independently billing clinical laboratories, specialty code 69.

The billing laboratory submits, on the same claim, tests referred to another (referral/rendered) laboratory, with modifier 90 reported on the line item and reports the referral laboratory's CLIA number in:

X12N 837 (HIPAA version) loop 2400, REF02. REF01 = F4

EXAMPLE: A physician has ordered the DEF independent laboratory to perform glucose testing and tissue typing for a patient. Since the DEF Laboratory is approved to perform only at the routine chemistry LC level (which includes glucose testing), it refers the tissue-typing test to the GHI laboratory.

The DEF laboratory submits a single claim for the glucose and tissue typing tests; the line item service for the glucose test is submitted without a '90' modifier since the DEF laboratory performed this test. The CLIA number for the DEF laboratory is entered in the electronic claim in:

X12N 837 (HIPAA version) loop 2300, REF02. REF01 = X4

On the same claim, the line item service for the tissue typing test is submitted with a '90' modifier and the referral/rendering GHI laboratory's CLIA number is entered on the electronic claim in:

X12N 837 (HIPAA version) loop 2400, REF02. REF01 = F4

Reference Laboratory's Address:

An electronic claim for laboratory testing requires the presence of the performing and billing laboratory's, name and address. The performing laboratory for a service with a line item CPT 90 modifier requires provider information for the appropriate 837 loop.

National Standard Format (NSF) Electronic Claims:

An independent clinical laboratory that submits claims in the NSF format) may not combine non-referred (i.e., self-performed) and referred services on the same NSF claim form. When the referring laboratory bills for both non-referred and referred tests, it shall submit two separate claims, one claim for non-referred tests, the other for referred tests. If billing for services that have been referred to more than one laboratory, the referring laboratory shall submit a separate claim for each laboratory to which services were referred. (unless one or more of the reference laboratories are separately billing Medicare). A NSF claim that contains both non-referred and referred tests is returned as unprocessable.

CLIA number:

An NSF claim for laboratory testing will require the presence of the performing laboratory's CLIA number: if tests are referred to another laboratory, the CLIA number of the laboratory where the testing is rendered must be on the claim. An NSF electronic claim for laboratory testing must be submitted using the following format:

The CLIA number reported on line items with modifier 90 will be the CLIA number of the performing clinical diagnostic laboratory. Referral laboratory claims are only permitted for independently billing clinical laboratories, specialty code 69.

The CLIA number shall be reported in:

FA0 – 34.0

Reference Laboratory's Address

An NSF electronic claim for laboratory testing requires the presence of the performing and billing laboratory's, name and address. The performing laboratory for a service with a line item CPT '90' modifier requires provider information to be submitted in the following NSF record and fields:

EA0 Field 39 Facility/Lab Name
EA1 Field 06 Facility/Lab ADDR1
EA1 Field 07 Facility/Lab ADDR1
EA1 Field 08 Facility/Lab City
EA1 Field 09 Facility/Lab State
EA1 Field 10 Facility/Lab Zip Code

40.2—Payment Limit for Purchased Services

(Rev. 16, 10-31-03)

For payment instructions for Physician purchased diagnostic tests refer to the Claims Processing Manual 100-04, Chapter 1, §30.2.9, Chapter 13 §20.2.4ff.

When an Independent Laboratory (IL) bills for the technical component (TC) of a physician pathology service purchased from a separate physician or supplier, the payment amount for the TC is based on the lower of the billed charge or the Medicare Physician Fee Schedule. The purchase diagnostic test payment provision does not apply, thus, the purchase service information shall not be entered on the claim.

All purchased diagnostic services are based on the Medicare Physician Fee Schedule and are subject to the jurisdiction rules for that fee schedule.

The IL must perform at least one of the component services. If they purchase both the PC and the TC services, only the physician or supplier that performed those services may bill.

40.3—Hospital Billing Under Part B

(Rev. 100, 02-13-04)

HO-437, A3-3628

Hospital laboratories, billing for either outpatient or nonpatient claims, bill the FI. Neither deductible nor coinsurance applies to laboratory tests paid under the fee schedule.

Hospital laboratories, billing for either outpatient or nonpatient claims, bill the FI. Neither deductible nor coinsurance applies to laboratory tests paid under the fee schedule.

Hospitals must follow requirements for submission of the Form CMS-1450 (see Chapter 25 for billing requirements).

When the hospital obtains laboratory tests for outpatients under arrangements with clinical laboratories or other hospital laboratories, only the hospital can bill for the arranged services.

If all tests are for a nonpatient, the hospital may submit one bill and be reimbursed at 60 percent. If the hospital is a sole community hospital identified in the PPS Provider Specific File with a qualified hospital laboratory identified on the hospital's certification; tests for outpatients are reimbursable at 62 percent. If tests are for an outpatient, those referred to a reference laboratory are considered nonpatient tests reimbursable at 60 percent.

If the hospital bills for both types of outpatient tests, it should prepare two bills: one for its own laboratory tests reimbursable at 62 percent, the other for the tests referred to the reference laboratory reimbursable at 60 percent. The CMS-1450 (UB-92) Type of Bill (TOB) code (FL4) for the nonpatient bill is 14X. The hospital includes fee schedule laboratory tests on the same bill with other outpatient services to the same beneficiary on the same day, unless it is billing for a reference laboratory as described above, in which case it submits a separate bill for the reference laboratory tests. Hospitals should not submit separate bills for laboratory tests performed in different departments on the same day.

Section 416 of the Medicare Prescription, Drug, Improvement, and Modernization Act (MMA) of 2003 also eliminates the application of the clinical laboratory fee schedule for hospital outpa-

tient laboratory testing by a hospital laboratory with fewer than 50 beds in a qualified rural area for cost reporting periods beginning during the 2-year period beginning on July 1, 2004. Payment for these hospital outpatient laboratory tests will be reasonable costs without coinsurance and deductibles during the applicable time period. A qualified rural area is one with a population density in the lowest quartile of all rural county populations.

The reasonable costs are determined using the ratio of costs to charges for the laboratory cost center multiplied by the PS&R's billed charges for outpatient laboratory services for cost reporting periods beginning on or after July 1, 2004 but before July 1, 2006.

In determining whether clinical laboratory services are furnished as part of outpatient services of a hospital, the same rules that are used to determine whether clinical laboratory services are furnished, as an outpatient critical access hospital service will apply.

40.3.1—Critical Access Hospital (CAH) Outpatient Laboratory Service

(Rev. 1, 10-01-03)

HO-437, A3-3628, PM A-01-31

Effective for services furnished on or after the enactment of Balanced Budget Refinement Act of 1999 (BBRA), Medicare beneficiaries are not liable for any coinsurance, deductible, co-payment, or other cost sharing amount with respect to clinical laboratory services furnished as a CAH outpatient service. This change is effective for claims with dates of service on or after November 29, 1999, that were received July 1, 2001 or later.

For CAH bill type 85X, the laboratory fees are paid at cost with no cost-sharing.

When the CAH electing the standard reimbursement method (see Chapter 3) bills a 14X bill type as a reference laboratory, it is paid the laboratory fee schedule rather than reasonable cost.

For CAHs billing as a reference laboratory (Bill Type 14X) and choosing the "Optional Method" of reimbursement (See Chapter 4) reimbursement is at reasonable cost for non-professional clinical laboratory services and at 115 percent of the fee schedule for professional clinical laboratory services.

40.4—Special Skilled Nursing Facility (SNF) Billing Exceptions for Laboratory Tests

(Rev. 1, 10-01-03)

SNF 541, A3-3137.1, HO-437, B3-5114.1

When a SNF furnishes laboratory services directly, it must have a Clinical Laboratory Improvement Act (CLIA) number or a CLIA certificate of waiver, and the laboratory itself must be in the portion of the facility so certified. Normally the FI makes payment under Part B for clinical laboratory tests only to the entity that performed the test. However, the law permits SNFs to submit a Part B claim to the FI for laboratory tests that it makes arrangements for another entity to perform on the SNF's behalf. Section 1833(h)(5) of the Act (as enacted by The Deficit Reduction Act of 1984, P.L. 98-369) requires the establishment of a fee schedule for clinical laboratory tests paid under Part B and also requires that, with certain exceptions, only the entity that performed the test may be paid.

The fee schedule applies to all SNF clinical laboratory services.

Where a SNF operates a laboratory that provides laboratory services to patients other than its own patients, it is functioning as a clinical laboratory. The billing for these laboratory services depends upon the HCPCS code as defined in the CMS annual fee schedule releases (laboratory and MPFS), and the arrangements made for payment with the referring entity (e.g., does the SNF or the referring entity bill under the agreement between the two). The SNF is responsible for ascertaining the necessary information for billing the FI. Any questions must be referred to the FI.

40.4.1—Which Contractor to Bill for Laboratory Services Furnished to a Medicare Beneficiary in a Skilled Nursing Facility (SNF)

(Rev. 1, 10-01-03)

Inpatient Part A beneficiary—SNF bills the FI under Part A. The service is included in SNF PPS payment.

Inpatient Part B beneficiary (benefits exhausted or no Part A entitlement)—SNFs may provide the service and bill the FI, may obtain the service under arrangement and bill the FI under Part B, or may have agreement with a reference laboratory for the reference laboratory to provide the service and have the reference laboratory bill the carrier under Part B. Regardless of who bills, CMS policy requires that the service be paid under the fee schedule, whether or not the beneficiary is in a Medicare certified bed.

Outpatient Part B—See inpatient Part B beneficiary (benefits exhausted or no Part A entitlement), immediately above.

40.5—Rural Health Clinic (RHC) Billing

(Rev. 1, 10-01-03)

B3-3628

For independent RHCs, laboratory services provided in the RHC's laboratory are not included in the all-inclusive rate payment to the RHC and may be billed separately to the carrier. This includes the six basic laboratory tests required for certification as well as any other laboratory tests provided in the RHC laboratory.

Note: If the RHC sends laboratory services to an outside laboratory, the outside laboratory bills the Part B carrier for the tests.

If the RHC laboratory becomes certified as a clinical laboratory, it bills all laboratory tests performed in its laboratory to the laboratory's Part B carrier. Laboratory tests are not included as RHC costs nor as part of the RHC all-inclusive rate payment.

For provider based RHCs the rules in the preceding paragraph apply with the following exception. The provider bills tests provided in its laboratory to the FI.

40.6—Billing for End Stage Renal Disease (ESRD) Related Laboratory Tests

(Rev. 1, 10-01-03)

PM AB-98-7, PRM 1 2711, B3-4270.2

Hemodialysis, Intermittent Peritoneal Dialysis (IPD), and Continuous Cycling Peritoneal Dialysis (CCPD) Tests

With some exceptions, laboratory tests for hemodialysis, intermittent peritoneal dialysis (IPD), and continuous cycling peritoneal dialysis (CCPD) are included in the ESRD composite rate.

For a particular date of service to a beneficiary, if 50 percent or more of the covered laboratory tests are noncomposite rate tests Medicare allows separate payment beyond that included in the composite rate

For a description of what laboratory tests and other tests are included in the composite rate and under what conditions such tests may qualify for additional payment in addition to the composite rate, see the Medicare Benefit Policy Manual Chapter 11, "End Stage Renal Disease (ESRD)," and Chapter 8 of this manual.

Clinical diagnostic laboratory tests included under the composite rate payment are paid through the composite rate paid by the FI.

40.6.1—Automated Multi-Channel Chemistry (AMCC) Tests for ESRD Beneficiaries—FIs

(Rev. 79, 02-06-04)

A-03-033

Medicare will apply the following rules to Automated Multi-Channel Chemistry (AMCC) tests for ESRD beneficiaries:

- Payment is at the lowest rate for test performed by the same provider, for the same beneficiary, for the same date of service.
- The facility must identify, for a particular date of service, the

AMCC tests ordered that are included in the composite rate and those that are not included. See Chapter 8 for the composite rate tests for Hemodialysis, Intermittent Peritoneal Dialysis (IPD), Continuous Cycling Peritoneal Dialysis (CCPD), Hemofiltration, and Continuous Ambulatory Peritoneal Dialysis (CAPD).

- If 50 percent or more of the covered tests are included under the composite rate payment, then all submitted tests are included within the composite payment. In this case, no separate payment in addition to the composite rate is made for any of the separately billable tests.
- If less than 50 percent of the covered tests are composite rate tests, all AMCC tests submitted for that Date of Service (DOS) for that beneficiary are separately payable.
- A noncomposite rate test is defined as any test separately payable outside of the composite rate or beyond the normal frequency covered under the composite rate that is reasonable and necessary.
- For carrier processed claims, all chemistries ordered for beneficiaries with chronic dialysis for ESRD must be billed individually and must be rejected when billed as a panel.

(See §100.6 for details regarding pricing modifiers.)

Implementation of this Policy:

ESRD facilities when ordering an ESRD-related AMCC must specify for each test within the AMCC whether the test:

a. Is part of the composite rate and not separately payable;

b. Is a composite rate test but is, on the date of the order, beyond the frequency covered under the composite rate and thus separately payable; or

c. Is not part of the ESRD composite rate and thus separately payable.

Laboratories must:

a. Identify which tests, if any, are not included within the ESRD facility composite rate payment

b. Identify which tests ordered for chronic dialysis for ESRD as follows:

1) Modifier CD: AMCC Test has been ordered by an ESRD facility or MCP physician that is part of the composite rate and is not separately billable.

2) Modifier CE: AMCC Test has been ordered by an ESRD facility or MCP physician that is a composite rate test but is beyond the normal frequency covered under the rate and is separately reimbursable based on medical necessity.

3) Modifier CF: AMCC Test has been ordered by an ESRD facility or MCP physician that is not part of the composite rate and is separately billable.

c. Bill all tests ordered for a chronic dialysis ESRD beneficiary individually and not as a panel.

The shared system must calculate the number of AMCC tests provided for any given date of service. Sum all AMCC tests with a CD modifier and divide the sum of all tests with a CD, CE, and CF modifier for the same beneficiary and provider for any given date of service.

If the result of the calculation for a date of service is 50 percent or greater, do not pay for the tests.

If the result of the calculation for a date of service is less than 50 percent, pay for all of the tests.

For FI processed claims, all tests for a date of service must be billed on the monthly ESRD bill. Providers that submit claims to a FI, must send in an adjustment if they identify additional tests that have not been billed.

Carrier standard systems shall adjust the previous claim when the incoming claim for a date of service is compared to a claim on history and the action is adjust payment. Carrier standard systems shall spread the payment amount over each line item on both claims (the claim on history and the incoming claim).

The organ and disease oriented panels (80048, 80051, 80053, and 80076) are subject to the 50 percent rule. However, clinical diagnostic laboratories shall not bill these services as panels, they must be billed individually. Laboratory tests that are not covered under the composite rate and that are furnished to CAPD end stage renal disease (ESRD) patients dialyzing at home are billed in the same way as any other test furnished home patients.

Business Requirements for ESRD Reimbursement of AMCC Tests:

Requirement Number	Requirements	Responsibility
1.1	The FI shared system must RTP a claim for AMCC tests when a claim for that date of service has already been submitted.	Shared system
1.2	Based upon the presence of the CD, CE and CF payment modifiers, identify the AMCC tests ordered that are included and not included in the composite rate payment	Shared system
1.3	Based upon the determination of requirement 1.2, if 50 percent or more of the covered tests are included under the composite rate, no separate payment is made.	Shared system
1.4	Based upon the determination of requirement 1.2, if less than 50 percent are covered tests included under the composite rate, all AMCC tests for that date of service are payable.	Shared system
1.5	Reject line items that contain a procedure (identified in exhibit 1 and 2) with a modifier CE and a modifier 91 and no line item on the claim with modifier CE and no modifier 91.	Shared system
1.6	Reject line items that contain a procedure (identified in exhibits 1 and 2) with a modifier CF and a modifier 91 and no line item on the claim with modifier CF and no modifier 91.	Shared system
1.7	FI must return any claims for additional tests for any date of service within the billing period when the provider has already submitted a claim. Instruct the provider to adjust the first claim.	FI or Shared system
1.8	Do not apply the 50/50 rule to line items for one of the chemistries in exhibits 1 or 2 that contain modifiers CE or CF and modifier 91 on the line item.	Shared system

Carrier Business Requirements for ESRD Reimbursement of AMCC Tests:

Requirement #	Requirements	Responsibility
1	The standard systems shall calculate payment at the lowest rate for these automated tests even if reported on separate claims for services performed by the same provider, for the same beneficiary, for the same date of service	Standard Systems
2	Standard Systems shall identify the AMCC tests ordered that are included and are not included in the composite rate payment based upon the presence of the "CD," "CE" and "CF" modifiers.	Standard Systems
3	Based upon the determination of requirement 2 if 50 percent or more of the covered services are included under the composite rate payment, Standard Systems shall indicate that no separate payment is provided for the services submitted for that date of service.	Standard Systems
4	Based upon the determination of requirement 2 if less than 50 percent are covered services include under the composite rate, Standard Systems shall indicate that all AMCC tests for that date of service are payable under the 50/50 rule.	Standard Systems
5	Standard Systems/local carriers shall return as unprocessable line items that contain a procedure reported with modifier "CE" and modifier 91 and no line item on the claim or a claim in history or in cycle for that date of service with modifier "CE" only.	Standard Systems/ Carriers
6	Standard Systems/local carriers shall return as unprocessable line items that contain a procedure reported with modifier "CF" and modifier 91 and no line item on the claim or a claim in history or in cycle for that date of service with modifier "CF" only.	Carriers
7	Standard Systems shall not apply the 50/50 rule to line items for one of the chemistries that contain modifiers "CE" or "CF" and modifier 91 on the line item.	Standard Systems
8	Standard Systems shall adjust the previous claim when the incoming claim is compared to the claim on history and the action is to deny the previous claim. Spread the payment amount over each line item on both claims (the adjusted claim and the incoming claim).	Standard Systems
9	Standard Systems shall spread the adjustment across the incoming claim unless the adjusted amount would exceed the submitted amount of the services on the claim.	Standard System
10	Local carriers shall return as unprocessable claims submitted as outlined in business rules 5 and 6. When returning as unprocessable line items based upon the requirements of 5 and 6, local carriers shall use remittance advice remark code M78, reason code 125.	Carriers
11	Local carriers shall return an unprocessable lab panel codes billed with the "CD", "CE", and "CF" modifiers. When returning an unprocessable these lab panel codes use remittance advice remark code N56, reason code 4.	Carriers

Require- ment #	Requirements	Responsibility
12	Local carriers shall return as un-processable line items submitted with a "CD" modifier and "91" modifier on the same line item. When returning an unprocessa-ble line items that contain a "CD" modifier and a " 91" mod-ifier, local carriers shall use re-mittance advice remark code M78, reason code 125.	Carriers

Examples of the Application of the 50/50 Rule

The following examples are to illustrate how claims should be paid. The percentages in the action section represent the number of composite rate tests over the total tests. If this percentage is 50 percent or greater, no payment should be made for the claim.

Example 1:

Provider Name: Jones Hospital

DOS 2/1/02

Claim/Services 82040 Mod CD*
82310 Mod CD
82374 Mod CD
82435 Mod CD
82947 Mod CF
84295 Mod CF
82040 Mod CD (Returned as duplicate)
84075 Mod CE
82310 Mod CE
84155 Mod CE

ACTION: 9 services total, 2 non-composite rate tests, 3 composite rate tests beyond the frequency, 4 composite rate tests; 4/9 = 44.4% < 50% pay at ATP 09

Example 2:

Provider Name: Bon Secours Renal Facility

DOS 2/15/02

Claim/Services 82040 Mod CE and Mod 91
84450 Mod CE
82310 Mod CE
82247 Mod CF
82465 No modifier present
82565 Mod CE
84550 Mod CF
82040 Mod CD
84075 Mod CE
82435 Mod CE
82550 Mod CF
82947 Mod CF
82977 Mod CF

ACTION: 11 services total, 6 non-composite rate tests, 4 compos-ite rate tests beyond the frequency, 1 composite rate test; 1/11 = .09.4% < 50% pay at ATP 12

Example 3:

Provider Name: Sinai Hospital Renal Facility

DOS 4/02/02

Claim/Services 82565 Mod CD*
83615 Mod CD
82247 Mod CF
82248 Mod CF
82040 Mod CD
84450 Mod CD
82565 Mod CE
84550 Mod CF
82248 Mod CF (Duplicate)

ACTION: 8 services total, 4 composite rate tests; 4/8 = 50%, therefore no payment is made

Example 4:

Provider Name: Dr. Andrew Ross

DOS 6/01/02

Claim/Services 84460 Mod CF
82247 Mod CF
82248 Mod CF
82040 Mod CD
84075 Mod CD
84450 Mod CD

ACTION: 6 services total, 3 non-composite rate tests and 3 com-posite rate tests; 3/6 = 50%, therefore no payment.

Example 5: (Carrier Processing Example Only)

Payment for first claim, second creates a no payment for either claim

Provider Name: Dr. Andrew Ross

DOS 6/01/02

84460 Mod CF
82247 Mod CF
82248 Mod CF

ACTION: 3 services total, 3 non-composite rate tests, 0 compos-ite rate tests beyond the frequency, and 0 composite rate tests, 0/3 = 0%, therefore ATP 03

Second Claim: No payment.

Provider Name: Dr. Andrew Ross

DOS 6/01/02

82040 Mod CD
84075 Mod CD
84450 Mod CD

ACTION: An additional 3 services are billed, 0 non-composite rate tests, 8 composite rate test beyond the frequency, 3 compos-ite rate tests. For both claims there are 6 services total, 3 non-composite rate tests and 3 composite rate tests; 3/6 = 50% ≥ 50%, therefore no payment. An overpayment should be recovered for the ATP 03 payment

40.6.2—Claims Processing for Separately Billable Tests for ESRD Beneficiaries

(Rev. 1, 10-01-03)

Clinical laboratory tests can be performed individually or in pre-determined groups on automated profile equipment. If a test pro-file is performed see §40.6.1. If a clinical laboratory test is per-formed individually, see §40.6.2.1 or §40.6.2.2 depending upon whether the patient is treated in a hospital-based or independent dialysis facility

40.6.2.1—Separately Billable ESRD Laboratory Tests Furnished by Hospital-Based Facilities

(Rev. 1, 10-01-03)

Hospital-based facilities are reimbursed for the separately billable ESRD laboratory tests furnished to their outpatients following the same rules that apply to all other Medicare covered outpatient laboratory services furnished by a hospital.

40.6.2.2—Separately Billable ESRD Laboratory Tests Furnished to Patients of Independent Dialysis Facilities—FIs

(Rev. 1, 10-01-03)

In accord with Medicare program rules, the FI pays the labora-tory that provided the service for all separately billable ESRD clinical laboratory services furnished to patients of independent dialysis. Independent dialysis facilities with appropriate clinical laboratory certification may bill their FI for any separately billable clinical laboratory tests they perform. The FI pays both laborato-ries and independent dialysis facilities for separately billable clini-

---

*CPT only © 2004. *Current Procedural Terminology, 2005, Professional Edition,* American Medical Association. All Rights Reserved.

cal laboratory tests according to the Medicare clinical laboratory fee schedule.

40.6.2.3—Skilled Nursing Facility (SNF) Consolidated Billing (CB) Editing and Separately Billed ESRD Laboratory Test Furnished to Patients of Independent Dialysis Facilities—Carriers

(Rev. 69, 01-23-04)

Effective April 1, 2003, for DOS on or after April 1, 2001, CWF will not apply the SNF CB edits to line items that contain the CB modifier. A provider or supplier may use the "CB" modifier only when it has determined that: (a) the beneficiary has ESRD entitlement, (b) the test is related to the dialysis treatment for ESRD, (c) the test is ordered by a doctor providing care to patients in the dialysis facility, and (d) the test is not included in the dialysis facility's composite rate payment.

Those diagnostic tests that are presumptively considered to be dialysis-related and, therefore, appropriate for submission with the " CB" modifier are identified in Exhibit 3. This list was not designed as an all-inclusive list of Medicare covered diagnostic services. Additional diagnostic services related to the beneficiary's ESRD treatment/care may be considered dialysis-related. However, if these services are not included in our listing, the carrier may require supporting medical documentation.

Beneficiaries in a SNF Part A stay are eligible for a broad range of diagnostic services as part of the SNF Part A benefit. Physicians ordering medically necessary diagnostic test that are not directly related to the beneficiary's ESRD are subject to the SNF consolidated billing requirements. Physicians may bill the carrier for the professional component of these diagnostic tests. In most cases, however, the technical component of diagnostic tests is included in the SNF PPS rate and is not separately billable to the carrier. Physicians should coordinate with the SNF in ordering such tests since the SNF will be responsible for bearing the cost of the technical component.

40.7—Billing for Noncovered Clinical Laboratory Tests

(Rev. 1, 10-01-03)

B3-5114.1

Ordinarily, neither a physician nor a laboratory bills the Medicare Program for noncovered tests. However, if the beneficiary (or his/her representative) contends that a clinical laboratory test which a physician or laboratory believes is noncovered may be covered, the physician or laboratory must file a claim that includes the test to effectuate the beneficiary's right to a Medicare determination. The physician or laboratory annotates the claim that he/she believes that the test is noncovered and is submitting it at the beneficiary's insistence. Before furnishing a beneficiary a test which the physician or laboratory believes is excluded from coverage as not reasonable and necessary (rather than excluded from coverage as part of a routine physical check-up), the physician or laboratory must obtain a signed Advanced Beneficiary Notice (ABN) from the beneficiary (or representative) that the physician or laboratory has informed him/her of the noncoverage of the test and that there will be a charge for the test. This protects the physician or laboratory against possible liability for the test under the limitation of liability provision.

See Chapter 30, regarding Advance Beneficiary Notices (ABN) and demand bills.

104, Chapter 16

60—SPECIMEN COLLECTION FEE AND TRAVEL ALLOWANCE

(Rev. 1, 10-01-03)

B3-5114.1

60.1—Specimen Collection Fee

(Rev. 1, 10-01-03)

B3-5114.1, A3-3628

In addition to the amounts provided under the fee schedules, the Secretary shall provide for and establish a nominal fee to cover the appropriate costs of collecting the sample on which a clinical laboratory test was performed and for which payment is made with respect to samples collected in the same encounter.

A specimen collection fee is allowed in circumstances such as drawing a blood sample through venipuncture (i.e., inserting into a vein a needle with syringe or vacutainer to draw the specimen) or collecting a urine sample by catheterization. A specimen collection fee is not allowed for blood samples where the cost of collecting the specimen is minimal (such as a throat culture or a routine capillary puncture for clotting or bleeding time). This fee will not be paid to anyone who has not extracted the specimen. Only one collection fee is allowed for each type of specimen for each patient encounter, regardless of the number of specimens drawn. When a series of specimens is required to complete a single test (e.g., glucose tolerance test), the series is treated as a single encounter.

60.1.1—Physician Specimen Drawing

(Rev. 1, 10-01-03)

HO-437, A3-3628, B3-5114.1

Medicare allows a specimen collection fee for physicians only when (1) it is the accepted and prevailing practice among physicians in the locality to make separate charges for drawing or collecting a specimen, and (2) it is the customary practice of the physician performing such services to bill separate charges for drawing or collecting the specimen.

60.1.2—Independent Laboratory Specimen Drawing

(Rev. 1, 10-01-03)

B3-4110.4, HO-437, A3-3628

Medicare allows separate charges made by laboratories for drawing or collecting specimens whether or not the specimens are referred to hospitals or independent laboratories. The laboratory does not bill for routine handling charges where a specimen is referred by one laboratory to another.

Medicare allows a specimen collection fee when it is medically necessary for a laboratory technician to draw a specimen from either a nursing home patient or homebound patient. The technician must personally draw the specimen, e.g., venipuncture or urine sample by catheterization. Medicare does not allow a specimen collection fee to the visiting technician if a patient in a facility is (a) not confined to the facility, or (b) the facility has personnel on duty qualified to perform the specimen collection. Medical necessity for such services exists, for example, where a laboratory technician draws a blood specimen from a homebound or an institutionalized patient. A patient need not be bedridden to be homebound. However, where the specimen is a type that would require only the services of a messenger and would not require the skills of a laboratory technician, e.g., urine or sputum, a specimen pickup service would not be considered medically necessary. (See Chapters 7 and 15 of the Medicare Benefit Policy Manual for a discussion of "homebound" and a more complete definition of a medically necessary laboratory service to a homebound or an institutional patient.)

In addition to the usual information required on claim forms (including the name of the prescribing physician), all independent laboratory claims for such specimen drawing or EKG services prescribed by a physician should be appropriately annotated, e.g., "patient confined to home," "patient homebound," or "patient in nursing home, no qualified person on duty to draw specimen." Carriers must assure the validity of the annotation through scientific claims samples as well as through regular bill review techniques. (This could be done by use of the information in carrier files, and where necessary, contact with the prescribing physician.)

If a physician requests an independent laboratory to obtain specimens in situations which do not meet, or without regard to whether they meet, the medical necessity criteria in Chapter 15 of the Medicare Benefit Policy Manual, an educational contact with the prescribing physician is warranted and, where necessary, corroborating documentation should be obtained on claims until the carrier is assured that the physician prescribes such services only when the criteria are met.

60.1.3—Specimen Drawing for Dialysis Patients

(Rev. 1, 10-01-03)

A3 3644.1, PR 2711.1, B3-4270.2, PUB-29 322

See the Medicare Benefit Policy Manual, Chapter 11, for a description of laboratory services included in the composite rate.

Independent laboratories and independent dialysis facilities with the appropriate clinical laboratory certification in accordance with CLIA may be paid for ESRD clinical laboratory tests that are separately billable. The laboratories and independent dialysis facilities are paid for separately billable clinical laboratory tests according to the Medicare laboratory fee schedule for independent laboratories. Independent dialysis facilities billing for separately billable laboratory tests that they perform must submit claims to the FI. Independent laboratories must bill the carrier.

Hospital-based laboratories providing laboratory service to hospital dialysis patients of the hospital's dialysis facility are paid in accordance with the outpatient laboratory provisions. However, where the hospital laboratory does tests for an independent dialysis facility or for another hospital's facility, the nonpatient billing provisions apply (see §20.1).

Clinical laboratory tests can be performed individually or in predetermined groups on automated profile equipment. A specimen collection fee determined by CMS (as of this writing, up to $3.00) will be allowed only in the following circumstances:

- Drawing a blood sample through venipuncture (i.e., inserting into a vein a needle with a syringe or vacutainer to draw the specimen).
- Collecting a urine sample by catheterization.

Special rules apply when such services are furnished to dialysis patients. The specimen collection fee is not separately payable for y patients dialyzed in the facility or for patients dialyzed at home under reimbursement Method I. Payment for this service is included under the ESRD composite rate, regardless of whether the laboratory test itself is included in the composite rate or is separately billable.

Fees for taking specimens from home dialysis patients, who have elected reimbursement Method II may be paid separately, provided all other criteria for payment are met. Also, fees for taking specimens in the hospital setting, but outside of the dialysis unit, for use in performing laboratory tests not included in the ESRD composite rate may be paid separately.

60.1.4—Coding Requirements for Specimen Collection

(Rev. 1, 10-01-03)

The following HCPCS codes and terminology must be used:

- G0001—Routine venipuncture for collection of specimen(s).
- P9615—Catheterization for collection of specimen(s).

The allowed amount for specimen collection in each of the above circumstances is included in the laboratory fee schedule distributed annually by CMS.

60.2—Travel Allowance

(Rev. 1, 10-01-03)

HO-437, A3-3628.F, B3-5114.1K; PM-AB-99-49

In addition to a specimen collection fee allowed under §60.1, Medicare, under Part B, covers a specimen collection fee and travel allowance for a laboratory technician to draw a specimen from either a nursing home patient or homebound patient under §1833(h)(3) of the Act and payment is made based on the clinical laboratory fee schedule. The travel allowance is intended to cover the estimated travel costs of collecting a specimen and to reflect the technician's salary and travel costs.

The additional allowance can be made only where a specimen collection fee is also payable, i.e., no travel allowance is made where the technician merely performs a messenger service to pick up a specimen drawn by a physician or nursing home personnel. The travel allowance may not be paid to a physician unless the trip to the home, or to the nursing home was solely for the purpose of drawing a specimen. Otherwise travel costs are considered to be associated with the other purposes of the trip.

The travel allowance is not distributed by CMS. Instead, the carrier must calculate the travel allowance for each claim using the following rules for the particular Code. The following HCPCS codes are used for travel allowances:

Per Mile Travel Allowance (P9603)

- The minimum "per mile travel allowance" is 75 cents. The per mile travel allowance is to be used in situations where the average trip to patients' homes is longer than 20 miles round trip, and is to be pro-rated in situations where specimens are drawn or picked up from non-Medicare patients in the same trip.—one way, in connection with medically necessary laboratory specimen collection drawn from homebound or nursing home bound patient; prorated miles actually traveled (carrier allowance on per mile basis); or
- The per mile allowance was computed using the Federal mileage rate plus an additional 44 cents a mile to cover the technician's time and travel costs. Contractors have the option of establishing a higher per mile rate in excess of the minimum (75 cents a mile in cy 2000) if local conditions warrant it. The minimum mileage rate will be reviewed and updated in conjunction with the clinical lab fee schedule as needed. At no time will the laboratory be allowed to bill for more miles than are reasonable or for miles not actually traveled by the laboratory technician.

Example 1: In CY 2000, a laboratory technician travels 60 miles round trip from a lab in a city to a remote rural location, and back to the lab to draw a single Medicare patient's blood. The total reimbursement would be $45.00 (60 miles x .75 cents a mile), plus the specimen collection fee of $3.00.

Example 2: In CY 2000, a laboratory technician travels 40 miles from the lab to a Medicare patient's home to draw blood, and then travels an additional 10 miles to a non-Medicare patient's home and then travels 30 miles to return to the lab. The total miles traveled would be 80 miles. The claim submitted would be for one half of the miles traveled or $30.00 (40 x .75), plus specimen collection fee of $3.00.

Flat Rate (P9604)

The CMS will pay a minimum of $7.50 one way flat rate travel allowance. The flat rate travel allowance is to be used in areas where average trips are less than 20 miles round trip. The flat rate travel fee is to be pro-rated for more than one blood drawn at the same address, and for stops at the homes of Medicare and non-Medicare patients. The laboratory does the pro-ration when the claim is submitted based on the number of patients seen on that trip. The specimen collection fee will be paid for each patient encounter.

This rate is based on an assumption that a trip is an average of 15 minutes and up to 10 miles one way. It uses the Federal mileage rate and a laboratory technician's time of $17.66 an hour, including overhead. Contractors have the option of establishing a flat rate in excess of the minimum of $7.50, if local conditions warrant it. The minimum national flat rate will be reviewed and updated in conjunction with the clinical laboratory fee schedule, as necessitated by adjustments in the Federal travel allowance and salaries.

The claimant identifies round trip travel by use of the LR modifier

Example 3: A laboratory technician travels from the laboratory to a single Medicare patient's home and returns to the laboratory without making any other stops. The flat rate would be calculated as follows: 2 × $7.50 for a total trip reimbursement of $15.00, plus the specimen collection fee.

Example 4: A laboratory technician travels from the laboratory to the homes of five patients to draw blood, four of the patients are Medicare patients and one is not. An additional flat rate would be charged to cover the 5 stops and the return trip to the lab (6 × $7.50 = $45.00). Each of the claims submitted would be for $9.00 ($45.00/5 = $9.00). Since one of the patients is non-Medicare, four claims would be submitted for $9.00 each, plus the specimen collection fee for each.

Example 5: A laboratory technician travels from a laboratory to a nursing home and draws blood from 5 patients and returns to the laboratory. Four of the patients are on Medicare and one is not. The $7.50 flat rate is multiplied by two to cover the return trip to the laboratory (2 × $7.50 = $15.00) and then divided by five (1/5 of $15.00 = $3.00). Since one of the patients is non-Medicare, four claims would be submitted for $3.00 each, plus the specimen collection fee.

If a carrier determines that it results in equitable payment, the carrier may extend the former payment allowances for additional travel (such as to a distant rural nursing home) to all circumstances where travel is required. This might be appropriate, for example, if the carrier's former payment allowance was on a per mile basis. Otherwise, it should establish an appropriate allowance and inform the suppliers in its service area. If a carrier decides to establish a new allowance, one method is to consider developing a travel allowance consisting of:

• The current Federal mileage allowance for operating personal automobiles, plus a personnel allowance per mile to cover personnel costs based upon an estimate of average hourly wages and average driving speed.

Carriers must prorate travel allowance amounts claimed by suppliers by the number of patients (including Medicare and non-Medicare patients) from whom specimens were drawn on a given trip.

The carrier may determine that payment in addition to the routine travel allowance determined under this section is appropriate if:

• the patient from whom the specimen must be collected is in a nursing home or is homebound; and
• the clinical laboratory tests are needed on an emergency basis outside the general business hours of the laboratory making the collection.

70—CLINICAL LABORATORY IMPROVEMENT AMENDMENTS (CLIA) REQUIREMENTS

(Rev. 1, 10-01-03)

A3-3628.2, RHC-640, ESRD 322, HO-306, HHA-465, SNF 541, HO-437.2, PM B-97-3

70.1—Background

(Rev. 1, 10-01-03)

A3-3628.2, PM B-97-4

The Clinical Laboratory Improvements Amendments of 1988 (CLIA), Public Law 100-578, amended §353 of the Public Health Service Act (PHSA) to extend jurisdiction of the Department of Health and Human Services to regulate all laboratories that examine human specimens to provide information to assess, diagnose, prevent, or treat any disease or impairment. The purpose of the CLIA program is to assure that laboratories testing specimens in interstate commerce consistently provide accurate procedures and services. As a result of CLIA, any laboratory soliciting or accepting specimens in interstate commerce for laboratory testing is required to hold a valid license or letter of exemption from licensure issued by the Secretary of HHS. The term "interstate commerce" means trade, traffic, commerce, transportation, or communication between any state, possession of the United States, the Commonwealth of Puerto Rico, or the District of Columbia, and any place outside thereof, or within the District of Columbia.

CLIA mandates that virtually all laboratories, including physician office laboratories (POLs), meet applicable Federal requirements and have a CLIA certificate in order to receive reimbursement from Federal programs. CLIA also lists requirements for laboratories performing only certain tests to be eligible for a certificate of waiver or a certificate for Physician Performed Microscopy Procedures (PPMP). Since 1992, carriers have been instructed to deny clinical laboratory services billed by independent laboratories which did not meet the CLIA requirements. POLs were excluded from the 1992 instruction but included in 1997.

The CLIA number must be included on each Form CMS-1500 claim for laboratory services by any laboratory performing tests covered by CLIA.

70.2—Billing

(Rev. 1, 10-01-03)

The CLIA number is required in field 23 of the paper Form CMS-1500. The electronic formats have a field reserved for a CLIA number. See Chapter 26 for specific reporting requirements.

70.3—Verifying CLIA Certification

(Rev. 1, 10-01-03)

A3-3628.2

CWF edits Carrier claims to ascertain that the laboratory identified by the CLIA number is certified to perform the test. (CWF uses data supplied from the certification process.) See Chapter 27 for related specifications.

Providers that bill FIs are responsible for verifying CLIA certification prior to ordering laboratory services under arrangement. The survey process validates that these providers have procedures in place to insure that laboratory services are provided by CLIA approved laboratories. See the Medicare State Agency Manual for details.

70.4—CLIA Numbers

(Rev. 1, 10-01-03)

A3-3628.2.D

The structure of the CLIA number follows:

Positions 1 and 2 contain the State code (based on the laboratory's physical location at time of registration);

Position 3 contains the letter "D"; and

Positions 4-10 contain the unique CLIA system assigned number that identifies the laboratory. (No other laboratory in the country has this number.)

Initially, providers are issued a CLIA number when they apply to the CLIA program.

Independent dialysis facilities must obtain a CLIA certificate in order to perform clotting time tests.

70.5—CLIA Categories and Subcategories

(Rev. 1, 10-01-03)

A laboratory may be licensed or exempted from licensure in several major categories of procedures. These major categories are:

010	Histocompatibility
100	Microbiology
110	Bacteriology
115	Mycobacteriology
120	Mycology
130	Parasitology
140	Virology
150	Other Microbiology
200	Diagnostic Immunology
210	Syphilis Serology
220	General Immunology
300	Chemistry
310	Routine
320	Urinalysis
330	Endocrinology
340	Toxicology

350	Other
400	Hematology
500	Immuno-hematology
510	ABO Group and RH Type
520	Antibody Detection (Transfusion)
530	Antibody Detection (Non Transfusion)
540	Antibody Identification
550	Compatibility Testing
560	Other
600	Pathology
610	Histopathology
620	Oral Pathology
630	Cytology
800	Radioassay
900	Clinical Cytogenics

For a list of specific HCPCS codes see http://www.cms.hhs.gov/clia/default.asp

70.6—Certificate for Physician-Performed Microscopy Procedures

(Rev. 12, 10-24-03) See Business Requirements at http:/www.cms.hhs.gov/manuals/pm_trans/R12CP.pdf

A3-3628.2.E

Effective January 19, 1993, a laboratory that holds a certificate for physician-performed microscopy procedures may perform only those tests specified as physician-performed microscopy procedures and waived tests, as described below, and no others.

HCPCS Code	Test
Q0111	Wet mounts, including preparations of vaginal, cervical or skin specimens
Q0112	All potassium hydroxide (KOH) preparations
Q0113	Pinworm examinations
Q0114	Fern test
Q0115	Post-coital direct, qualitative examinations of vaginal or cervical mucous
81015	Urine sediment examinations

70.7—Deleted—Held for Expansion

(Rev. 1, 10-01-03)

70.8—Certificate of Waiver

(Rev. 102, 02-20-04)

A3-3628.2

Effective September 1, 1992, all laboratory testing sites (except as provided in 42 CFR 493.3(b)) must have either a CLIA certificate of waiver, certificate for provider-performed microscopy procedures, certificate of registration, certificate of compliance, or certificate of accreditation to legally perform clinical laboratory testing on specimens from individuals in the United States.

The Food and Drug Administration approves CLIA waived tests on a flow basis. The CMS identifies CLIA waived tests by providing an updated list of waived tests to the Medicare contractors on a quarterly basis via a Recurring Update Notification. To be recognized as a waived test, some CLIA waived tests have unique HCPCS procedure codes and some must have a QW modifier included with the HCPCS code.

For a list of specific HCPCS codes subject to CLIA see http://www.cms.hhs.gov/clia/waivetbl.pdf

70.9—CLIA License or Licensure Exemption

(Rev. 1, 10-01-03)

See the Medicare State Operations Manual.

70.10—CLIA Number Submitted on Form CMS-1500

(Rev. 1, 10-01-03)

Effective with services provided October 1, 1997, any independent laboratory performing tests covered by CLIA must submit the CLIA number on the Form CMS-1500 hardcopy or electronic claim form. The CLIA number is reported in:

- Field 23 of the paper CMS-1500,
- Record FAO, field 34 of the NSF,
- ASC X12 837 (3051) REF segment as REF02, with qualifier of "X4" in REF01
- ASC X12 837 (4010) REF segment as REF02, with qualifier of "X4" in REF01

The CLIA number is not required on UB 92 or its related data sets.

See Chapter 26 for detailed format instructions.

Laboratory claims submitted without the CLIA number are returned as unprocessable. If the CLIA number is submitted on the claim, but is inconsistent with the CLIA format, the carrier returns the claim as unprocessable. If more than one CLIA number is submitted on the claim, except when a reference laboratory is on the same claim, the carrier returns the claim as unprocessable.

If the tests on one claim have been performed in more than one Physician Office Laboratory (POL) by the same physician, the appropriate CLIA number should be associated with the test that was performed in each laboratory. In such a case, the physician must submit a separate claim for each location (CLIA number) where a test was performed.

70.10.1—Physician Notification of Denials

(Rev. 1, 10-01-03)

If there is no CLIA number on the claim, the carrier sends RA messages MA 120 and MA 130, which state:

MA 120—Did not complete or enter accurately the CLIA number.

MA 130—Your claim contains incomplete and/or invalid information, and no appeal rights are afforded because the claim in unprocessable. Please submit the correct information to the appropriate FI or carrier.

70.11—Reasons for Denial—Physician Office Laboratories Out-of-Compliance

(Rev. 1, 10-01-03)

Carriers use remittance advice (RA) message B7 to notify the provider of the reason for denial. The B7 message states: "This provider was not certified/eligible to be paid for this procedure/service on this date of service."

Carriers use MSN message #14.1, which states:

The laboratory is not approved for this type of test.

80—ISSUES RELATED TO SPECIFIC TESTS

(Rev. 1, 10-01-03)

80.1—Screening Services

(Rev. 1, 10-01-03)

See Chapter 18 for payment, edit and MSN requirements for the following screening services.

- Screening Pap Smear and Pelvic Examination
- Screening Prostate Tests
- Colorectal Cancer Screening

80.2—Anatomic Pathology Services

(Rev. 1, 10-01-03)

A3-3628.1, SNF 541.1, HO-437.1, RHC-437, CIM 50.20.1, PM AB-98-7, AB-98-22, B-98-16, A-98-6, R103.CIM, A3-4603.1

Clinical laboratory tests include some services described as anatomic pathology services in CPT (i.e., certain cervical, vaginal, or peripheral blood smears). The CPT code 85060* is used only

---

*CPT only © 2004. *Current Procedural Terminology, 2005, Professional Edition*, American Medical Association. All Rights Reserved.

when a physician interprets an abnormal peripheral blood smear for a hospital inpatient or a hospital outpatient, and the hospital is responsible for the technical component. When an independent laboratory bills a physician interpretation of an abnormal peripheral blood smear, the service is considered a complete or global service, and is not billed under the CPT code 85060*. A physician interpretation of an abnormal peripheral blood smear performed by an independent laboratory is considered a routine part of the ordered hematology service (i.e., those tests that include a different white blood count).

HCPCS code 88150 (cervical or vaginal smears) included both screening and interpretation in CPT 1986 terminology while the CPT 1987 terminology includes only screening. A new code, 88151, was added for those smears that require physician interpretation. Code 88151 is treated and priced in the same manner as code 88150 was previously treated and priced. Code 88151 with a "-26" modifier is paid when a physician performs an interpretation of an abnormal smear for a hospital inpatient or outpatient, and the hospital is responsible for the technical component. The "-26" modifier for code 88150 is no longer recognized. Code 88151(26) is priced as code 88150(26) would have been priced if the coding terminology had not been revised. Independent laboratories bill under code 88150 for normal smears and under code 88151 for abnormal smears. However, the fee schedule amount is equivalent.

80.2.1—Technical Component (TC) of Physician Pathology Services to Hospital Patients

(Rev. 1, 10-01-03)

PM AB-02-177

Section 542 of the Benefits Improvement and Protection Act of 2000 (BIPA) provides that the Medicare carrier can continue to pay for the TC of physician pathology services when an independent laboratory furnishes this service to an inpatient or outpatient of a covered hospital. This provision applies to TC services furnished during the 2-year period beginning on January 1, 2001.

For this provision, covered hospital means a hospital that had an arrangement with an independent laboratory that was in effect as of July 22, 1999, under which a laboratory furnished the TC of physician pathology services to fee-for-service Medicare beneficiaries who were hospital inpatients or outpatients and submitted claims for payment for the TC to a carrier. The TC could have been submitted separately or combined with the professional component and reported as a combined service.

The term "fee-for-service Medicare beneficiary" means an individual who is:

1. Is entitled to benefits under Part A or enrolled under Part B of title XVIII or both; and

2. Is not enrolled in any of the following:

a. A Medicare + Choice plan under Part C of such title;

b. A plan offered by an eligible organization under §1876 of the Act;

c. A program of all-inclusive care for the elderly under §1894 of the Act; or

d. A social health maintenance organization demonstration project established under §4108(b) of the Omnibus Budget Reconciliation Act of 1987.

The following examples illustrate the application of the statutory provision to arrangements between hospitals and independent laboratories.

In implementing §542, the carriers should consider as independent laboratories those entities that it has previously recognized and paid as independent laboratories.

An independent laboratory that has acquired another independent laboratory that had an arrangement on July 22, 1999, with a covered hospital, can bill the TC of physician pathology services for that hospital's inpatients and outpatients under the physician fee schedule.

EXAMPLE 1

Prior to July 22, 1999, independent laboratory A had an arrangement with a hospital in which this laboratory billed the carrier for the TC of physician pathology services. In July 2000, independent laboratory B acquires independent laboratory A. Independent laboratory B bills the carrier for the TC of physician pathology services for this hospital's patients in 2001 and 2002.

If a hospital is a covered hospital, any independent laboratory that furnishes the TC of physician pathology services to that hospital's inpatients or outpatients can bill the carrier for these services furnished in 2001 and 2002.

EXAMPLE 2:

As of July 22, 1999, the hospital had an arrangement with an independent laboratory, laboratory A, under which that laboratory billed the carrier for the TC of physician pathology service to hospital inpatients or outpatients. In 2001, the hospital enters into an arrangement with a different independent laboratory, laboratory B, under which laboratory B wishes to bill its carrier for the TC of physician pathology services to hospital inpatients or outpatients. Because the hospital is a "covered hospital," independent laboratory B can bill its carrier for the TC of physician pathology services to hospital inpatients or outpatients.

If the arrangement between the independent laboratory and the covered hospital limited the provision of TC physician pathology services to certain situations or at particular times, then the independent laboratory can bill the carrier only for these limited services.

An independent laboratory that furnishes the TC of physician pathology services to inpatients or outpatients of a hospital that is not a covered hospital may not bill the carrier for TC physician pathology services furnished to patients of that hospital in 2001 or 2002.

An independent laboratory that has an arrangement with a covered hospital should forward a copy of this agreement or other documentation to its carrier to confirm that an arrangement was in effect between the hospital and the independent laboratory as of July 22, 1999. This documentation should be furnished for each covered hospital the independent laboratory services. If the laboratory did not have an arrangement with the covered hospital as of July 22, 1999, but has subsequently entered into an arrangement, then it should obtain a copy of the arrangement between the predecessor laboratory and the covered hospital and furnish this to the carrier. The carrier maintains a hard copy of this documentation for postpayment reviews.

The hospital cannot bill under the OPPS for the TC of physician pathology services if the independent laboratory that services that hospital outpatients is receiving payment from its carrier under the physician fee schedule.

80.3—National Minimum Payment Amounts for Cervical or Vaginal Smear Clinical Laboratory Tests

(Rev. 1, 10-01-03)

PM AB-99-84, AB-99-99

For cervical or vaginal smear clinical laboratory tests, payment is the lesser of the local fee or the national limitation amount, but not less than the national minimum payment amount (NMPA). However, in no case may payment for these tests exceed actual charges. The Part B deductible and coinsurance do not apply.

For tests performed on or after January 1, 2000, a NMPA of $14.60 is established and applies for cervical or vaginal smear clinical laboratory tests in accordance with §224 of the Balanced Budget Refinement Act (Public Law 106-113). The affected CPT laboratory test codes for the NMPA are 88142, 88143, 88144, 88145, 88147, 88148, 88150, 88152, 88153, 88154, 88164, 88165,

88166, 88167, G0123, G0143, G 0144, G0145, G0147, G0148, and P3000.*

The NMPA will be reviewed and updated in conjunction with the clinical laboratory fee schedule, as required. Instructions for such updates will be sent to contractors through periodic temporary instructions.

80.4—Oximetry

(Rev. 1, 10-01-03)

B3-5114.1

Certain blood gas levels are determined either by invasive means through use of a blood specimen for a clinical laboratory test or by noninvasive means through ear or pulse oximetry, which is not considered a clinical laboratory test. CPT code 82792* is used for invasive oximetry. HCPCS code M0592 is used for ear and pulse oximetry. Code M0592 is not subject to fee schedules.

90—AUTOMATED PROFILE TESTS AND ORGAN/DISEASE ORIENTED PANELS

(Rev. 1, 10-01-03)

The term "profile" or "panel" means a grouping of laboratory tests, which is usually performed automatically on a single piece of testing equipment.

90.1—Laboratory Tests Utilizing Automated Equipment

(Rev. 1, 10-01-03)

B3-5114, HO-437, A3-3628

Clinical laboratory tests are covered under Medicare if they are reasonable and necessary for the diagnosis or treatment of an illness or injury. Because of the numerous technological advances and innovations in the clinical laboratory field and the increased availability of automated testing equipment, no distinction is generally made in determining payment for individual tests because of either (1) the sites where the service is performed, or (2) the method of the testing process used, whether manual or automated. Whether the test is actually performed manually or with automated equipment, the services are considered similar and the payment is the same.

However, where groups of tests that are billed individually may be done as a panel or profile, a determination must be made about whether payment should be made at the individual rate or at the panel or profile rate.

90.1.1—Automated Test Listing

(Rev. 1, 10-01-03)

B3-5114, HO-437, A3-3628, PMs AB-97-5, AB-97-7, AB-97-17

Profiles are specific groupings of blood chemistries that enable physicians to more accurately diagnose their patients' medical problems. While the component tests in automated profiles may vary somewhat from one laboratory to another, or from one physician's office or clinic to another, in order to develop appropriate payment amounts, contractors group together those profile tests that can be performed at the same time on the same equipment. The carrier or FI must group together the individual tests in the profile when billed separately and consider the price of the related automated profile test. Payment cannot exceed the lower of the profile price or the totals of the prices of all the individual tests. (This rule is applicable also if the tests are done manually.) The profile HCPCS code and each individual test is priced at the lower of the billed charge or the fee amount; and payment is made at the lower of the profile/panel price or the total of the prices for all covered components.

Payment is made only for those tests in an automated profile that meet Medicare coverage rules. Where only some of the tests in a profile of tests are covered, payment cannot exceed the amount that would have been paid if only the covered tests had been ordered. For example, the use of the 12-channel serum chemistry test to determine the blood sugar level in a proven case of diabetes is unreasonable because the results of a blood sugar test performed separately provide the essential information. Normally, the payment allowance for a blood sugar test is lower than the payment allowance for the automated profile of tests. In no event, however, may payment for the covered tests exceed the payment allowance for the profile.

However, the carrier prices and pays the 1-22 automated multi-channel chemistry tests tested in §90.2 at the lowest possible amount in accordance with §90.3.

APPENDIX B

COVERAGE ISSUES MANUAL (CIM), SELECT

CIM 30-1

310.1—Routine Costs in Clinical Trials

(Rev. 1, 10-03-03)

Effective for items and services furnished on or after September 19, 2000, Medicare covers the routine costs of qualifying clinical trials, as such costs are defined below, as well as reasonable and necessary items and services used to diagnose and treat complications arising from participation in all clinical trials. All other Medicare rules apply.

Routine costs of a clinical trial include all items and services that are otherwise generally available to Medicare beneficiaries (i.e., there exists a benefit category, it is not statutorily excluded, and there is not a national noncoverage decision) that are provided in either the experimental or the control arms of a clinical trial except:

The investigational item or service, itself;

Items and services provided solely to satisfy data collection and analysis needs and that are not used in the direct clinical management of the patient (e.g., monthly CT scans for a condition usually requiring only a single scan); and

Items and services customarily provided by the research sponsors free of charge for any enrollee in the trial.

Routine costs in clinical trials include:

Items or services that are typically provided absent a clinical trial (e.g., conventional care);

Items or services required solely for the provision of the investigational item or service (e.g., administration of a noncovered chemotherapeutic agent), the clinically appropriate monitoring of the effects of the item or service, or the prevention of complications; and

Items or services needed for reasonable and necessary care arising from the provision of an investigational item or service—in particular, for the diagnosis or treatment of complications.

This policy does not withdraw Medicare coverage for items and services that may be covered according to local medical review policies or the regulations on category B investigational device exemptions (IDE) found in 42 CFR 405.201-405.215, 411.115, and 411.406. For information about local medical review policies (LMRPs), refer to http://www.lmrp.net/, a searchable database of Medicare contractors' local policies.

For noncovered items and services, including items and services for which Medicare payment is statutorily prohibited, Medicare only covers the treatment of complications arising from the delivery of the noncovered item or service and unrelated reasonable and necessary care. (Refer to MCM §§2300.1 and MIM 3101.) However, if the item or service is not covered by virtue of a national noncoverage policy in the Coverage Issues Manual and is the focus of a qualifying clinical trial, the routine costs of the clinical trial (as defined above) will be covered by Medicare but the noncovered item or service, itself, will not. Requirements for Medicare Coverage of Routine Costs.—Any clinical trial receiving Medicare coverage of routine costs must meet the following three requirements:

The subject or purpose of the trial must be the evaluation of an item or service that falls within a Medicare benefit category (e.g., physicians' service, durable medical equipment, diagnostic test) and is not statutorily excluded from coverage (e.g., cosmetic surgery, hearing aids).

The trial must not be designed exclusively to test toxicity or disease pathophysiology. It must have therapeutic intent.

Trials of therapeutic interventions must enroll patients with diagnosed disease rather than healthy volunteers. Trials of diagnostic interventions may enroll healthy patients in order to have a proper control group.

The three requirements above are insufficient by themselves to qualify a clinical trial for Medicare coverage of routine costs. Clinical trials also should have the following desirable characteristics; however, some trials, as described below, are presumed to meet these characteristics and are automatically qualified to receive Medicare coverage:

The principal purpose of the trial is to test whether the intervention potentially improves the participants' health outcomes;

The trial is well-supported by available scientific and medical information or it is intended to clarify or establish the health outcomes of interventions already in common clinical use;

The trial does not unjustifiably duplicate existing studies;

The trial design is appropriate to answer the research question being asked in the trial;

The trial is sponsored by a credible organization or individual capable of executing the proposed trial successfully;

The trial is in compliance with Federal regulations relating to the protection of human subjects; and

All aspects of the trial are conducted according to the appropriate standards of scientific integrity.

Qualification Process for Clinical Trials:

Using the authority found in §1142 of the Act (cross-referenced in §1862(a)(1)(E) of the Act), the Agency for Healthcare Research and Quality (AHRQ) will convene a multi-agency Federal panel (the "panel") composed of representatives of the Department of Health and Human Services research agencies (National Institutes of Health (NIH), Centers for Disease Control and Prevention (CDC), the Food and Drug Administration (FDA), AHRQ, and the Office of Human Research Protection), and the research arms of the Department of Defense (DOD) and the Department of Veterans Affairs (VA) to develop qualifying criteria that will indicate a strong probability that a trial exhibits the desirable characteristics listed above. These criteria will be easily verifiable, and where possible, dichotomous. Trials that meet these qualifying criteria will receive Medicare coverage of their associated routine costs. This panel is not reviewing or approving individual trials. The multi-agency panel will meet periodically to review and evaluate the program and recommend any necessary refinements to HCFA.

Clinical trials that meet the qualifying criteria will receive Medicare coverage of routine costs after the trial's lead principal investigator certifies that the trial meets the criteria. This process will require the principal investigator to enroll the trial in a Medicare clinical trials registry, currently under development.

Some clinical trials are automatically qualified to receive Medicare coverage of their routine costs because they have been deemed by AHRQ, in consultation with the other agencies represented on the multi-agency panel to be highly likely to have the above-listed seven desirable characteristics of clinical trials. The principal investigators of these automatically qualified trials do not need to certify that the trials meet the qualifying criteria, but must enroll the trials in the Medicare clinical trials registry for administrative purposes, once the registry is established.

Effective September 19, 2000, clinical trials that are deemed to be automatically qualified are:

Trials funded by NIH, CDC, AHRQ, HCFA, DOD, and VA;

Trials supported by centers or cooperative groups that are funded by the NIH, CDC, AHRQ, HCFA, DOD and VA;

Trials conducted under an investigational new drug application (IND) reviewed by the FDA; and

Drug trials that are exempt from having an IND under 21 CFR 312.2(b)(1) will be deemed automatically qualified until the qualifying criteria are developed and the certification process is in place. At that time the principal investigators of these trials must certify that the trials meet the qualifying criteria in order to maintain Medicare coverage of routine costs. This certification process will only affect the future status of the trial and will not be used to retroactively change the earlier deemed status.

Medicare will cover the routine costs of qualifying trials that either have been deemed to be automatically qualified or have certified that they meet the qualifying criteria unless HCFA's Chief Clinical Officer subsequently finds that a clinical trial does not meet the qualifying criteria or jeopardizes the safety or welfare of Medicare beneficiaries.

Should HCFA find that a trial's principal investigator misrepresented that the trial met the necessary qualifying criteria in order to gain Medicare coverage of routine costs, Medicare coverage of the routine costs would be denied under §1862(a)(1)(E) of the Act. In the case of such a denial, the Medicare beneficiaries enrolled in the trial would not be held liable (i.e., would be held harmless from collection) for the costs consistent with the provisions of §§1879, 1842(l), or 1834(j)(4) of the Act, as applicable. Where appropriate, the billing providers would be held liable for the costs and fraud investigations of the billing providers and the trial's principal investigator may be pursued.

Medicare regulations require Medicare+Choice (M+C) organizations to follow HCFA's national coverage decisions. This NCD raises special issues that require some modification of most M+C organizations' rules governing provision of items and services in and out of network. The items and services covered under this NCD are inextricably linked to the clinical trials with which they are associated and cannot be covered outside of the context of those clinical trials. M+C organizations therefore must cover these services regardless of whether they are available through in-network providers. M+C organizations may have reporting requirements when enrollees participate in clinical trials, in order to track and coordinate their members' care, but cannot require prior authorization or approval.

CIM 35-3

240.3—Heat Treatment, Including the Use of Diathermy and Ultra-Sound for Pulmonary Conditions

(Rev. 1, 10-03-03)

Not Covered

There is no physiological rationale or valid scientific documentation of effectiveness of diathermy or ultrasound heat treatments for asthma, bronchitis, or any other pulmonary condition and for such purpose this treatment cannot be considered reasonable and necessary within the meaning of §1862(a)(1) of the Act.

Cross-reference: §150.5.

CIM 35-5

30.8—Cellular Therapy

(Rev. 1, 10-03-03)

Not Covered

Cellular therapy involves the practice of injecting humans with foreign proteins like the placenta or lungs of unborn lambs. Cellular therapy is without scientific or statistical evidence to document its therapeutic efficacy and, in fact, is considered a potentially dangerous practice. Accordingly, cellular therapy is not considered reasonable and necessary within the meaning of §1862(a)(1) of the Act.

CIM 35-10

20.29—Hyperbaric Oxygen Therapy

(Rev. 1, 10-03-03)

For purposes of coverage under Medicare, hyperbaric oxygen (HBO) therapy is a modality in which the entire body is exposed to oxygen under increased atmospheric pressure.

A—Covered Conditions

Program reimbursement for HBO therapy will be limited to that which is administered in a chamber (including the one man unit) and is limited to the following conditions:

1. Acute carbon monoxide intoxication, (ICD-9-CM diagnosis 986).

2. Decompression illness, (ICD-9-CM diagnosis 993.2, 993.3).

3. Gas embolism, (ICD-9-CM diagnosis 958.0, 999.1).

4. Gas gangrene, (ICD-9-CM diagnosis 0400).

5. Acute traumatic peripheral ischemia. HBO therapy is a valuable adjunctive treatment to be used in combination with accepted standard therapeutic measures when loss of function, limb, or life is threatened. (ICD-9-CM diagnosis 902.53, 903.01, 903.1, 904.0, 904.41.)

6. Crush injuries and suturing of severed limbs. As in the previous conditions, HBO therapy would be an adjunctive treatment when loss of function, limb, or life is threatened. (ICD-9-CM diagnosis 927.00-927.03, 927.09-927.11, 927.20-927.21, 927.8-927.9, 928.00-928.01, 928.10-928.11, 928.20-928.21, 928.3, 928.8-928.9, 929.0, 929.9, 996.90-996.99.)

7. Progressive necrotizing infections (necrotizing fasciitis), (ICD-9-CM diagnosis 728.86).

8. Acute peripheral arterial insufficiency, (ICD-9-CM diagnosis 444.21, 444.22, 444.81).

9. Preparation and preservation of compromised skin grafts (not for primary management of wounds), (ICD-9-CM diagnosis 996.52; excludes artificial skin graft).

10. Chronic refractory osteomyelitis, unresponsive to conventional medical and surgical management, (ICD-9-CM diagnosis 730.10-730.19).

11. Osteoradionecrosis as an adjunct to conventional treatment, (ICD-9-CM diagnosis 526.89).

12. Soft tissue radionecrosis as an adjunct to conventional treatment, (ICD-9-CM diagnosis 990).

13. Cyanide poisoning, (ICD-9-CM diagnosis 987.7, 989.0).

14. Actinomycosis, only as an adjunct to conventional therapy when the disease process is refractory to antibiotics and surgical treatment, (ICD-9-CM diagnosis 039.0-039.4, 039.8, 039.9).

15. Diabetic wounds of the lower extremities in patients who meet the following three criteria:

a. Patient has type I or type II diabetes and has a lower extremity wound that is due to diabetes;

b. Patient has a wound classified as Wagner grade III or higher; and

c. Patient has failed an adequate course of standard wound therapy.

The use of HBO therapy is covered as adjunctive therapy only after there are no measurable signs of healing for at least 30 days of treatment with standard wound therapy and must be used in addition to standard wound care. Standard wound care in patients with diabetic wounds includes: assessment of a patient's vascular status and correction of any vascular problems in the affected limb if possible, optimization of nutritional status, optimization of glucose control, debridement by any means to remove devitalized tissue, maintenance of a clean, moist bed of granulation tissue with appropriate moist dressings, appropriate off-loading, and necessary treatment to resolve any infection that might be present. Failure to respond to standard wound care occurs when there are no measurable signs of healing for at least 30 consecutive days. Wounds must be evaluated at least every 30 days during administration of HBO therapy. Continued treatment with HBO therapy is not covered if measurable signs of healing have not been demonstrated within any 30-day period of treatment.

B—Noncovered Conditions

All other indications not specified under §270.4(A) are not covered under the Medicare program. No program payment may be made for any conditions other than those listed in §270.4(A).

No program payment may be made for HBO in the treatment of the following conditions:

1. Cutaneous, decubitus, and stasis ulcers (ICD-9-CM diagnosis 707.0.)

2. Chronic peripheral vascular insufficiency (ICD-9-CM diagnosis 443.8, 459.81)

3. Anaerobic septicemia and infection other than clostridial (ICD-9-CM diagnosis 038.3)

4. Skin burns (thermal). (ICD-9-CM diagnosis 692.71, 692.76-692.79, 940—949.5)

5. Senility. (ICD-9-CM diagnosis 797)

6. Myocardial infarction. (ICD-9-CM diagnosis 410—4109.2)

7. Cardiogenic shock. (ICD-9-CM diagnosis 7855.1)

8. Sickle cell anemia. (ICD-9-CM diagnosis 2826.9)

9. Acute thermal and chemical pulmonary damage, i.e., smoke inhalation with pulmonary insufficiency (ICD-9-CM diagnosis 5188.2)

10. Acute or chronic cerebral vascular insufficiency. (ICD-9-CM diagnosis 434, 437.0, 437.4)

11. Hepatic necrosis.(ICD-9-CM diagnosis 537.8, 537.9)

12. Aerobic septicemia. (ICD-9-CM diagnosis 038.8, 038.9)

13. Nonvascular causes of chronic brain syndrome (Pick's disease, Alzheimer's disease, Korsakoff's disease) (ICD-9-CM diagnosis 291.2, 331.0, 331.1)

14. Tetanus. (ICD-9-CM diagnosis 037, 771.3)

15. Systemic aerobic infection. (ICD-9-CM diagnosis

16. Organ transplantation.

17. Organ storage.

18. Pulmonary emphysema. (ICD-9-CM diagnosis 492)

19. Exceptional blood loss anemia. (ICD-9-CM diagnosis 285)

20. Multiple Sclerosis. (ICD-9-CM diagnosis 340)

21. Arthritic Diseases. (ICD-9-CM diagnosis (711.0-711.99)

22. Acute cerebral edema. (ICD-9-CM diagnosis (348.5)

C—Reasonable Utilization Parameters

Make payment where HBO therapy is clinically practical. HBO therapy should not be a replacement for other standard successful therapeutic measures. Depending on the response of the individual patient and the severity of the original problem, treatment may range from less than 1 week to several months duration, the average being two to four weeks. Review and document the medical necessity for use of hyperbaric oxygen for more than two months, regardless of the condition of the patient, before further reimbursement is made.

D—Topical Application of Oxygen

This method of administering oxygen does not meet the definition of HBO therapy as stated above. Also, its clinical efficacy has not been established. Therefore, no Medicare reimbursement may be made for the topical application of oxygen.
Cross reference: §270.5 of this manual.

CIM 35-13

150.7—Prolotherapy, Joint Sclerotherapy, and Ligamentous Injections with Sclerosing Agents

(Rev. 1, 10-03-03)

Not Covered

The medical effectiveness of the above therapies has not been

verified by scientifically controlled studies. Accordingly, reimbursement for these modalities should be denied on the ground that they are not reasonable and necessary as required by §1862(a)(1) of the Act.

CIM 35-20

160.2—Treatment of Motor Function Disorders with Electric Nerve Stimulation

(Rev. 1, 10-03-03)

Not Covered

While electric nerve stimulation has been employed to control chronic intractable pain for some time, its use in the treatment of motor function disorders, such as multiple sclerosis, is a recent innovation, and the medical effectiveness of such therapy has not been verified by scientifically controlled studies. Therefore, where electric nerve stimulation is employed to treat motor function disorders, no reimbursement may be made for the stimulator or for the services related to its implantation since this treatment cannot be considered reasonable and necessary. See §§30.1 and 160.7.

NOTE: For Medicare coverage of deep brain stimulation for essential tremor and Parkinson's disease, see §160.25.

CIM 35-27

30.1—Biofeedback Therapy

(Rev. 1, 10-03-03)

Biofeedback therapy provides visual, auditory or other evidence of the status of certain body functions so that a person can exert voluntary control over the functions, and thereby alleviate an abnormal bodily condition. Biofeedback therapy often uses electrical devices to transform bodily signals indicative of such functions as heart rate, blood pressure, skin temperature, salivation, peripheral vasomotor activity, and gross muscle tone into a tone or light, the loudness or brightness of which shows the extent of activity in the function being measured.

Biofeedback therapy differs from electromyography which is a diagnostic procedure used to record and study the electrical properties of skeletal muscle. An electromyography device may be used to provide feedback with certain types of biofeedback. Biofeedback therapy is covered under Medicare only when it is reasonable and necessary for the individual patient for muscle re-education of specific muscle groups or for treating pathological muscle abnormalities of spasticity, incapacitating muscle spasm, or weakness, and more conventional treatments (heat, cold, massage, exercise, support) have not been successful. This therapy is not covered for treatment of ordinary muscle tension states or for psychosomatic conditions. (See the Medicare Benefit Policy Manual, Chapter 15, for general coverage requirements about physical therapy requirements.)

CIM 35-27.1

30.1.1—Biofeedback Therapy for the Treatment of Urinary Incontinence

(Rev. 1, 10-03-03)

Biofeedback Therapy for the Treatment of Urinary Incontinence

This policy applies to biofeedback therapy rendered by a practitioner in an office or other facility setting.

Biofeedback is covered for the treatment of stress and/or urge incontinence in cognitively intact patients who have failed a documented trial of pelvic muscle exercise (PME) training. Biofeedback is not a treatment, per se, but a tool to help patients learn how to perform PME. Biofeedback-assisted PME incorporates the use of an electronic or mechanical device to relay visual and/or auditory evidence of pelvic floor muscle tone, in order to improve awareness of pelvic floor musculature and to assist patients in the performance of PME.

A failed trial of PME training is defined as no clinically significant improvement in urinary incontinence after completing four weeks of an ordered plan of pelvic muscle exercises to increase periurethral muscle strength.

Contractors may decide whether or not to cover biofeedback as an initial treatment modality.

Home use of biofeedback therapy is not covered.

CIM 35-31

270.4—Treatment of Decubitus Ulcers

(Rev. 1, 10-03-03)

An accepted procedure for healing decubitus ulcers is to remove dead tissue from the lesions and to keep them clean to promote the growth of new tissue. This may be accomplished by hydrotherapy (whirlpool) treatments. Hydrotherapy (whirlpool) treatment for decubitus ulcers is a covered service under Medicare for patients when treatment is reasonable and necessary. Some other methods of treating decubitus ulcers, the safety and effectiveness of which have not been established, are not covered under the Medicare program. Some examples of these types of treatments are: ultraviolet light, low intensity direct current, topical application of oxygen, and topical dressings with Balsam of Peru in castor oil.

CIM 35-34

20.23—Fabric Wrapping of Abdominal Aneurysms

(Rev. 1, 10-03-03)

Not Covered

Fabric wrapping of abdominal aneurysms is not a covered Medicare procedure. This is a treatment for abdominal aneurysms which involves wrapping aneurysms with cellophane or fascia lata. This procedure has not been shown to prevent eventual rupture. In extremely rare instances, external wall reinforcement may be indicated when the current accepted treatment (excision of the aneurysm and reconstruction with synthetic materials) is not a viable alternative, but external wall reinforcement is not fabric wrapping. Accordingly, fabric wrapping of abdominal aneurysms is not considered reasonable and necessary within the meaning of §1862(a)(1) of the Act.

CIM 35-41

150.5—Diathermy Treatment

(Rev. 1, 10-03-03)

High energy pulsed wave diathermy machines have been found to produce some degree of therapeutic benefit for essentially the same conditions and to the same extent as standard diathermy. Accordingly, where the contractor's medical staff has determined that the pulsed wave diathermy apparatus used is one which is considered therapeutically effective, the treatments are considered a covered service, but only for those conditions for which standard diathermy is medically indicated and only when rendered by a physician or incident to a physician's professional services. (CPT-4 code 97024*, ICD-9-CM code 93.34).

Cross-reference: §240.3.

CIM 35-46

160.3—Assessing Patients Suitability for Electrical Nerve Stimulation

(Rev. 1, 10-03-03)

Electrical nerve stimulation is an accepted modality for assessing a patient's suitability for ongoing treatment with a transcutaneous or an implanted nerve stimulator. Accordingly, program payment may be made for the following techniques when used to determine the potential therapeutic usefulness of an electrical nerve stimulator:

A—Transcutaneous Electrical Nerve Stimulation (TENS)

This technique involves attachment of a transcutaneous nerve stimulator to the surface of the skin over the peripheral nerve to be stimulated. It is used by the patient on a trial basis and its effectiveness in modulating pain is monitored by the physician, or physical therapist. Generally, the physician or physical therapist is able to determine whether the patient is likely to derive a significant therapeutic benefit from continuous use of a transcutaneous stimulator within a trial period of 1 month; in a few cases this determination may take longer to make. Document the medical necessity for such services that are furnished beyond the first month. (See §160.13 for an explanation of coverage of medically necessary supplies for the effective use of TENS.)

If TENS significantly alleviates pain, it may be considered as primary treatment; if it produces no relief or greater discomfort than the original pain, electrical nerve stimulation therapy is ruled out. However, where TENS produces incomplete relief, further evaluation with percutaneous electrical nerve stimulation may be considered to determine whether an implanted peripheral nerve stimulator would provide significant relief from pain.

Usually, the physician or physical therapist providing the services will furnish the equipment necessary for assessment. Where the physician or physical therapist advises the patient to rent the TENS from a supplier during the trial period rather than supplying it himself/herself, program payment may be made for rental of the TENS as well as for the services of the physician or physical therapist who is evaluating its use. However, the combined program payment which is made for the physician's or physical therapist's services and the rental of the stimulator from a supplier should not exceed the amount which would be payable for the total service, including the stimulator, furnished by the physician or physical therapist alone.

B—Percutaneous Electrical Nerve Stimulation (PENS)

This diagnostic procedure which involves stimulation of peripheral nerves by a needle electrode inserted through the skin is performed only in a physician's office, clinic, or hospital outpatient department. Therefore, it is covered only when performed by a physician or incident to physician's service. If pain is effectively controlled by percutaneous stimulation, implantation of electrodes is warranted.

As in the case of TENS (described in subsection A), generally the physician should be able to determine whether the patient is likely to derive a significant therapeutic benefit from continuing use of an implanted nerve stimulator within a trial period of one month. In a few cases, this determination may take longer to make. The medical necessity for such diagnostic services that are furnished beyond the first month must be documented.

NOTE: Electrical nerve stimulators do not prevent pain but only alleviate pain as it occurs. A patient can be taught how to employ the stimulator, and once this is done, can use it safely and effectively without direct physician supervision. Consequently, it is inappropriate for a patient to visit his/her physician, physical therapist, or an outpatient clinic on a continuing basis for treatment of pain with electrical nerve stimulation. Once it is determined that electrical nerve stimulation should be continued as therapy and the patient has been trained to use the stimulator, it is expected that a stimulator will be implanted or the patient will employ the TENS on a continual basis in his/her home. Electrical nerve stimulation treatments furnished by a physician in his/her office, by a physical therapist or outpatient clinic are excluded from coverage by §1862(a)(1) of the Act. (See §160.8 for an explanation of coverage of the therapeutic use of implanted peripheral nerve stimulators under the prosthetic devices benefit. See §230.15 for an explanation of coverage of the therapeutic use of TENS under the durable medical equipment benefit.)

CIM 35-47

140.2—Breast Reconstruction Following Mastectomy

(Rev. 1, 10-03-03)

During recent years, there has been a considerable change in the treatment of diseases of the breast such as fibrocystic disease and cancer. While extirpation of the disease remains of primary importance, the quality of life following initial treatment is increasingly recognized as of great concern. The increased use of breast reconstruction procedures is due to several factors:

- A change in epidemiology of breast cancer, including an apparent increase in incidence;
- Improved surgical skills and techniques;
- The continuing development of better prostheses; and
- Increasing awareness by physicians of the importance of post-surgical psychological adjustment.

Reconstruction of the affected and the contralateral unaffected breast following a medically necessary mastectomy is considered a relatively safe and effective noncosmetic procedure. Accordingly, program payment may be made for breast reconstruction surgery following removal of a breast for any medical reason.

Program payment may not be made for breast reconstruction for cosmetic reasons. (Cosmetic surgery is excluded from coverage under §1862(a)(10) of the Act.)

CIM 35-48

150.2—Osteogenic Stimulator (Various Effective Dates Below)

(Rev.41, Issued: 06-24-05, Effective: 04-27-05, Implementation: 08-01-05)

Electrical Osteogenic Stimulators

A. General

Electrical stimulation to augment bone repair can be attained either invasively or noninvasively. Invasive devices provide electrical stimulation directly at the fracture site either through percutaneously placed cathodes or by implantation of a coiled cathode wire into the fracture site. The power pack for the latter device is implanted into soft tissue near the fracture site and subcutaneously connected to the cathode, creating a self-contained system with no external components. The power supply for the former device is externally placed and the leads connected to the inserted cathodes. With the noninvasive device, opposing pads, wired to an external power supply, are placed over the cast. An electromagnetic field is created between the pads at the fracture site.

B. Nationally Covered Indications

1. Noninvasive Stimulator

The noninvasive stimulator device is covered only for the following indications:

- Nonunion of long bone fractures;
- Failed fusion, where a minimum of 9 months has elapsed since the last surgery;
- Congenital pseudarthroses
- Effective July 1, 1996, as an adjunct to spinal fusion surgery for patients at high risk of pseudarthrosis due to previously failed spinal fusion at the same site or for those undergoing multiple level fusion. A multiple level fusion involves 3 or more vertebrae (e.g., L3-L5, L4-S1, etc.).
- Effective September 15, 1980, nonunion of long bone fractures is considered to exist only after 6 or more months have elapsed without healing of the fracture.
- Effective April 1, 2000, nonunion of long bone fractures is considered to exist only when serial radiographs have confirmed that fracture healing has ceased for 3 or more months prior to starting treatment with the electrical osteogenic stimulator. Serial radiographs must include a minimum of 2 sets of radiographs, each including multiple views of the fracture site, separated by a minimum of 90 days.

2. Invasive (Implantable) Stimulator

The invasive stimulator device is covered only for the following indications:

- Nonunion of long bone fractures;
- Effective July 1, 1996, as an adjunct to spinal fusion surgery for patients at high risk of pseudarthrosis due to previously failed spinal fusion at the same site or for those undergoing multiple level fusion. A multiple level fusion involves 3 or more vertebrae (e.g., L3-L5, L4-S1, etc.).
- Effective September 15, 1980, nonunion of long bone fractures is considered to exist only after 6 or more months have elapsed without healing of the fracture.
- Effective April 1, 2000, nonunion of long bone fractures is considered to exist only when serial radiographs have confirmed that fracture healing has ceased for 3 or more months prior to starting treatment with the electrical osteogenic stimulator. Serial radiographs must include a minimum of 2 sets of radiographs, each including multiple views of the fracture site, separated by a minimum of 90 days.

Ultrasonic Osteogenic Stimulators

A. General

An ultrasonic osteogenic stimulator is a noninvasive device that emits low intensity, pulsed ultrasound. The device is applied to the surface of the skin at the fracture site and ultrasound waves are emitted via a conductive coupling gel to stimulate fracture healing. The ultrasonic osteogenic stimulators are not be used concurrently with other non-invasive osteogenic devices.

B. Nationally Covered Indications

Effective January 1, 2001, ultrasonic osteogenic stimulators are covered as medically reasonable and necessary for the treatment of nonunion fractures. In demonstrating non-union fractures, CMS expects:

- A minimum of 2 sets of radiographs, obtained prior to starting treatment with the osteogenic stimulator, separated by a minimum of 90 days. Each radiograph set must include multiple views of the fracture site accompanied with a written interpretation by a physician stating that there has been no clinically significant evidence of fracture healing between the 2 sets of radiographs; and,
- Indications that the patient failed at least one surgical intervention for the treatment of the fracture.
- Effective April 27, 2005, upon reconsideration of ultrasound stimulation for nonunion fracture healing, CMS determines that the evidence is adequate to conclude that noninvasive ultrasound stimulation for the treatment of nonunion bone fractures prior to surgical intervention is reasonable and necessary. In demonstrating non-union fractures, CMS expects:
- A minimum of 2 sets of radiographs, obtained prior to starting treatment with the osteogenic stimulator, separated by a minimum of 90 days. Each radiograph set must include multiple views of the fracture site accompanied with a written interpretation by a physician stating that there has been no clinically significant evidence of fracture healing between the 2 sets of radiographs.

C. Nationally Non-Covered Indications

Nonunion fractures of the skull, vertebrae and those that are tumor-related are excluded from coverage.

Ultrasonic osteogenic stimulators may not be used concurrently with other non-invasive osteogenic devices.

Ultrasonic osteogenic stimulators for fresh fractures and delayed unions remains non-covered.

(This NCD last reviewed June 2005.)

CIM 35-61

140.3—Transsexual Surgery

(Rev. 1, 10-03-03)

Transsexual surgery, also known as sex reassignment surgery or intersex surgery, is the culmination of a series of procedures designed to change the anatomy of transsexuals to conform to their gender identity. Transsexuals are persons with an overwhelming desire to change anatomic sex because of their fixed conviction that they are members of the opposite sex. For the male-to-female, transsexual surgery entails castration, penectomy and vulva-vaginal construction. Surgery for the female-to-male transsexual consists of bilateral mammectomy, hysterectomy and salpingo-oophorectomy which may be followed by phalloplasty and the insertion of testicular prostheses. Transsexual surgery for sex reassignment of transsexuals is controversial. Because of the lack of well controlled, long term studies of the safety and effectiveness of the surgical procedures and attendant therapies for transsexualism, the treatment is considered experimental. Moreover, there is a high rate of serious complications for these surgical procedures. For these reasons, transsexual surgery is not covered.

CIM 35-64

20.21—Chelation Therapy for Treatment of Atherosclerosis

(Rev. 1, 10-03-03)

Chelation therapy is the application of chelation techniques for the therapeutic or preventive effects of removing unwanted metal ions from the body. The application of chelation therapy using ethylenediamine-tetra-acetic acid (EDTA) for the treatment and prevention of atherosclerosis is controversial. There is no widely accepted rationale to explain the beneficial effects attributed to this therapy. Its safety is questioned and its clinical effectiveness has never been established by well-designed, controlled clinical trials. It is not widely accepted and practiced by American physicians. EDTA chelation therapy for atherosclerosis is considered experimental. For these reasons, EDTA chelation therapy for the treatment or prevention of atherosclerosis is not covered. Some practitioners refer to this therapy as chemoendarterectomy and may also show a diagnosis other than atherosclerosis, such as arteriosclerosis or calcinosis. Claims employing such variant terms should also be denied under this section.

Cross-reference: §20.22.

CIM 35-65

100.6—Gastric Freezing

(Rev. 1, 10-03-03)

Gastric freezing for chronic peptic ulcer disease is a non-surgical treatment which was popular about 20 years ago but now is seldom done. It has been abandoned due to a high complication rate, only temporary improvement experienced by patients, and lack of effectiveness when tested by double-blind, controlled clinical trials. Since the procedure is now considered obsolete, it is not covered.

CIM 35-74

20.20—External Counterpulsation (ECP) for Severe Angina

(Rev. 1, 10-03-03)

Covered

External counterpulsation (ECP), commonly referred to as enhanced external counterpulsation, is a noninvasive outpatient treatment for coronary artery disease refractory to medical and/or surgical therapy. Although ECP devices are cleared by the Food and Drug Administration (FDA) for use in treating a variety of cardiac conditions, including stable or unstable angina pectoris, acute myocardial infarction and cardiogenic shock, the use of this device to treat cardiac conditions other than stable angina pectoris is not covered, since only that use has developed sufficient evidence to demonstrate its medical effectiveness. Noncoverage of hydraulic versions of these types of devices remains in force.

Coverage is provided for the use of ECP for patients who have been diagnosed with disabling angina (Class III or Class IV, Canadian Cardiovascular Society Classification or equivalent classification) who, in the opinion of a cardiologist or cardiothoracic surgeon, are not readily amenable to surgical intervention, such as PTCA or cardiac bypass because:

1. Their condition is inoperable, or at high risk of operative complications or post-operative failure;

2. Their coronary anatomy is not readily amenable to such procedures; or

3. They have co-morbid states that create excessive risk.

A full course of therapy usually consists of 35 one-hour treatments which may be offered once or twice daily, usually five days per week. The patient is placed on a treatment table where their lower trunk and lower extremities are wrapped in a series of three compressive air cuffs which inflate and deflate in synchronization with the patient's cardiac cycle.

During diastole, the three sets of air cuffs are inflated sequentially (distal to proximal) compressing the vascular beds within the muscles of the calves, lower thighs and upper thighs. This action results in an increase in diastolic pressure, generation of retrograde arterial blood flow and an increase in venous return. The cuffs are deflated simultaneously just prior to systole which produces a rapid drop in vascular impedance, a decrease in ventricular workload and an increase in cardiac output.

The augmented diastolic pressure and retrograde aortic flow appear to improve myocardial perfusion, while systolic unloading appears to reduce cardiac workload and oxygen requirements. The increased venous return coupled with enhanced systolic flow appears to increase cardiac output. As a result of this treatment, most patients experience increased time until onset of ischemia, increased exercise tolerance, and a reduction in the number and severity of anginal episodes. Evidence was presented that this effect lasted well beyond the immediate post-treatment phase, with patients symptom-free for several months to two years.

This procedure must be done under direct supervision of a physician.

CIM 35-77

150.4—Neuromuscular Electrical Stimulator (NMES) in the Treatment of Disuse Atrophy

(Rev. 1, 10-03-03)

Neuromuscular electrical stimulation (NMES) involves the use of a device which transmits an electrical impulse to the skin over selected muscle groups by way of electrodes. Coverage of NMES is limited to the treatment of disuse atrophy where nerve supply to the muscle is intact, including brain, spinal cord, and peripheral nerves, and other non-neurological reasons for disuse are causing atrophy. Some examples would be casting or splinting of a limb, contracture due to scarring of soft tissue as in burn lesions, and hip replacement surgery (until orthotic training begins). (See §160.13 for an explanation of coverage of medically necessary supplies for the effective use of NMES.)

CIM 45-25

160.13—Supplies Used in the Delivery of Transcutaneous Electrical Nerve Stimulation (TENS) and Neuromuscular Electrical Stimulation (NMES)

(Rev. 1, 10-03-03)

Transcutaneous Electrical Nerve Stimulation (TENS) and/or Neuromuscular Electrical Stimulation (NMES) can ordinarily be delivered to patients through the use of conventional electrodes, adhesive tapes and lead wires. There may be times, however, where it might be medically necessary for certain patients receiving TENS or NMES treatment to use, as an alternative to conventional electrodes, adhesive tapes and lead wires, a form-fitting conductive garment (i.e., a garment with conductive fibers which are separated from the patients' skin by layers of fabric).

A form-fitting conductive garment (and medically necessary related supplies) may be covered under the program only when:

1. It has received permission or approval for marketing by the Food and Drug Administration;

2. It has been prescribed by a physician for use in delivering covered TENS or NMES treatment; and

3. One of the medical indications outlined below is met:

- The patient cannot manage without the conductive garment because there is such a large area or so many sites to be stimulated and the stimulation would have to be delivered so frequently that it is not feasible to use conventional electrodes, adhesive tapes and lead wires;
- The patient cannot manage without the conductive garment for the treatment of chronic intractable pain because the areas or sites to be stimulated are inaccessible with the use of conventional electrodes, adhesive tapes and lead wires;
- The patient has a documented medical condition such as skin problems that preclude the application of conventional electrodes, adhesive tapes and lead wires;
- The patient requires electrical stimulation beneath a cast either to treat disuse atrophy, where the nerve supply to the muscle is intact, or to treat chronic intractable pain; or
- The patient has a medical need for rehabilitation strengthening (pursuant to a written plan of rehabilitation) following an injury where the nerve supply to the muscle is intact.

A conductive garment is not covered for use with a TENS device during the trial period specified in §160.3 unless:

4. The patient has a documented skin problem prior to the start of the trial period; and

5. The carrier's medical consultants are satisfied that use of such an item is medically necessary for the patient.

(See conditions for coverage of the use of TENS in the diagnosis and treatment of chronic intractable pain in §§160.3 and 160.13 and the use of NMES in the treatment of disuse atrophy in §150.4.)

CIM 35-90

20.5—Extracorporeal Immunoadsorption (ECI) Using Protein A Columns

(Rev. 1, 10-03-03)

Extracorporeal immunoadsorption (ECI), using Protein A columns, has been developed for the purpose of selectively removing circulating immune complexes (CIC) and immunoglobulins (IgG) from patients in whom these substances are associated with their diseases. The technique involves pumping the patient's anticoagulated venous blood through a cell separator from which 1-3 liters of plasma are collected and perfused over adsorbent columns, after which the plasma rejoins the separated, unprocessed cells and is retransfused to the patient.

For claims with dates of service on or after January 1, 2001, Medicare covers the use of Protein A columns for the treatment of ITP. In addition, Medicare will cover Protein A columns for the treatment of rheumatoid arthritis (RA) under the following conditions:

- Patient has severe RA. Patient disease is active, having >5 swollen joints, >20 tender joints, and morning stiffness >60 minutes; or
- Patient has failed an adequate course of a minimum of 3 Disease Modifying Anti-Rheumatic Drugs (DMARDs). Failure does not include intolerance.

Other uses of these columns are currently considered to be investigational and, therefore, not reasonable and necessary under the Medicare law. (See §1862(a)(1)(A) of the Act.)

CIM 35-93

240.1—Lung Volume Reduction Surgery (Reduction Pneumoplasty)

(Rev. 3, 11-04-03)

Lung volume reduction surgery (LVRS) or reduction pneumoplasty, also referred to as lung shaving or lung contouring, is performed on patients with severe emphysema in order to allow the remaining compressed lung to expand, and thus, improve respiratory function.

Covered Indications

Medicare-covered LVRS approaches are limited to bilateral excision of a damaged lung with stapling performed via median sternotomy or video-assisted thoracoscopic surgery.

1. National Emphysema Treatment Trial (NETT) participants (effective for services performed on or after August 11, 1997):

Medicare provides coverage to those beneficiaries who are participating in the NETT trial for all services integral to the study and for which the Medicare statute does not prohibit coverage.

2. Medicare will only consider LVRS reasonable and necessary when all of the following requirements are met (effective for services performed on or after January 1, 2004):

a. The patient satisfies all the criteria outlined below:

Assessment	Criteria
History and physical examination	Consistent with emphysema BMI, ≤31.1 kg/m² (men) or ≤32.3 kg/m² (women) Stable with ≤20 mg prednisone (or equivalent) qd
Radiographic	High Resolution Computer Tomography (HRCT) scan evidence of bilateral emphysema
Pulmonary function (pre-rehabilitation)	Forced expiratory volume in one second (FEV$_1$) ≤45% predicted (≥15% predicted if age ≥70 years) Total lung capacity (TLC) ≥100% predicted post-bronchodilator Residual volume (RV) ≥150% predicted post-bronchodilator
Arterial blood gas level (pre-rehabilitation)	PCO$_2$, ≤60 mm Hg (PCO$_2$, ≤55 mm Hg if 1-mile above sea level) PO$_2$ ≥45 mm Hg on room air (PO$_2$, ≥30 mm Hg if 1-mile above sea level)
Cardiac assessment	Approval for surgery by cardiologist if any of the following are present: Unstable angina; left-ventricular ejection fraction (LVEF) cannot be estimated from the echocardiogram; LVEF <45%; dobutamine-radionuclide cardiac scan indicates coronary artery disease or ventricular dysfunction; arrhythmia (>5 premature ventricular contractions per minute; cardiac rhythm other than sinus; premature ventricular contractions on EKG at rest)
Surgical assessment	Approval for surgery by pulmonary physician, thoracic surgeon, and anesthesiologist post-rehabilitation
Exercise	Post-rehabilitation 6-min walk of ≥140 m; able to complete 3 min unloaded pedaling in exercise tolerance test (pre- and post-rehabilitation)
Consent	Signed consents for screening and rehabilitation
Smoking	Plasma cotinine level ≤13.7 ng/mL (or arterial carboxyhemoglobin ≤2.5% if using nicotine products) Nonsmoking for 4 months prior to initial interview and throughout evaluation for surgery
Preoperative diagnostic and therapeutic program adherence	Must complete assessment for and program of preoperative services in preparation for surgery

b. In addition, the patient must have:

Severe upper lobe predominant emphysema (as defined by radiologist assessment of upper lobe predominance on CT scan), or

Severe non-upper lobe emphysema with low exercise capacity.

Patients with low exercise capacity are those whose maximal exercise capacity is at or below 25 watts for women and 40 watts

(w) for men after completion of the preoperative therapeutic program in preparation for LVRS. Exercise capacity is measured by incremental, maximal, symptom-limited exercise with a cycle ergometer utilizing 5 or 10 watt/minute ramp on 30% oxygen after 3 minutes of unloaded pedaling.

c. The surgery must be performed at facilities that were identified by the National Heart, Lung, and Blood Institute to meet the thresholds for participation in the NETT, and at sites that have been approved by Medicare as lung transplant facilities. These facilities are listed on our Web site at www.cms.hhs.gov/coverage/lvrsfacility.pdf. The CMS is currently working to develop accreditation standards for facilities to perform LVRS and when implemented, will consider LVRS to be reasonable and necessary only at accredited facilities.

d. The surgery must be preceded and followed by a program of diagnostic and therapeutic services consistent with those provided in the NETT and designed to maximize the patient's potential to successfully undergo and recover from surgery. The program must include a 6- to 10-week series of at least 16, and no more than 20, preoperative sessions, each lasting a minimum of 2 hours. It must also include at least 6, and no more than 10, postoperative sessions, each lasting a minimum of 2 hours, within 8 to 9 weeks of the LVRS. This program must be consistent with the care plan developed by the treating physician following performance of a comprehensive evaluation of the patient's medical, psychosocial and nutritional needs, be consistent with the preoperative and postoperative services provided in the NETT, and arranged, monitored, and performed under the coordination of the facility where the surgery takes place.

Noncovered Indications

1. LVRS is not covered in any of the following clinical circumstances:

a. Patient characteristics carry a high risk for perioperative morbidity and/or mortality;

b. The disease is unsuitable for LVRS;

c. Medical conditions or other circumstances make it likely that the patient will be unable to complete the preoperative and postoperative pulmonary diagnostic and therapeutic program required for surgery;

d. The patient presents with FEVi ≤ 20% of predicted value, and either homogeneous distribution of emphysema on CT scan, or carbon monoxide diffusing capacity of ≤ 20% of predicted value (high-risk group identified October 2001 by the NETT); or

e. The patient satisfies the criteria outlined above in section 2(a), and has severe, non-upper lobe emphysema with high exercise capacity. High exercise capacity is defined as a maximal workload at the completion of the preoperative diagnostic and therapeutic program that is above 25 w for women and 40 w for men (under the measurement conditions for cycle ergometry specified above).

2. All other indications for LVRS not otherwise specified remain noncovered.

CIM 35-96

230.9—Cryosurgery of Prostate

(Rev. 1, 10-03-03)

Cryosurgery of the prostate gland, also known as cryosurgical ablation of the prostate (CSAP), destroys prostate tissue by applying extremely cold temperatures in order to reduce the size of the prostate gland. It is safe and effective, as well as medically necessary and appropriate, as primary treatment for patients with clinically localized prostate cancer, Stages T1-T3.

Cryosurgery of the prostate as a salvage therapy is not covered for any services performed prior to June 30, 2001.

Salvage Cryosurgery Of Prostate After Radiation Failure. Salvage cryosurgery of the prostate for recurrent cancer is medically necessary and appropriate only for those patients with localized disease who:

1. Have failed a trial of radiation therapy as their primary treatment; and

2. Meet one of the following conditions: Stage T2B or below, Gleason score < 9, PSA < 8 ng/mL.

Cryosurgery as salvage therapy is therefore not covered under Medicare after failure of other therapies as the primary treatment. Cryosurgery as salvage is only covered after the failure of a trial of radiation therapy, under the conditions noted above.

CIM 35-103

160.25—Multiple Electroconvulsive Therapy (MECT)

(Rev. 1, 10-03-03)

The clinical effectiveness of the multiple-seizure electroconvulsive therapy has not been verified by scientifically controlled studies. In addition, studies have demonstrated an increased risk of adverse effects with multiple seizures. Accordingly, MECT cannot be considered reasonable and necessary and is not covered by the Medicare program. Effective for services provided on or after April 1, 2003.

CIM 45-4

150.6—Vitamin B12 Injections to Strengthen Tendons, Ligaments, etc., of the Foot

(Rev. 1, 10-03-03)

Not Covered

Vitamin B12 injections to strengthen tendons, ligaments, etc., of the foot are not covered under Medicare because (1) there is no evidence that vitamin B12 injections are effective for the purpose of strengthening weakened tendons and ligaments, and (2) this is nonsurgical treatment under the subluxation exclusion. Accordingly, vitamin B12 injections are not considered reasonable and necessary within the meaning of §1862(a)(1) of the Act.

Cross reference:

The Medicare Benefit Policy Manual, Chapter 1, "Inpatient Hospital Services," §30. The Medicare Benefit Policy Manual, Chapter 16, "General Exclusions from Coverage," §100.

CIM 45-7

80.1—Hydrophilic Contact Lens for Corneal Bandage

(Rev. 1, 10-03-03)

Some hydrophilic contact lenses are used as moist corneal bandages for the treatment of acute or chronic corneal pathology, such as bulbous keratopathy, dry eyes, corneal ulcers and erosion, keratitis, corneal edema, descemetocele, corneal ectasis, Mooren's ulcer, anterior corneal dystrophy, neurotrophic keratoconjunctivitis, and for other therapeutic reasons.

Payment may be made under §1861(s)(2) of the Act for a hydrophilic contact lens approved by the Food and Drug Administration (FDA) and used as a supply incident to a physician's service. Payment for the lens is included in the payment for the physician's service to which the lens is incident. Contractors are authorized to accept an FDA letter of approval or other FDA published material as evidence of FDA approval. (See §80.4 for coverage of a hydrophilic contact lens as a prosthetic device.) See the Medicare Benefit Policy Manual, Chapter 15, "Covered Medical and Other Health Services," and the Medicare Benefit Policy Manual, Chapter 6, "Hospital Services Covered Under Part B," §20.4.

CIM 45-10

30.7—Laetrile and Related Substances

(Rev. 1, 10-03-03)

Not Covered

Laetrile (and the other drugs called by the various terms mentioned below) have been used primarily in the treatment or control of cancer. Although the terms "Laetrile," "laetrile," "amygdalin," "Sarcarcinase," "vitamin B-17," and "nitriloside" have been used interchangeably, the chemical identity of the substances to which these terms refer has varied.

The FDA has determined that neither Laetrile nor any other drug called by the various terms mentioned above, nor any other product which might be characterized as a "nitriloside" is generally recognized (by experts qualified by scientific training and experience to evaluate the safety and effectiveness of drugs) to be safe and effective for any therapeutic use. Therefore, use of this drug cannot be considered to be reasonable and necessary within the meaning of §1862(a)(1) of the Act and program payment may not be made for its use or any services furnished in connection with its administration. A hospital stay only for the purpose of having laetrile (or any other drug called by the terms mentioned above) administered is not covered. Also, program payment may not be made for laetrile (or other drug noted above) when it is used during the course of an otherwise covered hospital stay.

CIM 45-15

70.3—Physician's Office Within an Institution—Coverage of Services and Supplies Incident to a Physician's Services

(Rev. 1, 10-03-03)

Coverage of Services and Supplies Incident to a Physician's Services

Where a physician establishes an office within a nursing home or other institution, coverage of services and supplies furnished in the office must be determined in accordance with the "incident to a physician's professional service" provision (see the Medicare Benefit Policy Manual, Chapter 6, "Hospital Services Covered Under Part B," §20.4.1 or the Medicare Benefit Policy Manual, Chapter 15, "Covered Medical and Other Health Services," §60.1) as in any physician's office. A physician's office within an institution must be confined to a separately identified part of the facility which is used solely as the physician's office and cannot be construed to extend throughout the entire institution. Thus, services performed outside the "office" area would be subject to the coverage rules applicable to services furnished outside the office setting.

In order to accurately apply the criteria in the Medicare Benefit Policy Manual, Chapters 6, §20.4.1, or Chapter 15, "Covered Medical and Other Health Services," §60.1, the contractor gives consideration to the physical proximity of the institution and physician's office. When his office is located within a facility, a physician may not be reimbursed for services, supplies, and use of equipment which fall outside the scope of services "commonly furnished" in physician's offices generally, even though such services may be furnished in his institutional office. Additionally, make a distinction between the physician's office practice and the institution, especially when the physician is administrator or owner of the facility. Thus, for their services to be covered under the criteria in the Medicare Benefit Policy Manual, Chapter 6, §20.4.1, or the Medicare Benefit Policy Manual, Chapter 15, "Covered Medical and Other Health Services," §60.1, the auxiliary medical personnel must be members of the office staff rather than of the institution's staff, and the cost of supplies must represent an expense to the physician's office practice. Finally, services performed by the employees of the physician outside the "office" area must be directly supervised by the physician; his presence in the facility as a whole would not suffice to meet this requirement. (In any setting, of course, supervision of auxiliary personnel in and of itself is not considered a "physician's professional service" to which the services of the auxiliary personnel could be an incidental part, i.e., in addition to supervision, the physician must perform or have performed a personal professional service to the patient to which the services of the auxiliary personnel could be considered an incidental part). Denials for failure to meet any of these requirements would be based on §1861(s)(2)(A) of the Act.

Establishment of an office within an institution would not modify rules otherwise applicable for determining coverage of the physician's personal professional services within the institution. However, in view of the opportunity afforded to a physician who maintains such an office for rendering services to a sizable number of patients in a short period of time or for performing fre-

quent services for the same patient, claims for physicians' services rendered under such circumstances would require careful evaluation by the carrier to assure that payment is made only for services that are reasonable and necessary.

Cross-reference:

The Medicare Benefit Policy Manual, Chapter 15, "Covered Medical and Other Health Services."

The Medicare Benefit Policy Manual, Chapter 6, "Hospital Services Covered Under Part B," §20.4.1.

CIM 45-16

110.2—Certain Drugs Distributed by the National Cancer Institute

(Rev. 1, 10-03-03)

Under its Cancer Therapy Evaluation, the Division of Cancer Treatment of the National Cancer Institute (NCI), in cooperation with the Food and Drug Administration, approves and distributes certain drugs for use in treating terminally ill cancer patients. One group of these drugs, designated as Group C drugs, unlike other drugs distributed by the NCI, are not limited to use in clinical trials for the purpose of testing their efficacy. Drugs are classified as Group C drugs only if there is sufficient evidence demonstrating their efficacy within a tumor type and that they can be safely administered.

A physician is eligible to receive Group C drugs from the Division of Cancer Treatment only if the following requirements are met:

- A physician must be registered with the NCI as an investigator by having completed an FD-Form 1573;
- A written request for the drug, indicating the disease to be treated, must be submitted to the NCI;
- The use of the drug must be limited to indications outlined in the NCIs guidelines; and
- All adverse reactions must be reported to the Investigational Drug Branch of the Division of Cancer Treatment.

In view of these NCI controls on distribution and use of Group C drugs, intermediaries may assume, in the absence of evidence to the contrary, that a Group C drug and the related hospital stay are covered if all other applicable coverage requirements are satisfied.

If there is reason to question coverage in a particular case, the matter should be resolved with the assistance of the Quality Improvement Organization (QIO), or if there is none, the assistance of the contractor's medical consultants. Information regarding those drugs which are classified as Group C drugs may be obtained from:

Office of the Chief, Investigational Drug Branch
Division of Cancer Treatment, CTEP, Landow Building
Room 4C09, National Cancer Institute
Bethesda, Maryland 20205

CIM 45-20

20.22—Ethylenediamine-Tetra-Acetic (EDTA) Chelation Therapy for Treatment of Atherosclerosis

(Rev. 1, 10-03-03)

The use of EDTA as a chelating agent to treat atherosclerosis, arteriosclerosis, calcinosis, or similar generalized condition not listed by the FDA as an approved use is not covered. Any such use of EDTA is considered experimental. See §20.21 for an explanation of this conclusion.

CIM 45-22

260.7—Lymphocyte Immune Globulin, Anti-Thymocyte Globulin (Equine)

(Rev. 1, 10-03-03)

The lymphocyte immune globulin preparations are biologic drugs not previously approved or licensed for use in the management of renal allograft rejection. A number of other lymphocyte immune globulin products of equine, lapine, and murine origin are currently under investigation for their potential usefulness in controlling allograft rejections in human transplantation. These biologic drugs are viewed as adjunctive to traditional immunosuppressive products such as steroids and anti-metabolic drugs. At present, lymphocyte immune globulin preparations are not recommended to replace conventional immunosuppressive drugs, but to supplement them and to be used as alternatives to elevated or accelerated dosing with conventional immunosuppressive agents.

The FDA has approved one lymphocyte immune globulin preparation for marketing, lymphocyte immune globulin, anti-thymocyte globulin (equine). This drug is indicated for the management of allograft rejection episodes in renal transplantation. It is covered under Medicare when used for this purpose. Other forms of lymphocyte globulin preparation which the FDA approves for this indication in the future may be covered under Medicare.

CIM 45-23

230.12—Dimethyl Sulfoxide (DMSO)

(Rev. 1, 10-03-03)

DMSO is an industrial solvent produced as a chemical byproduct of paper production from wood pulp. The Food and Drug Administration has determined that the only purpose for which DMSO is safe and effective for humans is in the treatment of the bladder condition, interstitial cystitis. Therefore, the use of DMSO for all other indications is not considered to be reasonable and necessary. Payment may be made for its use only when reasonable and necessary for a patient in the treatment of interstitial cystitis.

CIM 45-24

110.3—Anti-Inhibitor Coagulant Complex (AICC)

(Rev. 1, 10-03-03)

Anti-inhibitor coagulant complex, AICC, is a drug used to treat hemophilia in patients with factor VIII inhibitor antibodies. AICC has been shown to be safe and effective and has Medicare coverage when furnished to patients with hemophilia A and inhibitor antibodies to factor VIII who have major bleeding episodes and who fail to respond to other, less expensive therapies.

CIM 45-25

160.13—Supplies Used in the Delivery of Transcutaneous Electrical Nerve Stimulation (TENS) and Neuromuscular Electrical Stimulation (NMES)

(Rev. 1, 10-03-03)

Transcutaneous Electrical Nerve Stimulation (TENS) and/or Neuromuscular Electrical Stimulation (NMES) can ordinarily be delivered to patients through the use of conventional electrodes, adhesive tapes and lead wires. There may be times, however, where it might be medically necessary for certain patients receiving TENS or NMES treatment to use, as an alternative to conventional electrodes, adhesive tapes and lead wires, a form-fitting conductive garment (i.e., a garment with conductive fibers which are separated from the patients' skin by layers of fabric).

A form-fitting conductive garment (and medically necessary related supplies) may be covered under the program only when:

1. It has received permission or approval for marketing by the Food and Drug Administration;

2. It has been prescribed by a physician for use in delivering covered TENS or NMES treatment; and

3. One of the medical indications outlined below is met:

- The patient cannot manage without the conductive garment because there is such a large area or so many sites to be stimulated and the stimulation would have to be delivered so frequently that it is not feasible to use conventional electrodes, adhesive tapes and lead wires;

- The patient cannot manage without the conductive garment for the treatment of chronic intractable pain because the areas or sites to be stimulated are inaccessible with the use of conventional electrodes, adhesive tapes and lead wires;

- The patient has a documented medical condition such as skin problems that preclude the application of conventional electrodes, adhesive tapes and lead wires;

- The patient requires electrical stimulation beneath a cast either to treat disuse atrophy, where the nerve supply to the muscle is intact, or to treat chronic intractable pain; or

- The patient has a medical need for rehabilitation strengthening (pursuant to a written plan of rehabilitation) following an injury where the nerve supply to the muscle is intact.

A conductive garment is not covered for use with a TENS device during the trial period specified in §160.3 unless:

4. The patient has a documented skin problem prior to the start of the trial period; and

5. The carrier's medical consultants are satisfied that use of such an item is medically necessary for the patient.

(See conditions for coverage of the use of TENS in the diagnosis and treatment of chronic intractable pain in §§160.3 and 160.13 and the use of NMES in the treatment of disuse atrophy in §150.4.)

CIM 45-30

80.3—Photosensitive Drugs

(Rev. 1, 10-03-03)

Photosensitive drugs are the light-sensitive agents used in photodynamic therapy. Once introduced into the body, these drugs selectively identify and adhere to diseased tissue. The drugs remain inactive until they are exposed to a specific wavelength of light, by means of a laser, that corresponds to their absorption peak. The activation of a photosensitive drug results in a photochemical reaction which treats the diseased tissue without affecting surrounding normal tissue.

Verteporfin

Verteporfin, a benzoporphyrin derivative, is an intravenous lipophilic photosensitive drug with an absorption peak of 690 nm. This drug was first approved by the Food and Drug Administration (FDA) on April 12, 2000, and subsequently, approved for inclusion in the United States Pharmacopoeia on July 18, 2000, meeting Medicare's definition of a drug when used in conjunction with ocular photodynamic therapy (see §80.2, "Photodynamic Therapy") when furnished intravenously incident to a physician's service. For patients with age-related macular degeneration, Verteporfin is only covered with a diagnosis of neovascular age-related macular degeneration (ICD-9-CM 362.52) with predominately classic subfoveal choroidal neovascular (CNV) lesions (where the area of classic CNV occupies = 50 percent of the area of the entire lesion) at the initial visit as determined by a fluorescein angiogram (CPT code 92235*). Subsequent follow-up visits will require a fluorescein angiogram prior to treatment. OPT with verteporfin is covered for the above indication and will remain noncovered for all other indications related to AMD (see §80.2). OPT with Verteporfin for use in non-AMD conditions is eligible for coverage through individual contractor discretion.

80.3.1—Verteporfin—Effective April 1, 2004 (see also 80.2.1 Ocular Photodynamic Therapy (OPT))

(Rev 9, 04-01-04)

General

Verteporfin, a benzoporphyrin derivative, is an intravenous lipophilic photosensitive drug with an absorption peak of 690 nm. Verteporfin was first approved by the Food and Drug Administration on April 12, 2000, and subsequently approved for inclu-

---

*CPT only © 2004. *Current Procedural Terminology, 2005, Professional Edition*, American Medical Association. All Rights Reserved.

sion in the United States Pharmacopoeia on July 18, 2000, meeting Medicare's definition of a drug as defined under §1861(t)(1) of the Social Security Act. Verteporfin is only covered when used in conjunction with ocular photodynamic therapy OPT) when furnished intravenously incident to a physician's service.

Covered Indications

Effective April 1, 2004, OPT with verteporfin is covered for patients with a diagnosis of neovascular age-related macular degeneration (AMD) with:

- Predominately classic subfoveal choroidal neovascularization (CNV) lesions (where the area of classic CNV occupies ≥ 50% of the area of the entire lesion) at the initial visit as determined by a fluorescein angiogram. (CNV lesions are comprised of classic and/or occult components.) Subsequent follow-up visits require a fluorescein angiogram prior to treatment. There are no requirements regarding visual acuity, lesion size, and number of retreatments when treating predominantly classic lesions.
- Subfoveal occult with no classic associated with AMD.
- Subfoveal minimally classic CNV CNV (where the area of classic CNV occupies <50% of the area of the entire lesion) associated with AMD.
- The above 2 indications are considered reasonable and necessary only when:

1. The lesions are small (4 disk areas or less in size) at the time of initial treatment or within the 3 months prior to initial treatment; and,

2. The lesions have shown evidence of progression within the 3 months prior to initial treatment. Evidence of progression must be documented by deterioration of visual acuity (at least 5 letters on a standard eye examination chart), lesion growth (an increase in at least 1 disk area), or the appearance of blood associated with the lesion.

Noncovered Indications

Other uses of OPT with verteporfin to treat AMD not already addressed by CMS will continue to be noncovered. These include, but are not limited to, the following AMD indications: juxtafoveal or extrafoveal CNV lesions (lesions outside the fovea), inability to obtain a fluorescein angiogram, or atrophic or "dry" AMD.

Other

The OPT with verteporfin for other ocular indications, such as pathologic myopia or presumed ocular histoplasmosis syndrome, continue to be eligible for local coverage determinations through individual contractor discretion. (This NCD last reviewed March 2004.)

CIM 50-1

20.8.1—Cardiac Pacemaker Evaluation Services

(Rev. 1, 10-03-03)

Medicare covers a variety of services for the post-implant follow-up and evaluation of implanted cardiac pacemakers. The following guidelines are designed to assist contractors in identifying and processing claims for such services.

NOTE: These new guidelines are limited to lithium battery-powered pacemakers, because mercury-zinc battery-powered pacemakers are no longer being manufactured and virtually all have been replaced by lithium units. Contractors still receiving claims for monitoring such units should continue to apply the guidelines published in 1980 to those units until they are replaced.

There are two general types of pacemakers in current use—single-chamber pacemakers which sense and pace the ventricles of the heart, and dual-chamber pacemakers which sense and pace both the atria and the ventricles. These differences require different monitoring patterns over the expected life of the units involved. One fact of which contractors should be aware is that many dual-chamber units may be programmed to pace only the ventricles; this may be done either at the time the pacemaker is implanted or at some time afterward. In such cases, a dual-cham-

ber unit, when programmed or reprogrammed for ventricular pacing, should be treated as a single-chamber pacemaker in applying screening guidelines.

The decision as to how often any patient's pacemaker should be monitored is the responsibility of the patient's physician who is best able to take into account the condition and circumstances of the individual patient. These may vary over time, requiring modifications of the frequency with which the patient should be monitored. In cases where monitoring is done by some entity other than the patient's physician, such as a commercial monitoring service or hospital outpatient department, the physician's prescription for monitoring is required and should be periodically renewed (at least annually) to assure that the frequency of monitoring is proper for the patient. Where a patient is monitored both during clinic visits and transtelephonically, the contractor should be sure to include frequency data on both types of monitoring in evaluating the reasonableness of the frequency of monitoring services received by the patient. Since there are over 200 pacemaker models in service at any given point, and a variety of patient conditions that give rise to the need for pacemakers, the question of the appropriate frequency of monitoring is a complex one. Nevertheless, it is possible to develop guidelines within which the vast majority of pacemaker monitoring will fall and contractors should do this, using their own data and experience, as well as the frequency guidelines which follow, in order to limit extensive claims development to those cases requiring special attention.

CIM 50-1

20.8.1.1—Transtelephonic Monitoring of Cardiac Pacemakers

(Rev. 1, 10-03-03)

A—General

Transtelephonic monitoring of pacemakers is furnished by commercial suppliers, hospital outpatient departments and physicians offices.

Telephone monitoring of cardiac pacemakers as described below is medically efficacious in identifying early signs of possible pacemaker failure, thus reducing the number of sudden pacemaker failures requiring emergency replacement. All systems that monitor the pacemaker rate (bpm) in both the free-running and/or magnetic mode are effective in detecting subclinical pacemaker failure due to battery depletion. More sophisticated systems are also capable of detecting internal electronic problems within the pulse generator itself and other potential problems. In the case of dual chamber pacemakers in particular, such monitoring may detect failure of synchronization of the atria and ventricles, and the need for adjustment and reprogramming of the device.

NOTE: The transmitting device furnished to the patient is simply one component of the diagnostic system, and is not covered as durable medical equipment. Those engaged in transtelephonic pacemaker monitoring should reflect the costs of the transmitters in setting their charges for monitoring.

B—Definition of Transtelephonic Monitoring

In order for transtelephonic monitoring services to be covered, the services must consist of the following elements:

- A minimum 30-second readable strip of the pacemaker in the free-running mode;
- Unless contraindicated, a minimum 30-second readable strip of the pacemaker in the magnetic mode; and
- A minimum 30 seconds of readable ECG strip.

C—Frequency Guidelines for Transtelephonic Monitoring

The guidelines below constitute a system which contractors should use, in conjunction with their knowledge of local medical practices, to screen claims for transtelephonic monitoring prior to payment. It is important to note that they are not recommendations with respect to a minimum frequency for such monitorings, but rather a maximum frequency (within which payment may be made without further claims development). As with previous guidelines, more frequent monitorings may be covered in cases where contractors are satisfied that such monitorings are medically necessary; e.g., based on the condition of the patient, or with respect to pacemakers exhibiting unexpected defects or premature failure. Contractors should seek written justification for more frequent monitorings from the patient's physician and/or any monitoring service involved.

These guidelines are divided into two broad categories—Guideline I which will apply to the majority of pacemakers now in use, and Guideline II which will apply only to pacemaker systems (pacemaker and leads) for which sufficient long-term clinical information exists to assure that they meet the standards of the Inter-Society Commission for Heart Disease Resources (ICHD) for longevity and end-of-life decay. (The ICHD standards are: (l) 90 percent cumulative survival at 5 years following implant; and (2) an end-of-life decay of less than a 50 percent drop of output voltage and less than 20 percent deviation of magnet rate, or a drop of 5 beats per minute or less, over a period of 3 months or more.) Contractors should consult with their medical advisers and other appropriate individuals and organizations (such as the North American Society of Pacing and Electrophysiology which publishes product reliability information) should questions arise over whether a pacemaker system meets the ICHD standards.

The two groups of guidelines are then further broken down into two general categories—single chamber and dual-chamber pacemakers. Contractors should be aware that the frequency with which a patient is monitored may be changed from time to time for a number of reasons, such as a change in the patient's overall condition, a reprogramming of the patient's pacemaker, the development of better information on the pacemaker's longevity or failure mode, etc. Consequently, changes in the proper set of guidelines may be required. Contractors should inform physicians and monitoring services to alert contractors to any changes in the patient's monitoring prescription that might necessitate changes in the screening guidelines applied to that patient. (Of particular importance is the reprogramming of a dual-chamber pacemaker to a single-chamber mode of operation. Such reprogramming would shift the patient from the appropriate dual-chamber guideline to the appropriate single-chamber guideline.)

Guideline I

1. Single-chamber pacemakers
   1st month—every 2 weeks.
   2nd through 36th month—every 8 weeks.
   37th month to failure—every 4 weeks.

2. Dual-chamber pacemaker
   1st month—every 2 weeks.
   2nd through 6th month—every 4 weeks.
   7th through 36th month—every 8 weeks.
   37th month to failure—every 4 weeks.

Guideline II

1. Single-chamber pacemakers
   1st month—every 2 weeks.
   2nd through 48th month—every 12 weeks.
   49th through 72nd month—every 8 weeks.
   Thereafter—every 4 weeks.

2. Dual-chamber pacemaker
   1st month—every 2 weeks.
   2nd through 30th month—every 12 weeks.
   31st through 48th month—every 8 weeks.
   Thereafter—every 4 weeks.

D—Pacemaker Clinic Services

1. General

Pacemaker monitoring is also covered when done by pacemaker clinics. Clinic visits may be done in conjunction with transtelephonic monitoring or as a separate service; however, the services rendered by a pacemaker clinic are more extensive than those currently possible by telephone. They include, for example, physical examination of patients and reprogramming of pacemakers. Thus, the use of one of these types of monitoring does not preclude concurrent use of the other.

2. Frequency Guidelines

As with transtelephonic pacemaker monitoring, the frequency of clinic visits is the decision of the patient's physician, taking into account, among other things, the medical condition of the patient. However, contractors can develop monitoring guidelines that will prove useful in screening claims. The following are recommendations for monitoring guidelines on lithium-battery pacemakers:

- For single-chamber pacemakers—twice in the first 6 months following implant, then once every 12 months.
- For dual-chamber pacemakers—twice in the first 6 months, then once every 6 months.

20.15—Electrocardiographic Services

(Rev. 26, Issued: 12-10-04, Effective: 08-26-04, Implementation: 12-10-04)

A—General

1. An electrocardiogram (EKG) is a graphic representation of electrical activity within the heart. Electrodes placed on the body in predetermined locations sense this electrical activity, which is then recorded by various means for review and interpretation. EKG recordings are used to diagnose a wide range of heart disease and other conditions that manifest themselves by abnormal cardiac electrical activity.

EKG services are covered diagnostic tests when there are documented signs and symptoms or other clinical indications for providing the service. Coverage includes the review and interpretation of EKGs only by a physician. There is no coverage for EKG services when rendered as a screening test or as part of a routine examination unless performed as part of the one-time, "Welcome to Medicare" preventive physical examination under section 611 of the Medicare Prescription Drug, Improvement, and Modernization Act of 2003.

2. Ambulatory electrocardiography (AECG) refers to services rendered in an outpatient setting over a specified period of time, generally while a patient is engaged in daily activities, including sleep. AECG devices are intended to provide the physician with documented episodes of arrhythmia, which may not be detected using a standard 12-lead EKG. AECG is most typically used to evaluate symptoms that may correlate with intermittent cardiac arrhythmias and/or myocardial ischemia. Such symptoms include syncope, dizziness, chest pain, palpitations, or shortness of breath. Additionally, AECG is used to evaluate patient response to initiation, revision, or discontinuation of arrhythmic drug therapy.

3. The Centers for Medicare & Medicaid Services (CMS), through the national coverage determination (NCD) process, may create new ambulatory EKG monitoring device categories if published, peer-reviewed clinical studies demonstrate evidence of improved clinical utility, or equal utility with additional advantage to the patient, as indicated by improved patient management and/or improved health outcomes in the Medicare population (such as superior ability to detect serious or life-threatening arrhythmias) as compared to devices or services in the currently described categories below.

Descriptions of Ambulatory EKG Monitoring Technologies

1. Dynamic electrocardiography devices that continuously record a real-time EKG, commonly known as Holter™ monitors, typically record over a 24-hour period. The recording is captured either on a magnetic tape or other digital medium. The data is then computer-analyzed at a later time, and a physician interprets the computer-generated report. A 24-hour recording is generally adequate to detect most transient arrhythmias. Documentation of medical necessity is required for monitoring longer than 24 hours. The recording device itself is not covered as durable medical equipment (DME) separate from the total diagnostic service.

2. An event monitor, or event recorder, is a patient-activated or event-activated EKG device that intermittently records cardiac arrhythmic events as they occur. The EKG is recorded on magnetic tape or other digital medium.

Cardiac event monitor technology varies among different devices. For patient-activated event monitors, the patient initiates recording when symptoms appear or when instructed to do so by a physician (e.g., following exercise). For self-sensing, automatically triggered monitors, an EKG is automatically recorded when the device detects an arrhythmia, without patient intervention. Some devices permit a patient to transmit EKG data trans-telephonically (i.e., via telephone) to a receiving center where the data is reviewed. A technician may be available at these centers to review transmitted data 24-hours per day. In some instances, when the EKG is determined to be outside certain pre-set criteria by a technician or other non-physician, a physician is available 24-hours per day to review the transmitted data and to make clinical decisions regarding the patient. These services are known as "24-hour attended monitoring". In other instances, transmitted EKG data is reviewed at a later time and are, therefore, considered "non-attended."

Cardiac event monitors without trans-telephonic capability must be removed from the patient and taken to a location for review of the stored EKG data. Some devices also permit a "time sampling" mode of operation. The "time sampling" mode is not covered under ambulatory EKG monitoring technology. Some cardiac event monitoring devices with trans-telephonic capabilities require the patient to dial the phone number of a central EKG data reception center and initiate transmission of EKG data. Other devices use Internet-based in-home computers to capture and store EKG data. When such devices detect pre-programmed arrhythmias, data is automatically sent via modem and standard telephone lines to a central receiving center, or independent diagnostic testing facility (IDTF), where the data is reviewed. Internet-based in-home computer systems may also provide the receiving center with a daily computer-generated report that summarizes 24 hours of EKG data.

Certain cardiac event monitors capture electrical activity with a single electrode attached to the skin. Other devices may employ multiple electrodes in order to record more complex EKG tracings. Additionally, devices may be individually programmed to detect patient-specific factors, electrode malfunction, or other factors. Cardiac event monitors can be further categorized as either "pre-event" or "post-event" recorders, based on their memory capabilities:

a. Pre-symptom Memory Loop Recorder (MLR)

Upon detecting symptoms, the wearer presses a button, which activates the recorder to save (i.e., memorize) an interval of pre-symptom EKG data along with data during and subsequent to the symptomatic event. Self-sensing recorders (also known as event-activated or automatic trigger) do not require patient input to capture these data. Single or multiple events may be recorded. The device is worn at all times, usually for up to 30 days.

• Implantable (or Insertable Loop) Recorder (ILR)

Another type of pre-symptom MLR, it is implanted subcutaneously in a patient's upper left chest and may remain implanted for many months. An ILR is used when syncope is thought to be cardiac-related, but is too infrequent to be detected by either a Holter™ monitor or a traditional pre-symptom MLR.

b. Post-symptom Recorder

The patient temporarily places this device against the chest when symptoms occur and activates it by pressing a button. These recorders represent old technology, as they do not include a memory loop. The device transmits EKG data telephonically in real-time and is usually used for up to 30 days.

B—Nationally Covered Indications

The following indications are covered nationally unless otherwise indicated:

1. Computer analysis of EKGs when furnished in a setting and under the circumstances required for coverage of other EKG services.

2. EKG services rendered by an independent diagnostic testing facility (IDTF), including physician review and interpretation.

Separate physician services are not covered unless he/she is the patient's attending or consulting physician.

3. Emergency EKGs (i.e., when the patient is or may be experiencing a life-threatening event) performed as a laboratory or diagnostic service by a portable x-ray supplier only when a physician is in attendance at the time the service is performed or immediately thereafter.

4. Home EKG services with documentation of medical necessity.

5. Trans-telephonic EKG transmissions (effective March 1, 1980) as a diagnostic service for the indications described below, when performed with equipment meeting the standards described below, subject to the limitations and conditions specified below. Coverage is further limited to the amounts payable with respect to the physician's service in interpreting the results of such transmissions, including charges for rental of the equipment. The device used by the beneficiary is part of a total diagnostic system and is not considered DME separately. Covered uses are to:

a. Detect, characterize, and document symptomatic transient arrhythmias;

b. Initiate, revise, or discontinue arrhythmic drug therapy; or,

c. Carry out early post-hospital monitoring of patients discharged after myocardial infarction (MI); (only if 24-hour coverage is provided, see C.5. below).

Certain uses other than those specified above may be covered if, in the judgment of the local contractor, such use is medically necessary.

Additionally, the transmitting devices must meet at least the following criteria:

a. They must be capable of transmitting EKG Leads, I, II, or III; and,

b. The tracing must be sufficiently comparable to a conventional EKG.

24-hour attended coverage used as early post-hospital monitoring of patients discharged after MI is only covered if provision is made for such 24-hour attended coverage in the manner described below:

24-hour attended coverage means there must be, at a monitoring site or central data center, an EKG technician or other non-physician, receiving calls and/or EKG data; tape recording devices do not meet this requirement. Further, such technicians should have immediate, 24-hour access to a physician to review transmitted data and make clinical decisions regarding the patient. The technician should also be instructed as to when and how to contact available facilities to assist the patient in case of emergencies.

C—Nationally Non-covered Indications

The following indications are non-covered nationally unless otherwise specified below:

1. The time-sampling mode of operation of ambulatory EKG cardiac event monitoring/recording.

2. Separate physician services other than those rendered by an IDTF unless rendered by the patient's attending or consulting physician.

3. Home EKG services without documentation of medical necessity.

4. Emergency EKG services by a portable x-ray supplier without a physician in attendance at the time of service or immediately thereafter.

5. 24-hour attended coverage used as early post-hospital monitoring of patients discharged after MI unless provision is made for such 24-hour attended coverage in the manner described in section B.5. above.

6. Any marketed Food and Drug Administration (FDA)-approved ambulatory cardiac monitoring device or service that cannot be categorized according to the framework below.

D—Other

Ambulatory cardiac monitoring performed with a marketed, FDA-approved device, is eligible for coverage if it can be categorized according to the framework below. Unless there is a specific NCD for that device or service, determination as to whether a device or service that fits into the framework is reasonable and necessary is according to local contractor discretion.

Electrocardiographic Services Framework

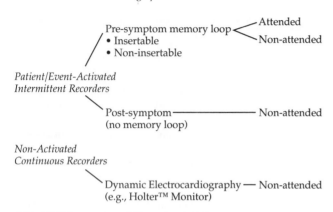

(This NCD last reviewed December 2004.)

CIM 50-17

190.10—Laboratory Tests—CRD Patients

(Rev. 1, 10-03-03)

Laboratory tests are essential to monitor the progress of CRD patients. The following list and frequencies of tests constitute the level and types of routine laboratory tests that are covered. Bills for other types of tests are considered nonroutine. Routine tests at greater frequencies must include medical justification. Nonroutine tests generally are justified by the diagnosis. The routinely covered regimen includes the following tests:

Per Dialysis

• All hematocrit or hemoglobin and clotting time tests furnished incident to dialysis treatments.

Per Week

• Prothrombin time for patients on anticoagulant therapy, and
• Serum Creatinine

Per Week or Thirteen Per Quarter

• BUN

Monthly

• CBC,
• Serum Calcium,
• Serum Chloride,
• Serum Potassium,
• Serum Bicarbonate,
• Serum Phosphorous,
• Total Protein,
• Serum Albumin,
• Alkaline Phosphatase,
• AST,
• SGOT, and
• LDH.

Guidelines for tests other than those routinely performed include:

• Serum Aluminum—one every 3 months, and
• Serum Ferritin—one every 3 months

The following tests for hepatitis B are covered when patients first enter a dialysis facility: hepatitis B surface antigen (HBsAg) and Anti-HBs. Coverage of future testing in these patients depends on their serologic status and on whether they have been successfully immunized against hepatitis B virus. The following table summa-

rizes the frequency of serologic surveillance for hepatitis B. Tests furnished according to this table do not require additional documentation and are paid separately because payment for maintenance dialysis treatments does not take them into account.

Frequency of Screening			
Vaccination and Serologic Status		**HBsAg Patients**	**Anti-HBs Patients**
Unvaccinated	Susceptible	Monthly	Semiannually
Unvaccinated	HBsAg Carrier	Annually	None
Unvaccinated	Anti-HBs-Positive (1)	None	Annually
Vaccinated	Anti-HBs-Positive (1)	None	Annually
Vaccinated	Low Level or No Anti-HBs	Monthly	Semiannually

(1) At least 10 sample ration units by radioimmunoassay or positive by enzyme immunoassay.

Patients who are in the process of receiving hepatitis B vaccines, but have not received the complete series, should continue to be routinely screened as susceptible. Between one and six months after the third dose, all vaccines should be tested for anti-HBs to confirm their response to the vaccine. Patients who have a level of anti-HBs of at least 10 sample ratio units (SRUs) by radioimmunoassay (RIA) or who are positive by enzyme immunoassay (EIA) are considered adequate responders to vaccine and need only be tested for anti-HBs annually to verify their immune status. If anti-HBs drops below 10 SRUs by RIA or is negative by EIA, a booster dose of hepatitis B vaccine should be given.

Laboratory tests are subject to the normal coverage requirements. If the laboratory services are performed by a free-standing facility, the facility must meet the conditions of coverage for independent laboratories.

CIM 50-20, CIM 50-20.1

190.2—Diagnostic Pap Smears

(Rev. 1, 10-03-03)

A diagnostic pap smear and related medically necessary services are covered under Medicare Part B when ordered by a physician under one of the following conditions:

• Previous cancer of the cervix, uterus, or vagina that has been or is presently being treated;
• Previous abnormal pap smear;
• Any abnormal findings of the vagina, cervix, uterus, ovaries, or adnexa;
• Any significant complaint by the patient referable to the female reproductive system; or
• Any signs or symptoms that might in the physician's judgment reasonably be related to a gynecologic disorder.

Screening Pap Smears and Pelvic Examinations for Early Detection of Cervical or Vaginal Cancer

(For screening pap smears, effective for services performed on or after July 1, 1990. For pelvic examinations including clinical breast examination, effective for services furnished on or after January 1, 1998.)

A screening pap smear (use HCPCS code P3000 Screening Papanicolaou smear, cervical or vaginal, up to three smears; by technician under physician supervision or P3001 Screening Papanicolaou smear, cervical or vaginal, up to three smears requiring interpretation by physician). (Use HCPCS codes G0123 Screening Cytopathology, cervical or vaginal (any reporting system), collected in preservative fluid, automated thin layer preparation, screening by cytotechnologist under physician supervision or G0124 Screening Cytopathology, cervical or vaginal (any reporting system) collected in preservative fluid, automated thin layer preparation, requiring interpretation by physician) and related medically necessary services provided to a woman for the early detection of cervical cancer (including collection of the sample of cells and a physician's interpretation of the test results) and pelvic examination (including clinical breast examination) (use

HCPCS code G0101 cervical or vaginal cancer screening; pelvic and clinical breast examination) are covered under Medicare Part B when ordered by a physician (or authorized practitioner) under one of the following conditions. She has not had such a test during the preceding three years or is a woman of childbearing age (§1861(nn) of the Act).

- There is evidence (on the basis of her medical history or other findings) that she is at high risk of developing cervical cancer and her physician (or authorized practitioner) recommends that she have the test performed more frequently than every 3 years.

High risk factors for cervical and vaginal cancer are:

- Early onset of sexual activity (under 16 years of age);
- Multiple sexual partners (five or more in a lifetime);
- History of sexually transmitted disease (including HIV infection);
- Fewer than three negative or any pap smears within the previous seven years; and
- DES (diethylstilbestrol)—exposed daughters of women who took DES during pregnancy.

NOTE: Claims for pap smears must indicate the beneficiary's low or high risk status by including the appropriate ICD-9-CM diagnosis code as required by claims processing instructions.

Definitions

A woman as described in §1861(nn) of the Act is a woman who is of childbearing age and has had a pap smear test during any of the preceding three years that indicated the presence of cervical or vaginal cancer or other abnormality, or is at high risk of developing cervical or vaginal cancer.

A woman of childbearing age is one who is premenopausal and has been determined by a physician or other qualified practitioner to be of childbearing age, based upon the medical history or other findings.

Other "qualified practitioner," as defined in 42CFR410.56(a) includes a certified nurse midwife (as defined in §1861(gg) of the Act), or a physician assistant, nurse practitioner, or clinical nurse specialist (as defined in §1861(aa) of the Act) who is authorized under State law to perform the examination.

Screening Pelvic Examination

Section 4102 of the Balanced Budget Act of 1997 provides for coverage of screening pelvic examinations (including a clinical breast examination) for all female beneficiaries, subject to certain frequency and other limitations. A screening pelvic examination (including a clinical breast examination) should include at least seven of the following eleven elements:

- Inspection and palpation of breasts for masses or lumps, tenderness, symmetry, or nipple discharge
- Digital rectal examination including sphincter tone, presence of hemorrhoids, and rectal masses. Pelvic examination (with or without specimen collection for smears and cultures) including:
- External genitalia (for example, general appearance, hair distribution, or lesions).
- Urethral meatus (for example, size, location, lesions, or prolapse).
- Urethra (for example, masses, tenderness, or scarring).
- Bladder (for example, fullness, masses, or tenderness).
- Vagina (for example, general appearance, estrogen effect, discharge lesions, pelvic support, cystocele, or rectocele).
- Cervix (for example, general appearance, lesions, or discharge).
- Uterus (for example, size, contour, position, mobility, tenderness, consistency, descent, or support).
- Adnexa/parametria (for example, masses, tenderness, organomegaly, or nodularity).
- Anus and perineum.

This description is from Documentation Guidelines for Evaluation and Management Services, published in May 1997 and was developed by the Centers for Medicare & Medicaid Services and the American Medical Association.

CIM 50-24

190.6—Hair Analysis

(Rev. 1, 10-03-03)

Not Covered

Hair analysis to detect mineral traces as an aid in diagnosing human disease is not a covered service under Medicare.

The correlation of hair analysis to the chemical state of the whole body is not possible at this time, and therefore this diagnostic procedure cannot be considered to be reasonable and necessary under §1862(a)(1) of the Act.

CIM 50-36

220.6—Positron Emission Tomography (PET) Scans

(Rev. 31, Issued: 04-04-05; Effective: 01-28-05; Implementation: 04-18-05)

I. General Description

Positron emission tomography (PET) is a noninvasive diagnostic imaging procedure that assesses the level of metabolic activity and perfusion in various organ systems of the [human] body. A positron camera (tomograph) is used to produce cross-sectional tomographic images, which are obtained from positron emitting radioactive tracer substances (radiopharmaceuticals) such as 2-[F-18] Fluoro-D-Glucose (FDG), that are administered intravenously to the patient.

The following indications may be covered for PET under certain circumstances. Details of Medicare PET coverage are discussed later in this section. Unless otherwise indicated, the clinical conditions below are covered when PET utilizes FDG as a tracer.

NOTE: This manual section 220.6 lists all Medicare-covered uses of PET scans. Except as set forth below in cancer indications listed as "Coverage with Evidence Development", a particular use of PET scans is not covered unless this manual specifically provides that such use is covered. Although this section lists some non-covered uses of PET scans, it does not constitute an exhaustive list of all non-covered uses.

Clinical Condition	Effective Date	Coverage
Solitary Pulmonary Nodules (SPNs)	January 1, 1998	Characterization
Lung Cancer (Non Small Cell)	January 1, 1998	Initial staging
Lung Cancer (Non Small Cell)	July 1, 2001	Diagnosis, staging, restaging
Esophageal Cancer	July 1, 2001	Diagnosis, staging, restaging
Colorectal Cancer	July 1, 1999	Determining location of tumors if rising CEA level suggests recurrence
Colorectal Cancer	July 1, 2001	Diagnosis, staging, restaging
Lymphoma	July 1, 1999	Staging and restaging only when used as alternative to Gallium scan
Lymphoma	July 1, 2001	Diagnosis, staging and restaging
Melanoma	July 1, 1999	Evaluating recurrence prior to surgery as alternative to Gallium scan
Melanoma	July 1, 2001	Diagnosis, staging, restaging; Non-covered for evaluating regional nodes

Clinical Condition	Effective Date	Coverage
Breast Cancer	October 1, 2002	As an adjunct to standard imaging modalities for staging patients with distant metastasis or restaging patients with loco-regional recurrence or metastasis; as an adjunct to standard imaging modalities for monitoring tumor response to treatment for women with locally advanced and metastatic breast cancer when a change in therapy is anticipated
Head and Neck Cancers (excluding CNS and thyroid	July 1, 2001	Diagnosis, staging, restaging
Thyroid Cancer	October 1, 2003	Restaging of recurrent or residual thyroid cancers of follicular cell origin previously treated by thyroidectomy and radioiodine ablation and have a serum thyroglobulin >10ng/ml and negative I-131 whole body scan performed
Myocardial Viability	July 1, 2001 to September 30, 2002	Only following inconclusive SPECT
Myocardial Viability	October 1, 2002	Primary or initial diagnosis, or following an inconclusive SPECT prior to revascularization. SPECT may not be used following an inconclusive PET scan
Refractory Seizures	July 1, 2001	Pre-surgical evaluation only
Perfusion of the heart using Rubidium 82* tracer	March 14, 1995	Noninvasive imaging of the perfusion of the heart
Perfusion of the heart using ammonia N-13* tracer	October 1, 2003	Noninvasive imaging of the perfusion of the heart

* Not FDG-PET.

EFFECTIVE JANUARY 28, 2005: This manual section lists Medicare-covered uses of PET scans effective for services performed on or after January 28, 2005. Except as set forth below in cancer indications listed as "coverage with evidence development", a particular use of PET scans is not covered unless this manual specifically provides that such use is covered. Although this section 220.6 lists some non-covered uses of PET scans, it does not constitute an exhaustive list of all non-covered uses.

For cancer indications listed as "coverage with evidence development" CMS determines that the evidence is sufficient to conclude that an FDG PET scan is reasonable and necessary only when the provider is participating in, and patients are enrolled in, one of the following types of prospective clinical studies that is designed to collect additional information at the time of the scan to assist in patient management:

• A clinical trial of FDG PET that meets the requirements of Food and Drug Administration (FDA) category B investigational device exemption (42 CFR 405.201);

• An FDG PET clinical study that is designed to collect additional information at the time of the scan to assist in patient management. Qualifying clinical studies must ensure that specific hypotheses are addressed; appropriate data elements are collected; hospitals and providers are qualified to provide the PET scan and interpret the results; participating hospitals and providers accurately report data on all enrolled patients not included in other qualifying trials through adequate auditing mechanisms; and, all patient confidentiality, privacy, and other Federal laws must be followed.

Effective January 28, 2005: For PET services identified as "Coverage with Evidence Development." Medicare shall notify providers and beneficiaries where these services can be accessed, as they become available, via the following:

• Federal Register Notice
• CMS coverage Web site at: www.cms.gov/coverage

Indication	Covered[1]	Nationally Non-covered[2]	Coverage with evidence development[3]
Brain			X
Breast			
—Diagnosis		X	
—Initial staging of axillary nodes		X	
—Staging of distant metastasis	X		
—Restaging, monitoring*	X		
Cervical			
—Staging as adjunct to conventional imaging	X		
—Other staging			X
—Diagnosis, restaging, monitoring*			X
Colorectal			
—Diagnosis, staging, restaging	X		
—Monitoring*			X
Esophagus			
—Diagnosis, staging, restaging	X		
—Monitoring*			X
Head and Neck (non-CNS/thyroid)			
—Diagnosis, staging, restaging	X		
—Monitoring*			X
Lymphoma			
—Diagnosis, staging, restaging	X		
—Monitoring*			X
Melanoma			
—Diagnosis, staging, restaging	X		
—Monitoring*			X
Non-Small Cell Lung			
—Diagnosis, staging, restaging	X		
—Monitoring*			X
Ovarian			X
Pancreatic			X
Small Cell Lung			X
Soft Tissue Sarcoma			X
Solitary Pulmonary Nodule (characterization)	X		
Thyroid			
—Staging of follicular cell tumors	X		
—Restaging of medullary cell tumors			X

Indication	Covered[1]	Nationally Non-covered[2]	Coverage with evidence development[3]
—Diagnosis, other staging & restaging			X
—Monitoring*			X
Testicular			X
All other cancers not listed herein (all indications)			X

[1] Covered nationally based on evidence of benefit. Refer to National Coverage Determination Manual Section 220.6 in its entirety for specific coverage language and limitations for each indication.
[2] Non-covered nationally based on evidence of harm or no benefit.
[3] Covered only in specific settings discussed above if certain patient safeguards are provided. Otherwise, non-covered nationally based on lack of evidence sufficient to establish either benefit or harm or no prior decision addressing this cancer. Medicare shall notify providers and beneficiaries where these services can be accessed, as they become available, via the following:
• Federal Register Notice
• CMS coverage Web site at: www.cms.gov/coverage
* Monitoring = monitoring response to treatment when a change in therapy is anticipated.

II. General Conditions of Coverage for FDG PET

III. Allowable FDG PET Systems

A. Definitions: For purposes of this section:

• "Any FDA-approved" means all systems approved or cleared for marketing by the Food and Drug Administration (FDA) to image radionuclides in the body.
• "FDA-approved" means that the system indicated has been approved or cleared for marketing by the FDA to image radionuclides in the body.
• "Certain coincidence systems" refers to the systems that have all the following features:
—Crystal at least 5/8-inch thick;
—Techniques to minimize or correct for scatter and/or random; and
—Digital detectors and iterative reconstruction.

Scans performed with gamma camera PET systems with crystals thinner than 5/8" will not be covered by Medicare. In addition, scans performed with systems with crystals greater than or equal to 5/8" in thickness, but that do not meet the other listed design characteristics are not covered by Medicare.

B. Allowable PET systems by covered clinical indication:

Covered Clinical Condition	Allowable Type of FDG PET System		
	Prior to July 1, 2001	July 1, 2001 through December 31, 2001	On or after January 1, 2002
Characterization of single pulmonary nodules	Effective 1/1/1998, any FDA-approved	Any FDA-approved	FDA-approved: Full/Partial ring certain co-incidence systems
Initial staging of lung cancer (non small cell)	Effective 1/1/1998, any FDA-approved	Any FDA-approved	FDA-approved: Full/Partial ring, certain coincidence systems
Determining location of colorectal tumors if rising CEA level suggests recurrence	Effective 7/1/1999, any FDA-approved	Any FDA-approved	FDA approved: Full/Partial ring, certain coincidence systems
Staging or restaging of lymphoma only when used as alternative to gallium scan	Effective 7/1/1999, any FDA-approved	Any FDA-approved	FDA-approved: Full/Partial ring, certain coincidence systems
Evaluating recurrence of melanoma prior to surgery as alternative to a gallium scan	Effective 7/1/1999, any FDA-approved	Any FDA-approved	FDA approved: Full/Partial ring, certain coincidence systems
Diagnosis, staging, restaging of colorectal cancer	Not covered by Medicare	Full ring	FDA-approved: Full/Partial ring
Diagnosis, staging, restaging of esophageal cancer	Not covered by Medicare	Full ring	FDA-approved: Full/Partial ring
Diagnosis, staging, restaging of head and neck cancers (excluding CNS and thyroid)	Not covered by Medicare	Full ring	FDA-approved: Full/Partial ring
Diagnosis, staging, restaging of lung cancer (non small cell)	Not covered by Medicare	Full ring	FDA-approved: Full/Partial ring
Diagnosis, staging, restaging of lymphoma	Not covered by Medicare	Full ring	FDA-approved: Full/Partial ring
Diagnosis, staging, restaging of melanoma (non-covered for evaluating regional nodes)	Not covered by Medicare	Full ring	FDA-approved: Full/Partial ring
Determination of myocardial viability only following inconclusive SPECT	Not covered by Medicare	Full ring	FDA-approved: Full/Partial ring
Pre-surgical evaluation of refractory seizures	Not covered by Medicare	Full ring	FDA-approved: Full ring
Breast Cancer	Not covered	Not covered	Effective October 1, 2002, Full/Partial ring
Thyroid Cancer	Not covered	Not covered	Effective October 1, 2003, Full/Partial ring
Myocardial Viability Primary or initial diagnosis prior to revascularization	Not covered	Not covered	Effective October 1, 2002, Full/Partial ring
All other oncology indications not previously specified	Not covered	Not covered	Effective January 28, 2005, Full/Partial ring

C. Regardless of any other terms or conditions, all uses of FDG PET scans, in order to be covered by the Medicare program, must meet the following general conditions prior to June 30, 2001:

- Submission of claims for payment must include any information Medicare requires to ensure the PET scans performed were: (a) medically necessary, (b) did not unnecessarily duplicate other covered diagnostic tests, and (c) did not involve investigational drugs or procedures using investigational drugs, as determined by the FDA.
- The PET scan entity submitting claims for payment must keep such patient records as Medicare requires on file for each patient for whom a PET scan claim is made.

Regardless of any other terms or conditions, all uses of FDG PET scans, in order to be covered by the Medicare program, must meet the following general conditions as of July 1, 2001:

- The provider of the PET scan should maintain on file the doctor's referral and documentation that the procedure involved only FDA-approved drugs and devices, as is normal business practice.
- The ordering physician is responsible for documenting the medical necessity of the study and ensuring that it meets the conditions specified in the instructions. The physician should have documentation in the beneficiary's medical record to support the referral to the PET scan provider.

III. Covered Indications for PET Scans and Limitations/Requirements for Usage

For all uses of PET relating to malignancies the following conditions apply:

A. Diagnosis: PET is covered only in clinical situations in which: (1) the PET results may assist in avoiding an invasive diagnostic procedure, or in which (2) the PET results may assist in determining the optimal anatomical location to perform an invasive diagnostic procedure. In general, for most solid tumors, a tissue diagnosis is made prior to the performance of PET scanning. PET scans following a tissue diagnosis are generally performed for the purpose of staging rather than diagnosis. Therefore, the use of PET in the diagnosis of lymphoma, esophageal, and colorectal cancers as well as in melanoma, should be rare.

PET is not covered as a screening test (i.e., testing patients without specific signs and symptoms of disease).

B. Staging: PET is covered for staging in clinical situations in which: (1)(a) the stage of the cancer remains in doubt after completion of a standard diagnostic workup, including conventional imaging (computed tomography (CT), magnetic resonance imaging (MRI), or ultrasound, or (1)(b) it could potentially replace one or more conventional imaging studies when it is expected that conventional study information is insufficient for the clinical management of the patient, and 2) clinical management of the patient would differ depending on the stage of the cancer identified.

C. Restaging: PET is covered for restaging: (1) after completion of treatment for the purpose of detecting residual disease, (2) for detecting suspected recurrence, (3) to determine the extent of a known recurrence, or (4) if it could potentially replace one or more conventional imaging studies when it is expected that conventional study information is insufficient for the clinical management of the patient.

D. Monitoring: This refers to use of PET to monitor tumor response to treatment during the planned course of therapy (i.e., when a change in therapy is anticipated)

NOTE: In the absence of national frequency limitations, contractors, should, if necessary, develop frequency requirements on any or all of the indications covered on and after July 1, 2001.

(This NCD last reviewed December 2004.)

(CIM 50-36)

220.6.1—PET for Perfusion of the Heart (Various Effective Dates Below)

(Rev. 31, Issued: 04-04-05; Effective: 01-28-05; Implementation: 04-18-05)

1. Rubidium 82 (Effective March 14, 1995)

Effective for services performed on or after March 14, 1995, PET scans performed at rest or with pharmacological stress used for noninvasive imaging of the perfusion of the heart for the diagnosis and management of patients with known or suspected coronary artery disease using the FDA-approved radiopharmaceutical Rubidium 82 (Rb 82) are covered, provided the requirements below are met:

- The PET scan, whether at rest alone, or rest with stress, is performed in place of, but not in addition to, a single photon emission computed tomography (SPECT); or
- The PET scan, whether at rest alone or rest with stress, is used following a SPECT that was found to be inconclusive. In these cases, the PET scan must have been considered necessary in order to determine what medical or surgical intervention is required to treat the patient. (For purposes of this requirement, an inconclusive test is a test(s) whose results are equivocal, technically uninterpretable, or discordant with a patient's other clinical data and must be documented in the beneficiary's file.)
- For any PET scan for which Medicare payment is claimed for dates of services prior to July 1, 2001, the claimant must submit additional specified information on the claim form (including proper codes and/or modifiers), to indicate the results of the PET scan. The claimant must also include information on whether the PET scan was performed after an inconclusive noninvasive cardiac test. The information submitted with respect to the previous noninvasive cardiac test must specify the type of test performed prior to the PET scan and whether it was inconclusive or unsatisfactory. These explanations are in the form of special G codes used for billing PET scans using Rb 82. Beginning July 1, 2001, claims should be submitted with the appropriate codes.

2. Ammonia N-13 (Effective October 1, 2003)

Effective for services performed on or after October 1, 2003, PET scans performed at rest or with pharmacological stress used for noninvasive imaging of the perfusion of the heart for the diagnosis and management of patients with known or suspected coronary artery disease using the FDA-approved radiopharmaceutical ammonia N-13 are covered, provided the requirements below are met:

- The PET scan, whether at rest alone, or rest with stress, is performed in place of, but not in addition to, a SPECT; or
- The PET scan, whether at rest alone or rest with stress, is used following a SPECT that was found to be inconclusive. In these cases, the PET scan must have been considered necessary in order to determine what medical or surgical intervention is required to treat the patient. (For purposes of this requirement, an inconclusive test is a test whose results are equivocal, technically uninterpretable, or discordant with a patient's other clinical data and must be documented in the beneficiary's file.)

(This NCD last reviewed April 2003.)

CIM 50-36

220.6.2—FDG PET for Lung Cancer (Various Effective Dates Below)

(Rev. 31, Issued: 04-04-05; Effective: 01-28-05; Implementation: 04-18-05)

1. Characterization of Single Pulmonary Nodules (SPNs) (Effective January 1, 1998)

Effective for services performed on or after January 1, 1998, Medicare covers regional FDG PET chest scans, on any FDA-approved scanner, for the characterization of SPNs. The primary purpose of such characterization should be to determine the likelihood of malignancy in order to plan future management and treatment for the patient.

Beginning July 1, 2001, documentation should be maintained in the beneficiary's medical record file at the referring physician's office to support the medical necessity of the procedure, as is normal business practice. The following documentation is required:

- There must be evidence of primary tumor. Claims for regional PET chest scans for characterizing SPNs should include evidence of the initial detection of a primary lung tumor, usually by computed tomography (CT). This should include, but is not restricted to, a report on the results of such CT or other detection method, indicating an indeterminate or possibly malignant lesion, not exceeding 4 centimeters (cm) in diameter.
- PET scan claims must include the results of concurrent thoracic CT (as noted above), which is necessary for anatomic information, in order to ensure that the PET scan is properly coordinated with other diagnostic modalities.
- In cases of serial evaluation of SPNs using both CT and regional PET chest scanning, such PET scans will not be covered if repeated within 90 days following a negative PET scan.

NOTE: A tissue sampling procedure (TSP) is not routinely covered in the case of a negative PET scan for characterization of SPNs, since the patient is presumed not to have a malignant lesion, based upon PET scan results. When there is a negative PET, the provider must submit additional information with the claim to support the necessity of a TSP, for review by the Medicare contractor.

2. Initial Staging of Non-Small-Cell Lung Carcinoma (LSCLC) (Effective January 1, 1998)

Effective for services performed from January 1, 1998, through June 30, 2001, Medicare approved coverage of FDG PET for initial staging of NSCLC.

Limitations: This service is covered only when the primary cancerous lung tumor has been pathologically confirmed; claims for PET must include a statement or other evidence of the detection of such primary lung tumor. The evidence should include, but is not restricted to, a surgical pathology report, which documents the presence of an NSCLC. Whole body PET scan results and results of concurrent CT and follow-up lymph node biopsy must be properly coordinated with other diagnostic modalities. Claims must include both:

- The results of concurrent thoracic CT, necessary for anatomic information, and
- The results of any lymph node biopsy performed to finalize whether the patient will be a surgical candidate. The ordering physician is responsible for providing this biopsy result to the PET facility.

NOTE: Where the patient is considered a surgical candidate, (given the presumed absence of metastatic NSCLC unless medical review supports a determination of medical necessity of a biopsy) a lymph node biopsy will not be covered in the case of a negative CT and negative PET. A lymph node biopsy will be covered in all other cases, i.e., positive CT + positive PET; negative CT + positive PET; positive CT + negative PET.

3. Diagnosis, Staging, and Restaging of NSCLC (Effective July 1, 2001)

Effective for serviced performed on or after July 1, 2001, Medicare covers FDG PET for diagnosis, staging, and restaging of NSCLC.

4. Monitoring response to treatment of NSCLC (Effective January 28, 2005)

Effective for services performed on or after January 28, 2005, Medicare only covers FDG PET for monitoring response to treatment for NSCLC as "coverage with evidence development".

Medicare shall notify providers and beneficiaries where these services can be accessed, as they become available, via the following:

- Federal Register Notice
- CMS coverage Web site at: www.cms.gov/coverage

Requirements: PET is covered in any/all of the following circumstances:

A. Diagnosis: PET is covered only in clinical situations in which: (1) the PET results may assist in avoiding an invasive diagnostic procedure, or in which (2) the PET results may assist in determining the optimal anatomical location to perform an invasive diagnostic procedure. In general, for most solid tumors, a tissue diagnosis is made prior to the performance of PET scanning. PET scans following a tissue diagnosis are generally performed for the purpose of staging, rather than diagnosis. Therefore, the use of PET in the diagnosis of lymphoma, esophageal, and colorectal cancers as well as in melanoma, should be rare.

B. Staging and/or Restaging: PET is covered for staging in clinical situations in which: (1)(a) the stage of the cancer remains in doubt after completion of a standard diagnostic workup, including conventional imaging (CT, magnetic resonance imaging, or ultrasound) or, (1)(b) the use of PET could potentially replace one or more conventional imaging studies when it is expected that conventional study information is insufficient for the clinical management of the patient, and (2) clinical management of the patient would differ depending on the stage of the cancer identified.

PET is covered for restaging after the completion of treatment for: (1) the purpose of detecting residual disease, (2) detecting suspected recurrence, (3) determining the extent of a known recurrence, or (4) potentially replacing one or more conventional imaging studies when it is expected that conventional study information is insufficient for the clinical management of the patient.

C. Monitoring Response to Treatment: PET is covered for monitoring response to treatment when a change in therapy is anticipated.

Documentation should be maintained in the beneficiary's medical record at the referring physician's office to support the medical necessity of the procedure, as is normal business practice.

(This NCD last reviewed March 2005.)

CIM 50-36

220.6.3—FDG PET for Esophageal Cancer (Various Effective Dates Below)

(Rev. 31, Issued: 04-04-05; Effective: 01-28-05; Implementation: 04-18-05)

Effective for services performed on or after July 1, 2001, Medicare covers FDG PET for the diagnosis, staging, and restaging of esophageal cancer.

Effective for services performed on or after January 28, 2005, Medicare only covers FDG PET for monitoring response to treatment for esophageal cancer as "coverage with evidence development".

Medicare shall notify providers and beneficiaries where these services can be accessed, as they become available, via the following:

- Federal Register Notice
- CMS coverage Web site at: www.cms.gov/coverage

Requirements: PET is covered in any/all of the following circumstances:

A. Diagnosis: PET is covered only in clinical situations in which: (1) the PET results may assist in avoiding an invasive diagnostic procedure, or (2) the PET results may assist in determining the optimal anatomical location to perform an invasive diagnostic procedure. In general, for most solid tumors, a tissue diagnosis is made prior to the performance of PET scanning. PET scans following a tissue diagnosis are generally performed for the purpose of staging rather than diagnosis. Therefore, the use of PET in the diagnosis of lymphoma, esophageal, and colorectal cancers as well as in melanoma, should be rare.

B. Staging and/or Restaging: PET is covered for staging in clinical situations in which: (1)(a) the stage of the cancer remains in doubt after completion of a standard diagnostic workup, including conventional imaging (CT, magnetic resonance imaging, or ultrasound), or (1)(b) the use of PET could potentially replace one or more conventional imaging studies when it is expected that conventional study information is insufficient for the clinical management of the patient, and (2) clinical management of the patient would differ depending on the stage of the cancer identified.

PET is covered for restaging after the completion of treatment for: (1) the purpose of detecting residual disease, (2) detecting suspected recurrence, (3) determining the extent of a known recurrence, or (4) potentially replacing one or more conventional imaging studies when it is expected that conventional study information is insufficient for the clinical management of the patient.

C. Monitoring Response to Treatment: PET is covered for monitoring response to treatment when a change in therapy is anticipated.

Documentation should be maintained in the beneficiary's medical record at the referring physician's office to support the medical necessity of the procedure, as is normal business practice.

(This NCD last reviewed March 2005.)

CIM 50-36

220.6.4—FDG PET for Colorectal Cancer (Various Effective Dates Below)

(Rev. 31, Issued: 04-04-05; Effective: 01-28-05; Implementation: 04-18-05)

1. Recurrent Colorectal Carcinoma With Rising Levels of Biochemical Tumor Marker Carcinoembryonic Antigen (CEA) (Effective July 1, 1999)

Effective for services performed on or after July 1, 1999, Medicare covers FDG PET for patients with recurrent colorectal carcinomas, suggested by rising levels of the biochemical tumor marker CEA.

Frequency Limitations: Whole body PET scans for assessment of recurrence of colorectal cancer cannot be ordered more frequently than once every 12 months unless medical necessity documentation supports a separate re-elevation of CEA within this period.

Limitations: Because this service is covered only in those cases in which there has been a recurrence of colorectal tumor, claims for PET should include a statement or other evidence of previous colorectal tumor, through June 30, 2001.

2. Diagnosis, Staging, and Re-Staging (Effective July 1, 2001)

Effective for services performed on or after July 1, 2001, Medicare covers FDG PET for colorectal carcinomas for diagnosis, staging, and re-staging. New medical evidence supports the use of FDG PET as a useful tool in determining the presence of hepatic/extrahepatic metastases in the primary staging of colorectal carcinoma, prior to selecting a treatment regimen. Use of FDG PET is also supported in evaluating recurrent colorectal cancer beyond the limited presentation of a rising CEA level where the patient presents clinical signs/symptoms of recurrence.

3. Monitoring Response to Treatment (Effective January 28, 2005)

Effective for services performed on or after January 28, 2005, Medicare only covers FDG PET for monitoring response to treatment for colorectal cancer as "coverage with evidence development".

Medicare shall notify providers and beneficiaries where these services can be accessed, as they become available, via the following:

• Federal Register Notice
• CMS coverage Web site at: www.cms.gov/coverage

Requirements: PET is covered in an/all of the following circumstances:

A. Diagnosis: PET is covered only in clinical situations in which: (1) the PET results may assist in avoiding an invasive diagnostic procedure, or in which (2) the PET results may assist in determining the optimal anatomical location to perform an invasive diagnostic procedure. In general, for most solid tumors, a tissue diagnosis is made prior to the performance of PET scanning. PET scans following a tissue diagnosis are generally performed for the purpose of staging rather than diagnosis.

B. Staging and/or Restaging: PET is covered for staging in clinical situations in which: (1)(a) the stage of the cancer remains in doubt after completion of a standard diagnostic workup, including conventional imaging (computed tomography, magnetic resonance imaging, or ultrasound), or (1)(b) the use of PET could potentially replace one or more conventional imaging studies when it is expected that conventional study information is insufficient for the clinical management of the patient, and (2) clinical management of the patient would differ depending on the stage of the cancer identified.

PET is covered for restaging after completion of treatment for the purpose of: (1) detecting residual disease, (2) detecting suspected recurrence, (3) determining the extent of a known recurrence, or (4) potentially replacing one or more conventional imaging studies when it is expected that conventional study information is insufficient for the clinical management of the patient.

C. Monitoring Response to Treatment: PET is covered for monitoring response to treatment when a change in therapy is anticipated.

Documentation that these conditions are met should be maintained by the referring physician in the beneficiary's medical record, as is normal business practice.

(This NCD last reviewed March 2005.)

CIM 50-36

220.6.5—FDG PET for Lymphoma (Various Effective Dates Below)

(Rev. 31, Issued: 04-04-05; Effective: 01-28-05; Implementation: 04-18-05)

1. Staging and Restaging as Alternative to Gallium Scan (Effective July 1, 1999)

Effective for services performed on or after July 1, 1999, FDG PET is covered for the staging and restaging of lymphoma.

Requirements:

• PET is covered only for staging or follow-up restaging of lymphoma. Claims must include a statement or other evidence of previous diagnosis of lymphoma when used as an alternative to a Gallium scan
• To ensure that the PET scan is properly coordinated with other diagnostic modalities, claims must include the results of concurrent computed tomography (CT) and/or other diagnostic modalities necessary for additional anatomic information.
• In order to ensure that the PET scan is covered only as an alternative to a Gallium scan, no PET scan may be covered in cases where it is performed within 50 days of a Gallium scan performed by the same facility where the patient has remained during the 50-day period. Gallium scans performed by another facility less than 50 days prior to the PET scan will not be counted against this screen. The purpose of this screen is to ensure that PET scans are covered only as an alternative to a Gallium scan within the same facility. The CMS is aware that, in order to ensure proper patient care, the treating physician may conclude that previously performed Gallium scans are either inconclusive or not sufficiently reliable.

Frequency Limitation for Restaging: PET scans will be allowed for restaging no sooner than 50 days following the last staging PET scan or Gallium scan, unless sufficient evidence is presented to convince the Medicare contractor that restaging at an earlier date is medically necessary. Since PET scans for restaging are generally performed following cycles of chemotherapy, and since such cycles usually take at least 8 weeks, CMS believes this screen will adequately prevent medically unnecessary scans while allowing some adjustments for unusual cases. In all cases, the determination of the medical necessity for a PET scan for re-staging lymphoma is the responsibility of the local Medicare contractor.

Effective for services performed on or after July 1, 2001, documentation should be maintained in the beneficiary's medical record at the referring physician's office to support the medical necessity of the procedure, as is normal business practice.

2. Diagnosis, Staging, and Restaging (Effective July 1, 2001)

Effective for services performed on or after July 1, 2001, Medicare covers FDG PET for the diagnosis, staging and restaging of lymphoma.

3. Monitoring Response to Treatment (Effective January 28, 2005)

Effective for services performed on or after January 28, 2005, Medicare only covers FDG PET for monitoring response to treatment for lymphoma as "coverage with evidence development".

Medicare shall notify providers and beneficiaries where these services can be accessed, as they become available, via the following:

• Federal Register Notice
• CMS coverage Web site at: www.cms.gov/coverage

Requirements: PET is covered in any/all of the following circumstances:

A. Diagnosis: PET is covered only in clinical situations in which: (1) the PET results may assist in avoiding an invasive diagnostic procedure, or (2) the PET results may assist in determining the optimal anatomical location to perform an invasive diagnostic procedure. In general, for most solid tumors, a tissue diagnosis is made prior to the performance of PET scanning. PET scans following a tissue diagnosis are generally performed for the purpose of staging rather than diagnosis.

B. Staging and/or Restaging: PET is covered for staging in clinical situations in which: (1)(a) the stage of the cancer remains in doubt after completion of a standard diagnostic workup, including conventional imaging (CT, magnetic resonance imaging, or ultrasound), or (1)(b) the use of PET could potentially replace one or more conventional imaging studies when it is expected that conventional study information is insufficient for the clinical management of the patient, and (2) clinical management of the patient would differ depending on the stage of the cancer identified.

PET is covered for restaging after completion of treatment for the purpose of: (1) detecting residual disease, (2) detecting suspected recurrence, (3) determining the extent of a known recurrence, or (4) potentially replacing one or more conventional imaging studies when it is expected that conventional study information is insufficient for the clinical management of the patient.

C. Monitoring Response to Treatment: PET is covered for monitoring response to treatment when a change in therapy is anticipated.

Documentation that these conditions are met should be maintained by the referring physician in the beneficiary's medical record, as is normal business practice.

(This NCD last reviewed March 2005.)

CIM 50-36

220.6.6—FDG PET for Melanoma (Various Effective Dates Below)

(Rev. 31, Issued: 04-04-05; Effective: 01-28-05; Implementation: 04-18-05)

1. Evaluation of Recurrent Melanoma Prior to Surgery As Alternative to Gallium Scan (Effective July 1, 1999)

Effective for services performed on or after July 1, 1999, FDG PET (when used as an alternative to a Gallium scan) is covered for patients with recurrent melanoma prior to surgery for tumor evaluation. FDG PET is not covered for the evaluation of regional nodes.

Frequency Limitations: Whole body PET scans cannot be ordered more frequently than once every 12 months, unless medical necessity documentation, maintained in the beneficiary's medical record, supports the specific need for anatomic localization of possible recurrent tumor within this period.

Limitations: The FDG PET scan is covered only as an alternative to a Gallium scan. PET scans can not be covered in cases where they are performed within 50 days of a Gallium scan performed by the same PET facility where the patient has remained under the care of the same facility during the 50-day period. Gallium scans performed by another facility less than 50 days prior to the PET scan will not be counted against this screen. The purpose of this screen is to ensure that PET scans are covered only as an alternative to a Gallium scan within the same facility. The CMS is aware that, in order to ensure proper patient care, the treating physician may conclude that previously performed Gallium scans are either inconclusive or not sufficiently reliable to make the determination covered by this provision. Therefore, CMS will apply this 50-day rule only to PET scans performed by the same facility that performed the Gallium scan.

Effective for services performed on or after July 1, 2001, documentation should be maintained in the beneficiary's medical file at the referring physician's office to support the medical necessity of the procedure, as is normal business practice.

2. Diagnosis, Staging, and Restaging (Effective July 1, 2001)

Effective for services performed on or after July 1, 2001, FDG PET is covered for the diagnosis, staging, and restaging of melanoma. FDG PET is not covered for the evaluation of regional nodes.

3. Monitoring Response to Treatment (Effective January 28, 2005)

Effective for services performed on or after January 28, 2005, Medicare only covers FDG PET for monitoring response to treatment for melanoma as "coverage with evidence development".

Medicare shall notify providers and beneficiaries where these services can be accessed, as they become available, via the following:

• Federal Register Notice
• CMS coverage Web site at: www.cms.gov/coverage

Requirements: PET is covered in any/all of the following circumstances:

A. Diagnosis: PET is covered only in clinical situations in which: (1) the PET results may assist in avoiding an invasive diagnostic procedure, or (2) the PET results may assist in determining the optimal anatomical location to perform an invasive diagnostic procedure. In general, for most solid tumors, a tissue diagnosis is made prior to the performance of PET scanning. PET scans following a tissue diagnosis are generally performed for the purpose of staging rather than diagnosis.

B. Staging and/or Restaging: PET is covered for staging in clinical situations in which: (1) (a) the stage of the cancer remains in doubt after completion of a standard diagnostic workup, including conventional imaging (computed tomography, magnetic resonance imaging, or ultrasound), or (1)(b) the use of PET could potentially replace one or more conventional imaging studies when it is expected that conventional study information is insufficient for the clinical management of the patient, and (2) clinical management of the patient would differ depending on the stage of the cancer identified.

PET is covered for restaging after the completion of treatment for the purpose of: (1) detecting residual disease, (2) detecting suspected recurrence, (3) determining the extent of a known recurrence, or (4) potentially replacing one or more conventional imaging studies when it is expected that conventional study information is insufficient for the clinical management of the patient.

C. Monitoring Response to Treatment: PET is covered for monitoring response to treatment when a change in therapy is anticipated.

Documentation that these conditions are met should be maintained by the referring physician in the beneficiary's medical file, as is normal business practice.

(This NCD last reviewed March 2005.)

CIM 50-36

220.6.7—FDG PET for Head and Neck Cancers (Various Effective Dates Below)

(Rev. 31, Issued: 04-04-05; Effective: 01-28-05; Implementation: 04-18-05)

Effective for services performed on or after July 1, 2001, Medicare covers FDG PET for diagnosis, staging and restaging of cancer of the head and neck, excluding the central nervous system (CNS) and thyroid. The head and neck cancers encompass a diverse set of malignancies of which the majority is squamous cell carcinomas. Patients may present with metastases to cervical lymph nodes but conventional forms of diagnostic imaging fail to identify the primary tumor. Patients that present with cancer of the head and neck are left with two options—either to have a neck dissection or to have radiation of both sides of the neck with random biopsies. PET scanning attempts to reveal the site of primary tumor to prevent the adverse effects of random biopsies or unnecessary radiation.

Limitations: PET scans for head and neck cancers are not covered for CNS or thyroid cancers prior to October 1, 2003. Refer to section 220.6.11 for coverage for thyroid cancer effective October1,2003.

Effective for services performed on or after January 28, 2005, Medicare only covers FDG PET for monitoring response to treatment for head and neck cancers as "coverage with evidence development".

Medicare shall notify providers and beneficiaries where these services can be accessed, as they become available, via the following:

• Federal Register Notice
• CMS coverage Web site at: www.cms.gov/coverage

Requirements: PET is covered in any/all both of the following circumstances:

A. Diagnosis: PET is covered only in clinical situations in which: (1) the PET results may assist in avoiding an invasive diagnostic procedure, or (2) the PET results may assist in determining the optimal anatomical location to perform an invasive diagnostic procedure. In general, for most solid tumors a tissue diagnosis is made prior to the performance of PET scanning. PET scans following a tissue diagnosis are generally performed for the purpose of staging rather than diagnosis.

B. Staging and/or Restaging: PET is covered for staging in clinical situations in which: (1)(a) the stage of the cancer remains in doubt after completion of a standard diagnostic workup, including conventional imaging (computed tomography, magnetic resonance imaging, or ultrasound), or (1)(b) the use of PET could potentially replace one or more conventional imaging studies when it is expected that conventional study information is insufficient for the clinical management of the patient, and (2) clinical management of the patient would differ depending on the stage of the cancer identified.

PET is covered for restaging after completion of treatment for the purpose of: (1) detecting residual disease, (2) detecting suspected recurrence, (3) determining the extent of a known recurrence, or (4) potentially replacing one or more conventional imaging studies when it is expected that conventional study information is insufficient for the clinical management of the patient.

C. Monitoring Response to Treatment: PET is covered for monitoring response to treatment when a change in therapy is anticipated.

Documentation that these conditions are met should be maintained by the referring physician in the beneficiary's medical record, as is normal business practice.

(This NCD last reviewed March 2005.)

CIM 50-36

220.6.8—FDG PET for Myocardial Viability (Various Effective Dates Below)

(Rev. 31, Issued: 04-04-05; Effective: 01-28-05; Implementation: 04-18-05)

The identification of patients with partial loss of heart muscle movement or hibernating myocardium is important in selecting candidates with compromised ventricular function to determine appropriateness for revascularization. Diagnostic tests such as FDG PET distinguish between dysfunctional but viable myocardial tissue and scar tissue in order to affect management decisions in patients with ischemic cardiomyopathy and left ventricular dysfunction.

1. FDG PET is covered for the determination of myocardial viability following an inconclusive single photon emission computed tomography (SPECT) test from July 1, 2001, through September 30, 2002. Only full ring PET scanners are covered from July 1, 2001, through December 31, 2001. However, as of January 1, 2002, full and partial ring scanners are covered.

2. Beginning October 1, 2002, Medicare covers FDG PET for the determination of myocardial viability as a primary or initial diagnostic study prior to revascularization, or following an inconclusive SPECT. Studies performed by full and partial ring scanners are covered.

Limitations: In the event a patient receives a SPECT test with inconclusive results, a PET scan may be covered. However, if a patient receives a FDG PET study with inconclusive results, a follow up SPECT test is not covered.

Documentation that these conditions are met should be maintained by the referring physician in the beneficiary's medical record, as is normal business practice.

(See §220.12 for SPECT coverage)

(This NCD last reviewed September 2002.)

CIM 50-36

220.6.9—FDG PET for Refractory Seizures (Effective July 1, 2001)

(Rev. 31, Issued: 04-04-05; Effective: 01-28-05; Implementation: 04-18-05)

Beginning July 1, 2001, Medicare covers FDG-PET for pre-surgical evaluation for the purpose of localization of a focus of refractory seizure activity.

Limitations: Covered only for pre-surgical evaluation.

Documentation that these conditions are met should be maintained by the referring physician in the beneficiary's medical record, as is normal business practice.

(This NCD last reviewed June 2001.)

CIM 50-36

220.6.10—FDG PET for Breast Cancer (Effective October 1, 2002)

(Rev. 31, Issued: 04-04-05; Effective: 01-28-05; Implementation: 04-18-05)

Effective for services performed on or after October 1, 2002, Medicare covers FDG PET only as an adjunct to other imaging modalities for: (1) staging breast cancer patients with distant metastasis, (2) restaging patients with loco-regional recurrence or metastasis, or (3) monitoring tumor response to treatment for women with locally advanced and metastatic breast cancer when a change in therapy is contemplated.

Limitations: Medicare continues to nationally non-cover initial diagnosis of breast cancer and staging of axillary lymph nodes.

Documentation that these conditions are met should be maintained by the referring physician in the beneficiary's medical record, as is normal business practice.

(This NCD last reviewed September 2002.)

CIM 50-36

220.6.11—FDG PET for Thyroid Cancer (Various Effective Dates Below)

(Rev. 31, Issued: 04-04-05; Effective: 01-28-05; Implementation: 04-18-05)

1. Effective for services performed on or after October 1, 2003, Medicare covers the use of FDG PET for thyroid cancer only for restaging of recurrent or residual thyroid cancers of follicular cell origin that have been previously treated by thyroidectomy and radioiodine ablation and have a serum thyroglobulin >10ng/ml and negative I-131 whole body scan performed.

2. Effective for services performed on or after January 28, 2005, Medicare only covers FDG PET for diagnosis, other staging and restaging, restaging of medullary cell tumors, and monitoring response to treatment as "coverage with evidence development"

Medicare shall notify providers and beneficiaries where these services can be accessed, as they become available, via the following:

• Federal Register Notice
• CMS coverage Web site at: www.cms.gov/coverage

Requirements: PET is covered in any/all of the following circumstances:

A. Diagnosis: PET is covered only in clinical situations in which; (1) the PET results may assist in avoiding an invasive diagnostic procedure, or (2) the PET results may assist in determining the optimal anatomical location to perform an invasive diagnostic procedure. In general, for most solid tumors a tissue diagnosis is made prior to the performance of PET scanning. PET scans following a tissue diagnosis are generally performed for staging rather than diagnosis.

B. Staging and/or Restaging: PET is covered for staging in clinical situations in which: (1)(a) the stage of the cancer remains in doubt after completion of a standard diagnostic workup, including conventional imaging (computed tomography, magnetic resonance imaging, or ultrasound), or (1)(b) the use of PET could potentially replace one or more conventional imaging studies when it is expected that conventional study information is insufficient for the clinical management of the patient, and (2) clinical management of the patient would differ depending on the stage of the cancer identified.

PET is covered for restaging after completion of treatment for the purpose of: (1) detecting residual disease, (2) detecting suspected recurrence, (3) determining the extent of a known recurrence, or (4) potentially replacing one or more conventional imaging studies when it is expected that conventional study information is insufficient for the clinical management of the patient.

C. Monitoring Response to Treatment: PET is covered for monitoring response to treatment when a change in therapy is anticipated.

Documentation that these conditions are met should be maintained by the referring physician in the beneficiary's medical record, as is normal business practice.

(This NCD last reviewed March 2005.)

CIM 50-36

220.6.12—FDG PET for Soft Tissue Sarcoma (Various Effective Dates Below)

(Rev. 31, Issued: 04-04-05; Effective: 01-28-05; Implementation: 04-18-05)

Following a thorough review of the scientific literature, including a technology assessment on the topic, Medicare maintains its national non-coverage determination for all uses of FDG PET for soft tissue sarcoma.

1. Effective for services performed on or after October 1, 2003, FDG PET for soft tissue sarcoma is nationally non-covered.

2. Effective for services performed on or after January 28, 2005, Medicare only covers FDG PET for soft tissue sarcoma as "coverage with evidence development". Medicare shall notify providers and beneficiaries where these services can be accessed, as they become available, via the following:

• Federal Register Notice
• CMS coverage Web site at: www.cms.gov/coverage

(This NCD last reviewed March 2005.)

CIM 50-36

220.6.13—FDG PET for Dementia and Neurodegenerative Diseases (Effective September 15, 2004)

(Rev. 31, Issued: 04-04-05; Effective: 01-28-05; Implementation: 04-18-05)

A. General

Medicare covers FDG-PET scans for either the differential diagnosis of fronto-temporal dementia (FTD) and Alzheimer's disease (AD) under specific requirements; OR, its use in a Centers for Medicare & Medicaid Services (CMS)-approved practical clinical trial focused on the utility of FDG-PET in the diagnosis or treatment of dementing neurodegenerative diseases. Specific requirements for each indication are clarified below:

B. Nationally Covered Indications

1. FDG-PET Requirements for Coverage in the Differential Diagnosis of AD and FTD

An FDG-PET scan is considered reasonable and necessary in patients with a recent diagnosis of dementia and documented cognitive decline of at least 6 months, who meet diagnostic criteria for both AD and FTD. These patients have been evaluated for specific alternate neurodegenerative diseases or other causative factors, but the cause of the clinical symptoms remains uncertain.

The following additional conditions must be met before an FDG-PET scan will be covered:

a. The patient's onset, clinical presentation, or course of cognitive impairment is such that FTD is suspected as an alternative neurodegenerative cause of the cognitive decline. Specifically, symptoms such as social disinhibition, awkwardness, difficulties with language, or loss of executive function are more prominent early in the course of FTD than the memory loss typical of AD;

b. The patient has had a comprehensive clinical evaluation (as defined by the American Academy of Neurology (AAN)) encompassing a medical history from the patient and a well-acquainted informant (including assessment of activities of daily living), physical and mental status examination (including formal documentation of cognitive decline occurring over at least 6 months) aided by cognitive scales or neuropsychological testing, laboratory tests, and structural imaging such as magnetic resonance imaging (MRI) or computed tomography (CT);

c. The evaluation of the patient has been conducted by a physician experienced in the diagnosis and assessment of dementia;

d. The evaluation of the patient did not clearly determine a specific neurodegenerative disease or other cause for the clinical symptoms, and information available through FDG-PET is reasonably expected to help clarify the diagnosis between FTD and AD and help guide future treatment;

e. The FDG-PET scan is performed in a facility that has all the accreditation necessary to operate nuclear medicine equipment. The reading of the scan should be done by an expert in nuclear medicine, radiology, neurology, or psychiatry, with experience interpreting such scans in the presence of dementia;

f. A brain single photon emission computed tomography (SPECT) or FDG-PET scan has not been obtained for the same indication. (The indication can be considered to be different in patients who exhibit important changes in scope or severity of cognitive decline, and meet all other qualifying criteria listed above and below (including the judgment that the likely diagnosis remains uncertain). The results of a prior SPECT or FDG-PET scan must have been inconclusive or, in the case of SPECT, difficult to interpret due to immature or inadequate technology. In these instances, an FDG-PET scan may be covered after 1 year has passed from the time the first SPECT or FDG-PET scan was performed.)

g. The referring and billing provider(s) have documented the appropriate evaluation of the Medicare beneficiary. Providers should establish the medical necessity of an FDG-PET scan by ensuring that the following information has been collected and is maintained in the beneficiary medical record:

- Date of onset of symptoms;
- Diagnosis of clinical syndrome (normal aging; mild cognitive impairment or MCI; mild, moderate or severe dementia);
- Mini mental status exam (MMSE) or similar test score;
- Presumptive cause (possible, probable, uncertain AD);
- Any neuropsychological testing performed;
- Results of any structural imaging (MRI or CT) performed;
- Relevant laboratory tests (B12, thyroid hormone); and,
- Number and name of prescribed medications.

The billing provider must furnish a copy of the FDG-PET scan result for use by CMS and its contractors upon request. These verification requirements are consistent with federal requirements set forth in 42 Code of Federal Regulations section 410.32 generally for diagnostic x-ray tests, diagnostic laboratory tests, and other tests. In summary, section 410.32 requires the billing physician and the referring physician to maintain information in the medical record of each patient to demonstrate medical necessity [410.32(d) (2)] and submit the information demonstrating medical necessity to CMS and/or its agents upon request [410.32(d)(3)(I)] (OMB number 0938-0685).

2. FDG-PET Requirements for Coverage in the Context of a CMS-approved Practical Clinical Trial Utilizing a Specific Protocol to Demonstrate the Utility of FDG-PET in the Diagnosis, and Treatment of Neurodegenerative Dementing Diseases

An FDG-PET scan is considered reasonable and necessary in patients with mild cognitive impairment or early dementia (in clinical circumstances other than those specified in subparagraph 1) only in the context of an approved clinical trial that contains patient safeguards and protections to ensure proper administration, use and evaluation of the FDG-PET scan.

The clinical trial must compare patients who do and do not receive an FDG-PET scan and have as its goal to monitor, evaluate, and improve clinical outcomes. In addition, it must meet the following basic criteria:

a. Written protocol on file;

b. Institutional Review Board review and approval;

c. Scientific review and approval by two or more qualified individuals who are not part of the research team; and,

d. Certification that investigators have not been disqualified.

C. Nationally Non-covered Indications

All other uses of FDG-PET for patients with a presumptive diagnosis of dementia-causing neurodegenerative disease (e.g., possible or probable AD, clinically typical FTD, dementia of Lewy bodies, or Creutzfeld-Jacob disease) for which CMS has not specifically indicated coverage continue to be non-covered.

D. Other

Not applicable.

(This NCD last reviewed September 2004.)

220.6.14—FDG PET for Brain, Cervical, Ovarian, Pancreatic, Small Cell Lung, and Testicular Cancers (Effective January 28, 2005)

(Rev. 31, Issued: 04-04-05; Effective: 01-28-05; Implementation: 04-18-05)

A. Staging for Invasive Cervical Cancer as an Adjunct to Conventional Imaging

The CMS has determined that there is sufficient evidence to conclude that an FDG PET scan is reasonable and necessary for the detection of metastases during the pre-treatment management phase (i.e., staging) in patients with newly diagnosed and locally advanced cervical cancer with no extra-pelvic metastasis on conventional imaging tests, such as computed tomography (CT) or magnetic resonance imaging (MRI). Use of FDG PET as an adjunct may more accurately assist in the non-invasive detection of para-aortic, pelvic nodal involvement and other metastases in the pre-treatment phase of disease. The following conditions must be met:

- A pathologic diagnosis of cervical cancer must have already been made before the FDG PET scan is performed,
- The results of other imaging procedures used (e.g., MRI or CT) must be reported, and,
- The available conventional imaging tests are negative for extra-pelvic metastasis.

NOTE: Other staging utilizing FDG PET (e.g., as a substitute for conventional structural imaging; when a previous MRI or CT is positive or inconclusive for para-aortic metastasis and negative for supra-clavicular nodal metastasis) are only covered as "coverage with evidence development".

Medicare shall notify providers and beneficiaries where these services can be accessed, as they become available, via the following:

- Federal Register Notice
- CMS coverage Web site at: www.cms.gov/coverage

B. Brain, Ovarian, Pancreatic, Small Cell Lung, and Testicular Cancers, and other indications of Cervical Cancer not mentioned in Section A above

"Coverage with evidence development" applies to all FDG PET indications for brain, ovarian, pancreatic, small cell lung, testicular cancers, and other indications of cervical cancer not mentioned in Section A above.

For cancer indications listed as "coverage with evidence development" CMS determines that the evidence is sufficient to conclude that an FDG PET scan is reasonable and necessary only when the provider is participating in, and patients are enrolled in, one of the following types of prospective clinical studies that is designed to collect additional information at the time of the scan to assist in patient management:

- A clinical trial of FDG PET that meets the requirements of Food and Drug Administration (FDA) category B investigational device exemption (42 CFR 405.201); or
- An FDG PET clinical study that is designed to collect additional information at the time of the scan to assist in patient management. Qualifying clinical studies must ensure that specific hypotheses are addressed; appropriate data elements are collected; hospitals and providers are qualified to provide the PET scan and interpret the results; participating hospitals and providers accurately report data on all enrolled patients not included in other qualifying trials through adequate auditing mechanisms; and, all patient confidentiality, privacy, and other Federal laws must be followed.

Medicare shall notify providers and beneficiaries where these services can be accessed, as they become available, via the following:

- Federal Register Notice
- CMS coverage Web site at: www.cms.gov/coverage

(This NCD last reviewed March 2005.)

220.6.15—FDG PET for All Other Cancer Indications Not Previously Specified (Effective January 28, 2005)

(Rev. 31, Issued: 04-04-05; Effective: 01-28-05; Implementation: 04-18-05)

Effective for services performed on or after January 28, 2005: "coverage with evidence development" applies to all FDG PET indications for all other cancers not previously specified in Section 220.6 above in its entirety.

For cancer indications listed as "coverage with evidence development" CMS has determined that the evidence is sufficient to conclude that an FDG PET scan is reasonable and necessary only when the provider is participating in, and patients are enrolled in, one of the following types of prospective clinical studies that is designed to collect additional information at the time of the scan to assist in patient management:

- A clinical trial of FDG PET that meets the requirements of Food and Drug Administration (FDA) category B investigational device exemption (42 CFR 405.201); or
- An FDG PET clinical study that is designed to collect additional information at the time of the scan to assist in patient management. Qualifying clinical studies must ensure that specific hypotheses are addressed; appropriate data elements are collected; hospitals and providers are qualified to provide the PET scan and interpret the results; participating hospitals and providers accurately report data on all enrolled patients not included in other qualifying trials through adequate auditing mechanisms; and, all patient confidentiality, privacy, and other Federal laws must be followed.

Medicare shall notify providers and beneficiaries where these services can be accessed, as they become available, via the following:

- Federal Register Notice
- CMS coverage Web site at: www.cms.gov/coverage

(This NCD last reviewed March 2005.)

CIM 50-44

150.3—Bone (Mineral) Density Studies

(Rev. 1, 10-03-03)

Bone (mineral) density studies are used to evaluate diseases of bone and/or the responses of bone diseases to treatment. The studies assess bone mass or density associated with such diseases as osteoporosis, osteomalacia, and renal osteodystrophy. Various single or combined methods of measurement may be required to: (a) diagnose bone disease, (b) monitor the course of bone changes with disease progression, or (c) monitor the course of bone changes with therapy. Bone density is usually studied by using photodensitometry, single or dual photon absorptiometry, or bone biopsy.

The Following Bone (Mineral) Density Studies Are Covered Under Medicare

A—Single Photon Absorptiometry

A noninvasive radiological technique that measures absorption of a monochromatic photon beam by bone material. The device is placed directly on the patient, uses a low dose of radionuclide, and measures the mass absorption efficiency of the energy used. It provides a quantitative measurement of the bone mineral of cortical and trabecular bone, and is used in assessing an individual's treatment response at appropriate intervals. Single photon absorptiometry is covered under Medicare when used in assessing changes in bone density of patients with osteodystrophy or osteoporosis when performed on the same individual at intervals of 6 to 12 months.

B—Bone Biopsy

A physiologic test which is a surgical, invasive procedure. A small sample of bone (usually from the ilium) is removed, generally by a biopsy needle. The biopsy sample is then examined histologically, and provides a qualitative measurement of the bone mineral of trabecular bone. This procedure is used in ascertaining a differential diagnosis of bone disorders and is used primarily to differentiate osteomalacia from osteoporosis.

Bone biopsy is covered under Medicare when used for the qualitative evaluation of bone no more than four times per patient, unless there is special justification given. When used more than four times on a patient, bone biopsy leaves a defect in the pelvis and may produce some patient discomfort.

C—Photodensitometry (radiographic absorptiometry)

A noninvasive radiological procedure that attempts to assess bone mass by measuring the optical density of extremity radiographs with a photodensitometer, usually with a reference to a standard density wedge placed on the film at the time of exposure. This procedure provides a quantitative measurement of the bone mineral of cortical bone, and is used for monitoring gross bone change.

The Following Bone (Mineral) Density Study Is Not Covered Under Medicare:

D—Dual Photon Absorptiometry

A noninvasive radiological technique that measures absorption of a dichromatic beam by bone material. This procedure is not covered under Medicare because it is still considered to be in the investigational stage.

CIM 50-50

20.24—Displacement Cardiography

(Rev. 1, 10-03-03)

Displacement cardiography, including cardiokymography and photokymography, is a noninvasive diagnostic test used in evaluating coronary artery disease.

A—Cardiokymography

Cardiokymography is covered for services rendered on or after October 12, 1988.

Cardiokymography is a covered service only when it is used as an adjunct to electrocardiographic stress testing in evaluating coronary artery disease and only when the following clinical indications are present:

- For male patients, atypical angina pectoris or nonischemic chest pain; or
- For female patients, angina, either typical or atypical.

B—Photokymography—Not Covered

Photokymography remains excluded from coverage.

20.16—Cardiac Output Monitoring By Thoracic Electrical Bioimpedance (TEB)

(Rev. 6, 01-23-04)

Thoracic electrical bioimpedance (TEB) devices, a form of plethysmography, monitor cardiac output by noninvasively measuring hemodynamic parameters, including: stroke volume, systemic vascular resistance, and thoracic fluid status. Under the previous coverage determination, effective July 1, 1999, use of TEB was covered for the "noninvasive diagnosis or monitoring of hemodynamics in patients with suspected or known cardiovascular disease." In reconsidering this policy, CMS concluded that this use was neither sufficiently defined nor supported by available clinical literature to offer the guidance necessary for practitioners to determine when TEB would be covered for patient management. Therefore, CMS revised its coverage policy language in response to a request for reconsideration to offer more explicit guidance and clarity for coverage of TEB based on a complete and updated literature review.

A. Covered Indications

1. TEB is covered for the following uses:

a. Differentiation of cardiogenic from pulmonary causes of acute dyspnea when medical history, physical examination, and standard assessment tools provide insufficient information, and the treating physician has determined that TEB hemodynamic data are necessary for appropriate management of the patient.

b. Optimization of atrioventricular (A/V) interval for patients with A/V sequential cardiac pacemakers when medical history, physical examination, and standard assessment tools provide insufficient information, and the treating physician has determined that TEB hemodynamic data are necessary for appropriate management of the patient.

c. Monitoring of continuous inotropic therapy for patients with terminal congestive heart failure, when those patients have chosen to die with comfort at home, or for patients waiting at home for a heart transplant.

d. Evaluation for rejection in patients with a heart transplant as a predetermined alternative to a myocardial biopsy. Medical necessity must be documented should a biopsy be performed after TEB.

e. Optimization of fluid management in patients with congestive heart failure when medical history, physical examination, and standard assessment tools provide insufficient information, and the treating physician has determined that TEB hemodynamic data are necessary for appropriate management of the patient.

2. Contractors have discretion to determine whether the use of TEB for the management of drug-resistant hypertension is reasonable and necessary. Drug resistant hypertension is defined as failure to achieve goal BP in patients who are adhering to full doses of an appropriate three-drug regimen that includes a diuretic.

B. Noncovered Indications

1. TEB is noncovered when used for patients:

a. With proven or suspected disease involving severe regurgitation of the aorta;

b. With minute ventilation (MV) sensor function pacemakers, since the device may adversely affect the functioning of that type of pacemaker;

c. During cardiac bypass surgery; or

d. In the management of all forms of hypertension (with the exception of drug-resistant hypertension as outlined above).

2. All other uses of TEB not otherwise specified remain noncovered.

CIM 50-55

210.1—Prostate Cancer Screening Tests

(Rev. 1, 10-03-03)

Covered

A—General

Section 4103 of the Balanced Budget Act of 1997 provides for coverage of certain prostate cancer screening tests subject to certain coverage, frequency, and payment limitations. Medicare will cover prostate cancer screening tests/procedures for the early detection of prostate cancer. Coverage of prostate cancer screening tests includes the following procedures furnished to an individual for the early detection of prostate cancer:

• Screening digital rectal examination; and
• Screening prostate specific antigen blood test.

B—Screening Digital Rectal Examinations

Screening digital rectal examinations (HCPCS code G0102) are covered at a frequency of once every 12 months for men who have attained age 50 (at least 11 months have passed following the month in which the last Medicare-covered screening digital rectal examination was performed). Screening digital rectal examination means a clinical examination of an individual's prostate for nodules or other abnormalities of the prostate. This screening must be performed by a doctor of medicine or osteopathy (as defined in §1861(r)(1) of the Act), or by a physician assistant, nurse practitioner, clinical nurse specialist, or certified nurse midwife (as defined in §1861(aa) and §1861(gg) of the Act) who is

authorized under State law to perform the examination, fully knowledgeable about the beneficiary's medical condition, and would be responsible for using the results of any examination performed in the overall management of the beneficiary's specific medical problem.

C—Screening Prostate Specific Antigen Tests

Screening prostate specific antigen tests (code G0103) are covered at a frequency of once every 12 months for men who have attained age 50 (at least 11 months have passed following the month in which the last Medicare-covered screening specific antigen test was performed). Screening prostate specific antigen tests (PSA) means a test to detect the marker for adenocarcinoma of prostate. PSA is a reliable immunocytochemical marker for primary and metastatic adenocarcinoma of prostate. This screening must be ordered by the beneficiary's physician or by the beneficiary's physician assistant, nurse practitioner, clinical nurse specialist, or certified nurse midwife (the term "attending physician" is defined in §1861(r)(1) of the Act to mean a doctor of medicine or osteopathy and the terms "physician assistant, nurse practitioner, clinical nurse specialist, or certified nurse midwife" are defined in §1861(aa) and §1861(gg) of the Act) who is fully knowledgeable about the beneficiary's medical condition, and who would be responsible for using the results of any examination (test) performed in the overall management of the beneficiary's specific medical problem.

CIM 55-1

230.7—Water Purification and Softening Systems Used in Conjunction With Home Dialysis

(Rev. 1, 10-03-03)

A—Water Purification Systems

Water used for home dialysis should be chemically free of heavy trace metals and/or organic contaminants that could be hazardous to the patient. It should also be as free of bacteria as possible but need not be biologically sterile. Since the characteristics of natural water supplies in most areas of the country are such that some type of water purification system is needed, such a system used in conjunction with a home dialysis (either peritoneal or hemodialysis) unit is covered under Medicare.

There are two types of water purification systems that will satisfy these requirements:

• Deionization—The removal of organic substances, mineral salts of magnesium and calcium (causing hardness), compounds of fluoride and chloride from tap water using the process of filtration and ion exchange; or
• Reverse Osmosis—The process used to remove impurities from tap water utilizing pressure to force water through a porous membrane.

Use of both a deionization unit and reverse osmosis unit in series, theoretically to provide the advantages of both systems, has been determined medically unnecessary since either system can provide water which is both chemically and bacteriologically pure enough for acceptable use in home dialysis. In addition, spare deionization tanks are not covered since they are essentially a precautionary supply rather than a current requirement for treatment of the patient.

Activated carbon filters used as a component of water purification systems to remove unsafe concentrations of chlorine and chloramines are covered when prescribed by a physician.

B—Water Softening System

Except as indicated below, a water softening system used in conjunction with home dialysis is excluded from coverage under Medicare as not being reasonable and necessary within the meaning of §1862(a)(1) of the Act. Such a system, in conjunction with a home dialysis unit, does not adequately remove the hazardous heavy metal contaminants (such as arsenic) which may be present in trace amounts.

A water softening system may be covered when used to pretreat water to be purified by a reverse osmosis (RO) unit for home dialysis where:

The manufacturer of the RO unit has set standards for the quality of water entering the RO (e.g., the water to be purified by the RO must be of a certain quality if the unit is to perform as intended);

The patients water is demonstrated to be of a lesser quality than required; and

The softener is used only to soften water entering the RO unit, and thus, used only for dialysis. (The softener need not actually be built into the RO unit, but must be an integral part of the dialysis system.)

C—Developing Need When a Water Softening System is Replaced with a Water

Purification Unit in an Existing Home Dialysis System

The medical necessity of water purification units must be care fully developed when they replace water softening systems in existing home dialysis systems. A purification system may be ordered under these circumstances for a number of reasons. For example, changes in the medical community's opinions regarding the quality of water necessary for safe dialysis may lead the physician to decide the quality of water previously used should be improved, or the water quality itself may have deteriorated. Patients may have dialyzed using only an existing water softener previous to Medicare ESRD coverage because of inability to pay for a purification system. On the other hand, in some cases, the installation of a purification system is not medically necessary. Thus, when such a case comes to the contractor's attention, the contractor asks the physician to furnish the reason for the changes. Supporting documentation, such as the suppliers recommendations or water analysis, may be required. All such cases should be reviewed by the contractor's medical consultants.

Cross reference:

The Medicare Benefit Policy Manual, Chapter 15, "Covered Medical and Other Health Services," §110.

CIM 55-3

230.14—Ultrafiltration Monitor

(Rev. 1, 10-03-03)

The Ultrafiltration Monitor is designed to reduce the clinical risks of overfiltration and underfiltration during hemodialysis. Overfiltration is the removal of too much fluid from body tissues and underfiltration is removal of too little fluid.

Covered

Ultrafiltration and ultrafiltration monitoring as a component of hemodialysis has an established and critical role in maintaining the well-being of ESRD patients and is a covered service. The Ultrafiltration Monitor is covered under the Medicare program when it is used to calculate fluid rates for those recipients who present difficult fluid management problems. Determine the medical necessity of this device on a case-by-case basis.

Not Covered

Ultrafiltration, independent of conventional dialysis, is considered experimental, and technology exclusively designed for this purpose is not covered under Medicare.

CIM 60-3

280.2—White Cane for Use by a Blind Person

(Rev. 1, 10-03-03)

Not Covered

A white cane for use by a blind person is more an identifying and self-help device than an item which makes a meaningful contribution in the treatment of an illness or injury.

CIM 60-4

240.2—Home Use of Oxygen

(Rev. 1, 10-03-03)

A—General

Medicare coverage of home oxygen and oxygen equipment under the durable medical equipment (DME) benefit (see §1861(s)(6)of the Act) is considered reasonable and necessary only for patients with significant hypoxemia who meet the medical documentation, laboratory evidence, and health conditions specified in subsections B, C, and D. This section also includes special coverage criteria for portable oxygen systems. Finally, a statement on the absence of coverage of the professional services of a respiratory therapist under the DME benefit is included in subsection F.

B—Medical Documentation

Initial claims for oxygen services must include a completed Form CMS-484 (Certificate of Medical Necessity: Oxygen) to establish whether coverage criteria are met and to ensure that the oxygen services provided are consistent with the physician's prescription or other medical documentation. The treating physician's prescription or other medical documentation must indicate that other forms of treatment (e.g., medical and physical therapy directed at secretions, bronchospasm and infection) have been tried, have not been sufficiently successful, and oxygen therapy is still required. While there is no substitute for oxygen therapy, each patient must receive optimum therapy before long-term home oxygen therapy is ordered. Use Form CMS-484 for recertifications. (See the Medicare Program Integrity Manual, Chapter 5, for completion of Form CMS-484.)

The medical and prescription information in section B of Form CMS-484 can be completed only by the treating physician, the physician's employee, or another clinician (e.g., nurse, respiratory therapist, etc.) as long as that person is not the DME supplier. Although hospital discharge coordinators and medical social workers may assist in arranging for physician-prescribed home oxygen, they do not have the authority to prescribe the services. Suppliers may not enter this information. While this section may be completed by non-physician clinician or a physician employee, it must be reviewed and the Form CMS-484 signed by the attending physician.

A physician's certification of medical necessity for oxygen equipment must include the results of specific testing before coverage can be determined.

Claims for oxygen must also be supported by medical documentation in the patient's record. Separate documentation is used with electronic billing. This documentation may be in the form of a prescription written by the patient's attending physician who has recently examined the patient (normally within a month of the start of therapy) and must specify:

- A diagnosis of the disease requiring home use of oxygen;
- The oxygen flow rate; and
- An estimate of the frequency, duration of use (e.g., 2 liters per minute, 10 minutes per hour, 12 hours per day), and duration of need (e.g., 6 months or lifetime).

NOTE: A prescription for "Oxygen PRN" or "Oxygen as needed" does not meet this last requirement. Neither provides any basis for determining if the amount of oxygen is reasonable and necessary for the patient.

A member of the carrier's medical staff should review all claims with oxygen flow rates of more than four liters per minute before payment can be made.

The attending physician specifies the type of oxygen delivery system to be used (i.e., gas, liquid, or concentrator) by signing the completed Form CMS-484. In addition, the supplier or physician may use the space in section C for written confirmation of additional details of the physician's order. The additional order information contained in section C may include the means of oxygen delivery (mask, nasal, cannula, etc.), the specifics of varying flow rates, and/or the noncontinuous use of oxygen as appropriate.

The physician confirms this order information with their signature in section D.

New medical documentation written by the patient's attending physician must be submitted to the carrier in support of revised oxygen requirements when there has been a change in the patient's condition and need for oxygen therapy.

Carriers are required to conduct periodic, continuing medical necessity reviews on patients whose conditions warrant these reviews and on patients with indefinite or extended periods of necessity as described in the Medicare Program Integrity Manual, Chapter 5, "Items and Services Having Special DMERC Review Considerations." When indicated, carriers may also request documentation of the results of a repeat arterial blood gas or oximetry study.

NOTE: Section 4152 of OBRA 1990 requires earlier recertification and retesting of oxygen patients who begin coverage with an arterial blood gas result at or above a partial pressure of 55 or an arterial oxygen saturation percentage at or above 89. (See the Medicare Claims Processing Manual, Chapter 20, "Durable Medical Equipment, Prosthetics and Orthotics, and Supplies (DMEPOS)," §100.2.3, for certification and retesting schedules.)

C—Laboratory Evidence

Initial claims for oxygen therapy must also include the results of a blood gas study that has been ordered and evaluated by the attending physician. This is usually in the form of a measurement of the partial pressure of oxygen (PO_2) in arterial blood. A measurement of arterial oxygen saturation obtained by ear or pulse oximetry, however, is also acceptable when ordered and evaluated by the attending and performed under his or her supervision or when performed by a qualified provider or supplier of laboratory services.

When the arterial blood gas and the oximetry studies are both used to document the need for home oxygen therapy and the results are conflicting, the arterial blood gas study is the preferred source of documenting medical need. A DME supplier is not considered a qualified provider or supplier of laboratory services for purposes of these guidelines.

This prohibition does not extend to the results of blood gas test conducted by a hospital certified to do such tests. The conditions under which the laboratory tests are performed must be specified in writing and submitted with the initial claim, i.e., at rest, during exercise, or during sleep.

The preferred sources of laboratory evidence are, existing physician and/or hospital records that reflect the patient's medical condition. Since it is expected that virtually all patients who qualify for home oxygen coverage for the first time under these guidelines have recently been discharged from a hospital where they submitted to arterial blood gas tests, the carrier needs to request that such test results be submitted in support of their initial claims for home oxygen. If more than one arterial blood gas test is performed during the patient's hospital stay, the test result obtained closest to, but no earlier than two days prior to the hospital discharge date is required as evidence of the need for home oxygen therapy.

For those patients whose initial oxygen prescription did not originate during a hospital stay, blood gas studies should be done while the patient is in the chronic stable state, i.e., not during a period of an acute illness or an exacerbation of their underlying disease. Carriers may accept an attending physician's statement of recent hospital test results for a particular patient, when appropriate, in lieu of copies of actual hospital records.

A repeat arterial blood gas study is appropriate when evidence indicates that an oxygen recipient has undergone a major change in their condition relevant to home use of oxygen. If the carrier has reason to believe that there has been a major change in the patient's physical condition, it may ask for documentation of the results of another blood gas or oximetry study.

D—Health Conditions

Coverage is available for patients with significant hypoxemia in the chronic stable state, i.e, not during a period of acute illness or an exacerbation of their underlying disease, if:

1. The attending physician has determined that the patient has a health condition outlined in subsection D.1,

2. The patient meets the blood gas evidence requirements specified in subsection D.3, and

3. The patient has appropriately tried other treatment without complete success. (See subsection B.)

1—Conditions for Which Oxygen Therapy May Be Covered

- A severe lung disease, such as chronic obstructive pulmonary disease, diffuse interstitial lung disease, cystic fibrosis, bronchiectasis, widespread pulmonary neoplasm, or
- Hypoxia-related symptoms or findings that might be expected to improve with oxygen therapy. Examples of these symptoms and findings are pulmonary hypertension, recurring congestive heart failure due to chronic cor pulmonale, erythrocytosis, impairment of the cognitive process, nocturnal restlessness, and morning headache.

2—Conditions for Which Oxygen Therapy Is Not Covered

- Angina pectoris in the absence of hypoxemia. This condition is generally not the result of a low oxygen level in the blood, and there are other preferred treatments;
- Breathlessness without cor pulmonale or evidence of hypoxemia. Although intermittent oxygen use is sometimes prescribed to relieve this condition, it is potentially harmful and psychologically addicting;
- Severe peripheral vascular disease resulting in clinically evident desaturation in one or more extremities. There is no evidence that increased PO_2 improves the oxygenation of tissues with impaired circulation; or
- Terminal illnesses that do not affect the lungs.

3—Covered Blood Gas Values

If the patient has a condition specified in subsection D.1, the carrier must review the medical documentation and laboratory evidence that has been submitted for a particular patient (see subsections B and C) and determine if coverage is available under one of the three group categories outlined below.

(a)—Group I—Except as modified in subsection d, coverage is provided for patients with significant hypoxemia evidenced by any of the following:

- An arterial PO_2 at or below 55 mm Hg, or an arterial oxygen saturation at or below 88 percent, taken at rest, breathing room air.
- An arterial PO_2 at or below 55 mm Hg, or an arterial oxygen saturation at or below 88 percent, taken during sleep for a patient who demonstrates an arterial PO_2 at or above 56 mm Hg, or an arterial oxygen saturation at or above 89 percent, while awake; or a greater than normal fall in oxygen level during sleep (a decrease in arterial PO_2 more than 10 mm Hg, or decrease in arterial oxygen saturation more than 5 percent) associated with symptoms or signs reasonably attributable to hypoxemia (e.g., impairment of cognitive processes and nocturnal restlessness or insomnia). In either of these cases, coverage is provided only for use of oxygen during sleep, and then only one type of unit will be covered. Portable oxygen, therefore, would not be covered in this situation.
- An arterial PO_2 at or below 55 mm Hg or an arterial oxygen saturation at or below 88 percent, taken during exercise for a patient who demonstrates an arterial PO_2 at or above 56 mm Hg, or an arterial oxygen saturation at or above 89 percent, during the day while at rest. In this case, supplemental oxygen is provided for during exercise if there is evidence the use of oxygen improves the hypoxemia that was demonstrated during exercise when the patient was breathing room air.

(b)—Group II—Except as modified in subsection d, coverage is available for patients whose arterial PO_2 is 56-59 mm Hg or whose arterial blood oxygen saturation is 89 percent, if there is evidence of:

- Dependent edema suggesting congestive heart failure;
- Pulmonary hypertension or cor pulmonale, determined by measurement of pulmonary artery pressure, gated blood pool scan, echocardiogram, or "P" pulmonale on EKG (P wave greater than 3 mm in standard leads II, III, or AVF); or
- Erythrocythemia with a hematocrit greater than 56 percent.

(c)—Group III—Except as modified in subsection d, carriers must apply a rebuttable presumption that a home program of oxygen use is not medically necessary for patients with arterial PO_2 levels at or above 60 mm Hg, or arterial blood oxygen saturation at or above 90 percent. In order for claims in this category to be reimbursed, the carrier's reviewing physician needs to review any documentation submitted in rebuttal of this presumption and grant specific approval of the claims.

The CMS expects few claims to be approved for coverage in this category.

(d)—Variable Factors That May Affect Blood Gas Values—In reviewing the arterial PO_2 levels and the arterial oxygen saturation percentages specified in subsections D. 3.a, b and c, the carrier's medical staff must take into account variations in oxygen measurements that may result from such factors as the patient's age, the altitude level, or the patient's decreased oxygen carrying capacity.

E—Portable Oxygen Systems

A patient meeting the requirements specified below may qualify for coverage of a portable oxygen system either (1) by itself or (2) to use in addition to a stationary oxygen system. Portable oxygen is not covered when it is provided only as a backup to a stationary oxygen system. A portable oxygen system is covered for a particular patient if:

- The claim meets the requirements specified in subsections A-D, as appropriate; and
- The medical documentation indicates that the patient is mobile in the home and would benefit from the use of a portable oxygen system in the home. Portable oxygen systems are not covered for patients who qualify for oxygen solely based on blood gas studies obtained during sleep

F—Respiratory Therapists

Respiratory therapists' services are not covered under the provisions for coverage of oxygen services under the Part B durable medical equipment benefit as outlined above. This benefit provides for coverage of home use of oxygen and oxygen equipment, but does not include a professional component in the delivery of such services.

(See §280.1, and the Medicare Benefit Policy Manual, Chapter 15, "Covered Medical and Other Health Services," §110)

CIM 60-5 and 60-6

280.3—Mobility Assistive Equipment (MAE) (Effective May 5, 2005)

(Rev. 37, Issued: 06-03-05; Effective: 05-05-05; Implementation: 07-05-05)

A—General

The Centers for Medicare & Medicaid Services (CMS) addresses numerous items that it terms "mobility assistive equipment" (MAE) and includes within that category canes, crutches, walkers, manual wheelchairs, power wheelchairs, and scooters. This list, however, is not exhaustive.

Medicare beneficiaries may require mobility assistance for a variety of reasons and for varying durations because the etiology of the disability may be due to a congenital cause, injury, or disease. Thus, some beneficiaries experiencing temporary disability may need mobility assistance on a short-term basis, while in contrast, those living with chronic conditions or enduring disabilities will require mobility assistance on a permanent basis.

Medicare beneficiaries who depend upon mobility assistance are found in varied living situations. Some may live alone and independently while others may live with a caregiver or in a custodial care facility. The beneficiary's environment is relevant to the determination of the appropriate form of mobility assistance that should be employed. For many patients, a device of some sort is compensation for the mobility deficit. Many beneficiaries experience co-morbid conditions that can impact their ability to safely utilize MAE independently or to successfully regain independent function even with mobility assistance.

The functional limitation as experienced by a beneficiary depends on the beneficiary's physical and psychological function, the availability of other support, and the beneficiary's living environment. A few examples include muscular spasticity, cognitive deficits, the availability of a caregiver, and the physical layout, surfaces, and obstacles that exist in the beneficiary's living environment.

B—Nationally Covered Indications

Effective May 5, 2005, CMS finds that the evidence is adequate to determine that MAE is reasonable and necessary for beneficiaries who have a personal mobility deficit sufficient to impair their participation in mobility-related activities of daily living (MRADLs) such as toileting, feeding, dressing, grooming, and bathing in customary locations within the home. Determination of the presence of a mobility deficit will be made by an algorithmic process, Clinical Criteria for MAE Coverage, to provide the appropriate MAE to correct the mobility deficit.

Clinical Criteria for MAE Coverage

The beneficiary, the beneficiary's family or other caregiver, or a clinician, will usually initiate the discussion and consideration of MAE use. Sequential consideration of the questions below provides clinical guidance for the coverage of equipment of appropriate type and complexity to restore the beneficiary's ability to participate in MRADLs such as toileting, feeding, dressing, grooming, and bathing in customary locations in the home. These questions correspond to the numbered decision points on the accompanying flow chart. In individual cases where the beneficiary's condition clearly and unambiguously precludes the reasonable use of a device, it is not necessary to undertake a trial of that device for that beneficiary.

1. Does the beneficiary have a mobility limitation that significantly impairs his/her ability to participate in one or more MRADLs in the home? A mobility limitation is one that:

   a. Prevents the beneficiary from accomplishing the MRADLs entirely, or,

   b. Places the beneficiary at reasonably determined heightened risk of morbidity or mortality secondary to the attempts to participate in MRADLs, or,

   c. Prevents the beneficiary from completing the MRADLs within a reasonable time frame.

2. Are there other conditions that limit the beneficiary's ability to participate in MRADLs at home?

   a. Some examples are significant impairment of cognition or judgment and/or vision.

   b. For these beneficiaries, the provision of MAE might not enable them to participate in MRADLs if the comorbidity prevents effective use of the wheelchair or reasonable completion of the tasks even with MAE.

3. If these other limitations exist, can they be ameliorated or compensated sufficiently such that the additional provision of MAE will be reasonably expected to significantly improve the beneficiary's ability to perform or obtain assistance to participate in MRADLs in the home?

   a. A caregiver, for example a family member, may be compensatory, if consistently available in the beneficiary's home and willing and able to safely operate and transfer the beneficiary to and from the wheelchair and to transport the beneficiary using the wheelchair. The caregiver's need to use a wheelchair to assist the beneficiary in the MRADLs is to be considered in this determination.

b. If the amelioration or compensation requires the beneficiary's compliance with treatment, for example medications or therapy, substantive non-compliance, whether willing or involuntary, can be grounds for denial of MAE coverage if it results in the beneficiary continuing to have a significant limitation. It may be determined that partial compliance results in adequate amelioration or compensation for the appropriate use of MAE.

4. Does the beneficiary or caregiver demonstrate the capability and the willingness to consistently operate the MAE safely?

a. Safety considerations include personal risk to the beneficiary as well as risk to others. The determination of safety may need to occur several times during the process as the consideration focuses on a specific device.

b. A history of unsafe behavior in other venues may be considered.

5. Can the functional mobility deficit be sufficiently resolved by the prescription of a cane or walker?

a. The cane or walker should be appropriately fitted to the beneficiary for this evaluation.

b. Assess the beneficiary's ability to safely use a cane or walker.

6. Does the beneficiary's typical environment support the use of wheelchairs including scooters/power-operated vehicles (POVs)?

a. Determine whether the beneficiary's environment will support the use of these types of MAE.

b. Keep in mind such factors as physical layout, surfaces, and obstacles, which may render MAE unusable in the beneficiary's home.

7. Does the beneficiary have sufficient upper extremity function to propel a manual wheelchair in the home to participate in MRADLs during a typical day? The manual wheelchair should be optimally configured (seating options, wheelbase, device weight, and other appropriate accessories) for this determination.

a. Limitations of strength, endurance, range of motion, coordination, and absence or deformity in one or both upper extremities are relevant.

b. A beneficiary with sufficient upper extremity function may qualify for a manual wheelchair. The appropriate type of manual wheelchair, i.e. light weight, etc., should be determined based on the beneficiary's physical characteristics and anticipated intensity of use.

c. The beneficiary's home should provide adequate access, maneuvering space and surfaces for the operation of a manual wheelchair.

d. Assess the beneficiary's ability to safely use a manual wheelchair.

NOTE: If the beneficiary is unable to self-propel a manual wheelchair, and if there is a caregiver who is available, willing, and able to provide assistance, a manual wheelchair may be appropriate.

8. Does the beneficiary have sufficient strength and postural stability to operate a POV/scooter?

a. A POV is a 3- or 4-wheeled device with tiller steering and limited seat modification capabilities. The beneficiary must be able to maintain stability and position for adequate operation.

b. The beneficiary's home should provide adequate access, maneuvering space and surfaces for the operation of a POV.

c. Assess the beneficiary's ability to safely use a POV/scooter.

9. Are the additional features provided by a power wheelchair needed to allow the beneficiary to participate in one or more MRADLs?

a. The pertinent features of a power wheelchair compared to a POV are typically control by a joystick or alternative input device, lower seat height for slide transfers, and the ability to accommodate a variety of seating needs.

b. The type of wheelchair and options provided should be appropriate for the degree of the beneficiary's functional impairments.

c. The beneficiary's home should provide adequate access, maneuvering space and surfaces for the operation of a power wheelchair.

d. Assess the beneficiary's ability to safely use a power wheelchair.

NOTE: If the beneficiary is unable to use a power wheelchair, and if there is a caregiver who is available, willing, and able to provide assistance, a manual wheelchair is appropriate. A caregiver's inability to operate a manual wheelchair can be considered in covering a power wheelchair so that the caregiver can assist the beneficiary.

C—Nationally Non-Covered Indications

Medicare beneficiaries not meeting the clinical criteria for prescribing MAE as outlined above, and as documented by the beneficiary's physician, would not be eligible for Medicare coverage of the MAE.

D—Other

All other durable medical equipment (DME) not meeting the definition of MAE as described in this instruction will continue to be covered, or noncovered, as is currently described in the NCD Manual, in Section 280, Medical and Surgical Supplies. Also, all other sections not altered here and the corresponding policies regarding MAEs which have not been discussed here remain unchanged.

(This NCD last reviewed May 2005).

Cross-references: section 280.1 of the NCD Manual.

CIM 60-7

20.8.2—Self-Contained Pacemaker Monitors

(Rev. 1, 10-03-03)

Self-contained pacemaker monitors are accepted devices for monitoring cardiac pacemakers. Accordingly, program payment may be made for the rental or purchase of either of the following pacemaker monitors when a physician for a patient prescribes it with a cardiac pacemaker:

A—Digital Electronic Pacemaker Monitor

This device provides the patient with an instantaneous digital readout of his pacemaker pulse rate. Use of this device does not involve professional services until there has been a change of five pulses (or more) per minute above or below the initial rate of the pacemaker; when such change occurs, the patient contacts his physician.

B—Audible/Visible Signal Pacemaker Monitor

This device produces an audible and visible signal which indicates the pacemaker rate. Use of this device does not involve professional services until a change occurs in these signals; at such time, the patient contacts his physician.

NOTE: The design of the self-contained pacemaker monitor makes it possible for the patient to monitor his pacemaker periodically and minimizes the need for regular visits to the outpatient department of the provider.

Therefore, documentation of the medical necessity for pacemaker evaluation in the outpatient department of the provider should be obtained where such evaluation is employed in addition to the self-contained pacemaker monitor used by the patient in his home.

Cross-reference: §20.8.1

CIM 60-8

280.4—Seat Lift—(Rev. 1, 10-03-03)

Reimbursement may be made for the rental or purchase of a medically necessary seat lift when prescribed by a physician for a patient with severe arthritis of the hip or knee and patients with muscular dystrophy or other neuromuscular disease when it has been determined the patient can benefit therapeutically from use of the device. In establishing medical necessity for the seat lift, the evidence must show that the item is included in the physician's course of treatment, that it is likely to effect improvement, or arrest or retard deterioration in the patient's condition, and that the severity of the condition is such that the alternative would be chair or bed confinement.

Coverage of seat lifts is limited to those types which operate smoothly, can be controlled by the patient, and effectively assist a patient in standing up and sitting down without other assistance. Excluded from coverage is the type of lift which operates by a spring release mechanism with a sudden, catapult-like motion and jolts the patient from a seated to a standing position. Limit the payment for units which incorporate a recliner feature along with the seat lift to the amount payable for a seat lift without this feature.

Cross Reference:

The Medicare Claims Processing Manual, Chapter 20, "Durable Medical Equipment, Prosthetics and Orthotics, and Supplies (DMEPOS)," §90.

CIM 60-9

280.1—Durable Medical Equipment Reference List (Effective May 5, 2005)

(Rev. 37, Issued: 06-03-05; Effective: 05-05-05; Implementation: 07-05-05)

The durable medical equipment (DME) list that follows is designed to facilitate the contractor's processing of DME claims. This section is designed as a quick reference tool for determining the coverage status of certain pieces of DME and especially for those items commonly referred to by both brand and generic names. The information contained herein is applicable (where appropriate) to all DME national coverage determinations (NCDs) discussed in the DME portion of this manual. The list is organized into two columns. The first column lists alphabetically various generic categories of equipment on which NCDs have been made by the Centers for Medicare & Medicaid Services (CMS); the second column notes the coverage status.

In the case of equipment categories that have been determined by CMS to be covered under the DME benefit, the list outlines the conditions of coverage that must be met if payment is to be allowed for the rental or purchase of the DME by a particular patient, or cross-refers to another section of the manual where the applicable coverage criteria are described in more detail. With respect to equipment categories that cannot be covered as DME, the list includes a brief explanation of why the equipment is not covered. This DME list will be updated periodically to reflect any additional NDC that CMS may make with regard to other categories of equipment.

When the contractor receives a claim for an item of equipment which does not appear to fall logically into any of the generic categories listed, the contractor has the authority and responsibility for deciding whether those items are covered under the DME benefit.

These decisions must be made by each contractor based on the advice of its medical consultants, taking into account:

- The Medicare Claims Processing Manual, Chapter 20, "Durable Medical Equipment, Prosthetics and Orthotics, and Supplies (DMEPOS)."
- Whether the item has been approved for marketing by the Food and Drug Administration (FDA) and is otherwise generally considered to be safe and effective for the purpose intended; and
- Whether the item is reasonable and necessary for the individual patient.

The term durable medical equipment (DME) is defined as equipment which:

- Can withstand repeated use; i.e., could normally be rented, and used by successive patients;
- Is primarily and customarily used to serve a medical purpose;
- Generally is not useful to a person in the absence of illness or injury; and
- Is appropriate for use in a patient's home.

Durable Medical Equipment Reference List

Item	Coverage
Air Cleaners	Deny—environmental control equipment; not primarily medical in nature (§1861(n) of the Act).
Air Conditioners	Deny—environmental control equipment; not primarily medical in nature (§1861 (n) of the Act).
Air-Fluidized Beds	(See Air-Fluidized Beds §280.8 of this manual.)
Alternating Pressure Pads, Mattresses and Lambs Wool Pads	Covered if patient has, or is highly susceptible to, decubitus ulcers and the patient's physician specifies that he/she will be supervising the course of treatment.
Audible/Visible Signal/Pacemaker Monitor	(See Self-Contained Pacemaker Monitors.)
Augmentative Communication Device	(See Speech Generating Devices, §50.1 of this manual.)
Bathtub Lifts	Deny—convenience item; not primarily medical in nature (§1861(n) of the Act).
Bathtub Seats	Deny—comfort or convenience item; hygienic equipment; not primarily medical in nature (§1861(n) of the Act).
Bead Beds	(See §280.8.)
Bed Baths (home type)	Deny—hygienic equipment; not primarily medical in nature ((§1861(n) of the Act).
Bed Lifters (bed elevators)	Deny—not primarily medical in nature ((§1861(n) of the Act).
Bedboards	Deny—not primarily medical in nature ((§1861(n) of the Act).
Bed Pans (autoclavable hospital type)	Covered if patient is bed confined.
Bed Side Rails	(See Hospital Beds, §280.7 of this manual.)
Beds-Lounges (power or manual)	Deny—not a hospital bed; comfort or convenience item; not primarily medical in nature (§1861(n) of the Act).
Beds—Oscillating	Deny—institutional equipment; inappropriate for home use.
Bidet Toilet Seat	(See Toilet Seats.)
Blood Glucose Analyzers—Reflectance Colorimeter	Deny—unsuitable for home use (see §40.2 of this manual).
Blood Glucose Monitors	Covered if patient meets certain conditions (see §40.2 of this manual).
Braille Teaching Texts	Deny—educational equipment; not primarily medical in nature (§1861(n) of the Act).
Canes	Covered if patient meets Mobility Assistive Equipment clinical criteria (see §280.3 of this manual).
Carafes	Deny—convenience item; not primarily medical in nature (§1861(n) of the Act)
Catheters	Deny—nonreusable disposable supply (§1861(n) of the Act). (See The Medicare Claims Processing Manual, Chapter 20, DMEPOS

Item	Coverage
Commodes	Covered if patient is confined to bed or room. NOTE: The term "room confined" means that the patient's condition is such that leaving the room is medically contraindicated. The accessibility of bathroom facilities generally would not be a factor in this determination. However, confinement of a patient to his home in a case where there are no toilet facilities in the home may be equated to room confinement. Moreover, payment may also be made if a patient's medical condition confines him to a floor of his home and there is no bathroom located on that floor.
Communicator	(See §50.1 of this manual, "Speech Generating Devices.")
Continuous Passive Motion Devices	Continuous passive motion devices are devices Covered for patients who have received a total knee replacement. To qualify for coverage, use of the device must commence within 2 days following surgery. In addition, coverage is limited to that portion of the 3-week period following surgery during which the device is used in the patient's home. There is insufficient evidence to justify coverage of these devices for longer periods of time or for other applications.
Continuous Positive Airway Pressure (CPAP) Devices	(See §240.4 of this manual.)
Crutches	Covered if patient meets Mobility Assistive Equipment clinical criteria (see section 280.3 of this manual).
Cushion Lift Power Seats	(See Seat Lifts.)
Dehumidifiers (room or central heating system type)	Deny—environmental control equipment; not primarily medical in nature (§1861(n) of the Act.
Diathermy Machines (standard pulses wave types)	Deny—inappropriate for home use (see §150.5 of this manual).
Digital Electronic Pacemaker Monitors	(See Self-Contained Pacemaker Monitors.)
Disposable Sheets and Bags	Deny—nonreusable disposable supplies (§1861(n) of the Act)
Elastic Stockings	Deny—nonreusable supply; not rental-type items (§1861(n) of the Act) (See §270.5 of this manual)
Electric Air Cleaners	Deny—(See Air Cleaners.) (§1861(n) of the Act).
Electric Hospital Beds	(See Hospital Beds §280.7 of this manual.)
Electrical Stimulation for Wounds	Deny—inappropriate for home use. (See §270.1 of this manual)
Electrostatic Machines	Deny—(See Air Cleaners and Air Conditioners.) (§1861(n) of the Act).
Elevators	Deny—convenience item; not primarily medical in nature (§1861(n) of the Act).
Emesis Basins	Deny—convenience item; not primarily medical in nature (§1861(n) of the Act).
Esophageal Dilators	Deny—physician instrument; inappropriate for patient use.
Exercise Equipment	Deny—not primarily medical in nature (§1861(n) of the Act).
Fabric Supports	Deny—nonreusable supplies; not rental-type items (§1861(n) of the Act).

Item	Coverage
Face Masks (oxygen)	Covered if oxygen is Covered. (See §240.2 of this manual.)
Face Masks (surgical)	Deny—nonreusable disposable items (§1861(n) of the Act)
Flowmeters	(See Medical Oxygen Regulators.) (See §240.2 of this manual.)
Fluidic Breathing Assisters	(See Intermittent Positive Pressure Breathing Machines.)
Fomentation Device	(See Heating Pads.)
Gel Flotation Pads and Mattresses	(See Alternating Pressure Pads and Mattresses.)
Grab Bars	Deny—self-help device; not primarily medical in nature (§1861(n) of the Act).
Heat and Massage Foam Cushion Pads	Deny—not primarily medical in nature; personal comfort item (§1861(n) and 1862(a)(6) of the Act).
Heating and Cooling Plants	Deny—environmental control equipment not primarily; medical in nature (§1861(n) of the Act).
Heating Pads	Covered if the contractor's medical staff determines patient's medical condition is one for which the application of heat in the form of a heating pad is therapeutically effective.
Heat Lamps	Covered if the contractor's medical staff determines patient's medical condition is one for which the application of heat in the form of a heat lamp is therapeutically effective.
Hospital Beds	(See §280.7 of this manual.)
Hot Packs	(See Heating Pads.)
Humidifiers (oxygen)	(See Oxygen Humidifiers.)
Humidifiers (room or central heating system types)	Deny—environmental control equipment; not medical in nature (§1861(n) of the Act).
Hydraulic Lifts	(See Patient Lifts.)
Incontinent Pads	Deny—nonreusable supply; hygienic item (§1861(n) of the Act).
Infusion Pumps	For external and implantable pumps, see §40.2 of this manual. If the pump is used with an enteral or parenteral nutritional therapy system, see §180.2 of this manual for special coverage rules.
Injectors (hypodermic jet	Deny—not covered self-administered drug supply'essure powered devices (§1861(s)(2)(A) of the Act) for injection of insulin.
Intermittent Positive Pressure Breathing Machines	Covered if patient's ability to breathe is severely impaired.
Iron Lungs	(See Ventilators.)
Irrigating Kits	Deny—nonreusable supply; hygienic equipment (§1861(n) of the Act).
Lambs Wool Pads	(See Alternating Pressure Pads, Mattresses, and Lambs Wool Pads)
Leotards	Deny—(See Pressure Leotards.) (§1861(n) of the Act).
Lymphedema Pumps	Covered (See Pneumatic Compression Devices, §280.6 of this manual.)
Massage Devices	Deny—personal comfort items; not primarily medical in nature (§1861(n) and 1862(a)(6) of the Act).
Mattresses	Covered only where hospital bed is medically necessary. (Separate Charge for replacement mattress should not be allowed where hospital bed with mattress is rented.) (See §280.7 of this manual.)
Medical Oxygen Regulators	Covered if patient's ability to breathe is severely impaired. (See §240.2 of this manual.)

Item	Coverage
Mobile Geriatric Chairs	Covered if patient meets Mobility Assistive Equipment clinical criteria (see §280.3 of this manual). (See Rolling Chairs).
Motorized Wheelchairs	Covered if patient meets Mobility Assistive Equipment clinical criteria (see §280.3 of this manual).
Muscle Stimulators	Covered for certain conditions. (See §250.4 of this manual.)
Nebulizers	Covered if patient's ability to breathe is severely impaired.
Oscillating Beds	Deny—institutional equipment—inappropriate for home use.
Overbed Tables	Deny—convenience item; not primarily medical in nature (§1861(n) of the Act).
Oxygen	Covered if the oxygen has been prescribed for use in connection with medically necessary DME. (See §240.2 of this manual.)
Oxygen Humidifiers	Covered if the oxygen has been prescribed for use in connection with medically necessary DME for purposes of moisturizing oxygen. (See §240.2 of this manual.)
Oxygen Regulators (Medical)	(See Medical Oxygen Regulators.)
Oxygen Tents	(See §240.2 of this manual.)
Paraffin Bath Units (Portable)	(See Portable Paraffin Bath Units.)
Paraffin Bath Units (Standard)	Deny—institutional equipment; inappropriate for home use.
Parallel Bars	Deny—support exercise equipment; primarily for institutional use; in the home setting other devices (e.g., walkers) satisfy the patient's need.
Patient Lifts	Covered if contractor's medical staff determines patient's condition is such that periodic movement is necessary to effect improvement or to arrest or retard deterioration in his condition.
Percussors	Covered for mobilizing respiratory tract secretions in patients with chronic obstructive lung disease, chronic bronchitis, or emphysema, when patient or operator of powered percussor has receives appropriate training by a physician or therapist, and no one competent to administer manual therapy is available.
Portable Oxygen Systems	1. Regulated covered (adjustable covered under conditions specified in a flow rate). Refer all claims to medical staff for this determination. 2. Preset Deny (flow rate deny emergency, first-aid, or not adjustable) precautionary equipment; essentially not therapeutic in nature.
Portable Paraffin Bath Units	Covered when the patient has undergone a successful trial period of paraffin therapy ordered by a physician and the patient's condition is expected to be relieved by long term use of this modality.
Portable Room Heaters	Deny—environmental control equipment; not primarily medical in nature (§1861(n) of the Act).
Portable Whirlpool Pumps	Deny—not primarily medical in nature; personal comfort items (§§1861(n) and 1862(a)(6) of the Act).

Item	Coverage
Postural Drainage Boards	Covered if patient has a chronic pulmonary condition.
Preset Portable Oxygen Units	Deny—emergency, first-aid, or precautionary equipment; essentially not therapeutic in nature.
Pressure Leotards	Deny—non-reusable supply, not rental-type item (§1861(n) of the Act).
Pulse Tachometers	Deny—not reasonable or necessary for monitoring pulse of homebound patient with or without a cardiac pacemaker.
Quad-Canes	Covered if patient meets Mobility Assistive Equipment clinical criteria (see §280.3 of this manual).
Raised Toilet Seats	Deny—convenience item; hygienic equipment; not primarily medical in nature (§1861(n) of the Act).
Reflectance Colorimeters	(See Blood Glucose Analyzers.)
Respirators	(See Ventilators.)
Rolling Chairs	Covered if patient meets Mobility Assistive Equipment clinical criteria (see §280.3 of this manual). Coverage is limited to those roll-about chairs having casters of at least 5 inches in diameter and specifically designed to meet the needs of ill, injured, or otherwise impaired individuals. Coverage is denied for the wide range of chairs with smaller casters as are found in general use in homes, offices, and institutions for many purposes not related to the care/treatment of ill/injured persons. This type is not primarily medical in nature. (§1861(n) of the Act.)
Safety Rollers	Covered if patient meets Mobility Assistive Equipment clinical criteria (see §280.3 of this manual).
Sauna Baths	Deny—not primarily medical in nature; personal comfort items (§§1861(n) and (1862(a)(6) of the Act).
Seat Lifts	Covered under the conditions specified in §280.4 of this manual. Refer all to medical staff for this determination.
Self Contained Pacemaker Monitors	Covered when prescribed by a physician for a patient with a cardiac pacemaker. (See §§20.8.1 and 280.2 of this manual.)
Sitz Baths	Covered if the contractor's medical staff determines patient has an infection or injury of the perineal area and the item has been prescribed by the patient's physician as a part of his planned regimen of treatment in the patient's home.
Spare Tanks of Oxygen	Deny—convenience or precautionary supply.
Speech Teaching Machines	Deny—education equipment; not primarily medical in nature (§1861(n) of the Act).
Stairway Elevators	Deny—(See Elevators.) (§1861(n) of the Act).
Standing Tables	Deny—convenience item; not primarily medical in nature (§1861(n) of the Act).
Steam Packs	These packs are Covered under the same conditions as a heating pads. (See Heating Pads.)

Item	Coverage
Suction Machines	Covered if the contractor's medical staff determines that the machine specified in the claim is medically required and appropriate for home use without technical or professional supervision.
Support Hose	Deny (See Fabric Supports.) (§1861(n) of the Act).
Surgical Leggings	Deny—non-reusable supply; not rental-type item (§1861(n) of the Act).
Telephone Alert Systems	Deny—these are emergency communications systems and do not serve a diagnostic or therapeutic purpose.
Toilet Seats	Deny—not medical equipment (§1861(n) of the Act).
Traction Equipment	Covered if patient has orthopedic impairment requiring traction equipment that prevents ambulation during the period of use (Consider covering devices usable during ambulation; e.g., cervical traction collar, under the brace provision).
Trapeze Bars	Covered if patient is bed confined and the patient needs a trapeze bar to sit up because of respiratory condition, to change body position for other medical reasons, or to get in and out of bed.
Treadmill Exercisers	Deny—exercise equipment; not primarily medical in nature (§1861(n) of the Act).
Ultraviolet Cabinets	Covered for selected patients with generalized intractable psoriasis. Using appropriate consultation, the contractor should determine whether medical and other factors justify treatment at home rather than at alternative sites, e.g., outpatient department of a hospital.
Urinals autoclavable	Covered if patient is bed confined hospital type.
Vaporizers	Covered if patient has a respiratory illness.
Ventilators	Covered for treatment of neuromuscular diseases, thoracic restrictive diseases, and chronic respiratory failure consequent to chronic obstructive pulmonary disease. Includes both positive and negative pressure types. (See also §240.5 of this manual.)
Walkers	Covered if patient meets Mobility Assistive Equipment clinical criteria (see §280.3 of this manual).
Water and Pressure Pads and Mattresses	(See Alternating Pressure Pads, Mattresses and Lamb Wool Pads.)
Wheelchairs (manual)	Covered if patient meets Mobility Assistive Equipment clinical criteria (see §280.3 of this manual).
Wheelchairs (power operated)	Covered if patient meets Mobility Assistive Equipment clinical criteria (see §280.3 of this manual).
Wheelchairs (scooter/POV)	Covered if patient meets Mobility Assistive Equipment clinical criteria (see §280.3 of this manual).
Wheelchairs (specially-sized)	Covered if patient meets Mobility Assistive Equipment clinical criteria (see §280.3 of this manual).

Item	Coverage
Whirlpool Bath Equipment	Covered if patient is homebound and has a (standard)condition for which the whirlpool bath can be expected to provide substantial therapeutic benefit justifying its cost. Where patient is not homebound but has such a condition, payment is restricted to the cost of providing the services elsewhere; e.g., an outpatient department of a participating hospital, if that alternative is less costly. In all cases, refer claim to medical staff for a determination.
Whirlpool Pumps	Deny—(See Portable Whirlpool Pumps.) (§1861(n) of the Act).
White Canes	Deny—(See §280.2 of this manual.) (Not considered Mobility Assistive Equipment)

Cross-reference:

Medicare Benefit Policy Manual, Chapters 13, "Rural Health Clinic (RHC) and Federally Qualified Health Center (FQHC) Services," 15, "Covered Medical and Other Health Services."

Medicare Claims Processing Manual, Chapters 12, "Physician/Practitioner Billing," 20, "Durable Medical Equipment, Prosthetics and Orthotics, and Supplies (DMEPOS)," 23, "Fee Schedule Administration and Coding Requirements."

CIM 60-11

40.2—Home Blood Glucose Monitors

(Rev. 1, 10-03-03)

There are several different types of blood glucose monitors that use reflectance meters to determine blood glucose levels. Medicare coverage of these devices varies, with respect to both the type of device and the medical condition of the patient for whom the device is prescribed.

Reflectance colorimeter devices used for measuring blood glucose levels in clinical settings are not covered as durable medical equipment for use in the home because their need for frequent professional re-calibration makes them unsuitable for home use. However, some types of blood glucose monitors which use a reflectance meter specifically designed for home use by diabetic patients may be covered as durable medical equipment, subject to the conditions and limitations described below. Blood glucose monitors are meter devices that read color changes produced on specially treated reagent strips by glucose concentrations in the patient's blood. The patient, using a disposable sterile lancet, draws a drop of blood, places it on a reagent strip and, following instructions which may vary with the device used, inserts it into the device to obtain a reading. Lancets, reagent strips, and other supplies necessary for the proper functioning of the device are also covered for patients for whom the device is indicated. Home blood glucose monitors enable certain patients to better control their blood glucose levels by frequently checking and appropriately contacting their attending physician for advice and treatment. Studies indicate that the patient's ability to carefully follow proper procedures is critical to obtaining satisfactory results with these devices. In addition, the cost of the devices, with their supplies, limits economical use to patients who must make frequent checks of their blood glucose levels. Accordingly, coverage of home blood glucose monitors is limited to patients meeting the following conditions:

1. The patient has been diagnosed as having diabetes;

2. The patient's physician states that the patient is capable of being trained to use the particular device prescribed in an appropriate manner. In some cases, the patient may not be able to perform this function, but a responsible individual can be trained to use the equipment and monitor the patient to assure that the

intended effect is achieved. This is permissible if the record is properly documented by the patient's physician; and

3. The device is designed for home rather than clinical use.

There is also a blood glucose monitoring system designed especially for use by those with visual impairments. The monitors used in such systems are identical in terms of reliability and sensitivity to the standard blood glucose monitors described above. They differ by having such features as voice synthesizers, automatic timers, and specially designed arrangements of supplies and materials to enable the visually impaired to use the equipment without assistance.

These special blood glucose monitoring systems are covered under Medicare if the following conditions are met:

• The patient and device meet the three conditions listed above for coverage of standard home blood glucose monitors; and
• The patient's physician certifies that he or she has a visual impairment severe enough to require use of this special monitoring system.

The additional features and equipment of these special systems justify a higher reimbursement amount than allowed for standard blood glucose monitors. Separately identify claims for such devices and establish a separate reimbursement amount for them. For those carriers using HCPCS, the procedure code and definitions are E2100 (Blood glucose monitor with integrated voice synthesizer) and E2101 (Blood glucose monitor with integrated lancing/blood sample).

CIM 60-14

280.14—Infusion Pumps

(Rev. 27, Issued: 02-04-05, Effective: 12-17-04, Implementation: 02-18-05)

A—General

Infusion pumps are medical devices used to deliver solutions containing parenteral drugs under pressure at a regulated flow rate.

B—Nationally Covered Indications

The following indications for treatment using infusion pumps are covered under Medicare:

1. External Infusion Pumps

a. Iron Poisoning—Effective for Services Performed On or After September 26, 1984.

When used in the administration of deferoxamine for the treatment of acute iron poisoning and iron overload, only external infusion pumps are covered.

b. Thromboembolic Disease—Effective for Services Performed On or After September 26, 1984

When used in the administration of heparin for the treatment of thromboembolic disease and/or pulmonary embolism, only external infusion pumps used in an institutional setting are covered.

c. Chemotherapy for Liver Cancer—Effective for Services Performed On or After January 29, 1985.

The external chemotherapy infusion pump is covered when used in the treatment of primary hepatocellular carcinoma or colorectal cancer where this disease is unresectable or where the patient refuses surgical excision of the tumor.

d. Morphine for Intractable Cancer Pain—Effective for Services Performed On or After April 22, 1985.

Morphine infusion via an external infusion pump is covered when used in the treatment of intractable pain caused by cancer (in either an inpatient or outpatient setting, including a hospice).

e. Continuous Subcutaneous Insulin Infusion (CSII) Pumps (Effective for Services Performed On or after December 17, 2004)

Continuous subcutaneous insulin infusion (CSII) and related drugs/supplies are covered as medically reasonable and necessary in the home setting for the treatment of diabetic patients who: (1) either meet the updated fasting C-Peptide testing requirement, or, are beta cell autoantibody positive; and, (2) satisfy the remaining criteria for insulin pump therapy as described below. Patients must meet either Criterion A or B as follows:

Criterion A: The patient has completed a comprehensive diabetes education program, and has been on a program of multiple daily injections of insulin (i.e. at least 3 injections per day), with frequent self-adjustments of insulin dose for at least 6 months prior to initiation of the insulin pump, and has documented frequency of glucose self-testing an average of at least 4 times per day during the 2 months prior to initiation of the insulin pump, and meets one or more of the following criteria while on the multiple daily injection regimen:

• Glycosylated hemoglobin level (HbAlc) > 7.0 percent
• History of recurring hypoglycemia
• Wide fluctuations in blood glucose before mealtime
• Dawn phenomenon with fasting blood sugars frequently exceeding 200 mg/dl
• History of severe glycemic excursions

Criterion B: The patient with diabetes has been on a pump prior to enrollment in Medicare and has documented frequency of glucose self-testing an average of at least 4 times per day during the month prior to Medicare enrollment.

General CSII Criteria

In addition to meeting Criterion A or B above, the following general requirements must be met:

The patient with diabetes must be insulinopenic per the updated fasting C-peptide testing requirement, or, as an alternative, must be beta cell autoantibody positive.

Updated fasting C-peptide testing requirement:

• Insulinopenia is defined as a fasting C-peptide level that is less than or equal to 110% of the lower limit of normal of the laboratory's measurement method.
• For patients with renal insufficiency and creatinine clearance (actual or calculated from age, gender, weight, and serum creatinine) ≤50 ml/minute, insulinopenia is defined as a fasting C-peptide level that is less than or equal to 200% of the lower limit of normal of the laboratory's measurement method.
• Fasting C-peptide levels will only be considered valid with a concurrently obtained fasting glucose ≤225 mg/dL.
• Levels only need to be documented once in the medical records.

Continued coverage of the insulin pump would require that the patient has been seen and evaluated by the treating physician at least every three months.

The pump must be ordered by and follow-up care of the patient must be managed by a physician who manages multiple patients with CSII and who works closely with a team including nurses, diabetes educators, and dietitians who are knowledgeable in the use of CSII.

Other Uses of CSII

The CMS will continue to allow coverage of all other uses of CSII in accordance with the Category B investigational device exemption (IDE) clinical trials regulation (42 CFR 405.201) or as a routine cost under the clinical trials policy (Medicare National Coverage Determinations (NCD) Manual 310.1).

f. Other Uses

Other uses of external infusion pumps are covered if the contractor's medical staff verifies the appropriateness of the therapy and of the prescribed pump for the individual patient.

NOTE: Payment may also be made for drugs necessary for the effective use of a covered external infusion pump as long as the drug being used with the pump is itself reasonable and necessary for the patient's treatment.

2. Implantable Infusion Pumps

a. Chemotherapy for Liver Cancer

Effective for Services Performed On or After September 26, 1984.

The implantable infusion pump is covered for intra-arterial infusion of 5-FUdR for the treatment of liver cancer for patients with primary hepatocellular carcinoma or Duke's Class D colorectal cancer, in whom the metastases are limited to the liver, and where (1) the disease is unresectable or (2) where the patient refuses surgical excision of the tumor.

b. Anti-Spasmodic Drugs for Severe Spasticity

An implantable infusion pump is covered when used to administer anti-spasmodic drugs intrathecally (e.g., baclofen) to treat chronic intractable spasticity in patients who have proven unresponsive to less invasive medical therapy as determined by the following criteria:

As indicated by at least a 6-week trial, the patient cannot be maintained on noninvasive methods of spasm control, such as oral anti-spasmodic drugs, either because these methods fail to control adequately the spasticity or produce intolerable side effects, and

Prior to pump implantation, the patient must have responded favorably to a trial intrathecal dose of the anti-spasmodic drug.

c. Opioid Drugs for Treatment of Chronic Intractable Pain

An implantable infusion pump is covered when used to administer opioid drugs (e.g., morphine) intrathecally or epidurally for treatment of severe chronic intractable pain of malignant or non-malignant origin in patients who have a life expectancy of at least three months and who have proven unresponsive to less invasive medical therapy as determined by the following criteria:

The patient's history must indicate that he/she would not respond adequately to noninvasive methods of pain control, such as systemic opioids (including attempts to eliminate physical and behavioral abnormalities which may cause an exaggerated reaction to pain); and

A preliminary trial of intraspinal opioid drug administration must be undertaken with a temporary intrathecal/epidural catheter to substantiate adequately acceptable pain relief and degree of side effects (including effects on the activities of daily living) and patient acceptance.

d. Coverage of Other Uses of Implanted Infusion Pumps

Determinations may be made on coverage of other uses of implanted infusion pumps if the contractor's medical staff verifies that:

- The drug is reasonable and necessary for the treatment of the individual patient;
- It is medically necessary that the drug be administered by an implanted infusion pump; and
- The Food and Drug Administration (FDA) approved labeling for the pump must specify that the drug being administered and the purpose for which it is administered is an indicated use for the pump.

e. Implantation of Infusion Pump Is Contraindicated

The implantation of an infusion pump is contraindicated in the following patients:

- Patients with a known allergy or hypersensitivity to the drug being used (e.g., oral baclofen, morphine, etc.);
- Patients who have an infection;
- Patients whose body size is insufficient to support the weight and bulk of the device; and
- Patients with other implanted programmable devices since crosstalk between devices may inadvertently change the prescription.

NOTE: Payment may also be made for drugs necessary for the effective use of an implantable infusion pump as long as the drug being used with the pump is itself reasonable and necessary for the patient's treatment.

C—Nationally Noncovered Indications

The following indications for treatment using infusion pumps are not covered under Medicare:

1. External Infusion Pumps

    a. Vancomycin (Effective for Services Beginning On or After September 1, 1996)

Medicare coverage of vancomycin as a durable medical equipment infusion pump benefit is not covered. There is insufficient evidence to support the necessity of using an external infusion pump, instead of a disposable elastomeric pump or the gravity drip method, to administer vancomycin in a safe and appropriate manner.

2. Implantable Infusion Pump

    a. Thromboembolic Disease

Effective for Services Performed On or After September 26, 1984.

According to the Public Health Service, there is insufficient published clinical data to support the safety and effectiveness of the heparin implantable pump. Therefore, the use of an implantable infusion pump for infusion of heparin in the treatment of recurrent thromboembolic disease is not covered.

    b. Diabetes

An implanted infusion pump for the infusion of insulin to treat diabetes is not covered. The data does not demonstrate that the pump provides effective administration of insulin.

D—Other

Not applicable.

(This NCD last reviewed January 2005.)

CIM 60-16

280.6—Pneumatic Compression Devices

(Rev. 1, 10-03-03)

Pneumatic compression devices consist of an inflatable garment for the arm or leg and an electrical pneumatic pump that fills the garment with compressed air. The garment is intermittently inflated and deflated with cycle times and pressures that vary between devices. Pneumatic devices are covered for the treatment of lymphedema or for the treatment of chronic venous insufficiency with venous stasis ulcers.

Lymphedema

Lymphedema is the swelling of subcutaneous tissues due to the accumulation of excessive lymph fluid. The accumulation of lymph fluid results from impairment to the normal clearing function of the lymphatic system and/or from an excessive production of lymph. Lymphedema is divided into two broad classes according to etiology. Primary lymphedema is a relatively uncommon, chronic condition which may be due to such causes as Milroy's Disease or congenital anomalies. Secondary lymphedema which is much more common, results from the destruction of or damage to formerly functioning lymphatic channels, such as surgical removal of lymph nodes or post radiation fibrosis, among other causes.

Pneumatic compression devices are covered in the home setting for the treatment of lymphedema if the patient has undergone a four-week trial of conservative therapy and the treating physician determines that there has been no significant improvement or if significant symptoms remain after the trial. The trial of conservative therapy must include use of an appropriate compression bandage system or compression garment, exercise, and elevation of the limb. The garment may be prefabricated or custom-fabricated but must provide adequate graduated compression.

Chronic Venous Insufficiency With Venous Stasis Ulcers

Chronic venous insufficiency (CVI) of the lower extremities is a condition caused by abnormalities of the venous wall and valves, leading to obstruction or reflux of blood flow in the veins. Signs of CVI include hyperpigmentation, stasis dermatitis, chronic edema, and venous ulcers.

Pneumatic compression devices are covered in the home setting for the treatment of CVI of the lower extremities only if the patient has one or more venous stasis ulcer(s) which have failed to heal after a six month trial of conservative therapy directed by the treating physician. The trial of conservative therapy must include a compression bandage system or compression garment, appropriate dressings for the wound, exercise, and elevation of the limb.

General Coverage Criteria

Pneumatic compression devices are covered only when prescribed by a physician and when they are used with appropriate physician oversight, i.e., physician evaluation of the patient's condition to determine medical necessity of the device, assuring suitable instruction in the operation of the machine, a treatment plan defining the pressure to be used and the frequency and duration of use, and ongoing monitoring of use and response to treatment.

The determination by the physician of the medical necessity of a pneumatic compression device must include:

1. The patient's diagnosis and prognosis;

2. Symptoms and objective findings, including measurements which establish the severity of the condition;

3. The reason the device is required, including the treatments which have been tried and failed; and

4. The clinical response to an initial treatment with the device.

The clinical response includes the change in pretreatment measurements, ability to tolerate the treatment session and parameters, and ability of the patient (or caregiver) to apply the device for continued use in the home.

The only time that a segmented, calibrated gradient pneumatic compression device (HCPCS code E0652) would be covered is when the individual has unique characteristics that prevent them from receiving satisfactory pneumatic compression treatment using a nonsegmented device in conjunction with a segmented appliance or a segmented compression device without manual control of pressure in each chamber.

Cross Reference: §280.1.

CIM 60-17

240.4—Continuous Positive Airway Pressure (CPAP) Therapy For Obstructive Sleep Apnea (OSA) (Effective April 4, 2005)

(Rev.35, Issued: 05-06-05, Effective: 04-04-05, Implementation: 06-06-05)

A—General

Continuous positive airway pressure (CPAP) is a non-invasive technique for providing single levels of air pressure from a flow generator, via a nose mask, through the nares. The purpose is to prevent the collapse of the oropharyngeal walls and the obstruction of airflow during sleep, which occurs in obstructive sleep apnea (OSA).

B—Nationally Covered Indications

The use of CPAP is covered under Medicare when used in adult patients with moderate or severe OSA for whom surgery is a likely alternative to CPAP. The use of CPAP devices must be ordered and prescribed by the licensed treating physician to be used in adult patients with moderate to severe OSA if either of the following criterion using the Apnea-Hypopnea Index (AHI) are met:

• AHI greater than or equal to 15 events per hour, or
• AHI greater than or equal to 5 and less than or equal to 14 events per hour with documented symptoms of excessive daytime sleepiness, impaired cognition, mood disorders or insomnia, or documented hypertension, ischemic heart disease, or history of stroke.

The AHI is equal to the average number of episodes of apnea and hypopnea per hour and must be based on a minimum of 2 hours of sleep recorded by polysomnography using actual recorded hours of sleep (i.e., the AHI may not be extrapolated or projected). Apnea is defined as a cessation of airflow for at least 10 seconds. Hypopnea is defined as an abnormal respiratory event lasting at least 10 seconds with at least a 30 percent reduction in thoracoabdominal movement or airflow as compared to baseline, and with at least a 4 percent oxygen desaturation.

The polysomnography must be performed in a facility—based sleep study laboratory, and not in the home or in a mobile facility.

Initial claims must be supported by medical documentation (separate documentation where electronic billing is used), such as a prescription written by the patient's attending physician that specifies:

• A diagnosis of moderate or severe obstructive sleep apnea, and
• Surgery is a likely alternative.

The claim must also certify that the documentation supporting a diagnosis of OSA (described above) is available.

C—Nationally Non-covered Indications

Effective April 4, 2005, the Centers for Medicare & Medicaid Services determined that upon reconsideration of the current policy, there is not sufficient evidence to conclude that unattended portable multi-channel sleep study testing is reasonable and necessary in the diagnosis of OSA for CPAP therapy, and these tests will remain noncovered for this purpose.

D—Other

N/A

(This NCD last reviewed April 2005.)

CIM 60-18

280.7—Hospital Beds

(Rev. 1, 10-03-03)

A—General Requirements for Coverage of Hospital Beds

A physician's prescription, and such additional documentation as the contractors' medical staffs may consider necessary, including medical records and physicians' reports, must establish the medical necessity for a hospital bed due to one of the following reasons:

• The patient's condition requires positioning of the body; e.g., to alleviate pain, promote good body alignment, prevent contractures, avoid respiratory infections, in ways not feasible in an ordinary bed; or
• The patient's condition requires special attachments that cannot be fixed and used on an ordinary bed.

B—Physician's Prescription

The physician's prescription which must accompany the initial claim, and supplementing documentation when required, must establish that a hospital bed is medically necessary. If the stated reason for the need for a hospital bed is the patient's condition requires positioning, the prescription or other documentation must describe the medical condition, e.g., cardiac disease, chronic obstructive pulmonary disease, quadriplegia or paraplegia, and also the severity and frequency of the symptoms of the condition, that necessitates a hospital bed for positioning.

If the stated reason for requiring a hospital bed is the patient's condition requires special attachments, the prescription must describe the patient's condition and specify the attachments that require a hospital bed.

C—Variable Height Feature

In well documented cases, the contractors' medical staffs may determine that a variable height feature of a hospital bed, approved for coverage under subsection A above, is medically necessary and, therefore, covered, for one of the following conditions:

• Severe arthritis and other injuries to lower extremities; e.g., fractured hip—The condition requires the variable height feature to assist the patient to ambulate by enabling the patient to place his or her feet on the floor while sitting on the edge of the bed;

- Severe cardiac conditions—For those cardiac patients who are able to leave bed, but who must avoid the strain of "jumping" up or down;
- Spinal cord injuries, including quadriplegic and paraplegic patients, multiple limb amputee and stroke patients. For those patients who are able to transfer from bed to a wheelchair, with or without help; or
- Other severely debilitating diseases and conditions, if the variable height feature is required to assist the patient to ambulate.

D—Electric Powered Hospital Bed Adjustments

Electric powered adjustments to lower and raise head and foot may be covered when the contractor's medical staff determines that the patient's condition requires frequent change in body position and/or there may be an immediate need for a change in body position (i.e., no delay can be tolerated) and the patient can operate the controls and cause the adjustments. Exceptions may be made to this last requirement in cases of spinal cord injury and brain damaged patients.

E—Side Rails

If the patient's condition requires bed side rails, they can be covered when an integral part of, or an accessory to, a hospital bed.

CIM 60-19

280.8—Air-Fluidized Bed

(Rev. 1, 10-03-03)

Air fluidized beds are covered for services rendered on or after: July 30, 1990. An air-fluidized bed uses warm air under pressure to set small ceramic beads in motion which simulate the movement of fluid. When the patient is placed in the bed, his body weight is evenly distributed over a large surface area which creates a sensation of "floating." Medicare payment for home use of the air-fluidized bed for treatment of pressure sores can be made if such use is reasonable and necessary for the individual patient.

A decision that use of an air-fluidized bed is reasonable and necessary requires that:

- The patient has a stage 3 (full thickness tissue loss) or stage 4 (deep tissue destruction) pressure sore;
- The patient is bedridden or chair bound as a result of severely limited mobility;
- In the absence of an air-fluidized bed, the patient would require institutionalization;
- The air-fluidized bed is ordered in writing by the patient's attending physician based upon a comprehensive assessment and evaluation of the patient after completion of a course of conservative treatment designed to optimize conditions that promote wound healing. This course of treatment must have been at least one month in duration without progression toward wound healing. This month of prerequisite conservative treatment may include some period in an institution as long as there is documentation available to verify that the necessary conservative treatment has been rendered.
- Use of wet-to-dry dressings for wound debridement, begun during the period of conservative treatment and which continue beyond 30 days, will not preclude coverage of air-fluidized bed. Should additional debridement again become necessary, while a patient is using an air-fluidized bed (after the first 30-day course of conservative treatment) that will not cause the air-fluidized bed to become noncovered. In all instances documentation verifying the continued need for the bed must be available.
- A trained adult caregiver is available to assist the patient with activities of daily living, fluid balance, dry skin care, repositioning, recognition and management of altered mental status, dietary needs, prescribed treatments, and management and support of the air-fluidized bed system and its problems such as leakage;
- A physician directs the home treatment regimen, and reevaluates and recertifies the need for the air-fluidized bed on a monthly basis; and

- All other alternative equipment has been considered and ruled out.

Conservative treatment must include:

- Frequent repositioning of the patient with particular attention to relief of pressure over bony prominences (usually every 2 hours);
- Use of a specialized support surface (Group II) designed to reduce pressure and shear forces on healing ulcers and to prevent new ulcer formation;
- Necessary treatment to resolve any wound infection;
- Optimization of nutrition status to promote wound healing;
- Debridement by any means (including wet to dry dressings-which does not require an occlusive covering) to remove devitalized tissue from the wound bed;
- Maintenance of a clean, moist bed of granulation tissue with appropriate moist dressings protected by an occlusive covering, while the wound heals.

Home use of the air-fluidized bed is not covered under any of the following circumstances:

- The patient has coexisting pulmonary disease (the lack of firm back support makes coughing ineffective and dry air inhalation thickens pulmonary secretions);
- The patient requires treatment with wet soaks or moist wound dressings that are not protected with an impervious covering such as plastic wrap or other occlusive material;
- The caregiver is unwilling or unable to provide the type of care required by the patient on an air-fluidized bed;
- Structural support is inadequate to support the weight of the air-fluidized bed system (it generally weighs 1600 pounds or more);
- Electrical system is insufficient for the anticipated increase in energy consumption; or
- Other known contraindications exist.

Coverage of an air-fluidized bed is limited to the equipment itself. Payment for this covered item may only be made if the written order from the attending physician is furnished to the supplier prior to the delivery of the equipment. Payment is not included for the caregiver or for architectural adjustments such as electrical or structural improvement.

Cross reference:

The Medicare Claims Processing Manual, Chapter 23, "Fee Schedule Administration and Coding Requirements," §§60.

CIM 60-23

50.1—Speech Generating Devices

(Rev. 1, 10-03-03)

Effective January 1, 2001, augmentative and alternative communication devices or communicators which are hereafter referred to as "speech generating devices" are now considered to fall within the DME benefit category established by §1861(n) of the Social Security Act. They may be covered if the contractor's medical staff determines that the patient suffers from a severe speech impairment and that the medical condition warrants the use of a device based on the following definitions.

Definition of Speech Generating Devices

Speech generating devices are defined as speech aids that provide an individual who has a severe speech impairment with the ability to meet his functional speaking needs. Speech generating are characterized by:

- Being a dedicated speech device, used solely by the individual who has a severe speech impairment;
- May have digitized speech output, using prerecorded messages, less than or equal to 8 minutes recording time;
- May have digitized speech output, using prerecorded messages, greater than 8 minutes recording time;
- May have synthesized speech output which requires message formulation by spelling and device access by physical contact with the device-direct selection techniques;

- May have synthesized speech output which permits multiple methods of message formulation and multiple methods of device access; or
- May be software that allows a laptop computer, desktop computer or personal digital assistant (PDA) to function as a speech generating device.

Devices that would not meet the definition of speech generating devices and therefore, do not fall within the scope of §1861(n) of the Act are characterized by:

- Devices that are not dedicated speech devices, but are devices that are capable of running software for purposes other than for speech generation, e.g., devices that can also run a word processing package, an accounting program, or perform other than non-medical function.
- Laptop computers, desktop computers, or PDA's which may be programmed to perform the same function as a speech generating device, are noncovered since they are not primarily medical in nature and do not meet the definition of DME. For this reason, they cannot be considered speech-generating devices for Medicare coverage purposes.
- A device that is useful to someone without severe speech impairment is not considered a speech-generating device for Medicare coverage purposes.

CIM 60-24

230.8—Non-Implantable Pelvic Flood Electrical Stimulator

(Rev. 1, 10-03-03)

Non-implantable pelvic floor electrical stimulators provide neuromuscular electrical stimulation through the pelvic floor with the intent of strengthening and exercising pelvic floor musculature. Stimulation is generally delivered by vaginal or anal probes connected to an external pulse generator.

The methods of pelvic floor electrical stimulation vary in location, stimulus frequency (Hz), stimulus intensity or amplitude (mA), pulse duration (duty cycle), treatments per day, number of treatment days per week, length of time for each treatment session, overall time period for device use and between clinic and home settings. In general, the stimulus frequency and other parameters are chosen based on the patient's clinical diagnosis.

Pelvic floor electrical stimulation with a non-implantable stimulator is covered for the treatment of stress and/or urge urinary incontinence in cognitively intact patients who have failed a documented trial of pelvic muscle exercise (PME) training.

A failed trial of PME training is defined as no clinically significant improvement in urinary continence after completing 4 weeks of an ordered plan of pelvic muscle exercises designed to increase periurethral muscle strength.

CIM 65-1

80.4—Hydrophilic Contact Lenses

(Rev. 1, 10-03-03)

Hydrophilic contact lenses are eyeglasses within the meaning of the exclusion in §1862(a)(7) of the Act and are not covered when used in the treatment of nondiseased eyes with spherical ametrophia, refractive astigmatism, and/or corneal astigmatism. Payment may be made under the prosthetic device benefit, however, for hydrophilic contact lenses when prescribed for an aphakic patient.

Contractors are authorized to accept an FDA letter of approval or other FDA published material as evidence of FDA approval. (See §80.1 for coverage of a hydrophilic lens as a corneal bandage.)

Cross-references:

The Medicare Benefit Policy Manual, Chapter 15, "Covered Medical and Other Health Services," §100 and §120.

The Medicare Benefit Policy Manual, Chapter 16, "General Exclusions from Coverage," §20 and §90.

CIM 65.3

80.5—Scleral Shell

(Rev. 1, 10-03-03)

Scleral shell (or shield) is a catchall term for different types of hard scleral contact lenses.

A scleral shell fits over the entire exposed surface of the eye as opposed to a corneal contact lens which covers only the central non-white area encompassing the pupil and iris. Where an eye has been rendered sightless and shrunken by inflammatory disease, a scleral shell may, among other things, obviate the need for surgical enucleation and prosthetic implant and act to support the surrounding orbital tissue. In such a case, the device serves essentially as an artificial eye. In this situation, payment may be made for a scleral shell under §1861(s)(8) of the Act.

Scleral shells are occasionally used in combination with artificial tears in the treatment of "dry eye" of diverse etiology. Tears ordinarily dry at a rapid rate, and are continually replaced by the lacrimal gland. When the lacrimal gland fails, the half-life of artificial tears may be greatly prolonged by the use of the scleral contact lens as a protective barrier against the drying action of the atmosphere. Thus, the difficult and sometimes hazardous process of frequent installation of artificial tears may be avoided. The lens acts in this instance to substitute, in part, for the functioning of the diseased lacrimal gland and would be covered as a prosthetic device in the rare case when it is used in the treatment of "dry eye."

Cross-references:

The Medicare Benefit Policy Manual, Chapter 15, "Covered Medical and Other Health Services," §120 and §130

The Medicare Benefit Policy Manual, Chapter 1, "Inpatient Hospital Services," §40 and §120.1.

CIM 65-5

50.2—Electronic Speech Aids

(Rev. 1, 10-03-03)

Electronic speech aids are covered under Part B as prosthetic devices when the patient has had a laryngectomy or his larynx is permanently inoperative. There are two types of speech aids. One operates by placing a vibrating head against the throat; the other amplifies sound waves through a tube which is inserted into the user's mouth. A patient who has had radical neck surgery and/or extensive radiation to the anterior part of the neck would generally be able to use only the "oral tube" model or one of the more sensitive and more expensive "throat contact" devices.

Cross-reference:

The Medicare Benefit Policy Manual, Chapter 15, "Covered Medical and Other Health Services," §120.

CIM 65-7

80.12—Intraocular Lenses (IOLs)

(Rev. 1, 10-03-03)

An intraocular lens, or pseudophakos, is an artificial lens which may be implanted to replace the natural lens after cataract surgery. Intraocular lens implantation services, as well as the lens itself, may be covered if reasonable and necessary for the individual. Implantation services may include hospital, surgical, and other medical services, including preimplantation ultrasound (A-scan) eye measurement of one or both eyes.

Cross-reference:

The Medicare Benefit Policy Manual, Chapter 6, "Hospital Services Covered Under Part B," §10.

The Medicare Benefit Policy Manual, Chapter 15, "Covered Medical and Other Health Services," §120.

The Medicare Benefit Policy Manual, Chapter 16, "General Exclusions from Coverage," §20 and §90.

CIM 65-8

160.7—Electrical Nerve Stimulators

(Rev. 1, 10-03-03)

Two general classifications of electrical nerve stimulators are employed to treat chronic intractable pain: peripheral nerve stimulators and central nervous system stimulators.

A—Implanted Peripheral Nerve Stimulators

Payment may be made under the prosthetic device benefit for implanted peripheral nerve stimulators. Use of this stimulator involves implantation of electrodes around a selected peripheral nerve. The stimulating electrode is connected by an insulated lead to a receiver unit which is implanted under the skin at a depth not greater than 1/2 inch.

Stimulation is induced by a generator connected to an antenna unit which is attached to the skin surface over the receiver unit. Implantation of electrodes requires surgery and usually necessitates an operating room.

NOTE: Peripheral nerve stimulators may also be employed to assess a patient's suitability for continued treatment with an electric nerve stimulator. As explained in §160.7.1, such use of the stimulator is covered as part of the total diagnostic service furnished to the beneficiary rather than as a prosthesis.

B—Central Nervous System Stimulators (Dorsal Column and Depth Brain Stimulators)

The implantation of central nervous system stimulators may be covered as therapies for the relief of chronic intractable pain, subject to the following conditions:

1—Types of Implantations

There are two types of implantations covered by this instruction:

- Dorsal Column (Spinal Cord) Neurostimulation—The surgical implantation of neurostimulator electrodes within the dura mater (endodural) or the percutaneous insertion of electrodes in the epidural space is covered.
- Depth Brain Neurostimulation—The stereotactic implantation of electrodes in the deep brain (e.g., thalamus and periaqueductal gray matter) is covered.

2—Conditions for Coverage

No payment may be made for the implantation of dorsal column or depth brain stimulators or services and supplies related to such implantation, unless all of the conditions listed below have been met:

- The implantation of the stimulator is used only as a late resort (if not a last resort) for patients with chronic intractable pain;
- With respect to item a, other treatment modalities (pharmacological, surgical, physical, or psychological therapies) have been tried and did not prove satisfactory, or are judged to be unsuitable or contraindicated for the given patient;
- Patients have undergone careful screening, evaluation and diagnosis by a multidisciplinary team prior to implantation. (Such screening must include psychological, as well as physical evaluation);
- All the facilities, equipment, and professional and support personnel required for the proper diagnosis, treatment training, and follow up of the patient (including that required to satisfy item c) must be available; and
- Demonstration of pain relief with a temporarily implanted electrode precedes permanent implantation.

Contractors may find it helpful to work with Quality Improvement Organizatins (QIOs) to obtain the information needed to apply these conditions to claims.

See the Medicare Benefit Policy Manual, Chapter 15, "Covered Medical and Other Health Services," §120, and the following sections in this manual, §§160.2 and 30.1.

CIM 65-9

230.10—Incontinence Control Devices

(Rev. 1, 10-03-03)

A—Mechanical/Hydraulic Incontinence Control Devices

Mechanical/hydraulic incontinence control devices are accepted as safe and effective in the management of urinary incontinence in patients with permanent anatomic and neurologic dysfunctions of the bladder. This class of devices achieves control of urination by compression of the urethra. The materials used and the success rate may vary somewhat from device to device. Such a device is covered when its use is reasonable and necessary for the individual patient.

B—Collagen Implant

A collagen implant which is injected into the submucosal tissues of the urethra and/or the bladder neck and into tissues adjacent to the urethra, is a prosthetic device used in the treatment of stress urinary incontinence resulting from intrinsic sphincter deficiency (ISD). ISD is a cause of stress urinary incontinence in which the urethral sphincter is unable to contract and generate sufficient resistance in the bladder, especially during stress maneuvers.

Prior to collagen implant therapy, a skin test for collagen sensitivity must be administered and evaluated over a 4-week period.

In male patients, the evaluation must include a complete history and physical examination and a simple cystometrogram to determine that the bladder fills and stores properly. The patient then is asked to stand upright with a full bladder and to cough or otherwise exert abdominal pressure on his bladder. If the patient leaks, the diagnosis of ISD is established.

In female patients, the evaluation must include a complete history and physical examination (including a pelvic exam) and a simple cystometrogram to rule out abnormalities of bladder compliance and abnormalities of urethral support. Following that determination, an abdominal leak point pressure (ALLP) test is performed. Leak point pressure, stated in cm H2O, is defined as the intra-abdominal pressure at which leakage occurs from the bladder (around a catheter) when the bladder has been filled with a minimum of 150 cc fluid. If the patient has an ALLP of less than 100 cm H2O, the diagnosis of ISD is established.

To use a collagen implant, physicians must have urology training in the use of a cystoscope and must complete a collagen implant training program.

Coverage of a collagen implant, and the procedure to inject it, is limited to the following types of patients with stress urinary incontinence due to ISD:

- Male or female patients with congenital sphincter weakness secondary to conditions such as myelomeningocele or epispadias;
- Male or female patients with acquired sphincter weakness secondary to spinal cord lesions;
- Male patients following trauma, including prostatectomy and/or radiation; and
- Female patients without urethral hypermobility and with abdominal leak point pressures of 100 cm H2O or less.

Patients whose incontinence does not improve with five injection procedures (five separate treatment sessions) are considered treatment failures, and no further treatment of urinary incontinence by collagen implant is covered. Patients who have a reoccurrence of incontinence following successful treatment with collagen implants in the past (e.g., 6-12 months previously) may benefit from additional treatment sessions. Coverage of additional sessions may be allowed but must be supported by medical justification. See the Medicare Benefit Policy Manual, Chapter 15, "Covered Medical and Other Health Services," §120. (See §230.8.)

CIM 65-10

180.2—Enteral and Parenteral Nutritional Therapy

(Rev. 1, 10-03-03)

Covered As Prosthetic Device

There are patients who, because of chronic illness or trauma, cannot be sustained through oral feeding. These people must rely on either enteral or parenteral nutritional therapy, depending upon the particular nature of their medical condition.

Coverage of nutritional therapy as a Part B benefit is provided under the prosthetic device benefit provision which requires that the patient must have a permanently inoperative internal body organ or function thereof. Therefore, enteral and parenteral nutritional therapy are not covered under Part B in situations involving temporary impairments.

Coverage of such therapy, however, does not require a medical judgment that the impairment giving rise to the therapy will persist throughout the patient's remaining years. If the medical record, including the judgment of the attending physician, indicates that the impairment will be of long and indefinite duration, the test of permanence is considered met.

If the coverage requirements for enteral or parenteral nutritional therapy are met under the prosthetic device benefit provision, related supplies, equipment and nutrients are also covered under the conditions in the following paragraphs and the Medicare Benefit Policy Manual, Chapter 15, "Covered Medical and Other Health Services," §120.

Parenteral Nutrition Therapy

Daily parenteral nutrition is considered reasonable and necessary for a patient with severe pathology of the alimentary tract which does not allow absorption of sufficient nutrients to maintain weight and strength commensurate with the patient's general condition.

Since the alimentary tract of such a patient does not function adequately, an indwelling catheter is placed percutaneously in the subclavian vein and then advanced into the superior vena cava where intravenous infusion of nutrients is given for part of the day. The catheter is then plugged by the patient until the next infusion. Following a period of hospitalization which is required to initiate parenteral nutrition and to train the patient in catheter care, solution preparation, and infusion technique, the parenteral nutrition can be provided safely and effectively in the patient's home by nonprofessional persons who have undergone special training. However, such persons cannot be paid for their services, nor is payment available for any services furnished by nonphysician professionals except as services furnished incident to a physician's service.

For parenteral nutrition therapy to be covered under Part B, the claim must contain a physician's written order or prescription and sufficient medical documentation to permit an independent conclusion that the requirements of the prosthetic device benefit are met and that parenteral nutrition therapy is medically necessary. An example of a condition that typically qualifies for coverage is a massive small bowel resection resulting in severe nutritional deficiency in spite of adequate oral intake. However, coverage of parenteral nutrition therapy for this and any other condition must be approved on an individual, case-by-case basis initially and at periodic intervals of no more than three months by the carrier's medical consultant or specially trained staff, relying on such medical and other documentation as the carrier may require. If the claim involves an infusion pump, sufficient evidence must be provided to support a determination of medical necessity for the pump. Program payment for the pump is based on the reasonable charge for the simplest model that meets the medical needs of the patient as established by medical documentation.

Nutrient solutions for parenteral therapy are routinely covered. However, Medicare pays for no more than one month's supply of nutrients at any one time. Payment for the nutrients is based on the reasonable charge for the solution components unless the medical record, including a signed statement from the attending physician, establishes that the beneficiary, due to his/her physical or mental state, is unable to safely or effectively mix the solution and there is no family member or other person who can do so. Payment will be on the basis of the reasonable charge for more expensive premixed solutions only under the latter circumstances.

Enteral Nutrition Therapy

Enteral nutrition is considered reasonable and necessary for a patient with a functioning gastrointestinal tract who, due to pathology to, or nonfunction of, the structures that normally permit food to reach the digestive tract, cannot maintain weight and strength commensurate with his or her general condition. Enteral therapy may be given by nasogastric, jejunostomy, or gastrostomy tubes and can be provided safely and effectively in the home by nonprofessional persons who have undergone special training. However, such persons cannot be paid for their services, nor is payment available for any services furnished by nonphysician professionals except as services furnished incident to a physician's service.

Typical examples of conditions that qualify for coverage are head and neck cancer with reconstructive surgery and central nervous system disease leading to interference with the neuromuscular mechanisms of ingestion of such severity that the beneficiary cannot be maintained with oral feeding. However, claims for Part B coverage of enteral nutrition therapy for these and any other conditions must be approved on an individual, case-by-case basis. Each claim must contain a physician's written order or prescription and sufficient medical documentation (e.g., hospital records, clinical findings from the attending physician) to permit an independent conclusion that the patient's condition meets the requirements of the prosthetic device benefit and that enteral nutrition therapy is medically necessary. Allowed claims are to be reviewed at periodic intervals of no more than 3 months by the contractor's medical consultant or specially trained staff, and additional medical documentation considered necessary is to be obtained as part of this review.

Medicare pays for no more than one month's supply of enteral nutrients at any one time. If the claim involves a pump, it must be supported by sufficient medical documentation to establish that the pump is medically necessary, i.e., gravity feeding is not satisfactory due to aspiration, diarrhea, dumping syndrome. Program payment for the pump is based on the reasonable charge for the simplest model that meets the medical needs of the patient as established by medical documentation.

Nutritional Supplementation

Some patients require supplementation of their daily protein and caloric intake. Nutritional supplements are often given as a medicine between meals to boost protein-caloric intake or the mainstay of a daily nutritional plan. Nutritional supplementation is not covered under Medicare Part B.

CIM 65-11

230.16—Bladder Stimulators (Pacemakers)

(Rev. 1, 10-03-03)

Not Covered

There are a number of devices available to induce emptying of the urinary bladder by using electrical current which forces the muscles of the bladder to contract. These devices (commonly known as bladder stimulators or pacemakers) are characterized by the implantation of electrodes in the wall of the bladder, the rectal cones, or the spinal cord. While these treatments may effectively empty the bladder, the issue of safety involving the initiation of infection, erosion, placement, and material selection has not been resolved. Further, some facilities previously using electronic emptying have stopped using this method due to the pain experienced by the patient.

The use of spinal cord electrical stimulators, rectal electrical stimulators, and bladder wall stimulators is not considered reasonable and necessary. Therefore, no program payment may be made for these devices or for their implant.

CIM 65-14

50.3—Cochlear Implantation

(Rev. 1, 10-03-03)

A cochlear implant device is an electronic instrument, part of which is implanted surgically to stimulate auditory nerve fibers, and part of which is worn or carried by the individual to capture, analyze and code sound. Cochlear implant devices are available in single channel and multi-channel models. The purpose of implanting the device is to provide an awareness and identification of sounds and to facilitate communication for persons who are profoundly hearing impaired.

Medicare coverage is provided only for those patients who meet all of the following selection guidelines.

A—General

- Diagnosis of bilateral severe-to-profound sensorineural hearing impairment with limited benefit from appropriate hearing (or vibrotactile) aids;
- Cognitive ability to use auditory clues and a willingness to undergo an extended program of rehabilitation;
- Freedom from middle ear infection, an accessible cochlear lumen that is structurally suited to implantation, and freedom from lesions in the auditory nerve and acoustic areas of the central nervous system;
- No contraindications to surgery; and
- The device must be used in accordance with the FDA-approved labeling.

B—Adults

Cochlear implants may be covered for adults (over age 18) for prelinguistically, perilinguistically, and postlinguistically deafened adults. Postlinguistically deafened adults must demonstrate test scores of 30 percent or less on sentence recognition scores from tape recorded tests in the patient's best listening condition.

C—Children

Cochlear implants may be covered for prelinguistically and postlinguistically deafened children aged 2 through 17. Bilateral profound sensorineural deafness must be demonstrated by the inability to improve on age appropriate closed-set word identification tasks with amplification.

CIM 65-16

50.4—Tracheostomy Speaking Valve

(Rev. 1, 10-03-03)

A trachea tube has been determined to satisfy the definition of a prosthetic device, and the tracheostomy speaking valve is an add on to the trachea tube which may be considered a medically necessary accessory that enhances the function of the tube. In other words, it makes the system a better prosthesis. As such, a tracheostomy speaking valve is covered as an element of the trachea tube which makes the tube more effective.

CIM 65-18

230.18—Sacral Nerve Stimulation for Urinary Incontinence

(Rev. 1, 10-03-03)

Effective January 1, 2002, sacral nerve stimulation is covered for the treatment of urinary urge incontinence, urgency-frequency syndrome, and urinary retention. Sacral nerve stimulation involves both a temporary test stimulation to determine if an implantable stimulator would be effective and a permanent implantation in appropriate candidates. Both the test and the permanent implantation are covered.

The following limitations for coverage apply to all three indications:

- Patient must be refractory to conventional therapy (documented behavioral, pharmacologic and/or surgical corrective therapy) and be an appropriate surgical candidate such that implantation with anesthesia can occur.
- Patients with stress incontinence, urinary obstruction, and specific neurologic diseases (e.g., diabetes with peripheral nerve involvement) which are associated with secondary manifestations of the above three indications are excluded.
- Patient must have had a successful test stimulation in order to support subsequent implantation. Before a patient is eligible for permanent implantation, he/she must demonstrate a 50 percent or greater improvement through test stimulation. Improvement is measured through voiding diaries.
- Patient must be able to demonstrate adequate ability to record voiding diary data such that clinical results of the implant procedure can be properly evaluated.

CIM 70-1

280.11—Corset Used as Hernia Support

(Rev. 1, 10-03-03)

A hernia support (whether in the form of a corset or truss) which meets the definition of a brace is covered under Part B under §1861(s)(9) of the Act. See the Medicare Benefit Policy Manual, Chapter 15, "Covered Medical and Other Services," §130.

CIM 70-2

280.12—Sykes Hernia Control

(Rev. 1, 10-03-03)

Based on professional advice, it has been determined that the sykes hernia control (a spring-type, U-shaped, strapless truss) is not functionally more beneficial than a conventional truss. Make program reimbursement for this device only when an ordinary truss would be covered. (Like all trusses, it is only of benefit when dealing with a reducible hernia). Thus, when a charge for this item is substantially in excess of that which would be reasonable for a conventional truss used for the same condition, base reimbursement on the reasonable charges for the conventional truss. See the Medicare Benefit Policy Manual, Chapter 15, "Covered Medical and Other Services," §130.